6th Edition

Leadership Roles and Management Functions in Nursing

THEORY AND APPLICATION

■ **Bessie L. Marquis, RN, MSN**
Professor Emeritus of Nursing
California State University
Chico, California

■ **Carol J. Huston, RN, MSN, DPA, FAAN**
Professor of Nursing
California State University
Chico, California

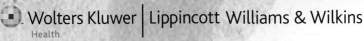
Wolters Kluwer | Lippincott Williams & Wilkins
Health
Philadelphia • Baltimore • New York • London
Buenos Aires • Hong Kong • Sydney • Tokyo

Senior Acquisitions Editor: Elizabeth Nieginski
Senior Managing Editor: Helen Kogut
Development Editor: Deedie McMahon
Editorial Assistant: Laura Scott
Production Project Manager: Cynthia Rudy
Director of Nursing Production: Helen Ewan
Senior Managing Editor / Production: Erika Kors
Design Coordinator: Joan Wendt
Manufacturing Coordinator: Karin Duffield
Production Services / Compositor: Aptara, Inc.

6th edition

9 8 7 6 5 4 3 2 1

Printed in China

Library of Congress Cataloging-in-Publication Data
Marquis, Bessie L.
 Leadership roles and management functions in nursing : theory and application / Bessie L. Marquis, Carol J. Huston. — 6th ed.
   p. ; cm.
 Includes bibliographical references and index.
 ISBN-13: 978-0-7817-7246-4
 ISBN-10: 0-7817-7246-X
 1. Nursing services—Administration. 2. Leadership. I. Huston, Carol Jorgensen. II. Title.
 [DNLM: 1. Leadership. 2. Nursing, Supervisory. 3. Nurse Administrators.
 4. Nursing–organization & administration.   WY 105 M357L 2009]
 RT89.M387 2009
 362.17'3068—dc22
                                                                    2007040508

Care has been taken to confirm the accuracy of the information presented and to describe generally accepted practices. However, the authors, editors, and publisher are not responsible for errors or omissions or for any consequences from application of the information in this book and make no warranty, expressed or implied, with respect to the currency, completeness, or accuracy of the contents of the publication. Application of this information in a particular situation remains the professional responsibility of the practitioner; the clinical treatments described and recommended may not be considered absolute and universal recommendations.

   The authors, editors, and publisher have exerted every effort to ensure that drug selection and dosage set forth in this text are in accordance with the current recommendations and practice at the time of publication. However, in view of ongoing research, changes in government regulations, and the constant flow of information relating to drug therapy and drug reactions, the reader is urged to check the package insert for each drug for any change in indications and dosage and for added warnings and precautions. This is particularly important when the recommended agent is a new or infrequently employed drug.

   Some drugs and medical devices presented in this publication have Food and Drug Administration (FDA) clearance for limited use in restricted research settings. It is the responsibility of the health care provider to ascertain the FDA status of each drug or device planned for use in his or her clinical practice.

I dedicate this book to the two most important partnerships in my life: my husband, Don Marquis, and my colleague, Carol Huston.

BESSIE L. MARQUIS

I dedicate this book to my son-in-law, Jason McKay. You bring so much happiness to Kristin's life as well as the whole family. We feel lucky to have you and we love you.

CAROL JORGENSEN HUSTON

Reviewers

Sonia Acorn, RN, PhD
Professor Emeritus
School of Nursing
University of British Columbia
Vancouver, British Columbia

Jo Azzarello, PhD, RN
Associate Professor
University of Oklahoma College of Nursing
Oklahoma City, Oklahoma

Mary Bjorklund, MSN, RN, CPN
Instructor
Kingwood College
Houston, Texas

Vicky Bowden, RN, DNSc
Professor, School of Nursing
Director of the Honors Program
Azusa Pacific University
Azusa, California

Diane Breckenridge, PhD, RN
Associate Research Director
Abington Memorial Hospital
Abington, Pennsylvania
Associate Professor
La Salle University
Philadelphia, Pennsylvania

Liane Connelly, PhD, MSN, BSN, RN,
    CNAA, BC, COI
Professor, Coordinator of Undergraduate and
    Graduate Nursing Studies
Fort Hays State University
Hays, Kansas

Rose E. Constantino, PhD, JD, RN,
    FAAN
Associate Professor
University of Pittsburgh School of Nursing
Pittsburgh, Pennsylvania

William D. Corser, PhD, RN, CNAA
Assistant Professor
Michigan State University
East Lansing, Michigan

Deborah L. Dalrymple, RN, MSN,
    CRNI
Professor of Nursing
Montgomery County Community College
Blue Bell, Pennsylvania

Bonnie DeSimone, EdD, RN, C
Associate Professor of Nursing
Coordinator of the ABSN Option
Dominican College
Orangeburg, New York

Angela M. Duncan, MNSc, APRN, BC,
    CEN, TNS, SANE
Clinical Instructor
University of Arkansas for Medical Sciences,
    College of Nursing
Little Rock, Arkansas

Sally K. Fauchald, PhD, RN
Assistant Professor of Nursing
The College of St. Scholastica
Duluth, Minnesota

Earl Goldberg, EdD, APRN, BC
Associate Professor of Nursing and Health
    Sciences
Track Director, MSN-MBA, Nursing
    Administration Track
La Salle University
Philadelphia, Pennsylvania

Catherine Grant, MSN, CRNP
Assistant Professor
Carlow University
Pittsburgh, Pennsylvania

Deborah A. Greenawald, RN, MSN, CSN
Assistant Professor of Nursing
Alvernia College
Reading, Pennsylvania

Kris Hale, RN, MSN
Assistant Professor of Nursing
San Diego City College
San Diego, California

Pamela G. Harrison, EdD, RN
Associate Professor
Division of Nursing
Indiana Wesleyan University
Marion, Indiana

Carol Keihn, MS, RN
Instructor
Ball State University School of Nursing
Muncie, Illinois

Vera G. Kling, DHSc, MSN, RN
Assistant Professor of Nursing
Derry Patterson Wingo School of Nursing
Charleston Southern University
Charleston, South Carolina

Maura MacPhee, RN, PhD
Lecturer
University of British Columbia, Nursing
Vancouver, British Columbia

Paula McWilliam, MS, ARNP
Assistant Professor
Department of Nursing, University of
   New Hampshire
Durham, New Hampshire

Mitzi Grace Mitchell, RN, GNC (C), BScN, BA (Sociology), MHSc, MN, DNS, PhD (c)
Lecturer
York University
Toronto, Ontario

Mary Ellen Murray, BA, BS, MS, PhD, RN
Associate Professor
University of Wisconsin–Madison
Madison, Wisconsin

Suzanne Palko, RN, BSN, MSN
Associate Professor of Nursing
California University of Pennsylvania
California, Pennsylvania

Harry Plummer, RN, PhD
Assistant Professor
University of Calgary
Calgary, Alberta

Gayle Preheim, RN, EdD, CNAA-BC, CNE
Associate Professor, Director, Baccalaureate
   Nursing Program
University of Colorado at Denver and Health
   Sciences Center
School of Nursing
Denver, Colorado

Brenda B. Rowe, RN, MN, JD
Associate Professor
Georgia Baptist College of Nursing of
   Mercer University
Atlanta, Georgia

Marilyn Rubin, EdM
Instructor
Fairleigh Dickinson University
Teaneck, New Jersey

Mary Elizabeth Sadler, PhD, RN
Faculty
Department of Nursing & Allied Health
   Professions
Indiana University of Pennsylvania
Indiana, Pennsylvania

Anna Marie Schmidt, MA, RN, PHN, CHPN
Instructor
Anoka-Ramsey Community College
Cambridge, Minnesota

Vaida Siga, RN, BScN, MN
Nursing Program Coordinator
Medicine Hat University
Medicine Hat, Alberta

Darlene Sredl, PhD, RN
Assistant Professor of Nursing
College of Nursing, University of Missouri
    at St. Louis
St. Louis, Missouri

Thelma Sword, MSN, RN
Assistant Professor of Nursing
Graceland University
Independence, Missouri

Karen S. Thacker, DNSc, RN
Dean of Professional Programs
Alvernia College
Reading, Pennsylvania

Doris C. Vallone, RN, PhD
Associate Professor
Widener University School of Nursing
Chester, Pennsylvania

JoAlice Vecchio, RN, MSN, CSN, CCM
Associate Professor of Nursing
California University of Pennsylvania
California, Pennsylvania

Linda R. Wagner, RN, CNS, MA
Assistant Professor
College of St. Scholastica
Duluth, Minnesota

Kendra Williams-Perez, EdD, MSN, RN
Professor
Allen College
Waterloo, Iowa

Michelle Willihnganz, RN, MS
Nursing Instructor
Rochester Community and Technical College
Rochester, Minnesota

Nashat Zuraikat, RN, PhD
Professor and Graduate Coordinator
School of Nursing, Indiana University
    of Pennsylvania
Indiana, Pennsylvania

Preface

This book's philosophy has evolved over the past 26 years of teaching leadership and management. We entered academe from the community sector of the health care industry, where we held nursing management positions. In our first effort as authors, *Management Decision Making for Nurses: 101 Case Studies*, published in 1987, we used an experiential approach and emphasized management functions appropriate for first- and middle-level managers. The primary audience for this text was undergraduate nursing students.

Our second book, *Retention and Productivity Strategies for Nurse Managers*, focused on leadership skills necessary for managers to decrease attrition and increase productivity. This book was directed at the nurse–manager rather than the student. The experience of completing research for the second book, coupled with our clinical observations, compelled us to incorporate more leadership content in our teaching and to write this book.

Leadership Roles and Management Functions in Nursing was also influenced by national events in business and finance that have led many to believe that a lack of leadership in management is widespread. It has become apparent that if managers are to function effectively in the rapidly changing health care industry, enhanced leadership and management skills are needed.

What we have attempted to do, then, is combine these two very necessary elements: leadership and management. We do not see leadership as merely one role of management, nor management as only one role of leadership. We view the two as equally important and necessarily integrated. We have attempted to show this interdependence by defining the leadership components and management functions inherent in all phases of the management process. Undoubtedly, a few readers will find fault with our divisions of management functions and leadership roles; however, we felt it was necessary to first artificially separate the two components for the reader, and then to reiterate the roles and functions. We do believe strongly, however, that adoption of this integrated role is critical for success in management.

The second concept that shaped this book was our commitment to developing critical thinking skills through the use of experiential learning exercises and the promotion of whole-brain thinking. We propose that integrating leadership and management and using whole-brain thinking can be accomplished through the use of learning exercises. The overwhelming majority of academic instruction continues to be conducted in a teacher-lecturer–student-listener format, which is the least effective of all teaching strategies. Few individuals learn best using this style. Instead, most people learn best by methods that utilize concrete, experiential, self-initiated, and real-world learning experiences.

In nursing, theoretical teaching is almost always accompanied by concurrent clinical practice that allows concrete and real-world learning experience. However, the exploration of leadership and management theory often has only limited practicum experience, so learners may have little first-hand opportunity to observe middle- and top-level managers in nursing practice. As a result, novice managers may have only a few chances to practice their skills before assuming their first management position, and much of their decision making reflects trial-and-error methodologies. For us, then, there is little question that vicarious learning, or learning through mock experience, provides students the opportunity to make significant leadership and management decisions in a safe environment and to learn from the decisions they make.

Having gradually moved away from the lecturer–listener format in our classes, we lecture for only a small portion of class time. Our students, once resistant to the experiential approach, are now our most enthusiastic supporters. We also find this enthusiasm for experiential learning apparent in the many workshops and seminars we provide for registered nurses. Experiential learning enables management and leadership theory to be fun and exciting, but most important, it facilitates retention of didactic material. The research we have completed on this teaching approach supports these findings.

Although many leadership and management texts are available, our book meets the need for an emphasis on both leadership and management and the use of an experiential approach. More than 240 learning exercises, taken from various health care settings and a wide variety of learning modes, are included to give readers many opportunities to apply theory, resulting in internalized learning. In Chapter 1 we provide guidelines for using the experiential learning exercises. We strongly urge readers to use them to supplement the text.

We also provide guidelines for instructors on thePoint, Wolters Kluwer Health's trademarked web-based course and content management system that is available to instructors who adopt the text. We recommend its use. The website includes a test bank, an image collection, suggestions for using the learning exercises, a glossary, and a large number of PowerPoint slides with images.

TEXT ORGANIZATION

The first edition of *Leadership Roles and Management Functions in Nursing* presented the symbiotic elements of leadership and management, with an emphasis on problem solving and critical thinking. This sixth edition maintains this precedent with a balanced presentation of a strong theory component along with a variety of real-world scenarios in the experiential Learning Exercises. Responding to reviewer recommendations, we have changed the organization of the text by combining chapters, adding chapters, and reordering the sequence of some chapters. For example, classical views of leadership and management are now combined in Chapter 2, and a new chapter (Chapter 3) on cutting-edge thinking about leadership and management has been added.

We have also retained the strengths of earlier editions, reflecting content and application exercises appropriate to the issues faced by nurse leader–managers as they practice in an era increasingly characterized by limited resources and emerging technologies. The sixth edition also includes contemporary research and theory to ensure accuracy of the didactic material.

Unit I provides a foundation for the decision-making, problem-solving, and critical-thinking skills, as well as management and leadership skills needed to address the management–leadership problems presented in the text. Unit II covers ethics, legal concepts, and advocacy, which we see as core components of leadership and management decision making. The remaining units are organized using the management processes of planning, organizing, staffing, directing, and controlling.

LEARNING TOOLS

The sixth edition contains many pedagogical features designed to benefit both the student and instructor:

Examining the Evidence, new to this edition and appearing in each chapter, depicts new research findings, evidence-based practice, and best practices in leadership and management.

Learning Exercises interspersed throughout each chapter foster readers' critical-thinking skills and promote interactive discussions. Additional Learning Exercises are also presented at the end of each chapter for further study and discussion.

Tables, displays, and illustrations are liberally supplied throughout the text to reinforce learning as well as to help clarify complex information.

Key Concepts summarize important information within every chapter.

Web Links at the end of each chapter guide the reader to new information on specific topics.

NEW AND EXPANDED CONTENT

Learning Exercises with new situations have been added, further strengthening the problem-based element of this text. A new chapter, Chapter 3: 21st Century Thinking About Leadership and Management, includes the latest thinking about emotional intelligence, quantum thinking, servant leadership, principal agent theory, human and social capital theory, authentic leadership, quantum leadership, thought leadership, and cultural bridging. Additional content that has been added or expanded includes:

- The need for evidence-based practice in all leadership and management decision making
- A review of traditional problem-solving and decision-making models as well as the addition of newer ones, including the IDEALS model and intuitive decision-making models
- New models for ethical problem solving
- A more detailed description of SWOT analysis, as well as an introduction to the Balanced Scorecard, both strategic planning tools
- An expanded discussion of chaos theory, systems theory, and nonlinear theories to explain organizational functioning and change
- Additional content on health care reimbursement, including public and private insurance as well as hybrid plans
- The importance of promoting evidence-based practice in career planning
- New clinical models for organizing patient care that recognize the RN as an expert clinician and leader
- A broadened discussion of the current nursing shortage and the impact of that shortage on patient outcomes and worker satisfaction
- An expanded discussion of the impact of new technologies on organizational communication and the ever-increasing challenges of maintaining client confidentiality
- An introduction to the Learning Organization as a means of enhancing productivity as well as developing human resources
- An expanded focus on creating work cultures that maximize patient and worker safety

- A more detailed examination of the application for and benefits of Magnet Certification
- New content on the use of interdisciplinary teams
- An expanded discussion of "bullying" and horizontal violence in the workplace

thePOINT

the**Point** (http://thepoint.lww.com), a trademark of Wolters Kluwer Health, is a web-based course and content management system providing every resource that instructors and students need in one easy-to-use site.

Instructor Resources

Advanced technology and superior content combine at thePoint to allow instructors to design and deliver on-line and off-line courses, maintain grades and class rosters, and communicate with students.

In addition, instructors will find the following content designed specifically for this edition:
- Test bank
- Image bank
- Instructor's Guide, including guidelines for using the experiential learning exercises in the text
- PowerPoint slides with images

Student Resources

Students can visit thePoint to access supplemental multimedia resources to enhance their learning experience, download content, upload assignments, and join an on-line study group. Students will also find a glossary that defines the italicized terms in the text.

Contents

UNIT I

THE CRITICAL TRIAD: DECISION MAKING, MANAGEMENT, AND LEADERSHIP 1

1 **Decision Making, Problem Solving, and Critical Thinking: Requisites for Successful Leadership and Management 1**

Decision Making, Problem Solving, and Critical Thinking 2
Vicarious Learning to Increase Problem-Solving and Decision-Making Skills 3
Theoretical Approaches to Problem Solving and Decision Making 5
Critical Elements in Problem Solving and Decision Making 9
Individual Variations in Decision Making 14
Overcoming Individual Vulnerability in Decision Making 17
Decision Making in Organizations 18
Pitfalls in Using Decision-Making Tools 25
Summary 25
Additional Learning Exercises and Applications 26

2 **Classical Views of Leadership and Management 31**

Managers 31
Leaders 32
Historical Development of Management Theory 33
Historical Development of Leadership Theory (1900–Present) 37
Integrating Leadership and Management 44
Summary 45
Additional Learning Exercises and Applications 46

3 **Twenty-First Century Thinking About Leadership and Management 51**

New Thinking About Leadership and Management 52
Transition From Industrial Age Leadership to Relationship Age Leadership 62
Leadership and Management for Nursing's Future 64
Additional Learning Exercises and Applications 65

UNIT II

FOUNDATION FOR EFFECTIVE LEADERSHIP AND MANAGEMENT: ETHICS, LAW, AND ADVOCACY 69

4 **Ethical Issues 69**

Types of Ethical Issues 70
Ethical Frameworks for Decision Making 72
Principles of Ethical Reasoning 73

American Nurses Association Code of Ethics and Professional Standards 77
Ethical Problem Solving and Decision Making 77
Ethical Dimensions in Leadership and Management 84
Integrating Leadership Roles and Management Functions in Ethics, Law,
    and Advocacy 88
Additional Learning Exercises and Applications 89

5   **Legal and Legislative Issues 93**
Sources of Law 94
Types of Laws and Courts 96
Legal Doctrines and the Practice of Nursing 97
Professional Negligence 98
Avoiding Malpractice Claims 100
Extending the Liability 102
Incident Reports 104
Intentional Torts 104
Other Legal Responsibilities of the Manager 105
Legal Considerations of Managing a Diverse Workforce 111
Professional Versus Institutional Licensure 112
Integrating Leadership Roles and Management Functions in Legal and
    Legislative Issues 113
Additional Learning Exercises and Applications 115

6   **Patient, Subordinate, and Professional Advocacy 119**
Becoming an Advocate 120
Patient Advocacy and Patient Rights 121
Whistle-Blowing as Advocacy 125
Professional Advocacy 127
Additional Learning Exercises and Applications 134

UNIT III

ROLES AND FUNCTIONS IN PLANNING 140

7   **Operational and Strategic Planning 140**
Proactive Planning 142
Strategic Planning 143
Looking to the Future 146
Organizational Planning: The Planning Hierarchy 148
Vision and Mission Statements 148
The Organization's Philosophy Statement 150
Societal Philosophies and Values 153
Individual Philosophies and Values 154
Goals and Objectives 156
Policies and Procedures 158
Rules 160

Overcoming Barriers to Planning 161
Integrating Leadership Roles and Management Functions in Operational and
    Strategic Planning 161
Additional Learning Exercises and Applications 163

8   Planned Change 166
The Development of Change Theory: Kurt Lewin 167
A Contemporary Adaptation of Lewin's Model 169
Lewin's Driving and Restraining Forces 170
Organizational Change Associated With Nonlinear Dynamics 171
Classic Change Strategies 174
Resistance: The Expected Response to Change 176
Planned Change as a Collaborative Process 177
The Leader–Manager as a Role Model During Planned Change 178
Organizational Aging: Change as a Means of Renewal 179
Is the Nursing Profession in Need of Renewal? 180
Integrating Leadership Roles and Management Functions in Planned Change 180
Additional Learning Experiences and Applications 182

9   Time Management 186
Three Basic Steps to Time Management 187
Managing Time at Work 192
Integrating Leadership Roles and Management Functions in Time Management 197
Additional Learning Exercises and Applications 200

10   Fiscal Planning 208
Balancing Costs and Quality 210
Responsibility Accounting and Forecasting 210
Basics of Budgets 211
Steps in the Budgetary Process 211
Types of Budgets 214
Budgeting Methods 219
Critical Pathways 221
Health Care Reimbursement 221
Medicare and Medicaid 223
The Prospective Payment System 223
The Managed Care Movement 224
Proponents and Critics of Managed Care Speak Up 226
The Future of Managed Care 228
Integrating Leadership Roles and Management Functions in Fiscal Planning 230
Additional Learning Exercises and Applications 232

11   Career Development: From New Graduate to Retirement 239
Justifications for Career Development 240
The Organization's Responsibility for Career Development 243
Career Coaching 244
Competency Assessment as Part of Career Development 247

Professional Specialty Certification 248
Employee Transfers 249
Promotions 251
Management Development 253
Résumé Preparation 254
Preparing a Professional Portfolio 256
Integrating Leadership Roles and Management Functions in Career Development 257
Additional Learning Exercises and Applications 259

UNIT IV

ROLES AND FUNCTIONS IN ORGANIZING 264

12 **Organizational Structure 264**
Organizational Theory 265
Components of Organizational Structure 267
Types of Organizational Structures 273
Decision Making Within the Organizational Hierarchy 275
Stakeholders 276
Limitations of Organization Charts 277
Organizational Culture 278
Shared Governance: Organizational Design for the 21st Century? 280
Organizations and Magnet Status 283
Committee Structure in an Organization 284
Responsibilities and Opportunities of Committee Work 285
Organizational Effectiveness 286
Integrating Leadership Roles and Management Functions Associated With Organizational Structure 287
Additional Learning Exercises and Applications 289

13 **Understanding Organizational, Political, and Personal Power 293**
Understanding Power 294
The Authority–Power Gap 297
Mobilizing the Power of Nursing 301
Strategies for Building a Personal Power Base 303
The Politics of Power 306
Integrating Leadership Roles and Management Functions in Understanding Organizational, Political, and Personal Power 309
Additional Learning Exercises and Applications 310

14 **Organizing Patient Care 315**
Traditional Modes of Organizing Patient Care 315
Disease Management and Case Management 325
Differentiated Nursing Practice 327
What the Future Holds for Patient Care Delivery Models 328
Selecting the Optimum Mode of Organizing Patient Care 329

Integrating Leadership Roles and Management Functions in Organizing
Patient Care 331
Additional Learning Exercises and Applications 332

UNIT V

ROLES AND FUNCTIONS IN STAFFING 335

15 Employee Recruitment, Selection, Placement, and Indoctrination 335
Predicting Staffing Needs 336
The Current Nursing Shortage 337
Supply Factors 338
Demand Factors 340
Recruitment 341
The Initial Contact 343
Interviewing as a Selection Tool 344
Tips for the Interviewee 352
Selection 354
Placement 357
Indoctrination 359
Integrating Leadership Roles and Management Functions in Employee Recruitment,
Selection, Placement, and Indoctrination 363
Additional Learning Exercises and Applications 364

16 Socializing and Educating Staff for Team Building 369
The Learning Organization 370
Staff Development 371
Theories of Learning 372
Assessing Staff Development Needs 376
Evaluation of Staff Development Activities 377
Shared Responsibility for Implementing Evidence-Based Practice 379
Socialization and Resocialization 379
Employees With Unique Socialization Needs 383
Meeting the Educational Needs of a Culturally Diverse Staff 389
Building Team Unity Through Staff Development and Socialization 390
Integrating Leadership and Management in Team Building Through Socializing
and Educating Staff for Team Building 391
Additional Learning Exercises and Applications 392

17 Staffing Needs and Scheduling Policies 397
Unit Manager's Responsibilities in Meeting Staffing Needs 397
Centralized and Decentralized Staffing 398
Managing a Diverse Staff 399
Complying With Staffing Mandates 400
Staffing and Scheduling Options 402
Workload Measurement Tools 405

The Relationship Between Nursing Care Hours, Staffing Mix, and Quality of Care 409
Generational Considerations for Staffing 410
The Impact of a Shortage of Nursing Staff Upon Staffing 411
Fiscal and Ethical Accountability for Staffing 412
Developing Staffing and Scheduling Policies 413
Integrating Leadership Roles and Management Functions in Staffing Needs and
    Scheduling Policies 415
Additional Learning Exercises and Applications 416

UNIT VI

ROLES AND FUNCTIONS IN DIRECTING 421

18 **Creating a Motivating Climate 421**
Intrinsic Versus Extrinsic Motivation 422
Motivational Theory 424
Creating a Motivating Climate 429
Finding Joy at Work: A Shared Responsibility 431
Strategies for Creating a Motivating Climate 432
Professional Support Systems for the Manager 433
Integrating Leadership Roles and Management Functions in Creating a
    Motivating Climate 434
Additional Learning Exercises and Applications 435

19 **Organizational, Interpersonal, and Group Communication 441**
The Communication Process 443
Variables Affecting Organizational Communication 445
Organizational Communication Strategies 446
The Impact of Technology on Contemporary Organizational Communication 447
Channels of Communication 448
Communication Modes 449
Written Communication Within the Organization 450
Elements of Nonverbal Communication 452
Verbal Communication Skills 454
Listening Skills 456
Group Communication 456
Group Dynamics 456
Communication and Confidentiality 459
Integrating Leadership and Management in Organizational, Interpersonal, and
    Group Communication 461
Additional Learning Exercises and Applications 462

20 **Delegation 468**
Common Delegation Errors 469
Effective Delegating 471
Delegation as a Function of Professional Nursing 473

Integrating Leadership Roles and Management Functions in Delegation 480
Additional Learning Exercises and Applications 482

21 **Managing Conflict 487**
The History of Conflict Management 488
Categories of Conflict 490
The Conflict Process 492
Conflict Management 493
Managing Unit Conflict 497
Negotiation 499
Alternative Dispute Resolution 504
Seeking Consensus 505
Integrating Leadership Skills and Management Functions in
    Managing Conflict 505
Additional Learning Exercises and Applications 507

22 **Understanding Collective Bargaining, Unionization, and
Employment Laws 513**
Unions and Collective Bargaining 514
Historical Perspective of Unionization in America 515
American Nurses Association and Collective Bargaining 517
Employee Motivation to Join or Reject Unions 518
Union-Organizing Strategies 521
Managers' Role During Union Organizing 521
Effective Labor–Management Relations 524
Employment Legislation 525
State Health Facilities Licensing Boards 533
Integrating Leadership Roles and Management Functions in Understanding
    Collective Bargaining, Unionization, and Employment Laws 533
Additional Learning Exercises and Applications 534

UNIT VII

ROLES AND FUNCTIONS IN CONTROLLING 537

23 **Quality Control 537**
Defining Quality Health Care 538
Quality Control as a Process 540
The Development of Standards 543
Audits as a Quality Control Tool 545
Quality Improvement Models 548
Who Should Be Involved in Quality Control? 550
Quality Measurement as an Organizational Mandate 550
Medical Errors: An Ongoing Threat to Quality of Care 557
Integrating Leadership Roles and Management Functions in Quality Control 560
Additional Learning Exercises and Applications 563

24 Performance Appraisal 569

Using the Performance Appraisal to Motivate Employees 570
Strategies to Ensure Accuracy and Fairness in the Performance Appraisal 572
Performance Appraisal Tools 575
Planning the Appraisal Interview 582
Overcoming Appraisal Interview Difficulties 583
Performance Management 585
Coaching: A Mechanism for Informal Performance Appraisal 586
Becoming an Effective Coach 586
Integrating Leadership Roles and Management Functions in Conducting Performance Appraisals 587
Additional Learning Exercises and Applications 588

25 Problem Employees: Rule Breakers, Marginal Employees, and the Chemically or Psychologically Impaired 593

Constructive Versus Destructive Discipline 594
Self-Discipline and Group Norms 596
Fair and Effective Rules 597
Discipline as a Progressive Process 598
Disciplinary Strategies for the Nurse–Manager 602
Grievance Procedures 606
Disciplining the Unionized Employee 607
The Marginal Employee 609
The Chemically Impaired Employee 610
Integrating Leadership Roles and Management Functions Through Dealing With Problem Employees 619
Additional Learning Exercises and Applications 620

APPENDIX
Solutions to Selected Learning Exercises 624

INDEX 634

1

Decision Making, Problem Solving, and Critical Thinking:
Requisites for Successful Leadership and Management

> . . . the successful nurse executive has the ability to make good decisions consistently.
>
> —*Thomas R. Clancy*

> . . . in any moment of decision the best thing you can do is the right thing, the next best thing is the wrong thing, and the worst thing you can do is nothing.
>
> —*Theodore Roosevelt*

Decision making is often thought to be synonymous with management and is one of the criteria on which management expertise is judged. Much of any manager's time is spent critically examining issues, solving problems, and making decisions. The quality of the decisions that leader–managers make is the factor that often weighs most heavily in their success or failure. As a character in J. K. Rowling's Harry Potter series says, "It is our choices . . . that show what we truly are, far more than our abilities" (*Beginner's Guide*, September 2005, para 2).

Decision making, then, is both the innermost leadership activity and the core of management. This chapter explores the primary requisites for successful management and leadership: decision making, problem solving, and critical thinking. Also, because it is the authors' belief that decision making, problem solving, and critical thinking are learned skills that improve with practice and consistency, an introduction to established tools, techniques, and strategies for effective decision making is included. This chapter introduces the learning exercise as a new approach for

1

vicariously gaining skill in management and leadership decision making. Finally, evidence-based decision making is introduced as an imperative for both individual and professional problem solving.

DECISION MAKING, PROBLEM SOLVING, AND CRITICAL THINKING

Decision making is a complex, cognitive process often defined as choosing a particular course of action. *Beginner's Guide* (September 2005) defines *decision making* as "the process of choosing one course of action over another" (para 1). Both definitions imply that there was *doubt* about several courses of action and that a choice was made that eliminated the uncertainty.

Problem solving is part of decision making. A systematic process that focuses on analyzing a difficult situation, *problem solving* always includes a decision-making step. Many educators use the terms *problem solving* and *decision making* synonymously, but there is a small yet important difference between the two. Although decision making is the last step in the problem-solving process, it is possible for decision making to occur without the full analysis required in problem solving. Because problem solving attempts to identify the root problem in situations, much time and energy are spent on identifying the real problem.

Decision making, on the other hand, is usually triggered by a problem but is often handled in a manner that does not focus on eliminating the underlying problem. For example, if a person decided to handle a conflict crisis when it occurred but did not attempt to identify the real problem causing the conflict, only decision-making skills would be used. The decision maker might later choose to address the real cause of the conflict or might decide to do nothing at all about the problem. The decision has been made *not* to problem solve. This alternative may be selected because of a lack of energy, time, or resources to solve the real problem adequately. In some situations, this is an appropriate decision. For example, assume a nursing supervisor has a staff nurse who has been absent a great deal over the last 3 months. Normally, the supervisor would feel compelled to intervene. However, the supervisor has reliable information that the nurse will be resigning soon to return to school in another state. Because the problem will soon no longer exist, the supervisor *decides* that the time and energy needed to correct the problem are not warranted.

Critical thinking, sometimes referred to as reflective thinking, is related to evaluation and has a broader scope than decision making and problem solving. "Critical thinking is a manner of thinking that moves from the general to specific, ever narrowing the focus until the logic of both the questions and arguments comes to the same conclusion (*Beginner's Guide*, November 2005, para 2). In other words, critical thinking can be seen as having two components: "1) a set of information and belief generating and processing skills, and 2) the habit, based on intellectual commitment, of using those skills to guide behavior" (Foundation for Critical Thinking, 2004, para 3).

Similarly, critical thinking consists of a mental process of analyzing or evaluating information, particularly statements or propositions that have been offered as true. It involves reflecting upon the meaning of statements, examining the offered evidence and reasoning, and forming judgments about facts. Whatever definition of critical thinking is used, most agree that it is more complex than problem solving or decision making, involves higher-order reasoning and evaluation, and has

DISPLAY 1.1   **Characteristics of a Critical Thinker**

Open to new ideas	Flexible	Creative
Intuitive	Empathetic	Insightful
Energetic	Caring	Willing to take action
Analytical	Observant	Outcome directed
Persistent	Risk taker	Willing to change
Assertive	Resourceful	Knowledgeable
Communicator	"Outside the box" thinker	

both a cognitive and affective component. The authors believe that insight, intuition, empathy, and the willingness to take action are additional components of critical thinking. These same skills are necessary to some degree in decision making and problem solving. See Display 1.1 for additional characteristics of a critical thinker.

 Insight, intuition, empathy, and the willingness to take action are components of critical thinking.

VICARIOUS LEARNING TO INCREASE PROBLEM-SOLVING AND DECISION-MAKING SKILLS

Decision making, one step in the problem-solving process, is an important task that relies heavily on critical thinking skills. How do people become successful problem solvers and decision makers? Although successful decision making can be learned through life experience, not everyone learns to solve problems and judge wisely by this trial-and-error method because much is left to chance. Some educators feel that people are not successful in problem solving and decision making because individuals are not taught how to reason insightfully from multiple perspectives. Moreover, information and new learning are seldom presented within the context of real-life situations.

Case Studies

Case studies may remedy both problems. Indeed, this was the case in research done by Bowers (2004), which concluded that case study learning provided a positive learning experience to promote clinical decision making and judgment in nursing students. Similarly, simulation models are increasingly being used by schools of nursing to allow the transference of textbook knowledge into a real-life situation where nursing students can function in their role without negatively affecting their clients (Robertson, 2006).

The Marquis-Huston Critical Thinking Teaching Model

The desired outcome for teaching and learning decision making and critical thinking in management is an interaction between learners and others that results in the ability to critically examine management and leadership issues. This is a learning of appropriate social/professional

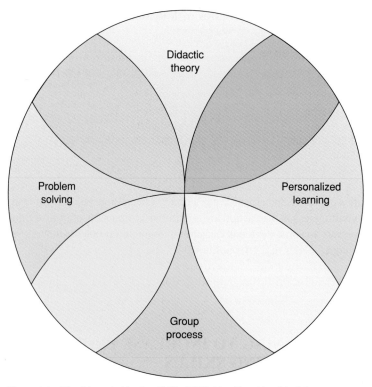

Figure 1.1   The Marquis-Huston Critical-Thinking Teaching Model.

behaviors rather than a mere acquisition of knowledge. This type of learning occurs best in groups. When teaching management and leadership, therefore, the group process should be used in some way.

Additionally, learners retain didactic material more readily when it is personalized or when they can relate to the material being presented. The use of case studies that learners can identify with assists in retention of didactic materials.

While formal instruction in critical thinking is important, using a formal decision-making process improves both the quality and consistency of decision making. Many new leaders and managers struggle to make quality decisions because their opportunity to practice making management and leadership decisions is very limited until they are appointed to a management position. These limitations can be overcome by creating opportunities for vicariously experiencing the problems that individuals would encounter in the real world of leadership and management.

The Marquis-Huston Model for Teaching Critical Thinking assists in achieving desired learner outcomes (Fig. 1.1). Basically, the model comprises four overlapping spheres, each being an essential component for teaching leadership and management. The first is a didactic theory component, such as the material that is presented in each chapter; second, a formalized approach to problem solving and decision making must be used. Third, there must be some use of the group process, which can be accomplished through large and small groups and classroom discussion. Finally, the material must be made real for the learner so that the learning is internalized. This can be accomplished through writing exercises, personal exploration, and values clarification, along with risk-taking, as case studies are examined.

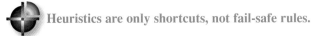 Experiential learning provides mock experiences that have tremendous value in applying leadership and management theory.

This book was developed with the perspective that experiential learning provides mock experiences that have tremendous value in applying leadership and management theory. The text includes numerous opportunities for readers to experience the real world of leadership and management. Some of these learning situations, called learning exercises, include case studies, writing exercises, specific management or leadership problems, staffing and budgeting calculations, group discussion or problem-solving situations, and assessment of personal attitudes and values. Some exercises include opinions, speculation, and value judgments. All of the learning exercises, however, require some degree of critical thinking, problem solving, or decision making.

Some of the case studies have been solved (solutions are found at the back of the book) so that readers can observe how a systematic problem-solving or decision-making model can be applied in solving problems common to nurse–managers. The authors feel strongly, however, that the problem solving suggested in the solved cases should not be considered the only plausible solution or "the right solution" to that learning exercise. Most of the learning exercises in the book have multiple solutions that could be implemented successfully to solve the problem.

THEORETICAL APPROACHES TO PROBLEM SOLVING AND DECISION MAKING

Most people make decisions too quickly and fail to systematically examine the problem or its alternatives for solution. Instead, most individuals rely on discrete, often unconscious processes known as *heuristics*. Heuristics involve "being able to recognize patterns and then being able to more rapidly solve a problem or come to a conclusion" (Pritchard, 2006, p. 128). Thus, it is "a way of thinking and solving problems, quickly, efficiently, and maximizing what is already known" (Heuristic Solutions, n.d., para 1). Heuristics also frequently refer to using a trial and error or rules of thumb approach to problem solving. Facione (2006) recognizes the value of heuristics in decision making but warns that heuristics are only shortcuts, not fail-safe rules, and that relying on heuristics may work most of the time but will not be the best all of the time.

 Heuristics are only shortcuts, not fail-safe rules.

Formal process and structure can benefit the decision-making process, as they force decision makers to be specific about options and to separate probabilities from values. A structured approach to problem solving and decision making increases critical reasoning and is the best way to learn how to make quality decisions because it eliminates trial and error and focuses the learning on a proven process. A structured or professional approach involves applying a theoretical model in problem solving and decision making.

A structured approach to problem solving and decision making increases critical reasoning.

To improve decision-making ability, it is important to use an adequate process model as the theoretical base for understanding and applying critical-thinking skills. Many acceptable problem-solving models exist, and most include a decision-making step; only four are reviewed here.

Traditional Problem-Solving Process

One of the most well-known and widely used problem-solving models is the *traditional problem-solving model*. The seven steps follow. (Decision-making occurs at step 5.)
1. Identify the problem.
2. Gather data to analyze the causes and consequences of the problem.
3. Explore alternative solutions.
4. Evaluate the alternatives.
5. Select the appropriate solution.
6. Implement the solution.
7. Evaluate the results.

Although the traditional problem-solving process is an effective model, its weakness lies in the amount of time needed for proper implementation. This process, therefore, is less effective when time constraints are a consideration. Another weakness is lack of an initial objective-setting step. Setting a decision goal helps to prevent the decision maker from becoming sidetracked.

Managerial Decision-Making Models

To address the weaknesses of the traditional problem-solving process, many contemporary models for management decision making have added an objective-setting step. These models are known as *managerial decision-making models*. One such model suggested by Sorach (2000) includes the following steps:
1. Determine the importance and the context of the decision.
2. Determine the objectives for the decision.
3. List all options.
4. Explore promising options.
5. Establish decision-making criteria.
6. Evaluate the options against the criteria.
7. Select the options to pursue.
8. Analyze the risks.

In the first step, problem solvers must consider the possible consequences of the decision, the time period involved, and who needs to be involved in the decision process. More important decisions require more careful consideration of context. Primary and secondary goals are outlined in the second step as well as desirable and undesirable outcomes. In step 3, problem solvers must attempt to identify as many alternatives as possible. Alternatives are then analyzed in step 4, often using some type of SWOT (strengths, weaknesses, opportunities, and threats) analysis. In step 5, objectives are rank ordered or quantified so that problem solvers are clear regarding which criteria will be weighted most heavily in making their decision. Step 6 then encourages decision makers to apply quantitative decision-making tools, such as decision-making grids or payoff tables (discussed further later in this chapter), to objectively review the desirability of alternatives. In step 7, desirable alternatives or combinations of alternatives are selected for implementation. In the final step, challenges to successful implementation of chosen alternatives are identified and strategies are developed to manage those risks.

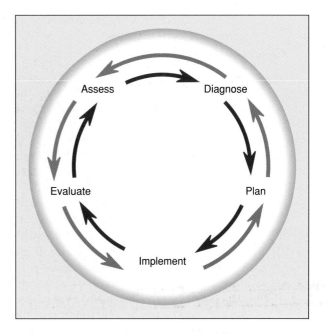

Figure 1.2 Feedback mechanism of the nursing process.

The Nursing Process

The *nursing process*, developed by Ida Jean Orlando in the late 1950s, provides another theoretical system for solving problems and making decisions. Originally a four-step model (assess, plan, implement, and evaluate), diagnosis was delineated as a separate step, and most contemporary depictions of this model now include at least five steps.

As a decision-making model, the greatest strength of the nursing process may be its multiple venues for feedback. The arrows in Figure 1.2 show constant input into the process. When the decision point has been identified, initial decision making occurs and continues throughout the process via a feedback mechanism.

Although the process was designed for nursing practice with regard to patient care and nursing accountability, it can easily be adapted as a theoretical model for solving leadership and management problems. Table 1.1 shows how closely the nursing process parallels the decision-making process.

The weakness of the nursing process, like the traditional problem-solving model, is in not requiring clearly stated objectives. Goals should be clearly stated in the planning phase of the process, but this step is frequently omitted or obscured. However, because nurses are familiar with this process and its proven effec-

TABLE 1.1 **Comparing the Decision-Making Process With the Nursing Process**

Decision–Making Process	Simplified Nursing Process
Identify the decision	Assess
Collect data	
Identify criteria for decision	Plan
Identify alternatives	
Choose alternative	Implement
Implement alternative	
Evaluate steps in decision	Evaluate

tiveness, it continues to be recommended as an adapted theoretical process for leadership and managerial decision making.

The IDEALS Model

A more contemporary model for effective thinking and problem solving, the *IDEALS model* was developed by Facione (2006) and includes six steps for effective thinking and problem solving. While similar to the models already presented, the mnemonic IDEALS makes this model easy to remember and use:

Identify the problem. "What's the real question we're facing here?"
Define the context. "What are the facts and circumstances that frame this problem?"
Enumerate choices. "What are our most plausible three or four options?"
Analyze options. "What is our best course of action, all things considered?"
List reasons explicitly. "Let's be clear: Why are we making this particular choice?"
Self-correct. "Okay, let's look at it again. What did we miss?" (p. 22).

Many other excellent problem analysis and decision models exist. The model selected should be one with which the decision maker is familiar and one appropriate for the problem to be solved. Using models or processes consistently will increase the likelihood that critical analysis will occur. Moreover, the quality of management/leadership problem solving and decision making will improve tremendously via a scientific approach.

 By cultivating a scientific approach, the quality of one's management/leadership problem solving and decision making will improve tremendously.

Intuitive Decision-Making Model

There are theorists who suggest that intuition should always be used as an adjunct to empirical or rational decision-making models. Andrews (2006) suggests that "one of the critical skills separating good leaders from great leaders is the conscious use of intuition in daily decision making. Great leaders actively call on their intuition to enhance decision making, whereas less effective leaders tend to rely too heavily on traditional approaches" (para 1).

Leaders in the field of intuitive decision-making research include Gary Klein. Dr. Klein and his colleagues developed the *Recognition-Primed Decision (RPD) model* for intuitive decision making in the mid-1980s to explain how people can make effective decisions under time pressure and uncertainty. Considered a part of *naturalistic decision making*, the RPD model attempts to understand how humans make relatively quick decisions in complex, real-world settings such as fire fighting or critical care nursing without having to compare options (Klein, 2004). Klein's work suggests that instead of using classical rational or systematic decision-making processes, many individuals act on their first impulse if the "imagined future" looks acceptable. If this turns out not to be the case, another idea or concept is allowed to emerge from their subconscious and is examined for probable successful implementation. Thus, the RPD model blends intuition and analysis, but pattern recognition and experience guide decision makers when time is limited or systematic rational decision making is not possible.

Aloi (2006) suggests that many expert nurses use intuition in solving problems. Experienced nurses often report that gut-level feelings encourage them to take appropriate strategic action that impacts patient outcomes. Alois warns, however, that the dark side of intuition is misjudgment and that intuition should serve only as an adjunct to decision making founded on nursing's scientific knowledge base.

LEARNING EXERCISE 1.1

Applying Scientific Models to Decision Making

You are an RN who graduated 3 years ago. During the last 3 years, your responsibilities in your first position have increased. Although you enjoy your family (spouse and one preschool-age child), you realize that you love your job and that your career is very important to you. Recently, you and your spouse decided to have another baby. At that time, you and your spouse reached a joint decision that if you had another baby, you wanted to reduce your work time and spend more time at home with the children. Last week, your supervisor told you that the charge nurse is leaving. You were thrilled and excited when she said that she wants to appoint you to the position. Yesterday, you found out that you and your spouse are expecting a baby.

Last night, you spoke with your spouse about your career future. Your spouse is an attorney whose practice has suddenly gained momentum. Although the two of you have shared child rearing equally until this point, your spouse is not sure how much longer this can be done if the law practice continues to expand. If you take the position, which you would like to do, it would mean full-time work. You want the decision that you and your spouse reach to be well thought out, as it has far-reaching consequences and concerns many people.

● ASSIGNMENT: Determine what you should do. After you have made your decision, get together in a group (four to six people) and share your resolutions. Were your decisions the same? How did you approach the problem solving differently from others in your group? Was a rational systematic problem-solving process used, or was the chosen solution based more on intuition? How many alternatives were generated? Did some of the group members identify alternatives that you had not considered? Was a goal(s) or objective identified? How did your personal values influence your decision?

CRITICAL ELEMENTS IN PROBLEM SOLVING AND DECISION MAKING

Because decisions may have far-reaching consequences, some problem solving and decision making must be of high quality. Using a scientific approach alone for problem solving and decision making does not, however, ensure a quality decision. Special attention must be paid to other critical elements. The following elements (Display 1.2), considered crucial in problem solving, must occur if a high-quality decision is to be made.

DISPLAY 1.2 Critical Elements in Decision Making

- Define objectives clearly.
- Gather data carefully.
- Generate many alternatives.
- Think logically.
- Choose and act decisively.

Define Objectives Clearly

Decision makers often forge ahead in their problem-solving process without first determining their goals or objectives. However, it is especially important to determine goals and objectives when problems are complex. Even when decisions must be made quickly, there is time to pause and reflect on the purpose of the decision. A decision that is made without a clear objective in mind or a decision that is inconsistent with one's philosophy is likely to be a poor-quality decision. Sometimes the problem has been identified but the wrong objectives are set.

 If a decision lacks a clear objective or if an objective is not consistent with the individual or organization's stated philosophy, a poor-quality decision is likely.

Gather Data Carefully

Because decisions are based on knowledge and information available to the problem solver at the time the decision must be made, one must learn how to process and obtain accurate information. The acquisition of information begins with identifying the problem or the occasion for the decision and continues throughout the problem-solving process. Often the information is unsolicited, but most information is sought actively. Acquiring information always involves people, and no tool or mechanism is infallible to human error. Girard (2005) suggests that an individual often must ask "why" five times to get to the root of a situation or problem. Questions that should be asked in data gathering are shown in Display 1.3.

In addition, human values tremendously influence our perceptions. Therefore, as problem solvers gather information, they must be vigilant that their own preferences and those of others are not mistaken for facts.

Keep in mind that facts can be misleading if they are presented in a seductive manner, if they are taken out of context, or if they are past oriented.

How many parents have been misled by the factual statement, "Johnny hit me"? In this case, the information seeker needs to do more fact finding. What was the accuser doing before Johnny hit him? What was he hit with? Where was he hit? When was he hit? Like the parent, the manager who becomes expert at acquiring adequate, appropriate, and accurate information will have a head start in becoming an expert decision maker and problem solver.

DISPLAY 1.3 Questions to Examine in Data Gathering

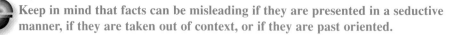

1. What is the setting?
2. What is the problem?
3. Where is it a problem?
4. When is it a problem?
5. Who is affected by the problem?
6. What is happening?
7. Why is it happening? What are the causes of the problem? Can the causes be prioritized?
8. What are the basic underlying issues? What are the areas of conflict?
9. What are the consequences of the problem? Which is the most serious?

LEARNING EXERCISE 1.2

Gathering Necessary Information
Identify a poor decision that you recently made because of faulty data gathering. Have you ever made a poor decision because necessary information was intentionally or unintentionally withheld from you?

Use an Evidence-Based Approach

To gain knowledge and insight into managerial and leadership decision making, individuals must reach outside their current sphere of knowledge in solving the problems presented in this text. Some data-gathering sources include textbooks, periodicals, experts in the field, colleagues, and current research. Indeed, "both *Evidence-Based Medicine* (EBM) and *Evidence-Based Practice* (EBP) assert that making clinical decisions based on best evidence, either from the research literature or clinical expertise, improves the quality of care and patients' quality of life" (Evidence-Based Practice Resource Center, 2006).

Nurses, then, must use an evidence-based approach in data gathering to make decisions regarding their nursing practice. Sigma Theta Tau International, the honor society for nurses, defines *evidence-based nursing practice* as:

> [T]he integration of the best evidence available, nursing expertise, and the values and preferences of the individuals, families and communities who are served. This assumes that optimal nursing care is provided when nurses and health care decision makers have access to a synthesis of the latest research, a consensus of expert opinion, and are thus able to exercise their judgment as they plan and provide care that takes into account cultural and personal values and preferences. (DiCenso et al., 2004, p. 69)

Yet Prevost (2006) suggests that many practicing nurses feel they do not have the time, access, or expertise needed to search and analyze the research literature to answer clinical questions. In addition, most staff nurses practicing in clinical settings have less than a baccalaureate degree and therefore may not have been exposed to a formal research course. Findings from research studies may also be technical, difficult to understand, and even more difficult to translate into practice. In addition, Clovis and Cobban (2006) suggest that health care practitioners may apply scientific evidence in their daily practices without any real appreciation of the theories or methodologies involved. Thus, an understanding of *why* certain practices are appropriate and *how* they came into being is needed to contribute to better application in practice (Clovis & Cobban, 2006). Strategies the new nurse might use to promote evidence-based practice are shown in Display 1.4

Evidence-based decision making and evidence-based practice should be viewed as imperatives for all nurses today as well as for the profession in general.

It is important to recognize that the implementation of evidence-based best practices is not just an individual, staff nurse–level pursuit (Prevost, 2006). Too few nurses understand what best practices and evidence-based practice are all about, and many organizational cultures do not support nurses who seek out and use research to change long-standing practices rooted in tradition rather than in science. "Administrative support is needed to access the resources, provide the support personnel, and sanction the necessary changes in policies, procedures, and practices" (Prevost,

DISPLAY 1.4   **Strategies for the New Nurse to Promote Evidence-Based Best Practice**

- Keep abreast of the evidence—subscribe to professional journals and read widely.
- Use and encourage use of multiple sources of evidence.
- Use evidence not only to support clinical interventions but also to support teaching strategies.
- Find established sources of evidence in your specialty—do not reinvent the wheel.
- Implement and evaluate nationally sanctioned clinical practice guidelines.
- Question and challenge nursing traditions, and promote a spirit of risk taking.
- Dispel myths and traditions not supported by evidence.
- Collaborate with other nurses locally and globally.
- Interact with other disciplines to bring nursing evidence to the table.

Source: Reprinted from Prevost, S. (2006). Defining evidence-based best practices. In C. Huston (Ed.), *Professional issues in nursing*. Philadelphia: Lippincott Williams & Wilkins.

2006, p. 54) for evidence-based data gathering to be a part of every nurse's practice. This approach to care is even being recognized as a standard expectation of accrediting bodies, such as the Joint Commission on Accreditation of Health Care Organizations (JCAHO) as well as an expectation for magnet hospital designation.

Generate Many Alternatives

The definition of *decision making* implies that there are at least two choices in every decision. Unfortunately, many problem solvers limit their choices to two when many more options usually are available.

> The greater the number of alternatives that can be generated, the greater the chance that the final decision will be sound.

Remember that one alternative in each decision should be the choice not to do anything. When examining decisions to be made by using a formal process, it is often found that the *status quo* is the right alternative.

Several techniques can help to generate more alternatives. Involving others in the process confirms the adage that two heads are better than one. Because everyone thinks uniquely, increasing the number of people working on a problem increases the number of alternatives that can be generated.

Brainstorming is another frequently used technique. The goal in brainstorming is to think of all possible alternatives, even those that may seem "off target." By not limiting the possible alternatives to only apparently appropriate ones, people can break through habitual or repressive thinking patterns and allow new ideas to surface. Although most often used by groups, people who make decisions alone also may use brainstorming.

LEARNING EXERCISE 1.3

Possible Alternatives in Problem Solving

In the personal-choice scenario presented in Learning Exercise 1.1, some of the following alternatives could have been generated:

- Do not take the new position.
- Hire a full-time housekeeper, and take the position.
- Ask your spouse to quit working.
- Have an abortion.
- Ask one of the parents to help.
- Take the position, and do not hire child care.
- Take the position, and hire child care.
- Have your spouse reduce the law practice and continue helping with child care.
- Ask the supervisor if you can work 4 days a week and still have the position.
- Take the position and wait and see what happens after the baby is born.

● ASSIGNMENT: How many of these alternatives did you or your group generate? What alternatives did you identify that are not included in this list?

Think Logically

During the problem-solving process, one must draw inferences from information. An *inference* is part of deductive reasoning. People must carefully think through the information and the alternatives. Faulty logic at this point may lead to poor-quality decisions. Primarily, people think illogically in three ways.

1. *Overgeneralizing*. This type of "crooked" thinking occurs when one believes that because A has a particular characteristic, every other A also has the same characteristic. This kind of thinking is exemplified when stereotypical statements are used to justify arguments and decisions.
2. *Affirming the consequences*. In this type of illogical thinking, one decides that if B is good and he or she is doing A, then A must not be good. For example, if a new method is heralded as the best way to perform a nursing procedure and the nurses on your unit are not using that technique, it is illogical to assume that the technique currently used in your unit is wrong or bad.
3. *Arguing from analogy*. This thinking applies a component that is present in two separate concepts and then states that because A is present in B, then A and B are alike in all respects. An example of this would be to argue that because intuition plays a part in clinical and managerial nursing, then any characteristic present in a good clinical nurse also should be present in a good nurse–manager. However, this is not necessarily true; a good nurse–manager does not necessarily possess all the same skills as a good nurse–clinician.

Various tools have been designed to assist managers with the important task of analysis. Several of these tools are discussed in this chapter. In analyzing possible solutions, individuals may want to look at the following questions:

1. What factors can you influence? How can you make the positive factors more important and minimize the negative factors?

2. What are the financial implications in each alternative? The political implications? Who else will be affected by the decision and what support is available?
3. What are the weighting factors?
4. What is the best solution?
5. What are the means of evaluation?
6. What are the consequences of each alternative?

Choose and Act Decisively

It is not enough to gather adequate information, think logically, select from among many alternatives, and be aware of the influence of one's values. In the final analysis, one must act. Many individuals delay acting because they don't want to face the consequences of their choices (e.g., if managers granted all employees' requests for days off, they would have to accept the consequences of dealing with short staffing).

 Many individuals choose to delay acting because they lack the courage to face the consequences of their choices.

It may help the reluctant decision maker to remember that even though decisions often have long-term consequences and far-reaching effects, they are not cast in stone. Often, judgments found to be ineffective or inappropriate can be changed. By later evaluating decisions, managers can learn more about their abilities and where the problem solving was faulty. However, decisions must continue to be made, although some are of poor quality, because through continued decision making, people develop increased decision-making skills.

INDIVIDUAL VARIATIONS IN DECISION MAKING

If each person receives the same information and uses the same scientific approach to solve problems, an assumption could be made that identical decisions would result. However, in practice, this is not true. Because decision making involves perceiving and evaluating, and people perceive by sensation and intuition and evaluate their perception by thinking and feeling, it is inevitable that individuality plays a part in decision making. Because everyone has different values and life experiences, and each person perceives and thinks differently, different decisions may be made given the same set of circumstances. No discussion of decision making would, therefore, be complete without a careful examination of the role of the individual in decision making.

Gender

New research suggests that gender may play a role in how individuals make decisions. Ripley (2005) reports that the two brain hemispheres appear to have more connections in women and that in certain brain regions, neuron density is higher in women than in men. Women also tend to use more areas of the brain to accomplish certain tasks, which is part of the reason that they tend to recover better from a stroke than men. Women also are able to see more colors and textures than men. In contrast, men tend to localize their thinking to more focused regions of the brain regardless of the type of problem solving they are engaged in or emotion they feel. Research by Hanlon also suggests, however, that the regions of the brain that deal with mechanical reasoning, visual targeting, and spatial reasoning mature more quickly in boys than in girls (Ripley, 2005).

Ripley reports that the adult male brain is approximately 10% larger than the adult female brain and that even when adjusted for body size, men's brains are still slightly larger. This difference does not appear, however, to be a predictor in terms of intellectual capacity or decision-making abilities. What does appear to matter is a section of the brain called the amygdale (i.e., *amygdala*). The connections between the amygdale and the regions of the brain that control language and higher-level functioning appears to be stronger in women. This may be one reason that women are more likely to talk about their emotions and to be verbal in their analysis (Ripley, 2005).

Values

Individual decisions are based on each person's value system. No matter how objective the criteria, value judgments will always play a part in a person's decision making, either consciously or subconsciously. The alternatives generated and the final choices are limited by each person's value system. For some, certain choices are not possible because of a person's beliefs. Because values also influence perceptions, they invariably influence information gathering, information processing, and final outcome. Values also determine which problems in one's personal or professional life will be addressed or ignored.

 No matter how objective the criteria, value judgments will always play a part in a person's decision making, either consciously or subconsciously.

Life Experience

Each person brings to the decision-making task past experiences that include education and decision-making experience. The more mature the person and the broader his or her background, the more alternatives he or she can identify. Each time a new behavior or decision is observed, that possibility is added to the person's repertoire of choices. This was clearly demonstrated in research completed by Bakalis and Watson (2005), where clinical experience was related to frequency of decision making (Examining the Evidence 1.1).

 EXAMINING THE EVIDENCE 1.1

Source: Bakalis, N. A., & Watson, R. (2005, February 16). Nurses' decision-making in clinical practice. *Nursing Standard, 19*(23), 33–39.

In this study, 60 nurses from three different clinical areas, completed a decision-making questionnaire. Most nurses, in all specialties, reported making regular clinical decisions on direct patient care, which included providing basic nursing care, psychological support, and teaching patients and/or family members. Critical care nurses reported that they regularly made decisions on their extended roles, such as acting in emergency situations and deciding to change patient medication, while medical and surgical nurses stated that they did this only occasionally. Length of clinical experience was significantly related to the frequency of decision making.

The authors concluded that decision making should be taught in both prenursing and nursing courses, that nurses should be encouraged to have greater autonomy in clinical decision making, and that clinical decision making should be research based.

In addition, people vary in their desire for autonomy, so some nurses may want more autonomy than others. It is likely that people seeking autonomy may have much more experience at making decisions than those who fear autonomy. Likewise, having made good or poor decisions in the past will influence a person's decision making.

Individual Preference

With all the alternatives a person considers in decision making, one alternative may be preferred over another. The decision maker, for example, may see certain choices as involving greater personal risk than others and therefore may choose the safer alternative. Physical, economic, and emotional risks and time and energy expenditures are types of personal risk and costs involved in decision making. For example, people with limited finances or a reduced energy level may decide to select an alternative solution to a problem that would not have been their first choice had they been able to overcome limited resources.

Brain Hemisphere Dominance and Thinking Styles

Our way of evaluating information and alternatives on which we base our final decision constitutes a thinking skill. Individuals think differently. Some think systematically—and are often called analytical thinkers—whereas others think intuitively. It is believed that most people have either right- or left-brain hemisphere dominance. Analytical, linear, *left-brain thinkers* process information differently from creative, intuitive, *right-brain thinkers*. Although the authors encourage whole-brain thinking, and studies have shown that people can strengthen the use of the less dominant side of the brain, most people continue to have a dominant side.

Some researchers, including Nobel Prize winner Roger Sperry, suggest that there are actually four different thinking styles based on brain dominance (Adams, 2003). Individuals with upper-left-brain dominance truly are analytical thinkers who like working with factual data and numbers. These individuals deal with problems in a logical and rational way. Individuals with lower-left-brain dominance are highly organized and detail oriented. They prefer a stable work environment and value safety and security over risk taking. Individuals with upper-right-brain dominance are big picture thinkers who look for hidden possibilities and are futuristic in their thinking. They also frequently rely on intuition to solve problems and are willing to take risks to seek new solutions to problems. Individuals with lower-right-brain dominance experience facts and problem solve in a more emotional way than the other three types. They are sympathetic, empathetic, and intuitive. They are more socially motivated in their interactions with others (Adams, 2003).

According to Adams (2003), 60% of the population have two dominant styles, 30% have three styles, 7% are single dominant, and 3% are whole brained, meaning that they employ all four problem-solving styles with ease.

 There is no evidence that any one thinking style or that having either right- or left-brain dominance is better.

In the past, some organizations more openly valued their logical, analytical thinkers but more recently have recognized that intuitive thinking is also a valuable managerial resource. Indeed, organizations need all types of thinkers. What may be most important is that individuals are self-aware about the thinking style(s) or brain hemisphere dominance that most typifies their behavior and that they recognize that how they think has an impact on how they relate to others and solve problems in their roles as leaders and managers (Adams, 2003).

LEARNING EXERCISE 1.4

Thinking Styles
In small groups, examine how each individual in the group thinks. Did you have a majority of individuals with right- or left-brain dominance? Did group members self-identify with one or more of the four thinking styles noted by Adams (2003)? Did gender seem to influence thinking style or brain hemisphere dominance? What types of thinkers were represented in group members' families? Did most group members view variances in a positive way?

OVERCOMING INDIVIDUAL VULNERABILITY IN DECISION MAKING

How do people overcome subjectivity in making decisions? This can never be completely overcome, nor should it. After all, life would be boring if everyone thought alike. However, managers and leaders must become aware of their own vulnerability and recognize how it influences and limits the quality of their decision making. Using the following suggestions will help to decrease individual subjectivity and increase objectivity in decision making.

Values

Being confused and unclear about one's values may affect decision-making ability. Overcoming a lack of self-awareness through values clarification decreases confusion. People who understand their personal beliefs and feelings will have a conscious awareness of the values on which their decisions are based. This awareness is an essential component of decision making and critical thinking. Therefore, to be successful problem solvers, managers must periodically examine their values. Values clarification exercises are included in Chapter 7.

Life Experience

It is difficult to overcome inexperience when making decisions. However, a person can do some things to decrease this area of vulnerability. First, use available resources, including current research and literature, to gain a fuller understanding of the issues involved. Second, involve other people, such as experienced colleagues, trusted friends, or superiors, to act as sounding boards and advisors. Third, analyze decisions later to assess their success. By evaluating decisions, people learn from mistakes and are able to overcome inexperience.

Individual Preference

Overcoming this area of vulnerability involves self-awareness, honesty, and risk taking. The need for self-awareness was discussed previously, but it is not enough to be self-aware; people also must be honest with themselves about their choices and their preferences for those choices.

Additionally, the successful decision maker must take some risks. Nearly every decision has some element of risk, and most decisions involve consequences and accountability.

> Those who can do the right but unpopular thing and who dare to stand alone will emerge as leaders.

Individual Ways of Thinking

People making decisions alone are frequently handicapped because they are not able to understand problems fully or make decisions from both an analytical and intuitive perspective. However, most organizations include both types of thinkers. Using group process, talking management problems over with others, and developing whole-brain thinking also are methods for ensuring that both intuitive and analytical approaches will be used in solving problems and making decisions. Use of heterogeneous rather than homogeneous groups will usually result in better-quality decision making. Indeed, learning to think "outside the box" is often accomplished by including a diverse group of thinkers when solving problems and making decisions.

Although not all experts agree, many consider the following to be qualities of a successful decision maker:

- *Courage*. Courage is particularly important and involves the willingness to take risks.
- *Sensitivity*. Good decision makers seem to have some sort of antenna that makes them particularly sensitive to situations and others.
- *Energy*. People must have the energy and desire to make things happen.
- *Creativity*. Successful decision makers tend to be creative thinkers. They develop new ways to solve problems.

DECISION MAKING IN ORGANIZATIONS

In the beginning of this chapter, the need for managers and leaders to make quality decisions was emphasized. The effect of the individual's values and preferences on decision making was discussed, but it is important for leaders and managers to also understand how the organization influences the decision-making process. Because organizations are made up of people with differing values and preferences, there is often conflict in organizational decision dynamics.

Effect of Organizational Power

Powerful people in organizations are more likely to have decisions made (by themselves or their subordinates) that are congruent with their own preferences and values. On the other hand, people wielding little power in organizations must always consider the preference of the powerful when they make management decisions. In organizations, choice is constructed and constrained by many factors, and therefore choice is not equally available to all people.

Additionally, not only do the preferences of the powerful influence decisions of the less powerful, but the powerful also can inhibit the preferences of the less powerful. This occurs because individuals who remain and advance in organizations are those who feel and express values and beliefs congruent with the organization. Therefore, a balance must be found between the limitations of choice posed by the power structure within the organization and totally independent decision making that could lead to organizational chaos.

The ability of the powerful to influence individual decision making in an organization often requires adopting a private personality and an organizational personality.

For example, some might believe they would have made a different decision had they been acting on their own, but they went along with the organizational decision. This "going along" in itself constitutes a decision. People choose to accept an organizational decision that differs from their own preferences and values. The concept of power in organizations is discussed more fully in Chapter 13

Rational and Administrative Decision Making

For many years, it was widely believed that most managerial decisions were based on a careful, scientific, and objective thought process and that managers made decisions in a rational manner. In the late 1940s, Herbert A. Simon's work revealed that most managers made many decisions that did not fit the objective rationality theory. Simon (1965) delineated two types of management decision makers: the *economic man* and the *administrative man*.

Managers who are successful decision makers often attempt to make rational decisions, much like the economic man described in Table 1.2. Because they realize that restricted knowledge and limited alternatives directly affect a decision's quality, these managers gather as much information as possible and generate many alternatives. Simon believed that the economic model of man, however, was an unrealistic description of organizational decision making. The complexity of information acquisition makes it impossible for the human brain to store and retain the amount of information that is available for each decision. Because of time constraints and the difficulty of assimilating large amounts of information, most management decisions are made using the administrative man model of decision making.

 Most management decisions are made by using the administrative man model of decision making.

TABLE 1.2   Comparing the Economic Man With the Administrative Man

Economic	Administrative
Makes decisions in a very rational manner	Makes decisions that are good enough
Has complete knowledge of the problem or decision situation	Because complete knowledge is not possible, knowledge is always fragmented.
Has a complete list of possible alternatives	Because consequences of alternatives occur in the future, they are impossible to predict accurately.
Has a rational system of ordering preference of alternatives	Usually chooses from among a few alternatives, not all possible ones
Selects the decision that will maximize utility function	The final choice is *satisficing* rather than maximizing

Source: Adapted from Simon, H. A. (1965). *The shape of automation for man and management.* New York: Harper Textbooks.

The administrative man never has complete knowledge and generates fewer alternatives. Simon argued that the administrative man carries out decisions that are only *satisficing*, a term used to describe decisions that may not be ideal but result in solutions that have adequate outcomes. These managers want decisions to be "good enough" so that they "work," but they are less concerned that the alternative selected is the optimal choice. The "best" choice for many decisions is often found to be too costly in terms of time or resources, so another less costly but workable solution is found.

DECISION-MAKING TOOLS

Clancy (2003) maintains that even the most experienced manager cannot eliminate all uncertainty when making decisions. However, to assist the manager in making decisions, management analysts have developed tools that provide order and direction in obtaining and using information or that are helpful in selecting who should be involved in making the decision. It is important to remember, though, that any decision-making tool always results in the need for the person to make a final decision and that all such tools are subject to human error. Because there are so many decision aids, this chapter presents selected technology that would be most helpful to beginning- or middle-level managers.

Decision Grids

A *decision grid* allows one to visually examine the alternatives and compare each against the same criteria. Although any criteria may be selected, the same criteria are used to analyze each alternative. An example of a decision grid is depicted in Figure 1.3. When many alternatives have been generated or a group or committee is collaborating on the decision, these grids are particularly helpful to the process. This tool, for instance, would be useful when changing the method of managing care on a unit or when selecting a candidate to hire from a large interview pool. The unit manager or the committee would evaluate all of the alternatives available using a decision grid. In this manner, every alternative is evaluated using the same criteria. It is possible to weight some of the criteria more heavily than others if some are more important. To do this, it is usually necessary to assign a number value to each criterion. The result would be a numeric value for each alternative considered.

Alternative	Financial effect	Political effect	Departmental effect	Time	Decision
#1					
#2					
#3					
#4					

Figure 1.3 A decision grid.

Payoff Tables

The decision aids known as *payoff tables* have a cost–profit–volume relationship and are very helpful when some quantitative information is available, such as an item's cost or predicted use. To use payoff tables, one must determine probabilities and use historical data, such as a hospital census or a report on the number of operating procedures performed. To illustrate, a payoff table might be appropriately used in determining how many participants it would take to make an in-service program break even in terms of costs.

If the instructor for the class costs $400, the in-service director would need to charge each of the 20 participants $20 for the class, but for 40 participants, the class would cost only $10 each. The in-service director would use attendance data from past classes and the number of nurses potentially available to attend to determine probable class size and thus how much to charge for the class. Payoff tables do not guarantee that a correct decision will be made, but they assist in visualizing data.

Decision Trees

Because decisions are often tied to the outcome of other events, management analysts have developed *decision trees.*

The decision tree in Figure 1.4 compares the cost of hiring regular staff to the cost of hiring temporary employees. Here, the decision is whether to hire extra nurses at regular salary to perform outpatient procedures on an oncology unit or to have nurses available to the unit on an on-call basis and pay them on-call and overtime wages. The possible consequences of a decreased

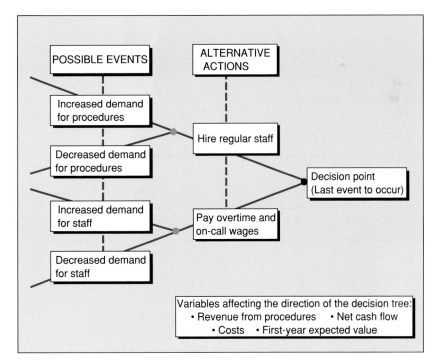

Figure 1.4   A decision tree.

EXAMINING THE EVIDENCE 1.2

Source: Matukaitis, J., Stillman, P, Wykpisz, E., & Ewen, E. (2005). Appropriate admissions to the appropriate unit: A decision tree approach. *American Journal of Medical Quality*, 20(2), 90–97.

This pilot project described the implementation of a decision-tree approach to problem solving in two acute-care hospitals of a large health care system in an effort to maximize their use of limited intermediate care beds. The impetus for the project was a study that found that only 42% of patients admitted to intermediate care beds actually met the criteria for such an admission. Thus, nursing resources were being overused in terms of nurse-to-patient ratios.

A multidisciplinary team was formed to develop the intermediate care decision tree to be used by the emergency department as a guide for admissions to the intermediate care unit. Emergency department staff were trained in its use.

Following implementation of the decision-tree approach, between 96% and 100% of patients admitted to the intermediate care unit from the emergency department met the criteria for such an admission. In addition, wait time in the emergency department was decreased from 5.5 hours to 2.5 hours, and the number of patients waiting daily in the emergency department for an intermediate care bed was reduced by approximately 80%.

volume of procedures and an increased volume must be considered. Initially, costs would increase in hiring a regular staff, but over a longer time, this move would mean greater savings if the volume of procedures does not dramatically decrease. A real-life example of the use of a decision tree to determine which hospital units patients should be admitted to is described in Examining the Evidence 1.2.

 Used to plot a decision over time, decision trees allow visualization of various outcomes.

Consequence Tables

Clancy (2003) used a *consequence table* to demonstrate how various alternatives create different consequences. A consequence table lists the objectives for solving a problem down one side of a table and rates how each alternative would meet the desired objective.

For example, consider this problem: "The number of patient falls has exceeded the benchmark rate for two consecutive quarters." After a period of analysis, the following alternatives were selected as solutions:

1. Provide a new educational program to instruct staff on how to prevent falls.
2. Implement a night check to ensure that patients have side rails up and beds in low position.
3. Implement a policy requiring soft restraints orders on all confused patients.

The decision maker then lists each alternative opposite the objectives for solving the problem, which for this problem might be (a) reduces the number of falls, (b) meets regulatory standards, (c) is cost-effective, and (d) fits present policy guidelines. The decision maker(s) then ranks each desired objective and examines each of the alternatives through a standardized key, which allows a fair comparison between alternatives and assists in eliminating undesirable choices. It is impor-

TABLE 1.3 A Consequence Table

Objectives for Problem Solving	Alternative 1	Alternative 2	Alternative 3
1. Reduces the number of falls	X	X	X
2. Meets regulatory standards	X	X	X
3. Is cost-effective		X	X
4. Fits present policy guidelines			X
Decision Score			

tant to examine long-term effects of each alternative as well as how the decision will affect others. See Table 1.3 for an example of a consequence table.

Logic Models

Logic models are schematics or pictures of how programs are intended to operate. The schematic typically includes resources, processes, and desired outcomes and depicts exactly what the relationships are between the three components. Longest (2005) says that logic models can improve a program's management in two ways: "1) the logic model can assist the manager in integrating the various management activities germane to effectively operating a program, and 2) the model can assist managers in establishing and maintaining good relationships with internal and external stakeholders" (p. 557).

Program Evaluation and Review Technique

Program evaluation and review technique (PERT) is a popular tool to determine the timing of decisions. Developed by the Booz-Allen-Hamilton organization and the U.S. Navy in connection with the Polaris missile program, PERT is essentially a flowchart that predicts when events and activities must take place if a final event is to occur. Figure 1.5 shows a PERT chart for devel-

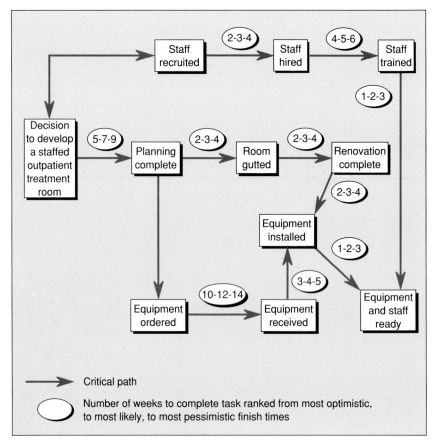

Figure 1.5 Example of a PERT flow diagram.

oping a new outpatient treatment room for oncology procedures. The number of weeks to complete tasks is listed in optimistic time, most likely time, and pessimistic time. The critical path shows something that must occur in the sequence before one may proceed. PERT is especially helpful when a group of people is working on a project. The flowchart keeps everyone up-to-date, and problems are easily identified when they first occur. Flowcharts are popular, and many people use them in their personal lives.

LEARNING EXERCISE 1.5

Using a Flowchart for Project Management

Think of a project that you are working on; it could be a dance, a picnic, remodeling your bathroom, or a semester schedule of activities in a class.

● ASSIGNMENT: Draw a flowchart, inserting at the bottom the date that activities for the event are to be completed. Working backward, insert critical tasks and their completion dates. Refer to your flowchart throughout the project to see if you are staying on target.

PITFALLS IN USING DECISION-MAKING TOOLS

Clancy (2003) maintains that there is a strong tendency for managers to favor first impressions when making a decision and that a second tendency called *confirmation biases* often follows. A confirmation bias has a tendency to affirm one's initial impression and preferences as other alternatives are evaluated. So, even the use of consequence tables, decision trees, and other quantitative decision tools will not guarantee a successful decision.

It is also human nature to focus on an event that leaves a strong impression, so individuals may have preconceived notions or biases that influence decisions. Too often, managers allow the past to influence current decisions. Managers often become too confident about their decision-making ability and remember their good decisions and forget the negative outcomes that resulted from some of their other decisions (Clancy, 2003).

 Many of the pitfalls associated with management decision-making tools can be reduced by choosing the correct decision-making style and involving others when appropriate.

Although there are times when others should be involved, it is not always necessary to involve others in decision making, and frequently a manager does not have time to involve a large group. However, it is important to separate out those decisions that need input from others and those that a manager can make alone.

SUMMARY

This chapter has discussed effective decision making, problem solving, and critical thinking as requisites for being a successful leader and manager. The effective leader–manager is aware of the need for sensitivity in decision making. The successful decision maker possesses courage, energy, and creativity. It is a leadership skill to recognize the appropriate people to include in decision making and to use a suitable theoretical model for the decision situation.

Managers who make quality decisions are effective administrators. The manager should develop a systematic, scientific approach to problem solving that begins with a fixed goal and ends with an evaluation step. Decision tools exist to help make more effective decisions; however, leader–managers must remember that they are not foolproof and that they often do not adequately allow for the human element in management. In addition, managers should strive to make decisions that reflect research-based best practices and nursing's scientific knowledge base. Yet the role of intuition as an adjunct to quality decision making should not be overlooked.

The integrated leader–manager understands the significance that gender, personal values, life experience, preferences, willingness to take risks, brain hemisphere dominance, and thinking styles have on selected alternatives in making the decision. The critical thinker pondering a decision is aware of the areas of vulnerability that hinder successful decision making and will expend his or her efforts to avoid the pitfalls of faulty logic and data gathering.

Both managers and leaders understand the impact that the organization has on decision making and that some of the decisions that will be made in the organization will be only *satisficing*. However, leaders will strive to problem solve adequately in order to reach optimal decisions as often as possible.

Key Concepts

* Successful decision makers are self-aware, courageous, sensitive, energetic, and creative.
* The rational approach to problem solving begins with a fixed goal and ends with an evaluation process.
* Naturalistic decision making blends intuition and analysis, but pattern recognition and experience guide decision makers when time is limited or systematic rational decision making is not possible.
* Evidence-based nursing practice integrates the best evidence available, nursing expertise, and the values and preferences of the individuals, families, and communities who are served.
* The successful decision maker understands the significance that gender, personal, individual values, life experience, preferences, willingness to take risks, brain hemisphere dominance, and predominant thinking style have on alternative identification and selection.
* The critical thinker is aware of areas of vulnerability that hinder successful decision making and makes efforts to avoid the pitfalls of faulty logic in his or her data gathering.
* The act of making and evaluating decisions increases the expertise of the decision maker.
* There are many models for improving decision making. Using a systematic decision-making or problem-solving model reduces *heuristic* trial and error or rule of thumb methods and increases the probability that appropriate decisions made will be made.
* Left- and right-brain dominance as well as thinking styles influence, at least to some degree, how individuals think.
* Two major considerations in organizational decision making are how power affects decision making and whether management decision making needs to be only *satisficing*.
* Management science has produced many tools to help decision makers make better and more objective decisions, but all are subject to human error, and many do not adequately consider the human element.

ADDITIONAL LEARNING EXERCISES AND APPLICATIONS

LEARNING EXERCISE 1.6

Evaluating Decision Making
Describe the two best decisions that you have made in your life and the two worst. What factors assisted you in making the wise decisions? What elements of critical thinking went awry in your poor decision making? How would you evaluate your decision-making ability?

LEARNING EXERCISE 1.7

Economic and Administrative Man
Examine the process that you used in your decision to become a nurse. Would you describe it as fitting a profile of the economic man or the administrative man?

LEARNING EXERCISE 1.8

Considering Critical Elements in Decision Making

You are a college senior and president of your nursing organization. You are on the committee to select a slate of officers for the next academic year. Several of the current officers will be graduating, and you want the new slate of officers to be committed to the organization. Some of the brightest members of the junior class involved in the organization are not well liked by some of your friends in the organization.

● ASSIGNMENT: Looking at the critical elements in decision making, compile a list of the most important points to consider in making the decision for selecting a slate of officers. What must you guard against, and how should you approach the data gathering to solve this problem?

LEARNING EXERCISE 1.9

Examining the Decision-Making Process

You have been a staff nurse for the 3 years since your graduation from nursing school. There is a nursing shortage in your area and many openings at other facilities. Additionally, you have been offered a charge nurse position by your present employer. Last, you have always wanted to do community health nursing and know that this is also a possibility. You are self-aware enough to know that it is time for a change, but which change, and how should you make the decision?

● ASSIGNMENT: Examine both the individual aspects of decision making and the critical elements in making decisions. Make a plan including a goal, a list of information, and data that you need to gather and areas where you may be vulnerable to poor decision making. Examine the consequences of each alternative available to you. After you have done this, as an individual, form a small group and share your decision-making planning with members of your group. How was your decision making like others in the group, and how was it different?

LEARNING EXERCISE 1.10

Using Models in Decision Making

Do you use a problem-solving or decision-making model to solve problems? Have you ever used an intuitive model? Think of a critical decision that you have made in the last year. What model, if any, did you use?

● ASSIGNMENT: Write a one-page essay about a problem that you solved or a decision that you made this year. Describe what theoretical model, if any, you used to assist you in the process. Determine if you consciously used the model or if it was purely by accident. Did you enlist the help of other experts in solving the problem?

LEARNING EXERCISE 1.11

Decision Making and Risk Taking

You are a new graduate nurse just finishing your 3-month probation period at your first job in acute-care nursing. You have been working closely with a preceptor; however, he has been gradually transitioning you to more independent practice. You now have your own patient care assignment and have been giving medications independently for several weeks. Today, your assignment included an elderly confused patient with severe coronary disease. Her medications include antihypertensives, antiarrhythmics, and beta blockers. It was a very busy morning, and you have barely had a moment to reorganize and collect your thoughts.

It is now 2:30 PM, and you are preparing your end-of-shift report. When you review the patient's 2:00 PM vital signs, you note a significant rise in this patient's blood pressure and heart rate. The patient, however, reports no distress. You remember that when you passed the morning medications, the patient was in the middle of her bath and asked that you just set the medications on the bedside table and that she would take them in a few minutes. You meant to return to see that she did but were sidetracked by a problem with another patient.

You now go to the patient's room to see if she indeed did take the pills. The pill cup and pills are not where you left them, and a search of the wastebasket, patient bed, and bedside table yields nothing. The patient is too confused to be an accurate historian regarding whether she took the pills. No one on your patient care team noticed the pills.

At this point, you are not sure what you should do next. You are frustrated that you did not wait to give the medications in person but cannot change this now. You charted the medications as being given this morning when you left them at the bedside. You are reluctant to report this as a medication error since you are still on probation and you are not sure that the patient did *not* take the pills as she said she would. Your probation period has not gone as smoothly as you would have liked anyway, and you are aware that reporting this incident will likely prolong your probation and that a copy of the error report will be placed in your personnel file. The patient's physician is also frequently short tempered and will likely be agitated when you report your uncertainty about whether the patient received her prescribed medications. The reality is that if you do nothing, it is likely that no one will ever know about the problem.

You do feel responsible, however, for the patient's welfare. The physician might want to give additional doses of the medication if indeed the patient did not take the pills. In addition, the rise in heart rate and blood pressure has only just become apparent, and you realize that her heart rate and blood pressure could continue to deteriorate over the next shift. The patient is not due to receive the medications again until 9 PM tonight (b.i.d. every 12 hours).

● ASSIGNMENT: Decide how you will proceed. Determine whether you will use a systematic problem-solving model, intuition, or both in making your choices. How did your values, preferences, life experiences, willingness to take risks, and individual ways of thinking influence your decision?

Web Links

Foundation and Center for Critical Thinking
http://www.criticalthinking.org/
Integrates the foundation's research and theoretical developments to create events and resources designed to help educators improve their instruction.

Society for Judgment and Decision Making
http://www.sjdm.org
Promotes the study of normative, descriptive theories of decision processes.

Mission Critical
http://www.sjsu.edu/depts/itl
This site creates a "virtual lab" capable of familiarizing users with the basic concepts of critical thinking in a self-paced, interactive environment.

Center for Rural Studies—Values Clarification Exercise
http://crs.uvm.edu/gopher/nerl/personal/growth/b.html
This document was posted by the New England Regional Leadership program for public use. The values clarification exercise works well for individual or small group classroom work.

Society for Medical Decision Making
http://www.smdm.org/main.html
This organization seeks to improve health outcomes through the advancement of proactive systematic approaches to clinical decision making and policy formation in health care by providing a scholarly forum that connects and educates researchers, providers, policy makers, and the public.

University of York—Centre for Evidence Based Nursing
http://www.york.ac.uk/healthsciences/centres/evidence/cebn.htm
The Centre for Evidence Based Nursing is concerned with furthering evidence-based nursing through education, research, and development.

Academic Center for Evidence-based Practice
http://www.acestar.uthscsa.edu/
This center of excellence for the University of Texas Health Science Center at San Antonio is dedicated to bridging research into practice by advancing cutting-edge, state-of-the-art, evidence-based nursing practice, research, and education within an interdisciplinary context.

References

Adams, J. (2003). *Whole brain thinking—Why bother? The whole brain in action.* Retrieved July 13, 2006, from *http://www.nzpf.ac.nz/resources/magazine/2003/aug/Whole%20Brain%20Thinking%20Article.htm.*

Aloi, J. A. (2006, May 8). The power of intuition: Is your "sixth sense" a viable, reliable nursing tool? *NurseWeek (South Central), 13*(10), 47.

Andrews, J. (2006). *Intuitive decision making profile.* Retrieved July 10, 2006, from *http://www.hrdq.com/products/idmp.htm.*

Bakalis, N. A., & Watson, R. (2005, February 16). Nurses' decision-making in clinical practice. *Nursing Standard, 19*(23), 33–39.

Beginners Guide (2005, September 21). *What is decision making?* Retrieved July 10, 2006, from *http://beginnersguide.com/executive-coaching/decision-making/what-is-decision-making.php.*

Beginners Guide (2005, November 18). *What is critical thinking?* Retrieved July 10, 2006, from *http://beginnersguide.com/leadership/critical-thinking/what-is-critical-thinking.php.*

Bowers, S. (2004). *The effect of problem-based learning on nursing students' clinical decision-making and learning satisfaction.* University of South Dakota (doctoral dissertation).

Clancy, T. R. (2003). The art of decision-making. *Journal of Nursing Administration, 33*(6), 343–349.

Clovis, J. B., & Cobban, S. J. (2006, January–February). The theory and method of disciplined inquiry. *Canadian Journal of Dental Hygiene, 40*(1), 26–32, 35.

DiCenso, A., Prevost, S., Benefield, L., Bingle, J., Ciliska, D., Driver, M., Lock, S., & Titler, M. (2004). Evidence-based nursing: Rationale and resources. *Worldviews on Evidence-Based Nursing, 1*(1), 69–75.

Evidence Based Practice Resource Center. Oncology Nursing Center. (2006). *Definitions.* Retrieved July 10, 2006, from *http://onsopcontent.ons.org/toolkits/ebp/definition/definition.htm.*

Facione, P. A. (2006). *2006 update. Critical thinking. What it is and why it counts.* Retrieved July 13, 2006, from *http://www.insightassessment.com/pdf_files/what&why2006.pdf.*

Foundation for Critical Thinking. (2004). *Defining critical thinking.* Retrieved July 13, 2006, from *http://www.criticalthinking.org/aboutCT/definingCT.shtml.*

Girard, N. J. (2005, December). Never underestimate the importance of asking "why?" *AORN Journal, 82*(6), 961–962.

Heuristic Solutions. (n.d.). *What is a heuristic?* Retrieved July 13, 2006, from *http://www.heuristics.net/html/whats.html.*

Klein, G. (2004). *The power of intuition. How to use your gut feelings to make better decisions at work.* New York: Random House.

Longest, B. B. (2005). Logic models as aids in managing health programs. *Journal of Nursing Administration, 35*(12), 557–562.

Prevost, S. (2006). Defining evidence-based best practices. In C. Huston (Ed.), *Professional issues in nursing.* Philadelphia: Lippincott Williams & Wilkins.

Pritchard, M. J. (2006). Professional development. Making effective clinical decisions: A framework for nurse practitioners. *British Journal of Nursing (BJN), 15*(3), 128–130.

Ripley, A. (2005, March 7). Who says a woman can't be Einstein? *Time, 165*(10), 50–60.

Robertson, B. (2006, March 31). An obstetric simulation experience in an undergraduate nursing curriculum. *Nurse Educator,* (2), 74–78.

Simon, H. A. (1965). *The shape of automation for man and management.* New York: Harper Textbooks.

Sorach Inc. (2000). *Decision-making fundamentals.* Retrieved July 12, 2006, from *http://www.sorach.com/decision.html.*

Bibliography

Anderson, D. J., & Shelton, W. 2005, October). Clarify your financial picture with staff management tools. *Journal of Nursing Administration,* (suppl), 23–24.

Bailey, S. (2006). Decision making in acute care: A practical framework supporting the "best interests" principle. *Nursing Ethics, 13*(3), 284–291.

Banning, M. (2006, March). Measures that can be used to instill critical thinking skills in nurse prescribers. *Nurse Education in Practice,* (2), 98–105.

Buckner M., & Nelson, M. S. (2006). A decision tree for anemia intervention: Nurses are key to improving clinical practice. *Oncology Nursing Forum, 33*(2), 429.

Farzaneh-Far, R., Schwarzberg T., & Mushlin, S. B. (2006). Clinical problem-solving. Thinking outside the box. *New England Journal of Medicine, 354*(22), 2376–2381.

Fesler-Birch, D. M. (2005). Critical thinking and patient outcomes: A review. *Nursing Outlook, 53*(2), 59–65.

Forrest, J. L., & Miller, S. A. (2005). Evidence-based decision making—A new term for a new concept. *Dimensions of Dental Hygiene, 3*(9), 12, 14, 16–17.

Geanellos, R . (2004). Nursing based evidence: Moving beyond evidence-based practice in mental health nursing. *Journal of Evaluation in Clinical Practice, 10*(2), 177–186.

Gerrish, K., & Clayton, J. (2004). Promoting evidence-based practice: An organizational approach. *Journal of Nursing Management, 12*(2), 114–123.

Goldenberg, M. J. (2006). On evidence and evidence-based medicine: Lessons from the philosophy of science. *Social Science and Medicine, 62*(11), 2621–2632.

Jamison, J. R. (2006, May 29). Teaching diagnostic decision making: Student evaluation of a diagnosis unit. *Journal of Manipulative and Physiological Therapeutics, 29*(4), 315.e1–e9.

Kiefer, L. (2005). Fostering evidence-based decision-making in Canada: Examining the need for a Canadian population and public health evidence centre and research network. *Canadian Journal of Public Health, 96*(3)(suppl), I1–I19.

Meadows, S., Baker, K., & Butler, J. (2005). The incident decision tree. National Patient Safety Agency. *Clinical Risk, 11*(2), 66–68.

Nathaniel, A. K. (2006). Moral reckoning in nursing. *Western Journal of Nursing Research, 28*(4), 419–438.

O'Neil, E. S., Dluhy, N. M., & Chin, E. (2005). Modelling novice clinical reasoning for a computerized decision support system. *Journal of Advanced Nursing, 49*(1), 68–77.

Snethen, J. A., Broome, M. E., Knafl, K., Deatrick, J. A., & Angst, D. B. (2006). Family patterns of decision-making in pediatric clinical trials. *Research in Nursing and Health, 29*(3), 223–232.

Thompson, P., Dowding, D., Swanson, V., Bland, R., Mair, C., Morrison, A, et al. (2006). Computerised guidance tree (decision aid) for hypertension, based on decision analysis: Development and preliminary evaluation. *European Journal of Cardiovascular Nursing, 5*(2), 146–149.

Wiest, D. A. (2006). Application of a decision-making model in clinical practice. *Topics in Emergency Medicine, 28*(2), 149–151.

2

Classical Views of Leadership and Management

. . . management is efficiency in climbing the ladder of success; leadership determines whether the ladder is leaning against the right wall.

—*Stephen R. Covey*

. . . no executive has ever suffered because his subordinates were strong and effective.

—*Peter Drucker*

The relationship between leadership and management continues to prompt some debate, although the literature demonstrates the need for both (Trent, 2003). Leadership is viewed by some as one of management's many functions; others maintain that leadership requires more complex skills than management and that management is only one role of leadership; still others delineate between the two. Others argue that management emphasizes *control*—control of hours, costs, salaries, overtime, use of sick leave, inventory, and supplies—whereas leadership increases productivity by maximizing workforce *effectiveness*.

But if a manager guides, directs, and motivates and a leader empowers others, then it could be said that every manager should be a leader. Similarly, leadership without management results in chaos and failure for both the organization and the individual executive. This chapter will first artificially differentiate between management and leadership, focusing on how theory development in each field of study has changed over time and then conclude with a discussion of how closely integrated the two roles must actually be for individuals in contemporary leadership or management roles.

MANAGERS

Wikipedia (2006, para 1) states that the term *management* comes from the old French term *ménagement* which means "the directing" and from the Latin term *manu agere*, which means "to

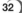

lead by the hand." Both word origins imply that management is the process of leading and direct-ing all or part of an organization, often a business, through the deployment and manipulation of resources. The act, manner, or practice of managing, handling, supervision, or control is another description of management. Managers then typically:

• Have an assigned position within the formal organization
• Have a legitimate source of power due to the delegated authority that accompanies their position
• Are expected to carry out specific functions, duties, and responsibilities
• Emphasize control, decision making, decision analysis, and results
• Manipulate people, the environment, money, time, and other resources to achieve organi-zational goals
• Have a greater formal responsibility and accountability for rationality and control than leaders
• Direct willing and unwilling subordinates

LEADERS

Although the term *leader* has been in use since the 1300s, the word *leadership* was not known in the English language until the first half of the 19th century. Despite its relatively new addition to the English language, leadership has many meanings. From Chapin's (1924) technical defini-tion of leadership as "a point of polarization for group cooperation" to Bitpipe's (2006) assertion that "leadership is a management skill that focuses on the development and deployment of vision, mission and strategy as well as the creation of a motivated workforce" (para 1), it becomes clear that there is no single definition broad enough to encompass the total leadership process. Because leadership researchers and theorists do not agree on exactly what leadership is, it is perhaps wiser to focus on what roles are inherent in leadership. Display 2.1 includes a par-tial list of common leadership roles.

To examine the word *leader*, however, is to note that leaders lead. A job title alone does not make a person a leader. Only a person's behavior determines if he or she occupies a leadership position. The manager is the person who brings things about—the one who accomplishes, has the responsibility, and conducts. A leader is the person who influences and guides direction, opinion, and course of action.

DISPLAY 2.1 **Leadership Roles**

Decision maker	Coach	Forecaster
Communicator	Counselor	Influencer
Evaluator	Teacher	Creative problem solver
Facilitator	Critical thinker	Change agent
Risk taker	Buffer	Diplomat
Mentor	Advocate	Role model
Energizer	Visionary	

Other characteristics of leaders include the following:
* Leaders often do not have delegated authority but obtain their power through other means, such as influence.
* Leaders have a wider variety of roles than do managers.
* Leaders may or may not be part of the formal organization.
* Leaders focus on group process, information gathering, feedback, and empowering others.
* Leaders emphasize interpersonal relationships.
* Leaders direct willing followers.
* Leaders have goals that may or may not reflect those of the organization.

Leaders are in the front, moving forward, taking risks, and challenging the status quo.

LEARNING EXERCISE 2.1

Leadership Roles and Management Functions
In small or large groups, discuss your views of management and leadership. Do you believe they are the same or different? If you believe that they are different, do you think that they have the same importance for the future of nursing? Do you feel that one is more important than the other? How can novice nurse–managers learn important management functions and develop leadership skills?

HISTORICAL DEVELOPMENT OF MANAGEMENT THEORY

Management science, like nursing, develops a theory base from many disciplines, such as business, psychology, sociology, and anthropology. Because organizations are complex and varied, theorists' views of what successful management is and what it should be have changed repeatedly in the last 100 years.

Theorists' views of what successful management is and what it should be have changed repeatedly in the last 100 years.

Scientific Management (1900–1930)

Frederick W. Taylor, the "father of scientific management," was a mechanical engineer in the Midvale and Bethlehem Steel plants in Pennsylvania in the late 1800s. Frustrated with what he called "systematic soldiering," where workers achieved minimum standards doing the least amount of work possible, Taylor postulated that if workers could be taught the "one best way to accomplish a task," productivity would increase. Borrowing a term coined by Louis Brandeis, a colleague of Taylor's, Taylor called these principles *scientific management*. The four overriding principles of scientific management as identified by Taylor (1911) are:
1. Traditional "rule of thumb" means of organizing work must be replaced with scientific methods. In other words, by using time and motion studies and the expertise of experienced workers, work could be scientifically designed to promote greatest efficiency of time and energy.

2. A scientific personnel system must be established so that workers can be hired, trained, and promoted based on their technical competence and abilities. Taylor thought that each employee's abilities and limitations could be identified so that the worker could be best matched to the most appropriate job.

3. Workers should be able to view how they "fit" into the organization and how they contribute to overall organizational productivity. This provides common goals and a sharing of the organizational mission. One way Taylor thought that this could be accomplished was by the use of financial incentives as a reward for work accomplished. Because Taylor viewed humans as "economic animals" motivated solely by money, workers were reimbursed according to their level of production rather than by an hourly wage.

4. The relationship between managers and workers should be cooperative and interdependent, and the work should be shared equally. Their roles, however, were not the same. The role of managers, or *functional foremen* as they were called, was to plan, prepare, and supervise. The worker was to do the work.

What was the result of scientific management? Productivity and profits rose dramatically. Organizations were provided with a rational means of harnessing the energy of the industrial revolution. Some experts have argued that Taylor lacked humanism and that his scientific principles were not in the best interest of unions or workers. However, it is important to remember the era in which Taylor did his work. During the Industrial Revolution, laissez-faire economics prevailed, optimism was high, and a Puritan work ethic prevailed. Taylor maintained that he truly believed managers and workers would be satisfied if financial rewards were adequate as a result of increased productivity. As the cost of labor rises in the United States, many organizations are taking a new look at scientific management with the implication that we need to think of new ways to do traditional tasks so that work is more efficient.

LEARNING EXERCISE 2.2

Strategies for Efficiency

In small groups, discuss some work routines carried out in health care organizations that seem to be inefficient. Could such routines or the time and motion involved to carry out a task be altered to improve efficiency without jeopardizing quality of care? Make a list of ways that nurses could work more efficiently. Do not limit your examination to only nursing procedures and routines, but examine the impact that other departments or the arrangement of the nurse's work area may have on preventing nurses from working more efficiently. Share your ideas with your peers.

About the same time that Taylor was examining worker tasks, Max Weber, a well-known German sociologist, began to study large-scale organizations to determine what made some workers more efficient than others. Weber saw the need for legalized, formal authority and consistent rules and regulations for personnel in different positions; he thus proposed *bureaucracy* as an organizational design. His essay "Bureaucracy" was written in 1922 in response to what he perceived as a need to provide more rules, regulations, and structure within organizations to increase efficiency. Much of Weber's work and bureaucratic organizational design are still evident today in many health care institutions. His work is discussed further in Chapter 12.

Management Functions Identified (1925)

Henri Fayol (1925) first identified the management functions of planning, organization, command, coordination, and control. Luther Gulick (1937) expanded on Fayol's management functions in his introduction of the "seven activities of management"—planning, organizing, staffing, directing, coordinating, reporting, and budgeting—as denoted by the mnemonic POSDCORB. Although often modified (either by including staffing as a management function or renaming elements), these functions or activities have changed little over time. Eventually, theorists began to refer to these functions as the management process.

The *management process*, shown in Figure 2.1, is this book's organizing framework. Brief descriptions of the five functions for each phase of the management process follow:

1. *Planning* encompasses determining philosophy, goals, objectives, policies, procedures, and rules; carrying out long- and short-range projections; determining a fiscal course of action; and managing planned change.
2. *Organizing* includes establishing the structure to carry out plans, determining the most appropriate type of patient care delivery, and grouping activities to meet unit goals. Other functions involve working within the structure of the organization and understanding and using power and authority appropriately.
3. *Staffing* functions consist of recruiting, interviewing, hiring, and orienting staff. Scheduling, staff development, employee socialization, and team building are also often included as staffing functions.
4. *Directing* sometimes includes several staffing functions. However, this phase's functions usually entail human resource management responsibilities, such as motivating, managing conflict, delegating, communicating, and facilitating collaboration.
5. *Controlling* functions include performance appraisals, fiscal accountability, quality control, legal and ethical control, and professional and collegial control.

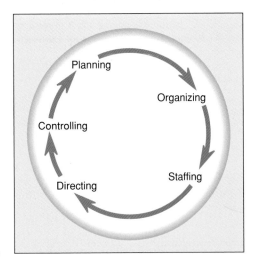

Figure 2.1   The management process.

Human Relations Management (1930–1970)

During the 1920s, worker unrest developed. The Industrial Revolution had resulted in great numbers of relatively unskilled laborers working in large factories on specialized tasks. Thus, management scientists and organizational theorists began to look at the role of worker satisfaction in production. This *human relations era* developed the concepts of participatory and humanistic management, emphasizing people rather than machines.

Mary Parker Follett was one of the first theorists to suggest basic principles of what today would be called *participative decision making* or *participative management*. In her essay "The Giving of Orders" (1926), Follett espoused her belief that managers should have authority with, rather than over, employees. Thus, solutions could be found that satisfied both sides without having one side dominate the other.

The human relations era also attempted to correct what was perceived as the major shortcoming of the bureaucratic system—a failure to include the "human element." Studies done at the Hawthorne Works of the Western Electric Company near Chicago between 1927 and 1932 played a major role in this shifting focus. The studies, conducted by Elton Mayo and his Harvard associates, began as an attempt to look at the relationship between light illumination in the factory and productivity.

Mayo and his colleagues discovered that when management paid special attention to workers, productivity was likely to increase, regardless of the environmental working conditions. This *Hawthorne effect* indicated that people respond to the fact that they are being studied, attempting to increase whatever behavior they feel will continue to warrant the attention. Mayo (1953) also found that informal work groups and a socially informal work environment were factors in determining productivity, and Mayo recommended more employee participation in decision making.

Douglas McGregor (1960) reinforced these ideas by theorizing that managerial attitudes about employees (and, hence, how managers treat those employees) can be directly correlated with employee satisfaction. He labeled this *Theory X* and *Theory Y*. Theory X managers believe that their employees are basically lazy, need constant supervision and direction, and are indifferent to organizational needs. Theory Y managers believe that their workers enjoy their work, are self-motivated, and are willing to work hard to meet personal and organizational goals.

Chris Argyris (1964) supported McGregor and Mayo by saying that managerial domination causes workers to become discouraged and passive. He believed that if self-esteem and independence needs are not met, employees will become discouraged and troublesome or may leave the organization. Argyris stressed the need for flexibility within the organization and employee participation in decision making.

The human relations era of management science brought about a great interest in the study of workers. Many sociologists and psychologists took up this challenge, and their work in management theory contributed to our understanding about worker motivation, which will be discussed in Chapter 18. Table 2.1

TABLE 2.1 **Management Theory Development 1900–1970**

Theorist	Theory
Taylor	Scientific management
Weber	Bureaucratic organizations
Fayol	Management functions
Gulick	Activities of management
Follett	Participative management
Mayo	Hawthorne effect
McGregor	Theory X and Theory Y
Argyris	Employee participation

summarizes the development of management theory up to 1970. By the late 1960s, however, there was growing concern that the human relations approach to management was not without its problems. Most people continued to work in a bureaucratic environment, making it difficult to always apply a participatory approach to management. The human relations approach was time-consuming and often resulted in unmet organizational goals. In addition, not every employee liked working in a less structured environment. This resulted in a greater recognition of the need to intertwine management and leadership than ever before.

HISTORICAL DEVELOPMENT OF LEADERSHIP THEORY (1900–PRESENT)

Because strong management skills were historically valued more than strong leadership skills, the scientific study of leadership did not begin until the 20th century. Early works focused on broad conceptualizations of leadership, such as the traits or behaviors of the leader. Contemporary research focuses more on leadership as a process of influencing others within an organizational culture and the interactive relationship of the leader and follower. To better understand newer views about leadership, it is necessary to look at how leadership theory has evolved over the last century.

Like management theory, leadership theory has been dynamic; that is, what is "known" and believed about leadership continues to change over time.

The Great Man Theory/Trait Theories (1900–1940)

The *Great Man theory* and *trait theories* were the basis for most leadership research until the mid-1940s. The Great Man theory, from Aristotelian philosophy, asserts that some people are born to lead whereas others are born to be led. It also suggests that great leaders will arise when the situation demands it.

Trait theories assume that some people have certain characteristics or personality traits that make them better leaders than others. To determine the traits that distinguish great leaders, researchers studied the lives of prominent people throughout history. The effect of followers and the impact of the situation were ignored. Contemporary opponents of these theories argue, however, that leadership skills can be developed, not just inherited.

Although trait theories have obvious shortcomings (e.g., they neglect the impact of others or the situation on the leadership role), they are worth examining. Many of the characteristics identified in trait theories (Display 2.2) are still used to describe successful leaders today.

LEARNING EXERCISE 2.3

Effective Leadership

In groups or individually, list additional characteristics that you believe an effective leader possesses. Which leadership characteristics do you have? Do you believe that you were born with leadership skills, or have you consciously developed them during your lifetime? If so, how did you develop them?

DISPLAY 2.2   **Characteristics Associated With Leadership**

Intelligence	Adaptability	Ability
Knowledge	Creativity	Able to enlist cooperation
Judgment	Cooperativeness	Interpersonal skills
Decisiveness	Alertness	Tact
Oral fluency	Self-confidence	Diplomacy
Emotional intelligence	Personal integrity	Prestige
Independence	Emotional balance and control	Social participation
Personable		

Behavioral Theories (1940–1980)

During the human relations era, many behavioral and social scientists studying management also studied leadership. For example, McGregor's (1960) theories had as much influence on leadership research as they did on management science. As leadership theory developed, researchers moved away from studying what traits the leader had and placed emphasis on what he or she did—the leader's style of leadership.

A major breakthrough occurred when Lewin (1951) and White and Lippitt (1960) isolated common *leadership styles*. Later, these styles came to be called authoritarian, democratic, and laissez-faire.

The *authoritarian* leader is characterized by the following behaviors:
- Strong control is maintained over the work group.
- Others are motivated by coercion.
- Others are directed with commands.
- Communication flows downward.
- Decision making does not involve others.
- Emphasis is on difference in status ("I" and "you").
- Criticism is punitive.

Authoritarian leadership results in well-defined group actions that are usually predictable, reducing frustration in the work group and giving members a feeling of security. Productivity is usually high, but creativity, self-motivation, and autonomy are reduced. Authoritarian leadership, useful in crisis situations, is frequently found in very large bureaucracies such as the armed forces.

The *democratic* leader exhibits the following behaviors:
- Less control is maintained.
- Economic and ego awards are used to motivate.
- Others are directed through suggestions and guidance.
- Communication flows up and down.
- Decision making involves others.
- Emphasis is on "we" rather than "I" and "you."
- Criticism is constructive.

Democratic leadership, appropriate for groups who work together for extended periods, promotes autonomy and growth in individual workers. This type of leadership is particularly effective when cooperation and coordination between groups are necessary.

Studies have shown, however, that democratic leadership is less efficient quantitatively than authoritative leadership.

 Because many people must be consulted, democratic leadership takes more time and, therefore, may be frustrating for those who want decisions made rapidly.

The *laissez-faire* leader is characterized by the following behaviors:
- Is permissive, with little or no control.
- Motivates by support when requested by the group or individuals.
- Provides little or no direction.
- Uses upward and downward communication between members of the group.
- Disperses decision making throughout the group.
- Places emphasis on the group.
- Does not criticize.

Because it is nondirected leadership, the laissez-faire style can be frustrating; group apathy and disinterest can occur. However, when all group members are highly motivated and self-directed, this leadership style can result in much creativity and productivity. Laissez-faire leadership is appropriate when problems are poorly defined and brainstorming is needed to generate alternative solutions.

A person's leadership style has a great deal of influence on the climate and outcome of the work group.

For some time, theorists believed that leaders had a predominant leadership style and used it consistently. During the late 1940s and early 1950s, however, theorists began to believe that most leaders did not fit a textbook picture of any one style but rather fell somewhere on a continuum between authoritarian and laissez-faire. They also came to believe that leaders moved dynamically along the continuum in response to each new situation. This recognition was a forerunner to what is known as *situational* or *contingency* leadership theory.

LEARNING EXERCISE 2.4

What's Your Leadership Style?
Define your predominant leadership style. Ask those who work with you if in their honest opinion this is indeed the leadership style that you use most often. What style of leadership do you work best under? What leadership style best describes your present or former managers?

Situational and Contingency Leadership Theories (1950–1980)

The idea that leadership style should vary according to the situation or the individuals involved was first suggested almost 100 years ago by Mary Parker Follett, one of the earliest management consultants and among the first to view an organization as a social system of contingencies. Her ideas, published in a series of books between 1896 and 1933, were so far ahead of their time that they did not gain appropriate recognition in the literature until the 1970s. Her *law of the situation,* which said that the situation should determine the directives given after allowing everyone to know the problem, was *contingency leadership* in its humble origins.

Fiedler's (1967) *contingency approach* reinforced these findings, suggesting that no one leadership style is ideal for every situation. Fiedler felt that the interrelationships between the group's leader and its members were most influenced by the manager's ability to be a good leader. The task to be accomplished and the power associated with the leader's position also were cited as key variables.

In contrast to the continuum from autocratic to democratic, Blake and Mouton's (1964) grid showed various combinations of concern or focus that managers had for or on productivity, tasks, people, and relationships. In each of these areas, the leader–manager may rank high or low, resulting in numerous combinations of leadership behaviors. Various formations can be effective depending on the situation and the needs of the worker.

Hersey and Blanchard (1977) also developed a situational approach to leadership. Their tridimensional leadership effectiveness model predicts which leadership style is most appropriate in each situation based on the level of the followers' maturity. As people mature, leadership style becomes less task focused and more relationship oriented.

Tannenbaum and Schmidt (1958) built on the work of Lewin and White, suggesting that managers need varying mixtures of autocratic and democratic leadership behavior. They believed that the primary determinants of leadership style should include the nature of the situation, the skills of the manager, and the abilities of the group members.

Although situational and contingency theories added necessary complexity to leadership theory and continue to be applied effectively by managers, by the late 1970s, theorists began arguing that effective leadership depended on an even greater number of variables, including organizational culture, the values of the leader and the followers, the work, the environment, the influence of the leader–manager, and the complexities of the situation. Efforts to integrate these variables are apparent in more contemporary interactional and transformational leadership theories.

Interactional Leadership Theories (1970–Present)

The basic premise of interactional theory is that leadership behavior is generally determined by the relationship between the leader's personality and the specific situation.

Schein (1970) was the first to propose a model of humans as complex beings whose working environment was an open system to which they responded. A *system* may be defined as a set of objects, with relationships between the objects and between their attributes. A system is considered open if it exchanges matter, energy, or information with its environment. Schein's model, based on systems theory, had the following assumptions:

- People are very complex and highly variable. They have multiple motives for doing things. For example, a pay raise might mean status to one person, security to another, and both to a third.
- People's motives do not stay constant but change over time.
- Goals can differ in various situations. For example, an informal group's goals may be quite distinct from a formal group's goals.
- A person's performance and productivity are affected by the nature of the task and by his or her ability, experience, and motivation.
- No single leadership strategy is effective in every situation.

To be successful, the leader must diagnose the situation and select appropriate strategies from a large repertoire of skills. Hollander (1978) was among the first to recognize that both leaders and followers have roles outside of the leadership situation and that both may be influenced by events occurring in their other roles. Indeed, Goleman, Boyatzis, and McKee (2002) suggest that followership is actually the mirror image of leadership.

With leader and follower contributing to the working relationship and both receiving something from it, Hollander (1978) saw leadership as a dynamic two-way process. According to Hollander, a leadership exchange involves three basic elements:

- The leader, including his or her personality, perceptions, and abilities
- The followers, with their personalities, perceptions, and abilities
- The situation within which the leader and the followers function, including formal and informal group norms, size, and density

Leadership effectiveness, according to Hollander, requires the ability to use the problem-solving process; maintain group effectiveness; communicate well; demonstrate leader fairness, competence, dependability, and creativity; and develop group identification.

Ouchi (1981) was a pioneer in introducing interactional leadership theory in his application of Japanese-style management to corporate America. *Theory Z*, the term Ouchi used for this type of management, is an expansion of McGregor's Theory Y and supports democratic leadership. Characteristics of Theory Z include consensus decision making, fitting employees to their jobs, job security, slower promotions, examining the long-term consequences of management decision making, quality circles, guarantee of lifetime employment, establishment of strong bonds of responsibility between superiors and subordinates, and a holistic concern for the workers (Ouchi, 1981). Ouchi was able to find components of Japanese-style management in many successful American companies.

In the 1990s, Theory Z lost favor with many management theorists. American managers are unable to put these same ideas into practice in the United States. Instead, they continue to boss-manage workers in an attempt to make them do what they do not want to do. Although Theory Z is more comprehensive than many of the earlier theories, it too neglects some of the variables that influence leadership effectiveness. It has the same shortcomings as situational theories in inadequately recognizing the dynamics of the interaction between worker and leader.

One of the pioneering leadership theorists of this time was Kanter (1977), who developed the theory that the structural aspects of the job shape a leader's effectiveness. She postulated that the leader becomes empowered through both formal and informal systems of the organization. A leader must develop relationships with a variety of people and groups within the organization in order to maximize job empowerment and be successful. The three major work empowerment structures within the organization are opportunity, power, and proportion. Kanter asserts that these work structures have the potential to explain differences in leader responses, behaviors, and attitudes in the work environment.

Nelson and Burns (1984) suggested that organizations and their leaders have four developmental levels and that these levels influence productivity and worker satisfaction. The first of these levels is *reactive*. The reactive leader focuses on the past, is crisis driven, and is frequently abusive to subordinates. In the next level, *responsive*, the leader is able to mold subordinates to work together as a team, although the leader maintains most decision-making responsibility. At the *proactive* level, the leader and followers become more future oriented and hold common driving values. Management and decision making are more participative. At the last level, *high-performance teams*, maximum productivity and worker satisfaction are apparent.

Brandt's (1994) interactive leadership model suggests that leaders develop a work environment that fosters autonomy and creativity through valuing and empowering followers. This leadership "affirms the uniqueness of each individual," motivating them to "contribute their unique talents to a common goal." The leader must accept the responsibility for quality of outcomes and quality of life for followers. Brandt states that this type of leadership affords the leader greater freedom while simultaneously adding to the burdens of leadership. The leader's responsibilities increase because priorities cannot be limited to the organization's goals, and authority confers not only power but also responsibility and obligation. The leader's concern for each worker decreases the need for competition and fosters an atmosphere of collegiality, freeing the leader from the burden of having to resolve follower conflicts.

Wolf, Boland, and Aukerman (1994) also emphasized an interactive leadership model in their creation of a *collaborative practice matrix*. This matrix highlights the framework for the development and ongoing support of relationships between and among professionals working together. The "social architecture" of the work group is emphasized, as is how expectations, personal values, and interpersonal relationships affect the ability of leaders and followers to achieve the vision of the organization. Similarly, Manojlovich's (2005) research suggested that nurses may be able to practice more professionally when they perceive that their unit leaders have strong leadership skills.

Kanter (1989) perhaps best summarized the work of the interactive theorists by her assertion that title and position authority were no longer sufficient to mold a workforce where subordinates are encouraged to think for themselves, and instead managers must learn to work synergistically with others.

Transactional and Transformational Leadership

Similarly, Burns (2003), a noted scholar in the area of leader–follower interactions, was among the first to suggest that both leaders and followers have the ability to raise each other to higher levels of motivation and morality. Identifying this concept as *transformational leadership*, Burns maintained that there are two primary types of leaders in management. The traditional manager, concerned with the day-to-day operations, was termed a *transactional leader*. "The transactional leader sets goals, gives directions, and uses rewards to reinforce employee behaviors associated with meeting or exceeding established goals" (McGuire & Kennerly, 2006, p. 180). The transactional leader then emphasizes process in setting goals and giving directions and seeks to control both situations and followers (McGuire and Kennerly, 2006).

The manager who is committed, has a vision, and is able to empower others with this vision, however, was termed a *transformational leader*. Transformational leaders are able to "motivate performance beyond expectations through their ability to influence attitudes" (McGuire & Kennerly, 2006, p. 179). Longnecker (2006) states that the transformational leader inspires and motivates followers not only as a role model but also by recognizing the uniqueness of their followers and being creative. A composite of the two different types of leaders is shown in Table 2.2.

Vision is the essence of transformational leadership.

TABLE 2.2   **Transactional and Transformational Leaders**

Transactional Leader	Transformational Leader
Focuses on management tasks	Identifies common values
Is a caretaker	Is committed
Uses trade-offs to meet goals	Inspires others with vision
Does not identify shared values	Has long-term vision
Examines causes	Looks at effects
Uses contingency reward	Empowers others

Transformational leaders "have a view of the future that will excite and convert potential followers" (ChangingMinds.org, 2002–2006, para 3). The transformational leader then "sells" this vision to followers. Indeed, the transformational leader "seeks to infect and reinfect the followers with a high level of commitment to the vision" (ChangingMinds.org, 2002–2006, para 3). This new shared vision provides the energy required to move an organizational unit toward the future.

Wolf, Boland, and Aukerman (1994) define *transformational leadership* as "an interactive relationship, based on trust, that positively impacts both the leader and the follower. The purposes of the leader and follower become focused, creating unity, wholeness and collective purpose" (p. 38). The high-performing transformational leader demonstrates a strong commitment to the profession and the organization and is willing to tackle obstacles by using group learning. This self-confidence comes from a strong sense of being in control. These transformational leaders also are able to create synergistic environments that enhance change. Change occurs because the transformational leader's futuristic focus values creativity and innovation. The transformational leader also values organizational culture and values strongly, perpetuating these same values and behaviors in their staff (Wolf et al., 1994).

Johns (2004) maintains that transformational leadership is a deliberate process of seeking insight into self and practice in order to create conditions that foster the realization of desirable practice. Three tasks essential to the learning process of the would-be transformational leader are (a) identifying the characteristics of this type of leader, (b) becoming aware of creative tension and factors that limit realization of goals and vision, and (c) breaking free of the constraints associated with transactional leadership.

Although the transformational leader is held as the current ideal, many management theorists, including Bass, Avoliio, and Goodheim (1987) and Dunham and Klafehn (1990), sound a warning about transformational leadership. Although transformational qualities are highly desirable, they must be coupled with the more traditional transactional qualities of the day-to-day managerial role.

> Although transformational qualities are highly desirable, they must be coupled with the more traditional transactional qualities of the day-to-day managerial role.

Both sets of characteristics need to be present in the same person in varying degrees. According to Bass and colleagues, the transformational leader will fail without traditional management skills. This was readily apparent in Johnson's (2005) research suggesting that highly effective managers need both vision as well as a specific plan able to carry out their plan if goals are to be achieved (Examining the Evidence 2.1).

In addition, Badaracco cautions that "because we admire heroes, it is easy to overlook the inconvenient fact that some leaders are effective without being either visionary or very inspiring. There must be a place for leading by example and other forms of quiet leadership" (McCrimmon, n.d., para 2). Similarly, ChangingMinds.org (2002–2006) warns that transformational leaders must be careful not to mistake passion and confidence for truth and reality. "Whilst it is true that great things have been achieved through enthusiastic leadership, it is also true that many passionate people have led the charge right over the cliff and into a bottomless chasm. Just because someone *believes* they are right, it does not mean they *are* right" (para 9).

Bennis (1989) sounds a different warning about the quest for transformational leadership in his assertion that "there is an unconscious conspiracy in contemporary society that prevents leaders—no matter what their original vision—from taking charge and making changes" (p . xii). Bennis elaborates by pointing out that entrenched bureaucracy and a commitment to the status quo undermine leaders and that tensions between individual rights and the common good discourage the emergence of leaders (Bennis, 1989). Similarly, McGuire and Kennerly (2006) suggest that "while transformational leadership is often considered to be more effective, nurse manager performance standards are often rooted in transactional characteristics" (p. 179). This

EXAMINING THE EVIDENCE 2.1

Source: Johnson, S. W. (2005, April–June). Characteristics of effective health care managers. *Health Care Manager, 24*(2), 124–128.

A survey of seven highly effective health care managers in a South Georgia community, using the *Scale of Transformational Leadership*, revealed that the technical skill or trust element—that is, the ability to follow through and deliver on plans and vision—was the skill or characteristic on which managers rated themselves highest. While all of the skills are necessary, the ability to carry out the vision, plan, and goals to achieve results seems to have the most value.

Mid-range skills were related to the self and feeling elements, or human skills. Perhaps due to the arena of uncertainty in a strained economy, risk taking was ranked as the lowest skills element by the managers. The study indicated that although conceptual skills (attention: vision, risk: chance, meaning: communication) have long been viewed as the "role" of the manager, technical skills (trust) to fulfill the services, goals, and visions were ranked by the managers as having more importance.

discourages the manager from pursuing a transformative leadership style. It is critical, then, to remember that the organization and the environment play a critical role in the development and support of the transformational and transactional leadership skills of its employees. The relationship must be symbiotic.

Finally, Kellerman (2004) maintains that in this age of leadership development, theorists have concluded that leaders are always good, when in reality flawed leaders are to be found everywhere. There is a need to remind ourselves that leaders are like the rest of us. Leaders may be deceitful and trustworthy, greedy and generous, cowardly and brave. To assume that all good leaders are good people is foolhardy and makes us blind to the human condition. It is only when we recognize and manage our failings that leaders achieve greatness (Kellerman, 2004). Future leadership theory may well focus on why leaders behave badly and why followers continue to follow bad leaders.

 To assume that all good leaders are good people is foolhardy and makes us blind to the human condition.

INTEGRATING LEADERSHIP AND MANAGEMENT

Because rapid, dramatic change will continue in nursing and the health care industry, it has grown increasingly important for nurses to develop skill in both leadership roles and management functions. For managers and leaders to function at their greatest potential, the two must be integrated.

Gardner (1990) asserted that *integrated leader–managers* possess six distinguishing traits:

1. *They think longer term.* They are visionary and futuristic. They consider the effect that their decisions will have years from now as well as their immediate consequences.
2. *They look outward, toward the larger organization.* They do not become narrowly focused. They are able to understand how their unit or department fits into the bigger picture.
3. *They influence others beyond their own group.* Effective leader–managers rise above an organization's bureaucratic boundaries.

TABLE 2.3 **Leadership Theorists and Theories**

Theorist	Theory
Aristotle	Great man theory
Lewin and White	Leadership styles
Follett	Law of the situation
Fiedler	Contingency leadership
Blake and Mouton	Task versus relationship in determining leadership style
Hersey and Blanchard	Situational leadership theory
Tannenbaum and Schmidt	Situational leadership theory
Kanter	Organizational structure shapes leader effectiveness
Gardner	The integrated leader–manager

4. *They emphasize vision, values, and motivation.* They understand intuitively the unconscious and often nonrational aspects that are present in interactions with others. They are very sensitive to others and to differences in each situation.
5. *They are politically astute.* They are capable of coping with conflicting requirements and expectations from their many constituencies.
6. *They think in terms of change and renewal.* The traditional manager accepts the structure and processes of the organization, but the leader–manager examines the ever-changing reality of the world and seeks to revise the organization to keep pace.

Leadership and management skills can and should be integrated as they are learned. Table 2.3 summarizes the development of leadership theory through the end of the 20th century. Newer (21st century) and emerging leadership theories are discussed in Chapter 3.

SUMMARY

In examining leadership and management, it becomes clear that these two concepts have a symbiotic or synergistic relationship. Every nurse is a leader and manager at some level, and the nursing role requires leadership and management skills.

The need for visionary leaders and effective managers in nursing precludes the option of stressing one role over the other. Highly developed management skills are needed to maintain healthy organizations. So too are the visioning and empowerment of subordinates through an organization's leadership team. Because rapid, dramatic change will continue in nursing and the health care industry, it continues to be critically important for nurses to develop skill in both leadership roles and management functions and to strive for the integration of leadership characteristics throughout every phase of the management process.

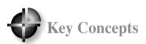 **Key Concepts**

* Management functions include *planning*, *organizing*, *staffing*, *directing*, and *controlling*. These are incorporated into what is known as the management process.

* *Classical*, or *traditional*, *management science* focused on production in the workplace and on delineating organizational barriers to productivity. Workers were assumed to be motivated solely by economic rewards, and little attention was given to worker job satisfaction.
* The *human relations era of management science* emphasized concepts of participatory and humanistic management.
* Three primary leadership styles have been identified: *authoritarian*, *democratic*, and *laissez-faire*.
* Research has shown that the leader–manager must assume a variety of leadership styles, depending on the needs of the worker, the task to be performed, and the situation or environment. This is known as *situational* or *contingency leadership theory*.
* *Leadership* is a process of persuading and influencing others toward a goal and is composed of a wide variety of roles.
* Early leadership theories focused on the traits and characteristics of leaders.
* *Interactional leadership theory* focuses more on leadership as a process of influencing others within an organizational culture and the interactive relationship of the leader and follower.
* The manager who is committed, has a vision, and is able to empower others with this vision is termed a *transformational leader*, whereas the traditional manager, concerned with the day-to-day operations, is called a *transactional leader*.
* Integrating leadership skills with the ability to carry out management functions is necessary if an individual is to become an effective leader–manager.

ADDITIONAL LEARNING EXERCISES AND APPLICATIONS

LEARNING EXERCISE 2.5

When Culture and Policy Clash

You are the nurse–manager of a medical unit. Recently, your unit admitted a 16-year-old East Indian boy who has been newly diagnosed with insulin-dependent diabetes. The nursing staff has been interested in his case and has found him to be a delightful young man—very polite and easygoing. However, his family has been visiting in increasing numbers and bringing him food that he should not have.

The nursing staff has come to you on two occasions and complained about the family's noncompliance with visiting hours and unauthorized food. Normally, the nursing staff on your unit has tried to develop a culturally sensitive nursing care plan for patients with special cultural needs, so their complaints to you have taken you by surprise.

Yesterday, two of the family members visited you and complained about hospital visitor policies and what they took to be rudeness by two different staff members. You spent time talking to the family, and when they left, they seemed agreeable and understanding.

Last night, one of the staff nurses told the family that according to hospital policy only two members could stay (this is true) and if the other family members did not leave, she would call hospital security. This morning the boy's mother and father have suggested that they will take him home if this matter is not resolved. The patient's diabetes is still not controlled, and you feel that it would be unwise for this to happen.

● ASSIGNMENT: Leadership is needed to keep this situation from deteriorating further. Divide into groups. Develop a plan of action for solving this problem. First, select three desired objectives for solving the problem and then proceed to determine what you would do that would enable you to meet your objectives. Be sure that you are clear as to who you consider your followers to be and what you expect from each of them.

LEARNING EXERCISE 2.6

Delineating Leadership Roles and Management Functions

Examine the scenario in Learning Exercise 2.5. How would you divide the management functions and leadership roles in this situation? For example, you might say that having the nurse–manager adhere to hospital policy was a management function and that counseling staff was a leadership role.

● ASSIGNMENT: List at least five management functions and five leadership roles that you could also delineate in this scenario. Share these with your group.

LEARNING EXERCISE 2.7

What's Your Management Style?

Recall times when you have been a manager. This does not only mean a nursing manager. Perhaps you were a head lifeguard or an evening shift manager at a fast-food restaurant. During those times, do you think you were a good manager? Did you involve others in your management decision making appropriately? How would you evaluate your decision-making ability? Make a list of your management strengths and a list of management skills that you felt you were lacking.

LEARNING EXERCISE 2.8

What Decision-Making Style Should Be Used?

● ASSIGNMENT: In the following scenarios, determine whether an autocratic, democratic, or laissez-faire decision-making style would be most appropriate. Provide rationale for your choice that includes a discussion of the individuals involved, the environment, and the task to be completed.

1. You are the evening shift charge nurse of the intensive care unit. Your supervisor is sending two nurses from each shift to an upcoming critical care conference in a nearby city. The supervisor wants each charge nurse to submit names of the selected nurses in 2 weeks. All of the 12 full-time evening shift nurses would like to go. From a staffing standpoint, there is no reason why any of them could not go. All are active in the local critical care organization. Financial resources, however, limit your choice to two. How do you resolve this situation? Select the most appropriate decision style.

(Learning Exercise continues on page 48)

2. You are the day shift charge nurse on a surgical unit. Because of your related expertise, your supervisor has asked you to select a new type of blood-warming unit. You want to be sure that you select the right one. Several companies have provided your staff with trial units. You have not received much feedback from the staff regarding their preferences, however, and you must submit your equipment request by 4 PM tomorrow. Select the most appropriate decision style.

3. You are the manager of a 30-bed medical unit. After consultation, you recently implemented a system for incorporating nursing diagnoses on the patient care plans. Although the system was expected to reduce report time between shifts and improve the quality of patient care, to everyone's surprise, including your own, you find that the system is not working. You do not think that there is anything wrong with your idea. Many other hospitals in the areas are using nursing diagnoses with success. You had a consultant come from another hospital and give an update to your nurses on use of the system. The consultant reported that your staff seemed knowledgeable and appeared to understand their responsibilities in implementing the system.

   You suspect that a few nurses might be sabotaging your efforts for planned change, but your charge nurses do not agree. They believe that the failure may be lack of proper incentives or poor staff morale. Your nursing administrator is anxious to implement the system in other patient care units but wants it to be working well in your unit first. You have just come from a manager's meeting where your administrator told you to solve the problem and report back to her within 1 week regarding the steps you had taken to solve your problem. You share your administrator's concern, but how should you solve this problem? Select the most appropriate decision style.

Web Links

Leadership Talks
http://www.regent.edu/acad/global/leadershiptalks/home.htm
This monthly audio e-newsletter provides fresh insights and perspectives from some of the top leadership scholars, practitioners, and presenters in the country. Benefit from case studies, practical lessons, and inspiring anecdotes provided by some of today's top leadership speakers.

International Leadership Association
http://www.ila-net.org
The International Leadership Association is the global network for all those who practice, study, and teach leadership and provides a forum where people can share ideas, research, and practices about leadership.

Reflections on Nursing Leadership
http://www.nursingsociety.org/RNL/Current/about_us/about_us.html
This magazine communicates nurses' contributions and relevance to the health of people worldwide. The magazine is published quarterly by the Honor Society of Nursing, Sigma Theta Tau International.

The Robert Wood Johnson Executive Nurse Fellows Program

Center for the Health Professions, San Francisco, CA
http://futurehealth.ucsf.edu/Program/rwj/
This is a three-year advanced leadership program for senior executive nurses seeking the experience and skills necessary to be leaders in the health care system.

References

Argyris, C. (1964). *Integrating the individual and the organization*. New York: John Wiley and Sons.

Bass, B. M., Avoliio, B. J., & Goodheim, L. (1987, January). Biography and the assessment of transformational leadership at the world-class level. *Journal of Management, 13(1)*, 7–19.

Bennis, W. (1989). *Why leaders can't lead*. San Francisco: Jossey-Boss.

Bitpipe.com. (2006). *Leadership (IT management leadership) definition*. Retrieved August 2, 2006, from *http://www.bitpipe.com/tlist/Leadership.html*.

Blake, R. R., & Mouton, J. S. (1964). *The managerial grid*. Houston, TX: Gulf Publishing.

Brandt, M. A. (1994). Caring leadership: Secret and path to success. *Nursing Management, 25(8)*, 68–72.

Burns, J. M. (2003). *Transforming leadership*. New York: Grove/Atlantic, Inc.

Chapin, F. S. (1924). Socialized leadership. *Social Forces, 3*, 57–60.

ChangingMinds.org. (2002–2006). *Transformational leadership*. Retrieved August 4, 2006, from *http://changingminds. org/disciplines/leadership/styles/transformational_leadership. htm*.

Dunham, J., & Klafehn, K. A. (1990). Transformational leadership and the nurse executive. *Journal of Nursing Administration, 20(4)*, 28–34.

Fayol, H. (1925). *General and industrial management*. London: Pittman and Sons.

Fiedler, F. (1967). *A theory of leadership effectiveness*. New York: McGraw-Hill.

Follett, M. P. (1926). The giving of orders. In H. C. Metcalf (Ed.), *Scientific foundations of business administration*. Baltimore: Williams & Wilkins.

Gardner, J. W. (1990). *On leadership*. New York: The Free Press.

Goleman, D., Boyatzis, R., & McKee, A. (2002). Primal leadership: The hidden driver in great performance. *Harvard Business Review on Breakthrough Leadership* (pp. 25–50). Boston: Harvard Business School Publishing Corporation.

Gulick, L. (1937). Notes on the theory of the organization. In L. Gulick & L. Urwick (Eds.), *Papers on the science of administration* (pp. 3–13). New York: Institute of Public Administration.

Hersey, P., & Blanchard, K. (1977). *Management of organizational behavior: Utilizing human resources* (3rd ed.). Englewood Cliffs, NJ: Prentice Hall.

Hollander, E. P. (1978). *Leadership dynamics: A practical guide to effective relationships*. New York: The Free Press.

Johns, C. (2004). Becoming a transformational leader through reflection. *Reflections on Nursing Leadership, 30(2)*, 24–26.

Johnson, S. W. (2005, April–June). Characteristics of effective health care managers. *Health Care manager, 24(2)*, 124–128.

Kanter, R. M. (1977). *Men and women of the corporation*. New York: Basic Books.

Kanter, R. M. (1989). The new managerial work. *Harvard Business Review, 67(6)*, 85–92.

Kellerman, B. (2004). Leadership, warts and all. *Harvard Business Review, 82(1)*, 40–45.

Lewin, K. (1951). *Field theory in social sciences*. New York: Harper & Row.

Longnecker, P. D. (2006). Evaluating transformational leadership skills of hospice executives. *American Journal of Hospice and Palliative Medicine, 23(3)*, 205–211.

Manojlovich, M. (2005). The effect of nursing leadership on hospital nurses' professional practice behaviors. *Journal of Nursing Administration, 35(7–8)*, 366–374.

Mayo, E. (1953). *The human problems of an industrialized civilization*. New York: Macmillan.

McCrimmin, M. (n.d.). *What's wrong with leadership theory?* Retrieved August 3, 2006, from *http://www.leadersdirect.com/ What%27s%20wrongV4.pdf*.

McGregor, D. (1960). *The human side of enterprise*. New York: McGraw-Hill.

McGuire, E., & Kennerly, S. M. (2006). Nurse managers as transformational and transactional leaders. *Nursing Economics, 24(4)*, 179–186.

Nelson, L., & Burns, F. (1984). High-performance programming: A framework for transforming organizations. In J. Adams (Ed.), *Transforming work* (pp. 225–242). Alexandria, VA: Miles River Press.

Ouchi, W. G. (1981). *Theory Z: How American business can meet the Japanese challenge*. Reading, MA: Addison-Wesley.

Schein, E. H. (1970). *Organizational psychology* (2nd ed.). Englewood Cliffs, NJ: Prentice-Hall.

Tannenbaum, R., & Schmidt, W. (1958). How to choose a leadership pattern. *Harvard Business Review, 36*, 95–102.

Taylor, F. W. (1911). *The principles of scientific management*. New York: Harper & Row.

Trent, B. A. (2003). Leadership myths. *Reflections on Nursing Leadership, 29(3)*, 8–9.

White, R. K., & Lippitt R. (1960). *Autocracy and democracy: An experimental inquiry*. New York: Harper & Row.

Wikipedia. (2006). *Definition-management*. Retrieved August 1, 2006 from *http://en.wikipedia.org/wiki/Management*.

Wolf, G. A., Boland, S., & Aukerman, M. (1994). A transformational model for the practice of professional nursing. Part II. *Journal of Nursing Administration, 24(5)*, 38–46.

Bibliography

Bennis, W. G. (2004). The seven ages of the leader. *Harvard Business Review, 82*(1), 46–53.

Bering, M. (2006, July). A personal journey into leadership. *Nursing Management UK, 13*(4), 20–25.

Canadian Nurses Association. (2005). Nursing leadership in a changing world. *Nursing Now: Issues and Trends in Canadian Nursing.* Ottawa, Canada: Canadian Nurses Association.

DeGroot, H. A. (2005). Evidence-based leadership: Nursing's new mandate. *Nurse Leader, 3*(2), 37–41.

Grayson, D., & Speckhart, R. (2006, Winter). The leader-follower relationship: Practitioner observations. *Leadership Advance Online.* Issue VI. Retrieved August 2, 2006, from *http://www.regent.edu/acad/global/publications/lao/issue_6/grayson_speckhart.htm.*

Grossman, S. C., & Valiga, T. M. (2005). *The new leadership challenge: Creating the future of nursing.* Philadelphia: F. A. Davis.

Leach, L. S. (2005). Nurse executive transformational leadership and organizational commitment. *Journal of Nursing Administration, 35*(5), 228–237.

Longnecker, P. D. (2006). Evaluating transformational leadership skills in hospice executives. *American Journal of Hospice and Palliative Medicine, 23*(3), 205–211.

Paliadelis, P. S. (2005). Rural nursing unit managers: Education and support for the role. *Rural and Remote Health, 5*(1), 1–8.

Parish, C. (2006). Good leadership needs a range of styles. *Nursing Management UK, 13*(4), 4.

Presutti, M. (2006, February). Is micromanagement killing your staff? The administrator who "has to do it all" can end up undoing everything. *Nursing Homes: Long Term Care Management, 55*(2), 34, 36–38, 59–60.

Scanlan, L. (2006). Leadership and management. Expectations without accomplishment. *Healthcare Financial Management, 60*(1), 100, 102.

Stanley, D. (2006). In command of care: Toward the theory of congruent leadership. Second of two papers. *Journal of Research in Nursing, 11*(2), 132–144.

The Free Dictionary. (2005). *Definition-Management.* Retrieved August 22, 2007 from *http://www.thefreedictionary.com/management.*

Winston, B., & Patterson, K. (2006). An integrative definition of leadership. *International Journal of Leadership Studies, 1*(2), 6–66.

Wolf, G. A., Bradle, J., & Greenhouse, P. (2006). Investment in the future: A 3-level approach for developing the healthcare leaders of tomorrow. *Journal of Nursing Administration, 36*(6), 331–336.

3

Twenty-First Century Thinking About Leadership and Management

. . . the roles of the nurse manager and nurse executive have evolved significantly in response to changes in the health care industry in the last 20 years.

—Carol S. Kleinman

. . . we are not creatures of circumstance; we are creators of circumstance.

—Benjamin Disraeli

Throughout history, nursing has been required to respond to changing technological and social forces. In the last few decades alone, the proliferation of managed care resulted in major redesign of most health care organizations. The locus of care shifted from acute-care hospitals to community and outpatient settings, innovation and technological advances transformed the workplace, and organizational cultures increasingly shifted to customer-focused care. All of these changes brought about a need for leader–managers to learn new roles and develop new skills.

The new managerial responsibilities placed on organized nursing services call for nurse administrators who are knowledgeable, skilled, and competent in all aspects of management. Now more than ever, there is a greater emphasis on the business of health care, with managers being involved in the financial and marketing aspects of their respective departments. Managers are expected to be skilled communicators, organizers, and team builders and to be visionary and proactive in preparing for emerging new threats such as terrorism, biological warfare, and global pandemics.

In addition, the need to develop nursing leadership skills has never been greater. At the national level, nurse–leaders and nurse–managers are actively involved in greatly needed health care reform and in addressing the ever-increasing international nursing shortage. At the organizational and unit levels, nurse–leaders are being directed to address high turnover rates by staff, a growing trend toward unionization, and new legislation directed at minimum staffing ratios and mandatory overtime in an effort to maintain cohesive and productive work environments. Moreover, ensuring successful recruitment, creating shared governance models, and maintaining high-quality practice depend on successful team building, another critical leadership skill in contemporary health care organizations. This challenging and changing health care system requires leader–managers to use their scarce resources appropriately and to be visionary and proactive in planning for challenges yet to come.

In confronting these expanding responsibilities and demands, many leader–managers turn to the experts for tools or strategies to meet these expanded role dimensions. What they have found is some new and innovative thinking about how best to manage organizations and lead people as well as some reengineered interactive leadership theories from the later 19th century. This emergent thinking about leadership "allows both private and public sector leaders to consider new understandings and research and then to practice leadership within current financial, societal and political realities" (Flumerfelt, 2006, para 1). This chapter explores contemporary thinking about leadership and management, with specific attention given to emergent 21st century thinking.

NEW THINKING ABOUT LEADERSHIP AND MANAGEMENT

Stanley (2006) suggests that there is a need to go beyond transformational leadership models, particularly in clinical leadership, as we enter the 21st century. Flumerfelt (2006) agrees, arguing that emerging leadership models have "evolved with thought development and within altering contextual frames" (para 1). Already in the 21st century, multiple new leadership and management concepts have emerged, many of which focus on the complexity of the relationship between the leader and the follower.

 Many recent leadership and management concepts focus on the complexity of the relationship between the leader and the follower.

In addition, contemporary leadership theorists have built upon the interactive leadership theories developed in the latter part of the 20th century. As a result, concepts such as servant leadership, principal agent theory, human and social capital theory, emotional intelligence, authentic leadership, quantum leadership, thought leadership, and cultural bridging have emerged as part of the leader–manager's repertoire for the 21st century.

Servant Leadership

Although Greenleaf (1977) developed the idea of servant leadership more than 30 years ago, it continues to greatly influence leadership thinking in the 21st century. In more than four decades of working as director of leadership development at AT&T, Greenleaf noticed that most successful managers lead in a different way from traditional managers. These managers, which he termed *servant leaders*, put serving others, including employees, customers, and the community, as the number-one priority.

 Greenleaf argued that to be a great leader, one must be a servant first.

Howatson-Jones (2004) also suggests that servant leadership is about "leaders serving the needs of followers, and empowering them rather than the organization" (p. 22). Thus, servant

DISPLAY 3.1 **Defining Qualities of Servant Leaders**

- The ability to listen on a deep level and to truly understand
- The ability to keep an open mind and hear without judgment
- The ability to deal with ambiguity, paradoxes, and complex issues
- The belief that honestly sharing critical challenges with all parties and asking for their input is more important than personally providing solutions
- Being clear on goals and good at pointing the direction toward goal achievement without giving orders
- The ability to be a servant, helper, and teacher first and then a leader
- Always thinking before reacting
- Choosing words carefully so as not to damage those being led
- The ability to use foresight and intuition
- Seeing things whole and sensing relationships and connections

leaders consider their followers' needs first and then empower them to achieve organizational goals (Howatson-Jones, 2004). This is very different from traditional management where the organizational goals and needs are paramount. In addition, Howatson-Jones says that trust is the cornerstone of servant leadership and that mutual respect and feedback are an essential part of the leader–follower relationship. So too is "direct in the field" access to leaders (p. 23). Other defining qualities of servant leadership are shown in Display 3.1.

LEARNING EXERCISE 3.1

Creating a Service Inclination
Greenleaf (1977) suggested that the true test of servant leadership is the servant leader's ability to create a service inclination in others. In doing so, more leaders are created for the organization.

● ASSIGNMENT: Identify servant leaders who you have worked with. Did they motivate followers to be service oriented? If so, what strategies did they use? Does servant leadership result in a greater number of leaders within an organization? If so, why do you think that this happens?

New Thinking about Leaders and Followers

Many contemporary scholars have expanded on Greenleaf's work, particularly in terms of how followers influence the actions of the leader. For example, Offermann (2004) postulated that followers influence leaders in both positive and negative ways. While the positive effect of followers on leaders has been fairly well described in most discussions of transformational leadership, less has been said about potential negative impacts. For example, followers can and do mislead leaders, whether intentionally or not.

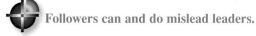 **Followers can and do mislead leaders.**

Leaders can counteract this, however, by keeping vision and values front and center, cultivating truth tellers, honoring one's intuition, making sure followers are allowed to disagree, setting a good ethical climate, and delegating appropriately. In doing so, the leader creates an atmosphere where follower influence will more likely result in positive rather than negative outcomes (Offermann, 2004).

Principal Agent Theory

Principal agent theory, which first emerged in the 1960s and 1970s, is another interactive leadership theory being actively explored in the 21st century. This theory suggests that not all followers (agents) are inherently motivated to act in the best interest of the principal (leader or employer). This is because followers may have an informational (expertise or knowledge) advantage over the leader as well as their own preferences, which may deviate from the principal's preferences. The risk then is that agents will pursue their own objectives or interests instead of that of their principal.

Principals then must identify and provide agents with appropriate incentives to act in the organization's best interest. For example, consumers with good health insurance and small out-of-pocket expenses may have little motivation to act prudently in accessing health care resources, since payment for services used will come primarily from the insurer. The insurer then must create incentives for agents who access only needed services.

Another example might be end-of-shift overtime. While most employees do not intentionally seek or want to work overtime after a long and busy shift, the reality is that doing so typically results in financial rewards. Employers then must either create incentives that reward employees who are able to complete their work in the allotted shift time or create disincentives for those who do not.

LEARNING EXERCISE 3.2

The Agent's Motives
You are a team leader for 10 patients on a busy medical unit. Your team includes Lori, an LVN passing medications and assisting with patient treatments, and Tom, an experienced CNA who provides basic care such as monitoring vital signs, ambulating patients, and assisting with hygiene. On several occasions in the past, Tom has failed to report significant changes in patients' vital signs to you until some time had elapsed or you discovered them yourself. Despite confronting Tom about the need to report these changes and the specific vital sign parameters that need to be reported, this behavior has continued. You have become concerned that patient harm might occur if this pattern of behavior is allowed to continue.

● ASSIGNMENT: Identify possible motives that Tom (the agent) may have for failing to share this information with you (the principal). What incentives might you employ to modify his behavior?

Principal agent dilemmas also occur at the organizational level. Santerre (2004) suggests that health care organizations with nonprofit status are actually more likely to face a principal–agent problem than their for-profit counterparts. He argues that this occurs because nonprofit organizations "must dispense all residual earnings for the expressed educational, charitable, or religious purposes for which they were formed" (p. 3). With less financial incentives, there may be fewer incentives to monitor the behavior of the organization and "unconstrained managers will be more inclined to pursue personal goals and objectives, which are likely to conflict with min-imum cost production" (p. 4). The result, Santerre says, is that the divergence between the inter-ests of the principal(s) and the agent(s) in this case can lead to inefficient production and provi-sion of medical care services.

Human and Social Capital Theory

Human capital refers to a group's collective knowledge, skills, and abilities. *Human capital the-ory* "recognizes that individuals and organizations invest in human capital in anticipation of gains in the forms of increased productivity and financial returns" (Jones, 2004, p. 563). For example, a health care organization that provides tuition reimbursement for nurses to go back to school to earn higher degrees is likely doing so in anticipation that a more highly educated nurs-ing staff will result in increased quality of care and higher retention rates—both of which should translate into higher productivity and financial return.

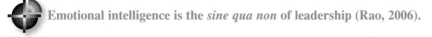 Human capital refers to a group's collective knowledge, skills, and abilities.

Jones (2004) suggests that human capital can be viewed from both an individual and an orga-nizational perspective. From the individual perspective, human capital includes the knowledge and skills that result from education, training, and experience. From an organizational perspec-tive, human capital refers to the collective group knowledge or experience. This aggregate of human capital, however, is sometimes called *social capital* (Jones, 2004, p. 565), although social capital tends to refer more to social connectedness within communities.

Simon and Norris (2004–2005) also differentiate between human and social capital in their assertion that "human capital is ultimately the property of the individual—it is what an employee can do. Social capital accrues within the organization. It determines what a group of employees can—and will—accomplish together" (para 3). Simon and Norris go on to say that social capi-tal is all about relationships and that relationships are increasingly important for contemporary organizations to achieve their goals.

This was apparent in a Lauder, Reel, Farmer, and Griggs (2006) discussion of social capital in rural health care settings. They suggested that because nurses in rural settings are often "immersed" or "embedded" in the social networks that make up the fabric of rural life, that they play an important role in developing social capital. Lauder and colleagues also emphasized that because social capital involves trust, social networks, and reciprocity within communities, rural nurses have a tremendous potential to positively influence health behaviors in rural residents—as much from these social relationships as from the knowledge and information that they impart.

Emotional Intelligence

Another leadership theory gaining prominence in the early 21st century is that of emotional intelligence (EI, also known as EQ). Reeves (2005) suggests that "cognitive intelligence is only half of the equation necessary for success in the workplace" (p. 172). The other half, and the most important half, she argues, is EI. Rao (2006) concurs, arguing that while IQ and technical skills are increasingly being recognized as critical to successful leadership and management, it is EI that is the "*sine qua non* of leadership."

Emotional intelligence is the *sine qua non* of leadership (Rao, 2006).

Broadly defined, *emotional intelligence* is the capacity to get optimal results from relationships with others (Six Seconds: The Emotional Intelligence Network, 2005). The Institute for Organizational Performance (IOP) (2006), however, defines EI as "the ability to use emotions effectively," noting that it is "the foundation of high-performing relationships" (para 2). The IOP says this is because "individual relationships create the workplace climate and, in turn, the climate shapes the ways employees and customers relate to each other and the organization" (para 2).

In their original work on EI in 1990, Salovey and Mayer (1997) suggested that EI develops with age and that it consists of three mental processes:
- Appraising and expressing emotions in the self and others
- Regulating emotion in self and others
- Using emotions in adaptive ways

In 1997, they further refined EI into four mental abilities: perceiving/identifying emotions, integrating emotions into thought processes, understanding emotions, and managing emotions (Vitello-Cicciu, 2003).

Goleman (1998), in his 1995 best seller *Emotional Intelligence*, built upon this work in his identification of five components of emotional intelligence: self-awareness, self-regulation, motivation, empathy, and social skills (Display 3.2). Goleman argued that all individuals have a rational thinking mind and an emotional feeling mind and that both influence action. The goal, then, in EI is *emotional literacy*—being self-aware about one's emotions and recognizing how they influence actions that are taken (Stuart, 2004).

Unlike Salovey and Mayer, however, Goleman argued that EI could be learned, although he too felt that it improves with age. Reeves (2005) suggests that developing EI begins with self-awareness enhanced by self-care behaviors. Then, the individual needs to develop an awareness of others. Finally is the development of empathy, which requires that the individual learn to actively listen to others. Reeves goes on to say that "it is important for nurses to cultivate these skills because the behaviors associated with emotional intelligence further nursing's mission by improving health outcomes" (p. 176).

In addition, most theorists studying EI agree that emotional intelligence is critical for building a cooperative and effective team. Leaders with EI possess the ability to identify emotions in themselves and others, use emotions in their thought processes, manage emotions in themselves and others, and understand and reason with emotions (Vitello-Cicciu, 2003). For example,

DISPLAY 3.2   Five Components of Emotional Intelligence

1. *Self-awareness*. The ability to recognize and understand one's moods, emotions, and drives as well as their effects on others
2. *Self-regulation*. The ability to control or redirect disruptive impulses or moods as well as the propensity to suspend judgment
3. *Motivation*. A passion to work for reasons that go beyond money or status; a propensity to pursue goals with energy and commitment
4. *Empathy*. The ability to understand and accept the emotional makeup of other people
5. *Social skills*. Proficiency in handling relationships and building networks; an ability to find common ground

Source: Adapted from Goleman, D. (1998). *Working with emotional intelligence.* New York: Bantam Books.

EXAMINING THE EVIDENCE 3.1

Source: Carson, K. D., Carson, P. P., Fontenot, G., & Burdin, J. J. (2005, July–September). Selecting productive, emotionally mature, and helpful employees. *The Health Care Manager, 24*(3), 209–215.

The researchers in this study distributed questionnaires to 152 employees of a nursing department in a rural hospital in the southeastern part of the United States. The employees were supervisors, RNs, LPNs, CNAs, technicians, and unit clerks. Seventy-five employees returned usable questionnaires, for a response rate of 49.3%.

Findings included that organizational citizenship behavior is positively correlated with emotional intelligence. Thus, emotionally intelligent employees are also likely to exhibit organizational citizenship behaviors. Because the literature suggests that individuals with high organizational citizenship behaviors generally exceed formal role expectations and positively influence organization outcomes, the researchers concluded that managers should consider an applicant's intelligence, emotional intelligence, and organizational citizenship behaviors as hiring variables. The researchers then provided behavioral description questions that could be used in a structured interview format to ascertain these characteristics.

Reeves (2005) says that the self-regulation component of EI is what allows nurses to work in a nondisruptive, calm, and professional manner during chaotic situations—regardless of their internal emotions—and that this leads to a calm and stable work environment. Carson, Carson, Fontenot, and Burdin (2005) also suggest that employees with high EI display high levels of organizational citizenship as well, fostering a positive work environment and team building (Examining the Evidence 3.1).

LEARNING EXERCISE 3.3

Emotions and Decision Making

Think back on a recent decision you made that was more emotionally laden than usual. Were you self-aware about what emotions were influencing your thinking and how your emotions might have influenced the course(s) of action you chose? Were you able to objectively identify the emotions that others were experiencing and how these emotions may have influenced their actions?

Authentic Leadership

Another emerging leadership theory for the contemporary leader–manager's arsenal is that of authentic leadership. The concept of *authentic leadership* emerged in the late 1990s as a part of *positive organizational scholarship*, a broad field of scientific inquiry that emphasizes positive organizational phenomena leading to enhanced human well-being (Cameron, Dutton, & Quinn, 2003). Authentic leadership suggests that in order to lead, leaders must be true to themselves and their values and act accordingly. Stanley (2006) calls this phenomenon *congruent leadership* and defines it as "a match (congruence) between the activities, actions, and deeds of the leader and the leader's values, principles, and beliefs" (p. 132).

DISPLAY 3.3   Five Distinguishing Characteristics of the Authentic Leader

1. *Purpose*. Authentic leaders understand their own purposes and passions as a result of ongoing self-reflection and self-awareness.
2. *Values*. Authentic leaders link between purpose and passion by having congruence in beliefs and actions.
3. *Heart*. Authentic leaders care for themselves and the people they lead, and their compassion is genuine.
4. *Relationships*. Authentic leaders value building relationships and establishing connections with others, not to receive rewards but rather to strengthen the human connection.
5. *Self-discipline*. Authentic leaders practice self-discipline by incorporating balance into their personal and professional lives.

Source: Shirey, M. R. (2006b). Fostering leadership through collaboration. *Reflections on Nursing Leadership* (third quarter). Sigma Theta Tau International. Retrieved October 2, 2006, from *http://www. nursingsociety. org/RNL/3Q_2006/features/feature5.html*.

Shirey (2006b) calls authentic leadership a positive leadership style and suggests that it creates lasting value that allows organizations and individuals to thrive over time. She goes on to say that there are five distinguishing characteristics of authentic leaders: purpose, values, heart, relationships, and self-discipline. These characteristics are further delineated in Display 3.3.

It is important to remember that authentic or congruent leadership theory differs somewhat from more traditional transformational leadership theories, which suggest that the leader's vision or goals are often influenced by external forces and that there must be at least some "buy-in" of that vision by followers. In authentic leadership, it is the leaders' principles and their conviction to act accordingly that inspire followers. Thus, authentic followers realize their own true nature.

 In authentic leadership, it is the leaders' principles and their conviction to act accordingly that inspire followers.

Authentic leadership then "is based on a leader's personal credibility and integrity. . . . It is about where the leader stands, not where they are going" (Stanley, 2006, p. 138). Williams (2005) calls this willingness to stick with one's values and principles about work and people, despite pressure to deliver results, *transparent integrity*. Williams goes on to say that what "appears to reinforce and project integrity are high personal authenticity and strong awareness of self and others, which are consciously and consistently acted upon" (p. 3).

Rogers (2005) agrees, arguing that nurse–managers with integrity act in ways that are consistent with their stated values. It takes great courage to be true to one's convictions when external forces or peer pressure encourage us to do something that we feel morally would be inappropriate. There are many examples of leaders who preach one message and then act in a different manner.

LEARNING EXERCISE 3.4

Inconsistency in Word and Action

There are many examples of internationally or nationally recognized leaders who have lost their followers because of actions being inconsistent with personally stated convictions. An example might be a world-class athlete and advocate for healthy lifestyles who is found to be using steroids to enhance physical performance. Or it might be a political figure who preaches morality and becomes involved in an extramarital affair or a religious leader who promotes celibacy and then becomes involved in a sex scandal.

● ASSIGNMENT: Think of a leader who espoused one message and then acted in a different manner. How did it affect the leader's ability to be an effective leader? How did it change how you personally felt about that leader? Do you feel that leaders who have lost their "authenticity" can ever regain the trust of their followers?

In 2005, the American Association of Critical Care Nurses released a landmark publication specifying six standards necessary to establish and sustain healthy work environments in health care (Shirey, 2006a). Authentic leadership was one of these standards. This publication expanded the definition of authentic leadership and its attributes to include genuineness, trustworthiness, reliability, compassion, and believability and suggested that authentic leaders can create healthy work environments for practice by engaging employees.

In addition, Ilies, Morgeson, & Nahrgang (2005) developed a four-component model of authentic leadership comprising self-awareness, unbiased processing, authentic behavior/acting and authentic relational orientation. *Self-awareness* refers to one's awareness of, and trust in, one's motives, feelings, cognitions, strengths, and weaknesses as well as one's emotions and personality (Ilies et al., 2005). *Unbiased processing* refers to the objective processing of self-relevant information, such as private knowledge, internal experiences, and external information. It also means being able to accurately interpret task feedback and estimate personal skill level in specific areas (Ilies et al., 2005). *Authentic behavior/acting* refers to acting in accord with your beliefs, values, preferences, and needs. *Authentic relational orientation*, the fourth component of the model, "involves valuing and striving for achieving openness and truthfulness in relationships" (Ilies et al., p. 381).

Ilies and associates (2005) argue that there are many reasons why employees who work for authentic leaders are generally more satisfied and motivated. "First, authentic leaders provide an atmosphere conducive to the experience of positive emotions. Second, leaders can serve as a positive behavioral model for personally expressive and authentic behaviors. Third, leaders can support the self-determination of followers, in part by providing opportunities for skill development and autonomy. Finally, through a process of social exchange, leaders can influence and elevate followers" (p. 382). Similarly, Rogers (2005) argues that trust between nurse–managers and staff nurses is integral to the attainment of an organization's desired outcomes.

Thought Leadership

Another relatively new leadership theory to emerge in the 21st century is that of *thought leadership*, which applies to a person who is recognized among his or her peers for innovative ideas and who demonstrates the confidence to promote those ideas. Thus, thought leadership refers to any situation in which one individual convinces another to consider a new idea, product, or way of looking at things.

Thought leaders always challenge the status quo and attract followers not by any promise of representation or empowerment, but by their risk taking and vision in terms of being innovative.

To be recognized as a thought leader, McGinity (2006) suggests that individuals must choose ideas that make a significant difference versus those that have marginal impact. In addition, she suggests that important ideas that solve some existing problem in the organization or that support organizational goals will always be more valued than those that do not.

The concept may also be applied to organizations. Halladay (2005) agrees, arguing that thought leadership challenges, prods, and instigates as well as encourages contribution and differing perspectives. Halladay suggests that thought leadership is defined by most organizations as innovation and that most market leaders were first thought leaders. For example, Blue Cross and Blue Shield were early thought leaders in the development of private health insurance in the late 1920s. Bauer (2003) agrees, suggesting that:

> A thought leader is a recognized leader in one's field. What differentiates a thought leader from any other knowledgeable company is the *recognition* from the outside world that the company deeply understands its business, the needs of its customers, and the broader marketplace in which it operates (para 2).

White (2006) suggests that organization thought leaders early in the 21st century will be those that lead in identifying and adopting innovative safety and quality improvement approaches. This is at least in part due to the series of public reports issued by the Institute of Medicine in the late 1990s and early 21st century, including *To Err is Human* and *Crossing the Quality Chasm*, that suggested medical errors were a leading cause of death in this country and that changes in culture and systems would be required to address the problem.

LEARNING EXERCISE 3.5

Technological Innovation and Thought Leadership
Technological innovations continue to change the face of health care, and the pace of such innovations continues to increase exponentially. For example, wireless communication, computerized charting, and the barcode scanning of medications have all greatly affected the practice of nursing.

● ASSIGNMENT: Choose at least one of the following technological innovations, and write a one-page report on how this technology is expected to impact nursing and health care in the coming decade. See if you can identify the thought leader(s) credited with developing these technologies, and explore the process that they used to both develop and market their innovations.
- Biometrics to assure patient confidentiality
- Computerized physician order entry (CPOE)
- Point of care testing (POC)
- Bluetooth technology
- Electronic health records
- Nursebots (prototype nurse robots)

Quantum Leadership

Quantum leadership is another relatively new leadership theory that is being used by leader–managers to better understand dynamics of environments, such as health care. This theory, which emerged in the 1990s, builds upon transformational leadership and suggests that leaders must work together with subordinates to identify common goals, exploit opportunities, and empower staff to make decisions for organizational productivity to occur. This is especially true during periods of rapid change and needed transition.

Building on quantum physics, which suggests that reality is often discontinuous and deeply paradoxical, quantum leadership suggests that the environment and context in which people work is complex and dynamic and that this has a direct impact on organizational productivity.

 Quantum leadership suggests that the environment and context in which people work is complex and dynamic and that this has a direct impact on organizational productivity.

The theory also suggests that change is constant. Porter-O'Grady (2003) goes so far as to suggest that currently, there is no permanent point of respite from change. A highly fluid, flexible, and mobile environment, which is today's workplace, calls for an entirely innovative set of interactions and relationships as well as the leadership necessary to create them (Malloch & Porter-O'Grady, 2005). Because the health care industry is characterized by rapid change, there is great potential for intraorganizational conflict. Porter-O'Grady and Malloch (2003) suggest that the quantum leader is able to address the unsettled space between present and future and resolve these conflicts appropriately, creating a better healing environment for both the providers and consumers of health care. Porter-O'Grady (2003), building on the work of a 20th century physicist named Schrodinger, says that this is because there are two prevailing realities at any given time: the actual reality and a potential reality. The actual reality is what we perceive at a given moment. The potential reality is "current and present to us at any given moment, but while present, has not yet been experienced" (p. 59). Porter-O'Grady suggests that it is the leader's role to "engage unfolding reality in advance of others experiencing it; to see it, note its demands and implications, translate it for others, and then guide others into processes that will act in concert with the demands of a reality that is not yet present but inexorably and continually becoming" (pp. 59–60).

Cultural Bridging

The final emerging leadership theory to be presented in this chapter is that of *cultural bridging*. The new role of the leader–manager as a *cultural bridge* has become a requirement as our society becomes more diverse.

 As society becomes more diverse, a new role of the leader–manager as a cultural bridge has become a requirement.

Cook (2003) sees *diversity* as the differences among groups or between individuals. Diversity then acknowledges that not everyone is alike and that for understanding and growth to occur, it is imperative to acknowledge our differences (Cook, 2003).

Increasing ethnic diversity, both in the population as a whole and in the workforce, has resulted in an increased need for nurse–leaders and nurse–managers to be cultural bridges. Indeed, current demographic data shows that the U.S. population continues to diversify ethnically, with minority populations increasing at a faster rate than the white non-Hispanic population (Huston, 2006). This is also true in the nursing workforce itself with the increasing global migration of nurses and international recruitment to solve the current nursing shortage. Ryan (2003) suggests that foreign nurses must be introduced to American jargon and variations in nursing-practice delivery, as language is commonly a barrier. In addition, many foreign nurses must be supported through a period of cultural, professional, and psychological dissonance that is associated with anxiety, homesickness, and isolation. Finally, these nurses must be integrated within the institution so that they develop a sense of community life on the nursing unit. All of these needs can be met by the leader–manager who serves as a cultural bridge.

Finally, *generational diversity* is occurring in all health care organizations. The whole idea of age has become the latest diversity issue, taking its place beside gender, race, and color. "Just as individuals from diverse racial, ethnic, and gender backgrounds need to learn to respect and value differing perspectives and contributions, so do people from various generational cohorts" (Weston, 2006, para 1). With four generations working side by side in the nursing workforce, there has never been a greater need for generational team building and conflict resolution. Weston suggests that members of each generation still operate as if their values and expectations are universal. As a result, their unquestioned assumptions often result in generational misinterpretation. Few organizations, however, have directly confronted the implications of how to deal with this diversity or to examine the impacts that it has on the quality of care provided (Huston, 2006).

 Few organizations have directly confronted the implications of how to deal with generational diversity among the staff.

Weston (2006) suggests, then, that contemporary leader–managers must appreciate the diverse points of view, leverage the strengths, and value the differences in colleagues from various generations so that individuals can form creative, adaptable, and cohesive work groups.

TRANSITION FROM INDUSTRIAL AGE LEADERSHIP TO RELATIONSHIP AGE LEADERSHIP

In considering all of these emerging leadership theories, it becomes apparent that a paradigm shift is taking place early in the 21st century—a transition from *industrial age leadership* to *relationship age leadership* (Scott, 2006).

Scott contends that industrial age leadership focused primarily on traditional hierarchical management structures, skill acquisition, competition, and control. These are the same skills traditionally associated with management. Relationship age leadership focuses primarily on the relationship between the leader and his or her followers, on discerning common purpose, working together cooperatively, and seeking information rather than wealth (Table 3.1). Servant leadership, authentic leadership, human and social capital, emotional intelligence, and cultural bridging are all relationship-centered theories that address the complexity of the leader–follower relationship.

TABLE 3.1 Comparing Industrial and Relationship Age Leadership

	Industrial Age Leadership	Relationship Age Leadership
Skills	Technical skills	People skills
Authority	Command and control	Invitation and interdependence
Strategy	Gaining advantage	Discerning purpose
Methodology	Competition	Cooperation
Focus	Gathering facts	Finding meaning
Value	What you have (wealth)	What you know (information)
Structure	Hierarchy (top down)	Circular (egalitarian)
Meaning of leadership	Leadership: position	Leadership: trusteeship

Source: Adapted from Scott (2006). © KiThoughtBridge, LLC 2000. Author, Katherine Taylor Scott. All rights reserved. Permission for use in this publication granted by KiThoughtBridge.

Yet the leader–manager in contemporary health care organizations can and must not focus solely on relationship building. Assuring productivity and achieving desired outcomes are essential to organizational success. The key, then, likely lies in integrating the two paradigms. Scott (2006) suggests that such integration is possible (Fig. 3.1).

> A paradigm shift is taking place early in the 21st century—a transition from *industrial age leadership* to *relationship age leadership.*

Technical skills and competence seeking must be balanced with the adaptive skills of influencing followers and encouraging their abilities. Performance and results priorities must be balanced with authentic leadership and character. In other words, leader–managers must seek the same tenuous balance between leadership and management that has existed since time began.

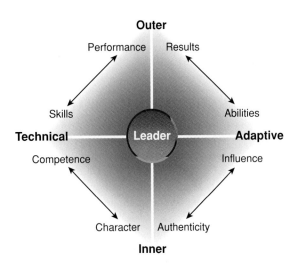

Figure 3.1 Integrated model of leadership. Reproduced with permission of KiThought-Bridge & Scott, K. T. (2006, September 29). *The gifts of leadership.* Keynote presented at the Sigma Theta Tau International Chapter Leader Academy, Indianapolis, IN.

LEARNING EXERCISE 3.6

Balancing the Focus Between Productivity and Relationships

You are a top-level nursing administrator in a large, urban medical center in California. As in many acute-care hospitals, your annual nursing turnover rate is more than 25%. At this point, you have many unfilled licensed nursing positions, and local recruitment efforts to fill these positions have been largely unsuccessful. The problem has been exacerbated by the recent passage of legislated minimum licensed staffing ratios in your state.

During a meeting with the CEO today, you are informed that the hospital vacancy rate for licensed nurses is expected to rise to 35% with the implementation of the new minimum staffing ratios in 3 months. The CEO states that you must reduce turnover or increase recruitment efforts immediately or the hospital will have to consider closing units or reducing available beds when the new ratios take effect.

You consider the following "industrial leadership" paradigm options:

1. You could aggressively recruit international nurses to solve at least the immediate staffing problem.
2. You could increase sign-on bonuses and offer other incentives for recruiting new nurses.
3. You could expand the job description for unlicensed assistive personnel and LVNs to relieve the RNs of some of their duties.
4. You could make newly recruited nurses sign a minimum 2-year contract upon hire.

You also consider the following "relationship leadership" paradigm options:

1. You could hold informal meetings with current staff to determine major variables affecting their current satisfaction levels and attempt to increase those variables that increase worker satisfaction.
2. You could develop an open-door policy in an effort to be more accessible to workers who wish to discuss concerns or issues about their work environment.
3. You could implement a shared governance model to increase worker participation in decision making on the units in which they work.
4. You could make daily rounds on all the units in an effort to get to know your nursing staff better on a one-to-one basis.

● ASSIGNMENT: Decide which of the options you would select. Rank order them in terms of what you would do first. Then look at your list. Did it reflect more of the industrial leadership paradigm or a relationship leadership paradigm? What inferences might you draw from your rank ordering in terms of your leadership skills? Do you think that your rank ordering might change with your age? Your experience?

LEADERSHIP AND MANAGEMENT FOR NURSING'S FUTURE

Seemingly insurmountable problems, a lack of resources to solve those problems, and individual apathy have been and will continue to be issues that contemporary leader–managers face. Effective leadership is absolutely critical to organizational success in the 21st century. Becoming a better leader–manager begins with a highly developed understanding of what leadership and management are and how these skills can be developed. The problem is that these skills are dynamic, and what we know and believe to be true about leadership and management changes constantly in response to new research and visionary thinking.

Contemporary leader–managers, then, are challenged not only to know and be able to apply classical leadership and management theory but also to keep abreast of new insights, new management decision-making tools, and new research in the field. It is more important than ever that leader–managers be able to integrate leadership roles and management functions and that some balance can be achieved between industrial age leadership and relationship age leadership skills. Leading and managing in the 21st century promises to be more complex than ever before, and leader–managers will be expected to have a greater skill set than ever before. The key to organizational success will likely be having enough highly qualified and visionary leader–managers to steer the course.

Key Concepts

* Many new leadership and management theories have emerged in the 21st century to explain the complexity of the leader–follower relationship and the environment in which work is accomplished and goals are achieved.
* *Servant leadership* is a contemporary leadership model that puts serving others as the first priority.
* Followers can and do influence leaders in both positive and negative ways.
* *Principal agent theory* suggests that followers may have an informational (expertise or knowledge) advantage over the leader as well as their own preferences, which may deviate from that of the principal. This may lead to a misalignment of goals.
* *Human capital* represents the capability of the individual. *Social capital* represents what a group can accomplish together.
* *Emotional intelligence* refers to the ability to use emotions effectively and is required by leader–managers in order to enhance their success.
* *Authentic leadership* suggests that in order to lead, leaders must be true to themselves and their values and act accordingly.
* *Thought leadership* refers to any situation whereby one individual convinces another to consider a new idea, product, or way of looking at things.
* *Thought leaders* attract followers not by any promise of representation or empowerment but by their risk taking and vision in terms of being innovative.
* *Quantum leadership* suggests that the environment and context in which people work is complex and dynamic and that this has a direct impact on organizational productivity.
* Leader–managers must adopt the role of *cultural bridge* in an increasingly diverse society and workplace.

ADDITIONAL LEARNING EXERCISES AND APPLICATIONS

LEARNING EXERCISE 3.7

Reflecting on Emotional Intelligence in Self
Do you feel that you have emotional intelligence? Do you express appropriate emotions such as empathy when taking care of patients? Are you able to identify and control your own emotions when you are in an emotionally charged situation?

● ASSIGNMENT: Describe a recent emotional experience. Write two to four paragraphs reporting on how you responded in this experience. Were you able to read the emotions of the other individuals involved? How did you respond, and were you later able to reflect on this incident?

LEARNING EXERCISE 3.8

Self-Regulation and Emotional Intelligence

You have just come from your 6-month performance evaluation as a new charge nurse. While your supervisor stated that he was very pleased in general with how you are performing in this new role, one area that he suggested you work on was to learn to be calmer in hectic clinical situations. He suggested that your anxiety could be transmitted to co-workers and subordinates who look to you to be their role model. He feels that you are especially anxious when staffing is short and that at times you vent your frustrations to your staff, which only adds to the general anxiety level on the unit.

● ASSIGNMENT: Create a specific plan of 6 to 10 things you can do to bolster your emotional intelligence in terms of self-regulation during stressful times.

LEARNING EXERCISE 3.9

Human and Social Capital

Examine the institution in which you work or go to school. Assess both the human capital and social capital present. Which is greater? Which do you believe contributes most to this institution in being able to accomplish its stated mission and goals?

Web Links

Williams, M. (2005). *Leadership for leaders*. London: Thorogood Publishers.
http://www.questia.com/PM.qst?a=o&d=110179030
This book, available online by Questia Media America Inc., explores relationships between leaders and followers in the 21st century and expounds upon contemporary leadership theories, including emotional intelligence and authentic leadership.

Center for Authentic Leadership
http://www.authenticleadership.com/
Founded in 1985 by Jan Smith, the Center for Authentic Leadership serves as a global leadership development community dedicated to self-discovery and to living life with profound meaning, purpose, passion, and fulfillment in a way that influences and inspires others to be their best.

How Important Is "Executive Intelligence" for Leaders?
http://hbswk.hbs.edu/item/5449.html
This article, authored by James Heskett in July 2006, defines executive intelligence and describes its role in leadership success.

Greenleaf Center for Servant-Leadership
http://www.greenleaf.org/
A nonprofit institution providing resources and opportunities to explore the principles and practices of servant leadership.

References

Bauer, E. (2003, November 10). *Be a thought leader!* Retrieved August 30, 2006, from *http://www.elise.com/web/a/ be_a_thought_leader.php.*

Cameron, K. S., Dutton, J. E., & Quinn, R. E. (2003). Foundations of positive organizational scholarship. In K. S. Cameron, J. E., Dutton, & R. E. Quinn (Eds.), *Positive organizational scholarship.* San Francisco: Berrett-Koehler.

Carson, K. D., Carson, P. P., Fontenot, G., & Burdin, J. J. (2005). Selecting productive, emotionally mature, and helpful employees. *The Health Care Manager, 24*(3), 209–215.

Cook, C. (2003, January 31). The many faces of diversity: Overview and summary. *Online Journal of Issues in Nursing, 8*(1). Retrieved July 7, 2004, from *http://www.nursingworld. org/ojin/topic20/tpc20ntr.htm.*

Flumerfelt, S. (2006, April). Understanding transformational leadership. *weLEAD Online Magazine.* Retrieved September 19, 2006, from *http://www.leadingtoday.org/Onmag/2006% 20Archives/april06/sf-april06.html.*

Goleman, D. (1998). *Working with emotional intelligence.* New York: Bantam Books.

Greenleaf, R. K. (1977). *Servant leadership: A journey in the nature of legitimate power and greatness.* New York: Paulist.

Halladay, H. (2005, October 24). *Thought leaders.* Leader Notes. Retrieved August 30, 2006, from *http://www.leadernotes.com/ topics/OpinionLeaders.html?gclid=CKCLsf2ViYcCFSk2GAod KXf_aA.*

Howatson-Jones, I. L. (2004). The servant leader. *Nursing Management UK, 11*(3), 20–24.

Huston, C. (2006). *Professional issues in nursing: Challenges and opportunities.* Philadelphia: Lippincott Williams &Wilkins.

Ilies, R., Morgeson, F. P., & Nahrgang, J. D. (2005). Authentic leadership and eudaemonic wellbeing: Understanding leader–follower outcomes. *Leadership Quarterly, 16,* 373–394.

Institute for Organizational Performance. (2006). *Emotional intelligence: At the heart of performance.* Retrieved August 8, 2006, from *http://www.eqperformance.com/pdf/EQ_ Business_Case.pdf.*

Jones, C. B. (2004). The costs of nurse turnover. Part 1: An economic perspective. *Journal of Nursing Administration, 34*(12), 562–570.

Lauder, W., Reel, S., Farmer, J., & Griggs, H. (2006). Social capital, rural nursing and rural nursing theory. *Nursing Inquiry, 13*(1), 73–79.

Malloch, K., & Porter-O'Grady, T. (2005). *The quantum leader: Applications for a new world of work.* Boston: Jones and Bartlett.

Mayer, J. D., & Salovey, P. (1997). What is emotional intelligence? In P. Salovey & D. Sluyter (Eds.), *Emotional development and emotional intelligence: Implications for educators* (pp. 3–31). New York: Basic Books.

McGinity, A. S. (2006). Turn new ideas into corporate visions. Executive extra. *Nursing Management, 37*(9), 50–52.

Offermann, L. R. (2004). When followers become toxic. *Harvard Business Review, 82*(1), 55–60.

Porter-O'Grady, T. (2003). Of hubris and hope. Transforming nursing for a new age. *Nursing Economics, 21*(2), 59–64.

Porter-O'Grady, T., & Malloch, K. (2003). *Quantum leadership: A textbook of new leadership.* Boston: Jones & Bartlett.

Rao, P. R. (2006). Emotional intelligence: The sine qua non for a clinical leadership toolbox. *Journal of Communication Disorders, 39*(4), 310–319.

Reeves, A. (2005). Emotional intelligence. *AOHN Journal, 53*(4), 172–176.

Rogers, L. G. (2005). Why trust matters. The nurse manager–staff nurse relationship. *Journal of Nursing Administration, 35*(10), 421–423.

Ryan, M. (2003). A buddy program for international nurses. *Journal of Nursing Administration, 33*(6), 350–352.

Santerre, R. E. (2004, September 16). *Testing for ownership mix efficiency: The case of the nursing home industry.* Retrieved September 20, 2006, from *http://www.business.uconn.edu/ healthcare/files/working-papers/Ownership%20Mix%20Efficiency.pdf.*

Salovey, P., & Mayer, J. D. (1990). Emotional intelligence. *Imagination, Cognition, and Personality, 9,* 185–211.

Scott, K. T. (2006, September 29). *The gifts of leadership.* Keynote presented at the Sigma Theta Tau International Chapter Leader Academy. Indianapolis, IN.

Shirey, M. R. (2006a). Authentic leaders creating healthy work environments for nursing practice. *American Journal of Critical Care, 15,* 256–267.

Shirey, M. R. (2006b). Promoting sustainability through collaboration. *Reflections on Nursing Leadership* (third quarter). Sigma Theta Tau International. Retrieved October 2, 2006, from *http://www.nursingsociety.org/RNL/3Q_2006/ features/feature5.html.*

Simon, M., & Norris, T. (2004–2005). *Social capital and the bottom line. Getting friendly with a key competitive advantage.* Workforce Engage. Retrieved September 21, 2006, from *http://www.workforceengage.com/social_capital. html.*

Six Seconds: The Emotional Intelligence Network. (2005). *Six Seconds' EQ model.* Retrieved August 8, 2006, from *http:// www.6seconds.org/modules.php?name=News&file=article&si d=2.*

Stanley, D. (2006). In command of care: Toward the theory of congruent leadership. *Journal of Research in Nursing, 11*(2),132–144.

Stuart, P. (2004, December). Emotional intelligence: Developing emotionally literate training in mental health. *Mental Health Practice, 8*(4), 12–15. Retrieved August 8, 2006, from *http://www.nursing-standard.co.uk/archives/mhp_pdfs/ mhpvol8-04/mhpv8n4p1215.pdf.*

Vitello-Cicciu, J. M. (2003). Exploring emotional intelligence. *Journal of Nursing Administration, 33(4),* 203–210.

Weston, M. J. (2006, May 31). Integrating generational perspectives in nursing. *The Online Journal of Issues in Nursing, 11*(2). Manuscript 1. Nursing World. Retrieved October 14, 2006, from *http://www.nursingworld.org/ojin/topic30/tpc30_1.htm.*

White, K. M. (2006). Be a best-in-class organization. *Nursing Management, 37*(9), 53–57.

Williams, M. (2005). *Leadership for leaders.* London: Thorogood Publishers. Retrieved September 21, 2006, from *http://www.questia.com/PM.qst?a=o&d=110179030.*

Bibliography

Avolio, B., & Gardner, W. L. (2005). Authentic leadership development. Getting to the root of positive forms of leadership. *The Leadership Quarterly, 16*(3), 315–338.

Barbuto, J. E., & Burbach, M. E. (2006). The emotional intelligence of transformational leaders: A field study of elected officials. *The Journal of Social Psychology, 146*(1), 51–64.

Bennis, W. G. (2004). The seven ages of the leader. *Harvard Business Review, 82*(1), 46–53.

Covey, S. R. (2004). *The 8th habit: From effectiveness to greatness.* New York: Free Press.

Dixon, D. L. (2005). Leadership: Servant leadership and more. *Caring for the Ages, 6*(12), 41–42.

Eagly, A. H. (2005). Achieving relational authenticity in leadership: Does gender matter? The Leadership Quarterly, 16(3), 459–474.

Ewing, B. (2006). A quantum leap for leadership. *Nursing Spectrum—New York and New Jersey Edition, 18A*(9), 15.

George, B. (2003). *Authentic leadership: Rediscovering the secrets to creating lasting value.* San Francisco: Jossey-Boss.

Layman, E. J. (2006). Coping with a turbulent health care environment: An integrative literature review. *Journal of Allied Health, 35*(1), 50–60.

Mattson, B., & Ludwig, G. (2005). Servant size . . . "Are you a servant leader?" (Leadership sector, June 2005 JEMS). *Journal of Emergency Medical Services, 30*(10), 14.

McCauley, K. (2005). President's note: All we needed was the glue. *AACN News, 22*(5), 2.

Michie, S., & Gooty, J. (2005). Values, emotions, and authenticity: Will the real leader please stand up? *The Leadership Quarterly, 16*(3), 441–457.

O'Dell, S. (2005). Thought leaders. Next-generation health plans: Managing the customer experience. *Health Management Technology, 26*(4), 47–48.

Schneider, H., & Mathios, A. (2006). Principal agency theory and health care utilization. *Economic Inquiry, 44,* 429–441.

Urch Druskat, V., Mount, G., & Sala, F. (2005). *Linking emotional intelligence and performance at work.* New Jersey: Lawrence Erlbaum Associates.

4

Ethical Issues

. . . when organizations and their leaders become fixated on the bottom line and ignore values, an environment conducive to ethics failure is nurtured.

—*J. G. Bruhn*

Unit II examines ethical, legal, and legislative issues affecting leadership and management as well as professional advocacy. This chapter focuses on applied ethical decision making as a critical leadership role for mangers. Chapter 5 examines the impact of legislation and the law on leadership and management, and Chapter 6 focuses on advocacy for patients and subordinates and for the nursing profession in general.

Ethics is the systematic study of what a person's conduct and actions should be with regard to self, other human beings, and the environment; it is the justification of what is right or good and the study of what a person's life and relationships should be, not necessarily what they are. Ethics is a system of moral conduct and principles that guide a person's actions in regard to right and wrong and in regard to oneself and society at large.

 Ethics is the systematic study of what a person's conduct and actions should be with regard to self, other humans, and the environment.

Applied ethics requires application of normative ethical theory to everyday problems. The normative ethical theory for each profession arises from the purpose of the profession. The values and norms of the nursing profession, therefore, provide the foundation and filter from which ethical decisions are made. The nurse–manager, however, has a different ethical responsibility than the clinical nurse and does not have as clearly defined a foundation to use as a base for ethical reasoning.

Because management is a discipline and not a profession, it does not have a defined purpose, such as medicine or the law; therefore, it lacks a specific set of norms to guide ethical decision

69

making. Instead, the organization reflects norms and values to the manager, and the personal values of managers are reflected through the organization. The manager's ethical obligation is tied to the organization's purpose, and the purpose of the organization is linked to the function that it fills in society and the constraints society places on it. So, the responsibilities of the nurse–manager emerge from a complex set of interactions. Society helps to define the purposes of various institutions, and the purposes, in turn, help to ensure that the institution fulfills specific functions. However, the specific values and norms in any particular institution determine the focus of its resources and shape its organizational life. The values of people within institutions influence actual management practice. In reviewing this set of complex interactions, it becomes evident that arriving at appropriate ethical management decisions is a difficult task.

Not only are nursing management ethics distinct from clinical nursing ethics, they are also distinct from other areas of management. Although there are many similar areas of responsibility between nurse–managers and non-nurse–managers, many leadership roles and management functions are specific to nursing. These differences require the nurse–manager to deal with unique obligations and ethical dilemmas that are not encountered in non-nursing management.

In addition, because personal, organizational, subordinate, and consumer responsibilities differ, there is great potential for nursing managers to experience intrapersonal conflict about the appropriate course of action. Bruhn (2005) maintains that frequently, ethics failures in organizations have been focused on leaders within that organization but that in reality it is the interaction of the culture of the organization and the character of the leader that creates ethical failure.

Multiple advocacy roles and accountability to the profession further increase the likelihood that all nurse–managers will be faced with ethical dilemmas in their practice. Nurses often find themselves viewed simultaneously as advocates for physicians, patients, and the organization—all of whose needs and goals may be dissimilar.

 Nurses are often placed in situations where they are expected to be agents for patients, physicians, and the organization simultaneously, all of which may have conflicting needs, wants, and goals.

To make appropriate ethical decisions, the manager must have knowledge of ethical principles and frameworks, use a professional approach that eliminates trial and error and focuses on proven decision-making models, and use available organizational processes to assist in making such decisions. Such organizational processes include institutional review boards, ethics committees, and professional codes of ethics. Using both a systematic approach and proven ethical tools and technology allows managers to make better decisions and increases the probability that they will feel confident about the decisions they have made. Leadership roles and management functions involved in management ethics are shown in Display 4.1.

TYPES OF ETHICAL ISSUES

In a review of nursing literature, Laabs (2005) found that there were many terms used to describe moral issues faced by nurses. The first of these, *moral uncertainty*, occurs when an individual is unsure which moral principles or values apply and may even include uncertainty as to what the moral problem is. This is also sometimes referred to as *moral conflict*, "when the duties and

DISPLAY 4.1 Leadership Roles and Management Functions Associated With Ethics

Leadership Roles

1. Is self-aware regarding own values and basic beliefs about the rights, duties, and goals of human beings
2. Accepts that some ambiguity and uncertainty must be a part of all ethical decision making
3. Accepts that negative outcomes occur in ethical decision making despite high-quality problem solving and decision making
4. Demonstrates risk taking in ethical decision making
5. Role models ethical decision making, which is congruent with the American Nurses Association Code of Ethics and Interpretive Statements and professional standards
6. Clearly communicates expected ethical standards of behavior

Management Functions

1. Uses a systematic approach to problem solving and decision making when faced with management problems with ethical ramifications
2. Identifies outcomes in ethical decision making that should always be sought or avoided
3. Uses established ethical frameworks to clarify values and beliefs
4. Applies principles of ethical reasoning to define what beliefs or values form the basis for decision making
5. Is aware of legal precedents that may guide ethical decision making and is accountable for possible liabilities should they go against the legal precedent
6. Continually reevaluates the quality of own ethical decision making, based on the process of decision making or problem solving used
7. Recognizes and rewards ethical conduct of subordinates
8. Takes appropriate action when subordinates use unethical conduct

obligations of health care providers or general guiding ethical principles are unclear" (Jormsri, 2004, p. 217).

On the other hand, *moral distress* is the result of the individual knowing the right thing to do but organizational constraints make it difficult to take the right course of action. *Moral outrage* occurs when an individual witnesses the immoral act of another but feels powerless to stop it. Last, the most difficult of all moral issues is termed a *moral* or *ethical dilemma* and occurs when two (or more) clear moral principles apply but they support inconsistent courses of action (Laabs, 2005). An ethical dilemma may also be described as choosing between two or more undesirable alternatives and attempting to select the least damaging from the choices available. In research examining moral problems, Laabs found that moral dilemmas created the most distress for nurse practitioners (Examining the Evidence 4.1).

In discussing such complex ethical decision making, Wueste (2005) states that "our task as ethical decision makers is to identify the best answer from among the available alternatives and to see to it that we are in a position to meet the challenge of justifying our ethical judgments" (p. 79). Because ethical dilemmas are so difficult to resolve, many of the learning exercises in this chapter are devoted to solving this type of moral issue.

EXAMINING THE EVIDENCE 4.1

Source: Laabs, C. A. (2005, February). Moral problems and distress among nurse practitioners in primary care. *Journal of the American Academy of Nurse Practitoners, 17*(2), 76–84.

The data source for this study was a convenience sample of 71 nurse practitioners (NPs). The descriptive study identified a number of ethical issues that NPs encountered in primary care. The issue encountered most frequently was patient refusal of appropriate treatment. Distress was reported most often over problems of moral dilemma, followed by moral distress, and least often, moral uncertainty and moral outrage. Conflict between patient autonomy and NP beneficence occurred most often as a moral dilemma. NPs reported encountering fewer ethical issues than a review of the literature would suggest. However, some NPs felt frustrated and powerless due to moral problems encountered in their practice.

> Individual values, beliefs, and personal philosophy play a major role in the moral or ethical decision making that is part of the daily routine of all managers.

How do managers decide what is right and what is wrong? What does the manager do if no right or wrong answer exists? What if all solutions generated seem to be wrong? Remember that the way managers approach and solve ethical issues is influenced by their values and basic beliefs about the rights, duties, and goals of all human beings. Self-awareness, then, is a vital leadership role in ethical decision making, just as it is in so many other aspects of management.

No rules, guidelines, or theories exist that cover all aspects of the ethical problems that managers face. However, it is the manager's responsibility to understand the ethical problem-solving process, to be familiar with ethical frameworks and principles, and to know ethical professional codes. It is these tools that will assist managers in effective problem solving and prevent ethical failure within their organization. Critical thinking occurs when managers are able to engage in an orderly process of ethical problem solving to determine the rightness or wrongness of courses of action.

ETHICAL FRAMEWORKS FOR DECISION MAKING

Ethical frameworks guide individuals in solving ethical dilemmas. These frameworks do not solve the ethical problem but assist the manager in clarifying personal values and beliefs. Four of the most commonly used ethical frameworks are utilitarianism, duty-based reasoning, rights-based reasoning, and intuitionism (Table 4.1).

The *teleological* theory of ethics is also called *utilitarianism* or *consequentialist* theory and consists of judging whether the consequences of an action are good or bad (Aita & Richer, 2005). Using an ethical framework of utilitarianism encourages the manager to make decisions based on what provides the greatest good for the greatest number of people. In doing so, the needs and wants of the individual are diminished. Utilitarianism also suggests that the end can justify the means. For example, a manager using a utilitarian approach might decide to use travel budget money to send many staff to local workshops rather than to fund one or two people to attend a

TABLE 4.1   **Ethical Frameworks**

Framework	Basic Premise
Utilitarian (teleological)	Provide the greatest good for the greatest number of people
Rights based (deontological)	Individuals have basic inherent rights that should not be interfered with
Duty based (deontological)	A duty to do something or to refrain from doing something
Intuitionist (deontological)	Each case weighed on a case-by-case basis to determine relative goals, duties, and rights

national conference. Another example would be an insurance program that meets the needs of many but refuses coverage for expensive organ transplants. In Learning Exercise 4.5, the organization uses utilitarianism to justify lying to employee applicants because their hiring would result in good for many employees by keeping several units in the hospital open.

Deontological ethical theory judges whether the action is right or wrong regardless of the consequences and is based on the philosophy of Emanuel Kant in the 18th century (Wueste, 2005). Primarily, this theory uses both *duty-based reasoning* and *rights-based reasoning* as the basis for its philosophy. Duty-based reasoning is an ethical framework stating that some decisions must be made because there is a duty to do something or to refrain from doing something. In Learning Exercise 4.5, the supervisor feels a duty to hire the most qualified person for the job, even if the personal cost is high.

Rights-based reasoning is based on the belief that some things are a person's just due (i.e., each individual has basic claims, or entitlements, with which there should be no interference). Rights are different from needs, wants, or desires. The supervisor in Learning Exercise 4.4 believes that both applicants have the right to fair and impartial consideration of their application. In Learning Exercise 4.5, Sam believes that all people have the right to truth and, in fact, that he has the duty to be truthful. The *intuitionist framework* allows the decision maker to review each ethical problem or issue on a case-by-case basis, comparing the relative weights of goals, duties, and rights. This weighting is determined primarily by intuition—what the decision maker believes is right for that particular situation. Recently, some ethical theorists have begun questioning the appropriateness of intuitionism as an ethical decision-making framework because of the potential for subjectivity and bias. All of the cases solved in this chapter involve some degree of decision making by intuition.

Other more recent theories of ethical philosophy include *ethical relativism* and *ethical universalism* (Aita & Richer, 2005). Ethical relativism is the belief that a specific culture's ethical principles cannot be generalized to individuals who do not share that culture. Conversely, the belief in universalism holds that ethical principles are universal and can be used to justify ethical decisions in all cultures.

PRINCIPLES OF ETHICAL REASONING

Both teleological and deontological theorists have developed a group of moral principles that are used for ethical reasoning. These principles of ethical reasoning further explore and define what beliefs or values form the basis for decision making. Respect for people is the most basic and

DISPLAY 4.2 Ethical Principles

Autonomy: Promotes self-determination and freedom of choice
Beneficence: Actions are taken in an effort to promote good
Nonmaleficence: Actions are taken in an effort to avoid harm
Paternalism: One individual assumes the right to make decisions for another
Utility: The good of the many outweighs the wants or needs of the individual
Justice: Seek fairness; treat "equals" equally and treat "unequals" according to their differences
Veracity: Obligation to tell the truth
Fidelity: Need to keep promises
Confidentiality: Keep privileged information private

universal ethical principle. The major ethical principles stemming from this basic principle are discussed in Display 4.2.

The most fundamental universal principle is respect for people.

Autonomy (Self-Determination)

A form of personal liberty, *autonomy* also is called freedom of choice or accepting the responsibility for one's choice. The legal right of self-determination supports this moral principle. The use of progressive discipline recognizes the autonomy of the employee. The employee, in essence, has the choice to meet organizational expectations or to be disciplined further. If the employee's continued behavior warrants termination, the principle of autonomy says that the employee has made the choice to be terminated by virtue of his or her actions, not by that of the manager.

Aita and Richer (2005) maintain that "this principle protects the ability of human beings to choose for themselves and determine their own course in life" (p. 121). Therefore, nurse–managers must be cognizant of the ethical component present whenever an individual's decisional capacity is in question. To take away a person's right to self-determination is a serious but sometimes necessary action.

Beneficence (Doing Good)

This principle states that the actions one takes should be done in an effort to promote good. The concept of *nonmaleficence*, which is associated with *beneficence*, says that if one cannot do good, then one should at least do no harm. For example, if a manager uses this ethical principle in planning performance appraisals, he or she is much more likely to view the performance appraisal as a means of promoting employee growth.

Aita and Richer (2005) state that beneficence and nonmaleficence rest in the ethical theory of utilitarianism. They maintain that an example of both principles can be represented in patient consent forms. That is, a consent form often shows benefits and risks with the underlying assumption that some harm is often considered unavoidable.

Paternalism

This principle is related to beneficence in that one person assumes the authority to make a decision for another. Because *paternalism* limits freedom of choice, most ethical theorists believe that paternalism is justified only to prevent a person from coming to harm. Unfortunately, some managers use the principle of paternalism in subordinates' career planning. In doing so, managers assume that they have greater knowledge of what an employee's short- and long-term goals should be than the employee does.

Utility

This principle reflects a belief in utilitarianism—what is best for the common good outweighs what is best for the individual. Utility justifies paternalism as a means of restricting individual freedom. Managers who use the principle of utility need to be careful not to become so focused on production that they become less humanistic.

Justice (Treating People Fairly)

This principle states that equals should be treated equally and that unequals should be treated according to their differences. This principle is frequently applied when there are scarcities or competition for resources or benefits. The manager who uses the principle of *justice* will work to see that pay raises reflect performance and not just time of service.

LEARNING EXERCISE 4.1

Are Some More Equal Than Others
Research suggests that individuals with health insurance in this country have better access to health care services and better health care outcomes than those who do not. This does not mean, however, that all individuals with health insurance receive "equal treatment." Medicaid recipients (the financially indigent) often complain that while they have public insurance, many private providers refuse to accept them as patients. Patients enrolled in managed care suggest that their treatment options are more limited than traditional private insurance because of the use of gatekeepers, required authorizations, and queuing. Even individuals with private insurance suggest that co-payments and out-of-pocket costs for deductibles place the cost of care beyond the reach of many.

● ASSIGNMENT: Using the ethical principle of justice, determine whether health care in this country should be a right or a privilege. Are the uninsured and the insured "unequals" that should be treated according to their differences? Does the type of health insurance that one has also create a system of "unequals"? If so, are the unequals being treated according to their differences?

Veracity (Truth Telling)

This principle is used to explain how people feel about the need for truth telling or the acceptability of deception. A manager who believes that deception is morally acceptable if it is done with the objective of beneficence may tell all rejected job applicants that they were highly considered whether they had been or not.

Fidelity (Keeping Promises)

Fidelity refers to the moral obligation that individuals should be faithful to their commitments and promises. Breaking a promise is believed by many ethicists to be wrong regardless of the consequences. In other words, even if there were no far-reaching negative results of the broken promise, it is still wrong because it would render the making of any promise meaningless. However, there are times when keeping a promise (fidelity) may not be in the best interest of the other party, as discussed below under confidentiality. Although nurses have multiple fidelity duties (patient, physician, organization, profession, and self) that at times may be in conflict, the American Nurses Association (ANA) Code of Ethics is clear that the nurse's primary commitment is to the patient (ANA, 2001).

Confidentiality (Respecting Privileged Information)

The obligation to observe the privacy of another and to hold certain information in strict confidence is a basic ethical principle and a foundation of both medical and nursing ethics. However, as in deception, there are times when the presumption against disclosing information must be overridden. For example, health care managers are required by law to report certain cases, such as drug abuse in employees, elder abuse, and child abuse.

LEARNING EXERCISE 4.2

Family Values

You are the evening-shift charge nurse of the recovery room. You have just admitted a 32-year-old woman who 2 hours ago was thrown from a Jeep in which she was a passenger. She was rushed to the emergency room and subsequently to surgery, where cranial burr holes were completed and an intracranial monitor was placed. No further cranial exploration was attempted because the patient sustained extensive and massive neurologic damage. She will probably not survive your shift. The plan is to hold her in recovery for 1 hour and, if she is still alive, transfer her to the intensive care unit.

Shortly after receiving the patient in the recovery room, you are approached by the evening house supervisor, who says that the patient's sister is pleading to be allowed into the recovery room. Normally, visitors are never allowed in the recovery room but occasionally exceptions are made. Tonight, the recovery room is empty except for this patient. You decide to bend the rules and allow the young woman's sister into the recovery room. The visiting sister is near collapse; it is obvious that she had been the driver of the Jeep. As the visitor continues to speak to the comatose patient, her behavior and words make you begin to wonder if she is indeed the sister.

Within 15 minutes, the house supervisor returns and states, "I have made a terrible mistake. The patient's family just arrived, and they say that the visitor we just allowed into the recovery room is not a member of the family but is the patient's lover. They are very angry and demand that this woman not be allowed to see the patient."

You approach the visitor and confront her in a kindly manner regarding the information that you have just received. She looks at you with tears streaming down her face and says, "Yes, it is true. Mary and I have been together for 6 years. Her family disowned her because of it, but we were everything to each other. She has been my life, and I have been hers. Please, please let me stay. I will never see her again. I know the family will not allow me to attend the funeral. I need to say my goodbyes. Please let me stay. It is not fair that they have the legal right to be family when I have been the one to love and care for Mary."

● ASSIGNMENT: You must decide what to do. Recognize that your own value system will play a part in your decision. List several alternatives that are available to you. Identify which ethical frameworks or principles most affected your decision making.

AMERICAN NURSES ASSOCIATION CODE OF ETHICS AND PROFESSIONAL STANDARDS

Another tool that managers can use for guidance in ethical problem solving is a *professional code of ethics*. A code of ethics is a set of principles, established by a profession, to guide the individual practitioner. The first code of ethics for nurses was adopted by the ANA in 1950 and has been revised five times since then.

The most recent revision, the 2001 Code of Ethics for Nurses, departs from previous versions in several important ways. The newest code returns to the use of the term *patient* rather than *client*, as *patient* more accurately reflects what the majority of nurses do—care for individuals with health problems. The code also explicitly details that the nurse's most fundamental accountability is to the patient, whether an individual, family, group, or community (No. 2). The 2001 code also addresses the responsibility of the nurse for assuring that the work environment is safe, even in an era of cutting costs and reduced revenues (No. 6). Finally, there is a new provision (No. 5) that addresses duties of nurses to themselves.

Although the Code of Ethics for Nurses consists of nine provisions and interpretive statements, Wueste (2005) states that three of them serve especially well in guiding a nurse's actions in ethical matters: "(1) subscribing to ethical theories; (2) adhering to ethical principles and (3) cultivating virtues" (p. 70). Professional codes of ethics do not have the power of law. They do, however, function as a guide to the highest ethical practice standards for nurses. The ANA Code of Ethics for Nurses (2001) is shown in Display 4.3.

> **Professional codes of ethics function as a guide to the highest standards of ethical practice for nurses.**

Another document that may be helpful specifically to the nurse–manager in creating and maintaining an ethical work environment is *The Scope and Standards for Nurse Administrators*. These standards are also used as the baseline for determining eligibility for magnet status for acute-care hospitals (Chapter 12). *The Scope and Standards for Nurse Administrators*, revised in 2004, specifically delineates professional standards in management ethics, and these appear in Display 4.4.

ETHICAL PROBLEM SOLVING AND DECISION MAKING

Ethical concepts and their utility in clinical practice must be taught along with the problem-solving skills that are a part of all decision making. Much of the difficulty that people have in making ethical decisions can be attributed to a lack of formal education about problem solving.

Because problem solving and decision making were discussed in Chapter 1, only a brief review is included here. Trial-and-error decision making helps some managers learn to make good decisions, but much is left to chance. The cost of poor ethical decisions is measured in terms of human and fiscal resources.

Another error made by managers in ethical problem solving is using the outcome of the decision as the sole basis for determining the quality of the decision making. Although decision

DISPLAY 4.3 American Nurses Association Code of Ethics for Nurses

The ANA House of Delegates approved these nine provisions of the new *Code of Ethics for Nurses* at its June 30, 2001, meeting in Washington, DC. In July 2001, the Congress of Nursing Practice and Economics voted to accept the new language of the interpretive statements resulting in a fully approved revised *Code of Ethics for Nurses with Interpretive Statements*.

1. The nurse, in all professional relationships, practices with compassion and respect for the inherent dignity, worth, and uniqueness of every individual, unrestricted by considerations of social or economic status, personal attributes, or the nature of health problems.
2. The nurse's primary commitment is to the patient, whether an individual, family, group, or community.
3. The nurse promotes, advocates for, and strives to protect the health, safety, and rights of the patient.
4. The nurse is responsible and accountable for individual nursing practice and determines the appropriate delegation of tasks consistent with the nurse's obligation to provide optimum patient care.
5. The nurse owes the same duties to self as to others, including the responsibility to preserve integrity and safety, to maintain competence, and to continue personal and professional growth.
6. The nurse participates in establishing, maintaining, and improving health care environments and conditions of employment conducive to the provision of quality health care and consistent with the values of the profession through individual and collective action.
7. The nurse participates in the advancement of the profession through contributions to practice, education, administration, and knowledge development.
8. The nurse collaborates with other health professionals and the public in promoting community, national, and international efforts to meet health needs.
9. The profession of nursing, as represented by associations and their members, is responsible for articulating nursing values, for maintaining the integrity of the profession and its practice, and for shaping social policy.

makers should be able to identify desirable and undesirable outcomes, outcomes alone cannot be used to assess the quality of the problem solving. Many variables affect outcome, and some of these are beyond the control or foresight of the problem solver. Even the most ethical courses of action can have undesirable and unavoidable consequences. The quality of ethical problem solving should be evaluated in terms of the process used to make the decision. The best possible decisions stem from structured problem solving, adequate data collection, and examination of multiple alternatives—even if outcomes are poor.

 If a structured approach to problem solving is used, data gathering is adequate, and multiple alternatives are analyzed, even with a poor outcome, the manager should accept that the best possible decision was made at that time with the information and resources available.

DISPLAY 4.4   Standards of Practice for Nurse Administrators

Standard 11. Ethics

The nurse administrator's decisions and actions are based on ethical principles.

Measurement Criteria

1. Advocates on behalf of recipients of services and personnel
2. Maintains privacy, confidentiality, and security of patient/client/resident, staff, and organization data
3. Adheres to the Code of Ethics for Nurses with Interpretive Statements (ANA, 2001)
4. Assures compliance with regulatory and professional standards as well as integrity in business practices
5. Fosters a nondiscriminatory climate in which care is delivered in a manner sensitive to sociocultural diversity
6. Assures a process to identify and address ethical issues within nursing and the organization

Source: American Nurses Association. (2004). *Scope and standards for nurse administrators* (2nd ed.). Washington, DC: American Nurses Publishing.

The Traditional Problem-Solving Process

Although not recognized specifically as an ethical problem-solving model, one of the oldest and most frequently used tools for problem solving is the traditional problem-solving process. This process, which was discussed in Chapter 1, consists of seven steps, with the actual decision being made at step five (review the seven steps under "Traditional Problem-Solving Process" in Chapter 1). Although many individuals use at least some of these steps in their decision making, they frequently fail to generate an adequate number of alternatives or to evaluate the results—two essential steps in the process.

LEARNING EXERCISE 4.3

A Nagging Uneasiness

You are a nurse on a pediatric unit. One of your patients is a 15-month-old girl with a diagnosis of failure to thrive. The mother says that the child is emotional, cries a lot, and does not like to be held. You have been taking care of the infant for 2 days since her admission, and she has smiled and laughed and held out her arms to everyone. She has eaten well. There is something about the child's reaction to the mother's boyfriend that bothers you. The child appears to draw away from him when he visits. The mother is very young and seems to be rather immature but appears to care for the child.

This is the second hospital admission for this child. Although you were not on duty for the first admission 6 weeks ago, you check the records and see that the child was admitted with the same diagnosis. While you are on duty today, the child's father calls and inquires about her condition. He lives several hundred miles away and requests that the child be hospitalized until

(Learning Exercise continues on page 80)

the weekend (it is Wednesday) so that he can "check things out." He tells you that he believes the child is mistreated. He says he also is concerned about his ex-wife's 4-year-old child from another marriage and is attempting to gain custody of that child in addition to his own child. From what little the father said, you are aware that the divorce was bitter and that the mother has full custody.

You talk with the physician at length. He says that after the last hospitalization, he requested that the community health agency and Child Protective Services call on the family. Their subsequent report to him was that the 4 year old appeared happy and well and that the 15 month old appeared clean, although underweight. There was no evidence to suggest child abuse. However, the community health agency plans to continue following the children. He says that the mother has been good about keeping doctor appointments and has kept the children's immunizations up to date. The pediatrician proceeds to write an order for discharge. He says that although he also feels somewhat uneasy, continued hospitalization is not justified, and the state medical aid will not pay for additional days.

When the mother and her boyfriend come to take the baby home, the baby clings to you and refuses to go to the boyfriend. She also seems reluctant to go to the mother. All during the discharge, you are extremely uneasy. When you see the car drive away, you feel very sad.

After returning to the unit, you talk with your supervisor, who listens carefully and questions you at length. Finally, she says, "It seems as if you have nothing concrete on which to act and are only experiencing feelings. I think you would be risking a lot of trouble for yourself and the hospital if you acted rashly at this time. Accusing people with no evidence and making them go through a traumatic experience is something I would hesitate to do."

You leave the supervisor's office still troubled. She did not tell you that you must do nothing, but you believe that she would disapprove of further action on your part. The doctor also felt strongly that there was no reason to do more than was already being done. The child will be followed by community health nurses. Perhaps the ex-husband was just trying to make trouble for his ex-wife and her new boyfriend. You would certainly not want anyone to have reported you or created problems regarding your own children. You remember how often your 5 year old bruised himself when he was that age. He often looked like an abused child. You go about your duties and try to shake off your feeling. What should you do?

● ASSIGNMENT:
1. Solve the case in small groups by using the traditional problem-solving process. Identify the problem and several alternative solutions to solving this ethical dilemma. What should you do and why? What are the risks? How does your value system play a part in your decision? Justify your solution. After completing this assignment, solve Part 2.
2. Assume that this was a real case. Twenty-four hours after the child's discharge, she is readmitted with critical head trauma. Police reports indicate that the child suffered multiple skull fractures after being thrown up against the wall by her mother's boyfriend. The child is not expected to live. Does knowing the outcome change how you would have solved the case? Does the outcome influence how you feel about the quality of your group's problem solving?

The Nursing Process

Another problem-solving model not specifically designed for ethical analysis but appropriate for it is the nursing process. Most nurses are aware of the nursing process and the cyclic nature of its components of assessment, diagnosis, planning, implementation, and evaluation (see Fig. 1.2). However, most nurses do not recognize its use as a decision-making tool. The cyclic nature of the process allows for feedback to occur at any step. It also allows the cycle to repeat until adequate information is gathered to make a decision. It does not, however, require clear problem identification. Learning Exercise 4.4 shows how the nursing process might be used as an ethical decision-making tool.

LEARNING EXERCISE 4.4

One Applicant Too Many

The reorganization of the public health agency has resulted in the creation of a new position of community health liaison. A job description has been written, and the job opening has been posted. As the chief nursing executive of this agency, it will be your responsibility to select the best person for the position. Because you are aware that all hiring decisions have some subjectivity, you want to eliminate as much personal bias as possible. Two people have applied for the position; one of them is a close personal friend.

Analysis

Assess: As the nursing executive, you have a responsibility to make personnel decisions as objectively as you can. This means that the hiring decision should be based solely on which employee is best qualified for the position. You do recognize, however, that there may be a personal cost in terms of the friendship.

Diagnose: You diagnose this problem as a potential intrapersonal conflict between your obligation to your friend and your obligation to your employer.

Plan: You must plan how you are going to collect your data. The tools you have selected are applications, résumés, references, and personal interviews.

Implement: Both applicants are contacted and asked to submit résumés and three letters of reference from recent employers. In addition, both are scheduled for structured formal interviews with you and two of the board members of the agency. Although the board members will provide feedback, you have reserved the right to make the final hiring decision.

Evaluate: As a result of your plan, you have discovered that both candidates meet the minimal job requirements. One candidate, however, clearly has higher-level communication skills, and the other candidate (your friend) has more experience in public health and is more knowledgeable regarding the resources in your community. Both employees have complied with the request to submit résumés and letters of reference; they are of similar quality.

Assess: Your assessment of the situation is that you need more information to make the best possible decision. You must assess whether strong communication skills or public health experience and familiarity with the community would be more valuable in this position.

Plan: You plan how you can gather more information about what the employee will be doing in this newly created position.

Implement: If the job description is inadequate in providing this information, it may be necessary to gather information from other public health agencies with a similar job classification.

Evaluate: You now believe that excellent communication skills are essential for the job. The candidate who had these skills has an acceptable level of public health experience and seems

(Learning Exercise continues on page 82)

motivated to learn more about the community and its resources. This means that your friend will not receive the job.

Assess: Now you must assess whether a good decision has been made.

Plan: You plan to evaluate your decision in 6 months, basing your criteria on the established job description.

Implement: You are unable to implement your plan because this employee resigns unexpectedly 4 months after she takes the position. Your friend is now working in a similar capacity in another state. Although you correspond infrequently, the relationship has changed as a result of your decision.

Evaluate: Did you make a good decision? This decision was based on a carefully thought-out process, which included adequate data gathering and a weighing of alternatives. Variables beyond your control resulted in the employee's resignation, and there was no apparent reason for you to suspect that this would happen. The decision to exclude or minimize personal bias was a conscious one, and you were aware of the possible ramifications of this choice. The decision making appears to have been appropriate.

The MORAL Decision-Making Model

Crisham (1985) developed a model for ethical decision making incorporating the nursing process and principles of biomedical ethics. This model is especially useful in clarifying ethical problems that result from conflicting obligations. This model is represented by the mnemonic MORAL:

Massage the dilemma. Collect data about the ethical problem and who should be involved in the decision-making process.

Outline options. Identify alternatives, and analyze the causes and consequences of each.

Review criteria and resolve. Weigh the options against the values of those involved in the decision. This may be done through a weighting or grid.

Affirm position and act. Develop the implementation strategy.

Look back. Evaluate the decision making.

Learning Exercise 4.5 demonstates the MORAL modeling in solving an ethical issue.

LEARNING EXERCISE 4.5

Little White Lies

Sam is the nurse recruiter for a metropolitan hospital that is experiencing an acute nursing shortage. He has been told to do or say whatever is necessary to recruit professional nurses so that the hospital will not have to close several units. He also has been told that his position will be eliminated if he does not produce a substantial number of applicants in the nursing career days to be held the following week. Sam loves his job and is the sole provider for his family. Because many organizations are experiencing severe personnel shortages, the competition for employees is keen. After his third career day without a single prospective applicant, he begins to feel desperate. On the fourth and final day, Sam begins making many promises to potential applicants regarding shift preference, unit preference, salary, and advancement that he is not sure he can keep. At the end of the day, Sam has a lengthy list of interested applicants but also feels a great deal of intrapersonal conflict.

Massage the Dilemma

In a desperate effort to save his job, Sam finds he has taken action that has resulted in high intrapersonal value conflict. Sam must choose between making promises he cannot keep and losing his job. This has far-reaching consequences for all involved. Sam has the ultimate responsibility for knowing his values and acting in a manner that is congruent with his value system. The organization is, however, involved in the value conflict in that its values and expectations conflict with those of Sam. Sam and the organization have some type of responsibility to these applicants, although the exact nature of this responsibility is one of the values in conflict. Because this is Sam's problem and an intrapersonal conflict, he must decide the appropriate course of action. His primary role is to examine his values and act in accordance.

Outline Options

Option 1. Quit his job immediately. This would prevent future intrapersonal conflict provided that Sam becomes aware of his value system and behaves in a manner consistent with that value system in the future. It does not, however, solve the immediate conflict about the action Sam has already taken. This action takes away Sam's livelihood.

Option 2. Do nothing. Sam could choose not to be accountable for his own actions. This will require Sam to rationalize that the philosophy of the organization is in fact acceptable or that he has no choice regarding his actions. Thus, the responsibility for meeting the needs and wants of the new employees is shifted to the organization. Although Sam will have no credibility with the new employees, there will be only a negligible impact on his ability to recruit at least on a short-term basis. Sam will continue to have a job and be able to support his family.

Option 3. If after value clarification Sam has determined that his values conflict with the organization's directive to do or say whatever is needed to recruit employees, he could approach his superior and share these concerns. Sam should be very clear about what his values are and to what extent he is willing to compromise them. He also should include in this meeting what, if any, action should be taken to meet the needs of the new employees. Sam must be realistic about the time and effort usually required to change the values and beliefs of an organization. He also must be aware of his bottom line if the organization is not willing to provide a compromise resolution.

Option 4. Sam could contact each of the applicants and tell them that certain recruitment promises may not be possible. However, he will do what he can to see that the promises are fulfilled. This alternative is risky. The applicants will probably be justifiably suspicious of both the recruiter and the organization, and Sam has little formal power at this point to fulfill their requests. This alternative also requires a time and energy commitment by Sam and does not prevent the problem from recurring.

Review the Options

In value clarification, Sam discovered that he valued truth telling. Alternative 3 allows Sam to present a recruiting plan to his supervisor that includes a bottom line that this value will not be violated.

Affirm Position and Act

Sam approached his superior and was told that his beliefs were idealistic and inappropriate in an age of severe worker shortages. Sam was terminated. Sam did, however, believe that he made an appropriate decision. He did become self-aware regarding his values and attempted to communicate these values to the organization in an effort to work out a mutually agreeable plan.

(Learning Exercise continues on page 84)

Look Back

Although Sam was terminated, he knew that he could find some type of employment to meet his immediate fiscal needs. He did become self-aware regarding his values and used what he had learned in this decision-making process, in that he planned to evaluate more carefully the recruitment philosophy of the organization in relation to his own value system before accepting another job.

The Wueste Approach to Ethical Problem Solving

Wueste (2005) uses a three-pronged approach to ethical decision making: *consequential ethics* (which is his term for a utilitarian theory), *deontological ethics*, and *aspirational ethics*. Aspirational ethics directs the decision maker to what one aspires to be or what one desires the organization to be. Wueste advises ethical decision makers to attempt to envision the most aspiring action that can be taken.

He maintains that if decision makers use all three of these approaches (solving the dilemma using consequential, utilitarian, and aspirational ethics frameworks), they should arrive at the same decision in at least two of the three frameworks and preferably all three. By using all three approaches, the decision is easily justified. Simplified, Wueste's four-step process is:

1. *Identification/recognition.* This step involves identifying all of the ethical issues and the stakeholders involved in the dilemma.
2. *Analysis.* This step examines the ethical issues and delineates the options.
3. *Justification.* Here, the decision maker must justify the decision by using all three types of ethical approaches. If the same decision is reached by at least two of the ethical theories, then the selected option is justified.
4. *Movement.* This final step moves the decision maker to action.

ETHICAL DIMENSIONS IN LEADERSHIP AND MANAGEMENT

The need for ethical decisions occurs in every phase of the management process, and many of the learning exercises in this book have an ethical component that must be considered in the problem solving. In fact, each section in this book could appropriately include a section on ethical issues, such as the following:

Unit III

- At what point do the needs of the organization become more important than those of the individual worker?
- Should employees ever be coerced into changing their stated values so that they more closely align with those of the organization?
- How can managers fairly allocate resources when virtually all resources are limited?

Unit IV

- Should quality or cost be the final determinant when selecting the most appropriate type of patient care delivery system?
- Should LVNs and LPNs be allowed to function in the primary nursing role?

- How should the manager protect clients from an inadequately trained nurse?
- Which should be more important to the organization—human relations or productivity?
- Which is more corrupting—power or powerlessness?

Unit V

- At what point does short staffing become unsafe?
- Should shift scheduling be used as a means of reward and punishment?
- Is luring or recruiting employees from other agencies ever ethical?
- How far can the truth be stretched in recruitment advertising before it becomes deceptive?
- Should pre-employment testing be required as a condition of employment?
- Is it ethical for employees to take a position in an organization if they know that they are planning to leave in a short time?
- Is it ever justified for an employee to lie in an interview?
- Who has the responsibility for socializing the new graduate into the professional nursing role—the nursing school, the hospital, or is it a joint process?
- What commitment does the organization have to the nurse who is re-entering the profession after not practicing for many years?

Unit VI

- To whom do managers owe their primary allegiance—the organization or their subordinates?
- When is it appropriate to use money as the primary motivator?
- If employees are producing at acceptable or higher levels, what new rewards and incentives should be introduced?
- Is it ethical to promote anti-union organizers to management to reduce the possibility of union formation?
- Is affirmative action hiring to compensate for past discrimination ethically justifiable, or does it promote reverse discrimination?
- Is it ethical for nurses to strike?
- Should the national nursing organization also be a collective bargaining agent?

Unit VII

- Is it necessary for each employee to be assisted to achieve at optimal levels? Can the manager be selective in determining which employees are assisted to reach optimal productivity?
- At what point does the power to evaluate the work of others become dangerous?
- Should the individual be allowed total self-determination in short- and long-term career planning?
- Is it ethical to promote or transfer a less-qualified person to keep a valuable employee on a unit?
- Does the organization have an obligation to reemploy the chemically impaired employee who seeks rehabilitation?
- When does the employee's right to privacy regarding drug or alcohol use stop and the manager's right to that information begin?
- Is it ever ethical to file a grievance against another person for the purpose of harassment?

- Can discipline administered in anger ever be fair?
- In pursuing beneficence, is it more appropriate to discipline marginal employees progressively or to terminate them?

Working Toward Ethical Behavior as the Norm

The concerns about ethical conduct in American institutions are documented by many news articles in the national press. Many individuals believe that organizational and institutional ethical failure has become the norm. Governmental agencies, both branches of Congress, the stock exchange, oil companies, and savings and loan institutions have all experienced problems with unethical conduct. Many members of society wonder what has gone wrong. Nurse–managers, then, have a responsibility to create a climate in their organizations in which ethical behavior is not only the expectation but the norm.

In an era of markedly limited physical, human, and fiscal resources, nearly all decision making by nurse–managers will involve some ethical component. Indeed, the following forces ensure that ethics will become an even greater dimension in management decision making in the future: increasing technology, regulatory pressures, and competitiveness among health care providers; national nursing shortages; reduced fiscal resources; spiraling costs of supplies and salaries; and the public's increasing distrust of the health care delivery system and its institutions. The following actions can help the manager in ethical problem solving.

Separate Legal and Ethical Issues

Although they are not the same, separating legal and ethical issues is sometimes difficult. Legal controls are generally clear and philosophically impartial; ethical controls are much less clear and individualized. In many ethical issues, courts have made a decision that may guide managers in their decision making. Often, however, these guidelines are not comprehensive, or they differ from the manager's own philosophy. Managers must be aware of established legal standards and cognizant of possible liabilities and consequences for actions that go against the legal precedent.

Legal precedents are frequently overturned later and often do not keep pace with the changing needs of society. Additionally, certain circumstances may favor an illegal course of action as the "right" thing to do. If a man were transporting his severely ill wife to the hospital, it might be morally correct for him to disobey traffic laws. Therefore, the manager should think of the law as a basic standard of conduct, whereas ethical behavior requires a greater examination of the issues involved.

The manager may confront several particularly sensitive legal–ethical issues, including termination or refusal of treatment, durable power of attorney, abortion, sterilization, child abuse, and human experimentation. Most health care organizations have legal counsel to assist managers in making decisions in such sensitive areas. Because legal aspects of management decision making are so important, Chapter 5 is devoted exclusively to this topic.

Collaborate to Solve Ethical Issues

The new manager must consult with others when solving sensitive legal–ethical questions because a person's own value system may preclude examining all possible alternatives. Jormsri (2004) posits that using collaboration and integrating the knowledge and training of various types of professionals when solving ethical problems will lead to more effective problem solving. Many institutions have ethics committees to assist with problem solving in ethical issues These ethics committees typically are multidisciplinary and are organized to consciously and reflectively consider significant and often difficult or ambiguous value issues related to patient care or organizational activities.

Ethics committees are a core element of collaborative ethical decision making and should include representatives of all stakeholders, including patients when they are involved in the ethical issue. Health care institutions should develop policies and procedural guidelines for such committees (Jormsri, 2004).

Create an Ethical Work Environment

Perhaps the most important thing a manager can do to create an ethical work environment is to model ethical behavior. Other important interventions, however, include encouraging staff to openly discuss ethical issues that they face daily in their practice. This allows subordinates to gain greater perspective on complex issues and provides a mechanism for peer support.

Raines (2000) also suggests the following proactive strategies for creating an ethical work environment and for reducing "ethics stress":

- Start a nursing ethics library or nursing ethics journal club at the workplace.
- Sponsor a nursing ethics committee and/or nursing research committee as a counterpart to the interdisciplinary ethics committee and/or institutional review board.
- Support a nursing ethics grand rounds and plan for interdisciplinary participation.
- Provide all staff an annual educational program that uses current issues for case discussion.
- Circulate a nursing ethics article of the month to all units, and encourage brief discussion at staff meetings or clinical rounds.
- Do a biannual survey of staff to assess what ethical issues they are facing most frequently or having most difficulty resolving.
- Send representatives from your nursing staff to other similar health care organizations to find out what their staff do related to ethical issues, ethics committees, nursing policies, educational programs, and the like.
- If there are no staff nurse representatives on the agency's ethics committee or institutional review board, take a nurse–manager or staff nurse to the regular meeting.

Use Institutional Review Boards Appropriately

Institutional Review Boards (IRB) are primarily formed to protect the rights and welfare of research subjects. They provide oversight to assure that individuals conducting research adhere to ethical principles that were articulated by the National Commission for the Protection of Human Subjects of Biomedical and Behavioral Research established in 1979 (Foss, 2005). The primary role of the manager regarding IRBs is to make sure that such a board is in place in the organization where the manager works and that any research performed within his or her sphere of responsibility has been approved by such a board.

Foss maintains that there is increasing controversy about research, program evaluation, and quality improvement. Although program evaluation has not historically been viewed as needing IRB's oversight, that apparently is changing, and there is a trend toward more ethical oversight in any project that collects data (Foss, 2005).

INTEGRATING LEADERSHIP ROLES AND MANAGEMENT FUNCTIONS IN ETHICS

Leadership roles in ethics focus on the human element involved in ethical decision making. Leaders are self-aware regarding their values and basic beliefs about the rights, duties, and goals of human beings. As self-aware and ethical people, they role model confidence in their decision making to subordinates. They also are realists and recognize that some ambiguity and uncertainty must be a part of all ethical decision making. Leaders are willing to take risks in their decision making despite the fact that negative outcomes can occur even with quality decision making.

In ethical issues, the manager is often the decision maker. Because ethical decisions are so complex and the cost of a poor decision may be high, management functions focus on increasing the chances that the best possible decision will be made at the least possible cost in terms of fiscal and human resources. This usually requires that the manager becomes expert at using systematic approaches to problem solving or decision making, such as theoretical models, ethical frameworks, and ethical principles. By developing expertise, the manager can identify universal outcomes that should be sought or avoided.

The integrated leader–manager recognizes that ethical issues pervade every aspect of leadership and management. Rather than being paralyzed by the complexity and ambiguity of these issues, the leader–manager seeks counsel as needed, accepts his or her limitations, and makes the best possible decision at that time with the information and resources available.

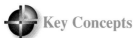 Key Concepts

* *Ethics* is the systematic study of what a person's conduct and actions should be with regard to self, other human beings, and the environment; it is the justification of what is right or good and the study of what a person's life and relationships should be—not necessarily what they are.

* In an era of markedly limited physical, human, and fiscal resources, nearly all decision making by nurse–managers involves some ethical component. Multiple advocacy roles and accountability to the profession further increase the likelihood that managers will be faced with ethical dilemmas in their practice.

* Many systematic approaches to ethical problem solving are appropriate. These include the use of theoretical problem-solving and decision-making models, ethical frameworks, and ethical principles.

* Outcomes should never be used as the sole criterion for assessing the quality of ethical problem solving, because many variables affect outcomes that have no reflection on whether the problem solving was appropriate. Quality, instead, should be evaluated both by the outcome and the process used to make the decision. If a structured approach to problem solving is used, data gathering is adequate, and multiple alternatives are analyzed, then, regardless of the outcome, the manager should feel comfortable that the best possible decision was made at that time with the information and resources available.

* Four of the most commonly used ethical frameworks for decision making are *utilitarianism*, *duty-based reasoning*, *rights-based reasoning*, and *intuitionism*. These frameworks

do not solve the ethical problem but assist individuals involved in the problem solving to clarify their values and beliefs.

* Principles of ethical reasoning explore and define what beliefs or values form the basis for our decision making. These principles include *autonomy*, *beneficence*, *nonmaleficence*, *paternalism*, *utility*, *justice*, *fidelity*, *veracity*, and *confidentiality*.

* Professional *codes of ethics* and *standards for practice* are guides to the highest standards of ethical practice for nurses.

* Sometimes it is very difficult to separate legal and ethical issues, although they are not the same. Legal controls are generally clear and philosophically impartial. Ethical controls are much more unclear and individualized.

ADDITIONAL LEARNING EXERCISES AND APPLICATIONS

LEARNING EXERCISE 4.6

The Impaired Employee

Beverly, a 35-year-old, full-time nurse on the day shift, has been with your facility for 10 years. There are rumors that she comes to work under the influence of alcohol. Staff report the smell of alcohol on her breath, unexcused absences from the unit, and an increase in medication errors. Although the unit supervisor suspected that Beverly was chemically impaired, she was unable to observe directly any of these behaviors.

After arriving at work last week, the supervisor walked into the nurses' lounge and observed Beverly covertly drinking from a dark-colored flask in her locker. She immediately confronted Beverly and asked her if she was drinking alcohol while on duty. Beverly tearfully admitted that she was drinking alcohol but stated this was an isolated incident and begged her to forget it. She promised never to consume alcohol at work again.

In an effort to reduce the emotionalism of the event and to give herself time to think, the supervisor sent Beverly home and scheduled a conference with her for later in the day. At this conference, Beverly was defensive and stated, "I do not have a drinking problem, and you are overreacting." The supervisor shared data that she had gathered supporting her impression that Beverly was chemically impaired. Beverly offered no explanation for these behaviors.

The plan for Beverly was a referral to the State Board of Nursing Diversion Program and a requirement that she complete the program as they direct her. Beverly again became very tearful and begged the supervisor to reconsider. She stated that she was the sole provider for her four small children and that her frequent sick days had taken up all available vacation and sick pay. The supervisor stated that she believed her decision was appropriate and again encouraged Beverly to seek guidance for her drinking. Four days later, the supervisor read in the newspaper that Beverly committed suicide the day after this meeting.

● ASSIGNMENT: Evaluate the problem solving of the supervisor. Would your actions have differed if you were the manager? Are there conflicting legal and ethical obligations? To whom does the manager have the greatest obligation—patients, subordinates, or the organization? Could the outcome have been prevented? Does this outcome reflect on the quality of the problem solving?

LEARNING EXERCISE 4.7

Everything Is Not What It Seems

You are a perinatal unit coordinator at a large teaching hospital. In addition to your management responsibilities, you have been asked to fill in as a member of the hospital promotion committee, which reviews petitions from clinicians for a step-level promotion on the clinical specialist ladder. You believe that you could learn a great deal on this committee and could be an objective and contributing member.

The committee has been convened to select the annual winner of the Outstanding Clinical Specialist Award. In reviewing the applicant files, you find that one file from a perinatal clinical specialist contains many overstatements and several misrepresentations. You know for a fact that this clinician did not accomplish all that she has listed, because she is a friend and close colleague. She did not, however, know that you would be a member of this committee and thus would be aware of this deception.

When the entire committee met, several members commented on this clinician's impressive file. Although you were able to dissuade them covertly from further considering her nomination, you are left with many uneasy feelings and some anger and sadness. You recognize that she did not receive the nomination and thus there is little real danger regarding the deceptions in the file being used inappropriately at this time. However, you will not be on this committee next year, and if she were to submit an erroneous file again, she could be highly considered for the award. You also recognize that even with the best of intentions and the most therapeutic of communication techniques, confronting your friend with her deception will cause her to lose face and will probably result in an unsalvageable friendship. Even if you do confront her, there is little you can do to stop her from doing the same in future nomination processes other than formally reporting her conduct.

● ASSIGNMENT: Determine what you will do. Do the potential costs outweigh the potential benefits? Be realistic about your actions.

LEARNING EXERCISE 4.8

The Valuable Employee

Gina has been the supervisor of a 16-bed intensive care unit/critical care unit (ICU/CCU) in a 200-bed urban hospital for 8 years. She is respected and well liked by her staff. Her unit's staff retention level and productivity are higher than any other unit in the hospital. For the last 6 years, Gina has relied heavily on Mark, her permanent charge nurse on the day shift. He is bright and motivated and has excellent clinical and managerial skills. Mark seems satisfied and challenged in his current position, although Gina has not had any formal career planning meetings with him to discuss his long-term career goals. It would be fair to say that Mark's work has greatly increased Gina's scope of power and has enhanced the reputation of the unit.

Recently, one of the physicians approached Gina about a plan to open an outpatient cardiac rehabilitation program. The program will require a strong leader and manager who is self-motivated. It will be a lot of work but also provides many opportunities for advancement. He suggests that Mark would be an excellent choice for the job, although he has given Gina full authority to make the final decision.

Gina is aware that Lynn, a bright and dynamic staff nurse from the open-heart surgery floor, also would be very interested in the job. Lynn has been employed at the hospital for only 1 year but has a proven track record and would probably be very successful in the job. In addition, there is a staffing surplus right now on the open-heart surgery floor because two of the surgeons have recently retired. It would be difficult and time-consuming to replace Mark as charge nurse in the ICU/CCU.

● ASSIGNMENT: What process should this supervisor pursue to determine who should be hired for the position? Should the position be posted? When does the benefit of using transfers/promotions as a means of reward outweigh the cost of reduced productivity?

LEARNING EXERCISE 4.9

To See or Not To See
For the last few days, you have been taking care of Mr. Cole, a 28-year-old patient with end-stage cystic fibrosis. You have developed a caring relationship with Mr. Cole and his wife. They are both aware of the prognosis of his disease and realize that he has only a short time left to live.

When Dr. Jones made rounds with you this morning, she told the Coles that Mr. Cole could be discharged today if his condition remains stable. They were both excited about the news because they had been urging the doctor to let him go home to enjoy his remaining time surrounded by things he loves.

When you bring in Mr. Cole's discharge orders to his room in order to review his medications and other treatments, you find Mrs. Cole assisting Mr. Cole as he coughs up bright red blood. When you confront them, they both beg you not to tell the doctor or chart the incident because this is the first time this has happened. They believe that it is their right to go home and let Mr. Cole die surrounded by his family. They said that they know that they can leave against their physician's wishes and go home AMA (against medical advice), but if they do, their insurance will not pay for home care.

● ASSIGNMENT: What is your duty in this case? What are Mr. Cole's rights? Is it ever justified to withhold information from the physician? Will you chart the incident, and will you report it to anyone? Solve this case, justifying your decision by using ethical principles.

Web Links

ANA: The Center for Ethics and Human Rights
http://www.nursingworld.org/ethics/index.htm
Established in 1990, this center is devoted to the study of ethics and nursing, including issue updates and policy development.

John Dossetor Health Ethics Centre, University of Alberta
http://www.ualberta.ca/BIOETHICS/
An interdisciplinary center committed to working in the area of health ethics.

International Code of Ethics (The International Council of Nurses)
http://www.icn.ch/icncode.pdf
The ICN Code of Ethics for Nurses, revised in 2000, is a guide for action based on social values and needs. The code has served as the standard for nurses worldwide since it was first adopted in 1953 (available in English, French, and Spanish).

Markkula Center for Applied Ethics—A Framework for Ethical Decision Making, Santa Clara University
http://www.scu.edu/ethics/practicing/decision/framework.html
Suggests a framework for ethical decision making as well as provides links on the scope of ethics or moral philosophy, on alternative frameworks for ethical decision making, and on ethical relativism.

References

Aita, M., & Richer, M. (2005). Essentials of research ethics for healthcare professionals. *Nursing and Health Sciences, 7*(2), 119–125.

American Nurses Association. (2001). *Code of ethics for nurses with interpretive statements.* Washington, DC: American Nurses Publishing.

American Nurses Association. (2004). *Scope and standards for nurse administrators* (2nd ed.). Washington, DC: American Nurses Publishing.

Bruhn, J. G. (2005). Looking good, but behaving badly: Leader accountability and ethics failure. *Health Care Manager, 24*(3), 191–199.

Crisham, P. (1985). MORAL: How can I do what is right? *Nursing Management, 16*(3), 42A–42N.

Foss, G. F. (2005). Modifications of graduate public community health nursing internships to facilitate compliance with institutional review board and health insurance portability and accountability act (HIPPAA) regulations. *Public Health Nursing, 22*(2), 172–179.

Jormsri, P. (2004). Moral conflict and collaborative mode as moral conflict resolution in health care. *Nursing and Health Sciences, 6*(3), 217–221.

Laabs, C. A. (2005). Moral problems and distress among nurse practitioners in primary care. *Journal of the American Academy of Nurse Practitioners, 17*(2), 76–84.

Raines, M. L. (2000). Ethical decision making in nurses. *JONA's Healthcare Law, Ethics, and Regulation, 2*(1), 29–41.

Wueste, D. E. (2005). A philosophical yet user-friendly framework for ethical decision making in critical care nursing. *Dimensions of Critical Care Nursing, 24*(2), 70–79.

Bibliography

Abma, T. A. (2005). Struggling with the fragility of life: A relational-narrative approach to ethics in palliative nursing. *Nursing Ethics, 12*(4), 337–348.

Bramstedt, K. A., Molnar, M., Carlson, K., & Bilyseu, S. M. (2005). When families complicate patient care: A case study with guidelines for approaching ethical dilemmas. *MEDSURG Nursing, 14*(2), 122–125.

Curtin, L. (2005). The long & short of it: Solving ethical dilemmas. Patients' rights: In whose best interests? *Healthcare Traveler, 12*(11), 14–16.

Davis, B. R. (2005). Coercion or collaboration? Nurses doing research with people who have severe mental health problems. *Journal of Psychiatric and Mental Health Nursing, 12*(1), 106–111.

Erlen, J. A. (2005). When patients and families disagree. *Orthopaedic Nursing, 24*(4), 279–282.

Fitzsimons, D., & McAloon, T. (2005). The ethics of non-intervention in a study of patients awaiting coronary artery bypass surgery. *Journal of Advanced Nursing, 46*(4), 395–402.

Fitzpatrick, J. J. (2004). From the editor. Naming and taming our ethical dilemmas. *Nursing Education Perspectives, 25*(2), 57.

Flicker, S., Haans, D., & Skinner, H. (2004). Ethical dilemmas in research on Internet communities. *Qualitative Health Research, 14*(1), 124–134.

Hoskins, S. A. (2005). Nurses and national socialism—A moral dilemma: One historical example of a route to euthanasia. *Nursing Ethics, 12*(1), 79–91.

Maze, C. D. M. (2005). Registered nurses' personal rights vs. professional responsibility in caring for members of underserved and disenfranchised populations. *Journal of Clinical Nursing, 14*(5), 546–554.

Snoxall, S., & Williamson, G. R. (2004). Assisted human reproduction, psychological and ethical dilemmas. *Journal of Advanced Nursing, 47*(2), 235.

5

Legal and Legislative Issues

. . . the medical malpractice crisis doesn't have to be permanent. Between legislation and nurse leader advocacy, the focus can return to patient care rather than defensive practice.

—*Kathleen White (2005)*

Chapter 4 presented ethics as an internal control of human behavior and nursing practice. Therefore, ethics has to do with actions that people should take, not necessarily actions that they are legally required to take. On the other hand, ethical behavior written into law is no longer just desired, it is mandated. This chapter focuses on the external controls of legislation and law. Since the first mandatory Nurse Practice Act was passed in North Carolina in 1903, nursing has been legislated, directed, and controlled to some extent.

The primary purpose of law and legislation is to protect the patient and the nurse. Laws and legislation define the scope of acceptable practice and protect individual rights. Nurses who are aware of their rights and duties in legal matters are better able to protect themselves against liability or loss of professional licensure.

This chapter has five sections. The first section presents the primary sources of law and how each affects nursing practice. The nurse's responsibility to be proactive in establishing and revising laws affecting nursing practice is emphasized. The second section presents the types of legal cases in which nurses may be involved and differentiates between the burden of proof and the consequences for each if the nurse is found guilty. The third section identifies specific doctrines used by the courts to define legal boundaries for nursing practice. The role of state boards in professional licensure and discipline is examined. The fourth section deals with the components of malpractice for the individual practitioner and the manager or supervisor. Legal terms are defined. The fifth section discusses issues such as informed consent, medical records, intentional torts, the Patient Self Determination Act, the Good Samaritan Act, and the Health Information Protection and Portability Act (HIPAA).

This chapter is not meant to be a complete legal guide to nursing practice. There are many excellent legal textbooks and handbooks that accomplish that function. The primary function of this chapter is to emphasize the widely varying and rapidly changing nature of laws and the

DISPLAY 5.1 Leadership Roles and Management Functions Associated With Legal and Legislative Issues

Leadership Roles

1. Serves as a role model by providing nursing care that meets or exceeds accepted standards of care
2. Updates knowledge and skills in the field of practice and seeks professional certification to increase expertise in a specific field
3. Reports substandard nursing care to appropriate authorities following established chain of command
4. Fosters nurse–patient relationships that are respectful, caring, and honest, thus reducing the possibility of future lawsuits
5. Creates an environment that encourages and supports cultural diversity and sensitivity
6. Prioritizes patient rights and patient welfare first in decision making
7. Demonstrates vision, risk taking, and energy in determining appropriate legal boundaries for nursing practice, thus defining what nursing is and should be in the future

Management Functions

1. Increases knowledge regarding sources of law and legal doctrines that affect nursing practice
2. Delegates to subordinates wisely, looking at the manager's scope of practice and that of the individuals he or she supervises
3. Understands and adheres to institutional policies and procedures
4. Minimizes the risk of product liability by assuring that all staff are appropriately oriented to the appropriate use of equipment and products
5. Monitors subordinates to ensure they have a valid, current, and appropriate license to practice nursing
6. Uses foreseeability of harm in delegation and staffing decisions
7. Increases staff awareness of intentional torts and assists them in developing strategies to reduce their liability in these areas
8. Provides educational and training opportunities for staff on legal issues affecting nursing practice

responsibility that each manager has to keep abreast of legislation and laws affecting both nursing and management practice. Leadership roles and management functions inherent in legal and legislative issues are shown in Display 5.1.

SOURCES OF LAW

The U.S. legal system can be somewhat confusing because there are not only four sources of the law but also parallel systems at the state and federal levels. The sources of law include constitutions, statutes, administrative agencies, and court decisions. A comparison is shown in Table 5.1.

TABLE 5.1 Sources of Law

Origin of Law	Use	Involvement with Nursing Practice
The Constitution	The highest law in the United States; interpreted by the U.S. Supreme Court; gives authority to other three sources of the law.	Little direct involvement in the area of malpractice.
Statutes	Also called *statutory law* or *legislative law;* laws that are passed by the state or federal legislators and that must be signed by the president or governor.	Before 1970s, very few state or federal laws dealt with malpractice. Since the malpractice crisis, many statutes affect malpractice.
Administrative agencies	The rules and regulations established by appointed agencies of the executive branch of the government (governor or president).	Some of these agencies, such as the National Labor Relations Board or health and safety boards, can effect nursing practice.
Court decisions	Also called *tort law;* this is court mode law and the courts interpret the statutes and set precedents; in the United States, there are two levels of court: trial court and appellate court.	Most malpractice law is addressed by the courts.

A *constitution* is a system of fundamental laws or principles that govern a nation, society, corporation, or other aggregate of individuals. The purpose of a constitution is to establish the basis of a governing system for the future and the present. The U.S. Constitution establishes the general organization of the federal government and grants and limits its specific powers. Each state also has a constitution that establishes the general organization of the state government and grants and limits its powers.

The second source of law is *statutes*—laws that govern. Legislative bodies, such as the U.S. Congress, state legislatures, and city councils, make these laws. Statutes are officially enacted (voted on and passed) by the legislative body and are compiled into codes, collections of statutes, and ordinances. The 51 nurse practice acts representing the 50 states and the District of Columbia are examples of statutes. These nurse practice acts define and limit the practice of nursing, thereby stating what constitutes authorized practice as well as what exceeds the scope of authority. Although nurse practice acts may vary among states, all must be consistent with provisions or statutes established at the federal level.

Administrative agencies, the third source of law, are given authority to act by the legislative bodies and create rules and regulations that enforce statutory laws. For example, state boards of nursing are administrative agencies set up to implement and enforce the state nurse practice act by writing rules and regulations and by conducting investigations and hearings to ensure the law's enforcement. Administrative laws are valid only to the extent that they are within the scope of the authority granted to them by the legislative body.

The fourth source of law is *court decisions*. Judicial or decisional laws are made by the courts to interpret legal issues that are in dispute. Depending on the type of court involved, judicial or decisional law may be made by a single justice, with or without a jury, or by a panel of justices. Generally, initial trial courts have a single judge or magistrate, intermediary appeal courts have three justices, and the highest appeal courts have nine justices.

TYPES OF LAWS AND COURTS

Although most nurses worry primarily about being sued for malpractice, they may actually be involved in three different types of court cases; criminal, civil, and administrative (Table 5.2). The court in which each is tried, the burden of proof required for conviction, and the resulting punishment associated with each is different.

In *criminal* cases, the individual faces charges generally filed by the state or federal attorney general for crimes committed against an individual or society. In criminal cases, the individual is always presumed to be innocent unless the state can prove his or her guilt beyond a reasonable doubt. Incarceration and even death are possible consequences for being found guilty in criminal matters. Nurses found guilty of intentionally administering fatal doses of drugs to patients would be charged in a criminal court.

In *civil* cases, one individual sues another for money to compensate for a perceived loss. The burden of proof required to be found guilty in a civil case is described as a *preponderance of the evidence*. In other words, the judge or jury must believe that it was more likely than not that the accused individual was responsible for the injuries of the complainant. Consequences of being found guilty in a civil suit are monetary. Most malpractice cases are tried in civil court.

In *administrative* cases, an individual is sued by a state or federal governmental agency assigned the responsibility of implementing governmental programs. State boards of nursing are one such governmental agency. When an individual violates the state nurse practice act, the board of nursing may seek to revoke licensure or institute some form of discipline. The burden of proof in these cases varies from state to state. When the *clear and convincing standard* is not used, the preponderance of the evidence standard may be used. Clear and convincing involves

TABLE 5.2 Types of Laws and Courts

Type	Burden of Proof Required for Guilty Verdict	Likely Consequences of a Guilty Verdict
Criminal	Beyond a reasonable doubt	Incarceration, probation, fines
Civil	Based on a preponderance of the evidence	Monetary damages
Administrative	Clear and convincing standard	Suspension or loss of licensure

higher burdens of proof than preponderance of evidence but significantly lower burdens of proof than beyond a reasonable doubt.

LEARNING EXERCISE 5.1

Both Guilty and Not Guilty
Think of celebrated cases where defendants have been tried in both civil and criminal courts. What were the verdicts in both cases? If the verdicts were not the same, analyze why this happened. Do you agree that taking away an individual's personal liberty by incarceration should require a higher burden of proof than assessing them monetary damages?

Then, do a literature search to see if you can find cases where a nurse faced both civil and administrative charges. Were you able to find cases where the nurse was found guilty in a civil court but did not lose his or her license? Did you find the opposite?

LEGAL DOCTRINES AND THE PRACTICE OF NURSING

Two important legal doctrines frequently guide all three courts in their decision making. The first of these, *stare decisis*, means to let the decision stand. *Stare decisis* uses precedents as a guide for decision making. This doctrine gives nurses insight into ways that the court has previously fixed liability in given situations. However, the nurse must avoid two pitfalls in determining if *stare decisis* should apply to a given situation.

The first is that the previous case must be within the jurisdiction of the court hearing the current case. For example, a previous Florida case decided by a state court does not set precedent for a Texas appellate court. Although the Texas court may model its decision after the Florida case, it is not compelled to do so. The lower courts in Texas, however, would rely on Texas appellate decisions.

The other pitfall is that the court hearing the current case can depart from the precedent and set a landmark decision. Landmark decisions generally occur because societal needs have changed, technology has become more advanced, or following the precedent would further harm an already injured person. *Roe* v. *Wade*, the 1973 landmark decision to allow a woman to seek and receive a legal abortion during the first two trimesters of pregnancy, is an example. Given changes in societal views about abortion, this precedent may change again in the future.

The second doctrine that guides courts in their decision making is *res judicata*, which means a "thing or matter settled by judgment." It applies only when a competent court has decided a legal dispute and when no further appeals are possible. This doctrine keeps the same parties in the original lawsuit from retrying the same issues that were involved in the first lawsuit.

When using doctrines as a guide for nursing practice, the nurse must remember that all laws are fluid and subject to change. An example of changing law regarding professional nursing recently occurred in an Illinois Supreme Court case when the law finally recognized nursing as an independent profession with its own unique body of knowledge. In this case (*Sullivan* v. *Edward Hospital*), the Illinois Supreme Court decided that physicians could not serve as expert witnesses regarding nursing standards (Murphy, 2004). The above demonstrates how the law is ever evolving. Laws cannot be static; they must change to reflect the growing autonomy and responsibility desired by nurses. It is critical that all nurses be aware of and sensitive to rapidly changing laws and legislation that affect their practice. Nurses also must recognize that state laws may differ from federal laws and that legal guidelines for nursing practice in the organization may differ from state or federal guidelines.

Boundaries for practice are defined in the nurse practice act of each state. These acts are general in most states to allow for some flexibility in the broad roles and varied situations in which nurses practice. Because this allows for some interpretation, many employers have established guidelines for nursing practice in their own organization. These guidelines regarding scope of practice cannot, however, exceed the requirements of the state nursing practice acts. Managers need to be aware of their organization's specific practice interpretations and ensure that subordinates are aware of the same and follow established practices. All nurses must understand the legal controls for nursing practice in their state.

PROFESSIONAL NEGLIGENCE

Historically, physicians were the health care providers most likely to be held liable for nursing care. As nurses have gained authority, autonomy, and accountability, they have assumed responsibility, accountability, and liability for their own practice. As roles have expanded, nurses have begun performing duties traditionally reserved for medical practice. As a result of an increased scope of practice, many nurses now carry individual malpractice insurance. This is a double-edged sword. Nurses need malpractice insurance in basic practice as well as in expanded practice roles. They do incur a greater likelihood of being sued however, if they have malpractice insurance, since injured parties will always seek damages from as many individuals with financial resources as possible.

Both the enhanced role of nurses and the increase in the number of insured nurses has led to a great increase in the number of liability suits seeking damages from nurses as individuals over the past few decades. In particular, malpractice has become of great concern to advanced practice nurses such as nurse practitioners and nurse midwives. Nurse practitioners are not only paying more for their premiums, but often they are losing their places of employment due to the high cost of insurance (Klutz, 2004).

All liability suits involve a plaintiff and a defendant. In malpractice cases, the *plaintiff* is the injured party and the *defendant* is the professional who is alleged to have caused the injury. *Negligence* is the omission to do something that a reasonable person, guided by the considerations that ordinarily regulate human affairs, would do—or as doing something that a reasonable and prudent person would not do. *Reasonable and prudent* generally means the average judgment, foresight, intelligence, and skill that would be expected of a person with similar training and experience. *Malpractice*—the failure of a person with professional training to act in a reasonable and prudent manner—also is called *professional negligence*. Five elements must be present for a professional to be held liable for malpractice (Table 5.3).

First, a *standard of care* must have been established that outlines the level or degree of quality considered adequate by a given profession. Standards of care outline the duties a defendant has to a plaintiff or a nurse to a client. These standards represent the skills and learning commonly possessed by members of the profession and generally are the minimal requirements that define an acceptable level of care. Standards of care, which guarantee clients safe nursing care, include organizational policy and procedure statements, job descriptions, and student guidelines.

TABLE 5.3   **Components of Professional Negligence**

Elements of Liability	Explanation	Example: Giving Medications
1. Duty to use due care (defined by the standard of care)	The care that should be given under the circumstances (what the reasonably prudent nurse would have done).	A nurse should give medications accurately, completely, and on time.
2. Failure to meet standard of care (breach of duty)	Not giving the care that should be given under the circumstances.	A nurse fails to give medications accurately, completely, or on time.
3. Forseeability of harm	The nurse must have reasonable access to information about whether the possibility of harm exists.	The drug handbook specifies that the wrong dosage or route may cause injury.
4. A direct relationship between failure to meet the standard of care (breach) and injury can be proved	Patient is harmed because proper care is not given.	Wrong dosage causes patient to have a convulsion.
5. Injury	Actual harm results to patient.	Convulsion or other serious complication occurs.

Second, after the standard of care has been established, it must be shown that the standard was violated—there must have been a *breach of duty*. This breach is shown by calling other nurses who practice in the same specialty area as the defendant to testify as expert witnesses.

Third, the nurse must have had the knowledge or availability of information that not meeting the standard of care could result in harm. This is called *foreseeability of harm*. If the average, reasonable person in the defendant's position could have anticipated the plaintiff's injury as a result of his or her actions, then the plaintiff's injury was foreseeable. Ignorance is not an excuse, but lack of information may have a negative effect on the ability to foresee harm.

Being ignorant is not a justifiable excuse, but not having all the information in a situation may impede one's ability to foresee harm.

For example, a charge nurse assigns another RN to care for a critically ill patient. The assigned RN makes a medication error that injures the patient in some way. If the charge nurse had reason to believe that the RN was incapable of adequately caring for the patient or failed to provide adequate supervision, foreseeability of harm is apparent, and the charge nurse also could be held liable. If the charge nurse was available as needed and had good reason to believe that the RN was fully capable, he or she would probably not be held liable.

A number of recent malpractice cases have hinged on whether the nurse was persistent enough in attempting to notify health care providers of changes in a patient's conditions or to convince the providers of the seriousness of a patient's condition (Nursing Malpractice, 2003). Because the nurse has foreseeability of harm in these situations, the nurse who is not persistent can be held liable for failure to intervene because the intervention was below what was expected of him or her as a patient advocate (Nursing Malpractice, 2003).

The fourth element is that *failure to meet the standard of care must have the potential to injure the patient*. There must be a provable correlation between improper care and injury to the patient.

The final element is that *actual patient injury* must occur. This injury must be more than transitory. The plaintiff must show that the action of the defendant directly caused the injury and that the injury would not have occurred without the defendant's actions. It is important to remember here, however, that not taking action is an action. Nurses can be held liable even if the patient injures him or herself because the nurse did not appropriately safeguard the patient from harm (Nursing Malpractice, 2003).

LEARNING EXERCISE 5.2

Who's Guilty? You Decide

You are a surgical nurse at Memorial Hospital. At 4 PM, you receive a patient from the recovery room who has had a total hip replacement. You note that the hip dressings are saturated with blood but are aware that total hip replacements frequently have some postoperative oozing from the wound. There is an order on the chart to reinforce the dressing as needed, and you do so. When you next check the dressing at 6 PM, you find the reinforcements saturated and drainage on the bed linen. You call the physician and tell her that you believe the patient is bleeding too heavily. The physician reassures you that the amount of bleeding you have described is not excessive but encourages you to continue to monitor the patient closely. You recheck the patient's dressings at 7 PM and 8 PM. You again call the physician and tell her that the bleeding still looks too heavy. She again reassures you and tells you to continue to watch the patient closely. At 10 PM, the patient's blood pressure becomes nonpalpable, and she goes into shock. You summon the doctor, and she comes immediately.

● ASSIGNMENT: What are the legal ramifications of this case? Using the components of professional negligence outlined in Table 5.3, determine who in this case is guilty of malpractice. Justify your answer. At what point in the scenario should each character have altered his or her actions to reduce the probability of a negative outcome?

AVOIDING MALPRACTICE CLAIMS

Interactions between nurses and clients that are less businesslike and more personal are more satisfying to both. It has been shown that despite technical competence, nurses who have difficulty establishing positive interpersonal relationships with patients and their families are at greater risk of being sued. Communication that proceeds in a caring and professional manner has been shown repeatedly to be a major reason that people do not sue, despite adequate grounds for a successful lawsuit. The importance of working to create open communication is listed as one of the major recommendations of The Joint Commission (formerly known as Joint Commission on Accreditation of Healthcare Organizations [JCAHO]) in its strategies for improving the medical liability system and preventing patient injury report (JCAHO, 2005).

Smith (2005) argues effectively that malpractice claims and resulting regulatory consequences have occurred because of failed leadership at all levels of health care. She cites several foreseeable "accidents waiting to happen" in regard to nursing practice. For example, even though there are unit-dose systems in play, nurse–leaders often look the other way when staff dump all the medications into a soufflé cup and hand them to patients, thus preventing patients from possibly identifying medication errors. She concludes by saying, "while many of the recommendations in the Joint Commission's call-to-action require policy change at the national level, the locus of power for their already evidence-based recommendations lies in the hands of every leader in every hospital" (p. 99). The strategies recommended by the Joint Commission can be viewed in Display 5.2,

DISPLAY 5.2   **Summary of Recommendations From the Executive Summary of "Healthcare in the Crossroads: Strategies for Improving the Medical Liability System and Preventing Injury"**

1. *Pursue patient safety initiatives that prevent medical injury by:*
   - Strengthening oversight and accountability mechanisms to better ensure the competencies of physicians and nurses
   - Encouraging appropriate adherence to clinical guidelines to improve quality and reduce liability risk
   - Supporting team development through team training
   - Continuing to leverage patient safety initiatives through regulatory and oversight bodies
   - Building an evidence-based information and technology system that impacts patient safety and pursue proposals to offset implementation costs
   - Promoting the creation of cultures of patient safety in health care organizations
   - Establishing a federal leadership locus for advocacy of patient safety and health care quality
   - Pursuing "pay-for-performance" strategies that provide incentives to improve patient safety and health care quality
2. *Promote open communication between patients and practitioners by:*
   - Involving health care consumers as active members of the health care team
   - Encouraging open communication between practitioners and patients when adverse events occur
   - Pursuing legislation that protects disclosure and apology from being used as evidence against practitioners in litigation
   - Encouraging nonpunitive reporting of errors to third parties that promote information and data analysis as a basis for developing safety improvement
   - Enacting federal safety legislation that provides legal protection for when information is reported to patient safety organizations
3. *Create an injury compensation system that is patient centered and serves the common good by:*
   - Conducting demonstration projects of alternatives to medical liability that promote patient safety and transparency and provide swift compensation for injured patients
   - Encouraging continued development of mediation and early-offer initiatives
   - Prohibiting confidential settlements that prevent learning from events
   - Redesigning the National Practitioner Data Bank
   - Advocating for court-appointed, independent expert witnesses to mitigate bias in expert witness testimony

Source: Joint Commission on Accreditation of Healthcare Organizations. (2005). *Health care in the crossroads: Strategies for improving the medical liability system and preventing patient injury.* Oakbrook Terrace, IL: Author.

which summarizes the three major areas of focus in the call-to-action to prevent injuries, improve communication, and examine mechanisms for injury compensation.

Nurses can reduce the risk for malpractice claims by taking the following actions:
- Practice within the scope of the nurse practice act.
- Observe agency policies and procedures.
- Model practice after established standards by using evidence-based practice.
- Always put patient rights and welfare first.
- Be aware of relevant law and legal doctrines and combine such with the biological, psychological, and social sciences that form the basis of all rational nursing decisions.
- Practice within the area of individual competence.
- Upgrade technical skills consistently by attending continuing education programs and seeking specialty certification.

Nurses should also purchase their own liability insurance and understand the limits of their policies. Although this will not prevent a malpractice suit, it will help to protect a nurse from financial ruin should there be a malpractice claim.

LEARNING EXERCISE 5.3

Discussing Lawsuits and Liability
In small groups, discuss the following questions:
1. Do you believe that there are unnecessary lawsuits in the health care industry? What criteria can be used to distinguish between appropriate and unnecessary lawsuits?
2. Have you ever advised a friend or family member to sue to recover damages that you believed they suffered as a result of poor-quality health care? What motivated you to encourage them to do so?
3. Do you think that you will make clinical errors in judgment as a nurse? If so, what types of errors should be considered acceptable (if any), and what types are not acceptable?
4. Do you believe that the recent national spotlight on medical error identification and prevention will encourage the reporting of medical errors when they do occur?

EXTENDING THE LIABILITY

In recent years, the concept of *joint liability*, in which the nurse, physician, and employing organization are all held liable, has become the current position of the legal system. This probably more accurately reflects the higher level of accountability now present in the nursing profession. Before 1965, nurses were rarely held accountable for their own acts, and hospitals were usually exempt due to charitable immunity. However, following precedent-setting cases in the 1960s, employers are now held liable for the nurse's acts under a concept known as *vicarious liability*. One form of vicarious liability is called *respondeat superior*, which means "the master is responsible for the acts of his servants." The theory behind the doctrine is that an employer should be held legally liable for the conduct of employees whose actions he or she has a right to direct or control.

The difficulty in interpreting *respondeat superior* is that many exceptions exist. The first and most important exception is related to the state in which the nurse practices. In some states, the *doctrine of charitable immunity* applies, which holds that a charitable (nonprofit) hospital cannot be sued by a person who has been injured as a result of a hospital employee's negligence. Thus, liability is limited to the employee.

Another exception to *respondeat superior* occurs when the state or federal government employs the nurse. The common-law rule of *governmental immunity* provides that governments cannot be held liable for the negligent acts of their employees while carrying out government activities. Some states have changed this rule by statute, however, and in these particular jurisdictions, *respondeat superior* continues to apply to the acts of nurses employed by the state government.

Nurses must remember that the purpose of *respondeat superior* is not to shift the burden of blame from the employee to the organization but rather to share the blame, increasing the possibility of larger financial compensation to the injured party. Some nurses erroneously assume that they do not need to carry malpractice insurance because their employer will in all probability be sued as well and thus will be responsible for financial damages. Under the doctrine of *respondeat superior*, any employer required to pay damages to an injured person because of an employee's negligence may have the legal right to recover or be reimbursed that amount from the negligent employee.

One rule that all nurses must know and understand is that of *personal liability*, which says that every person is liable for his or her own conduct. The law does not permit a wrongdoer to avoid legal liability for his or her own wrongdoing, even though someone else also may be sued and held legally liable. For example, if a manager directs a subordinate to do something that both know to be improper, the injured party can recover damages against the subordinate even if the supervisor agreed to accept full responsibility for the delegation at the time. In the end, each nurse is always held liable for his or her own negligent practice.

Managers are not automatically held liable for all acts of negligence on the part of those they supervise, but they may be held liable if they were negligent in the supervision of those employees at the time that they committed the negligent acts. Brooke (2006a) states that nurses remain responsible for all delegated tasks and are legally and professionally responsible for directing and supervising the activities of other staff. Liability for negligence is generally based on the manager's failure to determine which of the patient needs can be assigned safely to a subordinate or the failure to supervise a subordinate adequately for the assigned task (Huston, 2006a). Both the abilities of the staff member and the complexity of the task assigned must be considered when determining the type and amount of direction and supervision warranted.

Hospitals have also been found liable for assigning personnel who were unqualified to perform duties as shown by their evaluation reports. Managers, therefore, need to be cognizant of their responsibilities in assigning and appointing personnel because they could be found liable for ignoring organizational policies or for assigning employees duties that they are not capable of performing. In such cases, though, the employee must provide the supervisor with the information that he or she is not qualified for the assignment. The manager does have the right to reassign employees as long as they are capable of discharging the anticipated duties of the assignment.

In addition, there has been a push to have more in-depth background checks when health care employees are hired, with some states already mandating such checks. In addition, federal legislation has recently been introduced along these lines. Indeed, some states are now requiring a criminal background check on all license renewals (Nursing News, 2004).

At present, except in a few states, personnel directors in hospitals (those making hiring decisions) are required to request information from the National Practitioner Data Bank only for those individuals who seek clinical privileges, and many states even require nursing students to be fingerprinted before they are allowed to work with vulnerable populations. In the future, hiring someone without an adequate background check, who later commits a crime involving a patient, could be another area of liability for the manager. This is an example of the type of pending legislation with which a manager must keep abreast so that if it becomes law, its impact on future management practices will be minimized.

LEARNING EXERCISE 5.4

Understanding Limitations and Rules
Have you ever been directed in your nursing practice to do something that you believed might be unsafe or that you felt inadequately trained or prepared to do? What did you do? Would you act differently if the situation occurred now? What risks are inherent in refusing to follow the direct orders of a physician or superior? What are the risks of performing a task that you believe may be unsafe?

INCIDENT REPORTS

Incident reports are records of unusual or unexpected incidents that occur in the course of a client's treatment. Because attorneys use incident reports to defend the health agency against lawsuits brought by clients, the reports are generally considered confidential communications and cannot be subpoenaed by clients or used as evidence in their lawsuits in most states. (Be sure, however, that you know the law for the state in which you live, as this does vary.) However, incident reports that are inadvertently disclosed to the plaintiff are no longer considered confidential and can be subpoenaed in court. Thus, a copy of an incident report should not be left in the chart. In addition, no entry should be made in the patient's record about the existence of an incident report. The chart should, however, provide enough information about the incident or occurrence so that appropriate treatment can be given.

INTENTIONAL TORTS

Torts are legal wrongs committed against a person or property, independent of a contract, that render the person who commits them liable for damages in a civil action. Whereas professional negligence is considered to be an *unintentional tort,* assault, battery, false imprisonment, - invasion of privacy, defamation, and slander are intentional torts. *Intentional torts* are a direct invasion of someone's legal rights. Managers are responsible for seeing that staff members are aware of and adhere to laws governing intentional torts. In addition, the manager must clearly delineate policies and procedures about these issues in the work environment.

Nurses can be sued for assault and battery. *Assault* is conduct that makes a person fearful and produces a reasonable apprehension of harm, and *battery* is an intentional and wrongful physical contact with a person that entails an injury or offensive touching (Nursing Malpractice, 2003). Unit managers must be alert to patient complaints of being handled in a rough manner or complaints of excessive force in restraining patients. In fact, performing any treatment without patient permission or without receiving an informed consent might constitute both assault and battery. In addition, many battery suits have been won based on the use of restraints when dealing with confused patients.

The use of physical restraints also has led to claims of *false imprisonment*. False imprisonment describes any unlawful confinement within fixed boundaries, and this confinement can be produced by physical, emotional, or chemical means (Nursing Malpractice, 2003). Practitioners are liable for false imprisonment when they unlawfully restrain the movement of their patients. Physical restraints should be applied only with a physician's direct order. Likewise, the patient who wishes to sign out against medical advice should not be held against his or her will. This tort also is frequently applicable to involuntary commitments to mental health facilities. Managers in mental health settings must be careful to institutionalize patients in accordance with all laws governing commitment. Finally, false imprisonment by chemical confinement occurs when drugs are given, not for their therapeutic value but to keep a patient within an institution (Nursing Malpractice, 2003).

Another intentional tort is defamation. *Defamation* is communicating to a third party false information that injures a person's reputation; causes economic damage; diminishes the esteem, respect, goodwill, or confidence that others have for the person; or causes adverse, derogatory, or unpleasant opinions of him (Nursing Malpractice, 2003). Being truthful reduces the risk of charges of defamation; however, "truth is no defense against charges of invasion of privacy, breach of confidentiality, or inflicting emotional distress" (p. 11).

OTHER LEGAL RESPONSIBILITIES OF THE MANAGER

Managers also have some legal responsibility for the quality control of nursing practice at the unit level, including such duties as reporting dangerous understaffing, checking staff credentials and qualifications, and carrying out appropriate discipline. Health care facilities may also be held responsible for seeing that staff know how to operate equipment safely. Bross (2005) says that there are many sources of liability within a health care facility, and they vary from facility to facility and from position to position.

For example, standards of care as depicted in policies and procedures may pose a liability for the nurse if such policies and procedures are not followed. The chain of command in reporting inadequate care by a physician is another area in which management liability may occur if employees are not taught proper protocols. Managers have a responsibility to see that written protocols, policies, and procedures are followed in order to reduce liability.

Additionally, the manager, like all professional nurses, is responsible for reporting improper or substandard medical care, child and elder abuse, and communicable diseases, as specified by the Centers for Disease Control and Prevention. Individual nurses also may be held liable for *product liability*. When a product is involved, negligence does not have to be proved. This strict liability is a somewhat gray area of nursing practice. Essentially, strict liability holds that a product may be held to a higher level of liability than a person. In other words, if it can be proved that the equipment or product had a defect that caused an injury, then it would be debated in court by using all the elements essential for negligence, such as duty or breach. Therefore, equipment and other products fall within the scope of nursing responsibility. In general, if they are aware that equipment is faulty, nurses have a duty to refuse to use the equipment. If the fault in the equipment is not readily apparent, risks are low that the nurse will be found liable for the results of its use.

Informed Consent

Many nurses erroneously believe that they have obtained informed consent when they witness a patient's signature on a consent form for surgery or procedure. Strictly speaking, *informed consent* (outlined in Display 5.3) can be given only after the patient has received a complete explanation of the surgery, procedure, or treatment and indicates that he or she understands the risks and benefits related to it.

 Informed consent is obtained only after the patient receives full disclosure of all pertinent information regarding the surgery or procedure and only if the patient understands the potential benefits and risks associated with doing so.

The information must be in a language that the patient can understand and should be conveyed by the individual who will be performing the procedure. Patients must be invited to ask questions and have a clear understanding of the options as well. "An informed consent is a process, not a paper" (Brooke, 2006b, p. 67).

Only a competent adult can legally sign the form that shows informed consent. To be considered competent, patients must be capable of understanding the nature and consequences of the decision and of communicating their decision. Spouses or other family members cannot legally sign unless there is an approved guardianship or conservatorship or unless they hold a durable power of attorney for health care. If the patient is under age 16 (18 in some states), a parent or guardian must generally give consent.

In an emergency, the physician can invoke *implied consent*, in which the physician states in the progress notes of the medical record that the patient is unable to sign but that treatment is

DISPLAY 5.3 Guidelines for Informed Consent

The person(s) giving consent must fully comprehend:

1. The procedure to be performed
2. The risks involved
3. Expected or desired outcomes
4. Expected complications or side effects that may occur as a result of treatment
5. Alternative treatments that are available

Consent may be given by:

1. A competent adult
2. A legal guardian or individual holding durable power of attorney
3. An emancipated or married minor
4. Mature minor (varies by state)
5. Parent of a minor child
6. Court order

EXAMINING THE EVIDENCE 5.1

Source: Barrett, R. (2005). Quality of informed consent: Measuring understanding among participants in oncology clinical trials. *Oncology Nursing Forum*, *32*(4), 751–755.

This descriptive, correlation study was carried out to describe subjects' knowledge and understanding of consent to a clinical trial.

The findings indicated that the subjects had a good overall understanding of the basic elements of informed consent but failed to understand the full implication of a clinical trial. The implications for nursing were a need to focus on the development of reliable tools to measure participants' understanding of informed consent and on nursing interventions that improve the informed consent process.

immediately needed and is in the patient's best interest. Usually, this type of implied consent must be validated by another physician.

Nurses frequently seek *express consent* from patients by witnessing patients sign a standard consent form. In express consent, the role of the nurse is to be sure that the patient has received informed consent and to seek remedy if he or she has not.

Informed consent does pose ethical issues for nurses. Although nurses are obligated to provide teaching and to clarify information given to patients by their physicians, nurses must be careful not to give new information that contradicts information given by the physician, thus interfering in the physician–patient relationship. The nurse is not responsible for explaining the procedure to be performed. The role, rather, is to advocate for patients by protecting their rights, preserving their dignity, identifying their fears, and determining their level of understanding and approval of the care to be given (Barrett, 2005). At times, this can be a cloudy issue both legally and ethically. Examining the Evidence 5.1 examines the quality of understanding of informed consent.

LEARNING EXERCISE 5.5

Is it Really Informed Consent?

You are a staff nurse on a surgical unit. Shortly after reporting for duty, you make rounds on all your patients. Mrs. Jones is a 36-year-old woman scheduled for a bilateral salpingo-oophorectomy and hysterectomy. In the course of conversation, Mrs. Jones comments that she is glad she will not be undergoing menopause as a result of this surgery. She elaborates by stating that one of her friends had surgery that resulted in "surgical menopause" and that it was devastating to her. You return to the chart and check the surgical permit and doctor's progress notes. The operating room permit reads "bilateral salpingo-oophorectomy and hysterectomy," and it is signed by Mrs. Jones. The physician has noted "discussed surgery with patient" in the progress notes.

You return to Mrs. Jones's room and ask her what type of surgery she is having. She states, "I'm having my uterus removed." You phone the physician and relate your information to the surgeon who says, "Mrs. Jones knows that I will take out her ovaries if necessary; I've discussed it with her. She signed the permit. Now, please get her ready for surgery—she is the next case."

● ASSIGNMENT: Discuss what you should do at this point. Why did you select this course of action? What issues are involved here? Be able to discuss legal ramifications of this case.

Medical Records

One source of information that people seek to help them make decisions about their health care is their medical record. Resnick (2005) maintains that "thorough and thoughtful documentation provides evidence against miscommunication and misunderstanding, and may guard against a lengthy litigation process" (p. 17). Nurses have a legal responsibility for accurately recording appropriate information in the client's medical record. The alteration of medical records can result in license suspension or revocation.

Although the patient owns the information in that medical record, the actual record belongs to the facility that originally made the record and is storing it. Although patients must have "reasonable access" to their records, the method for retrieving the record varies greatly from one institution to another. Generally, a patient who wishes to inspect his or her records must make a written request and pay reasonable clerical costs to make such records available. The health care provider generally permits such inspection during business hours within several working days of the inspection request. Nurses should be aware of the procedure for procuring medical records for patients at the facilities where they work. Often, a patient's attempt to procure medical records results from a lack of trust or a need for additional teaching and education. Nurses can do a great deal to reduce this confusion and foster an open, trusting relationship between the patient and his or her health care providers. Collaboration between health care providers and patients, and documentation thereof, is a good indication of well-provided clinical care.

 Successful clinical care is a collaborative effort with the provider and the patient. Documentation should reflect this shared effort. (Renick, 2005, p. 17)

LEARNING EXERCISE 5.6

Mrs. Brown's Chart

Mrs. Brown has been diagnosed with invasive cancer. She has been having daily radiation treatments. Her husband is a frequent visitor and seems to be a devoted husband. They are both very interested in her progress and prognosis. Although they have asked many questions and you have given truthful answers, you know little because the physician has not shared much with the staff. Today, you walk into Mrs. Brown's room and find Mr. Brown sitting at Mrs. Brown's bedside reading her chart. The radiation orderly had inadvertently left the chart in the room when Mrs. Brown returned from the x-ray department.

● ASSIGNMENT: Identify several alternatives that you have. Discuss what you would do and why. Is there a problem here? What follow-up is indicated? Attempt to solve this problem on your own before reading the sample analysis that follows.

Analysis

The nurse needs to determine the most important goal in this situation. Possible goals include (a) getting the chart away from Mr. Brown as soon as possible, (b) protecting the privacy of Mrs. Brown, (c) gathering more information, or (d) becoming an advocate for the Browns.

In solving the case, it is apparent that not enough information has been gathered. Mr. Brown now has the chart, and it seems pointless to take it away from him. Usually, the danger in patients' families reading the chart lies in the direction of their not understanding the chart and thereby obtaining confusing information or the patient's privacy being invaded because the patient has not consented to family members' access to the chart.

Using this as the basis for rationale, the nurse should use the following approach:

1. Clarify that Mr. Brown has Mrs. Brown's permission to read the chart by asking her directly.
2. Ask Mr. Brown if there is anything in the chart that he did not understand or anything that he questions. You may even ask him to summarize what he has read. Clarify the things that are appropriate for the nurse to address, such as terminology, procedures, or nursing care.
3. Refer questions that are inappropriate for the nurse to answer to the physician, and let Mr. Brown know that you will help him in talking with the physician regarding the medical plan and prognosis.
4. When finished talking with Mr. Brown, the nurse should request the chart and place it in the proper location. The incident should be reported to the immediate supervisor.
5. The nurse should follow through by talking with the physician about the incident and Mr. Brown's concerns and by assisting the Browns to obtain the information that they have requested.

Conclusion

The nurse first gathered more information before becoming the adversary or advocate. It is possible that the Browns had only simple questions to ask and that the problem was a lack of communication between staff and their patients rather than a physician–patient communication deficit. Legally, patients have a right to understand what is happening to them, and that should be the basis for the decisions in this case.

The Patient Self Determination Act

The Patient Self Determination Act (PSDA), enacted in 1991, required health care organizations that received federal funding to provide education for staff and patients on issues concerning treatment and end-of-life issues. This education included the use of *advanced directives* (AD), where written instructions regarding end-of-life care are completed by competent individuals, to be implemented should they become incapacitated in the future (Salmond & David, 2005).

The PSDA requires acute-care facilities to document on the medical record whether a patient has an advance directive and to provide written information to patients who do not. However, despite mechanisms within most health care institutions to provide this information, the AD completion rate remains low (Salmond & David, 2005). Therefore, the intent of the statute may be lost, and recent studies indicate that the low rate of completed ADs among the population, especially among ethnically diverse individuals, may indicate that the ADs as currently designed and implemented are not appropriate for all groups (Salmond & David, 2005). Examining the Evidence 5.2 reveals evidence found in one study.

Good Samaritan Laws

Good Samaritan laws state that health care providers are protected from potential liability if they volunteer their nursing skills away from the workplace, provided that actions taken are not grossly negligent. The focus of Good Samaritan laws, however, is limited to emergencies and does not cover nonemergent care or advice given to family, friends, and neighbors, even if unpaid (Brooke, 2004).

EXAMINING THE EVIDENCE 5.2

Source: Salmond, S. W., & David, E. (2005). Attitudes toward advance directives and advance directive completion rates. *Orthopaedic Nursing, 24*(2), 28–34.

This research was a descriptive correlation design using a survey of a convenience sample of patients admitted to a medical–surgical unit during a 2-month period. Although all patients received information on advance directives (AD), only 82% of the sample identified having received such information. Only 18% of the sample had completed an AD prior to admission, and another 8% completed an AD after an interview.

Implications were that low AD completion rates among the majority of the population—and even lower among ethnically diverse individuals despite favorable attitudes toward ADs—suggested that there are factors beyond access to information that may influence the decision not to complete an AD. The results of this study are congruent with other research, raising the question of whether ADs as currently designed are appropriate for all groups.

Most states have Good Samaritan laws to encourage health care providers to help victims in an emergency, although protection under these laws varies tremendously from state to state. In some states, the law grants immunity to RNs but does not protect LVNs or LPNs. Other states offer protection to anyone who offers assistance, even if they do not have a health care background. Nurses should be familiar with the Good Samaritan laws in their state. "All licensed nurses are expected to know their scope of practice and act within it unless the victim is in imminent danger of dying" (Brooke, 2004, p. 22).

Health Insurance Portability and Accountability Act of 1996

Another area of the law that nurses must understand is the right to confidentiality. "Privacy and confidentiality are basic rights in our society. Safeguarding those rights, with respect to an individual's personal health information, is our ethical and legal obligation as health care providers" (Erickson & Millar, 2005, p. 7). Unauthorized release of information or photographs in medical records may make the person who discloses the information civilly liable for invasion of privacy, defamation, or slander. Written authorization by the patient to release information is needed to allow such disclosure. Many nurses have been caught unaware by the telephone call requesting information about a patient's condition. It is extremely important that the nurse does not give out unauthorized information, regardless of the urgency of the person making the request. Likewise, managers must ensure that unauthorized people do not have access to patient charts or medical records and that unauthorized people are not allowed to observe procedures.

Efforts to preserve patient confidentiality increased tremendously with the passage of the *Health Insurance Portability and Accountability Act of 1996* (HIPAA; also known as the Kassebaum–Kennedy Act). HIPAA gave Congress a deadline of August 1999 to pass legislation protecting the privacy of health information and to improve the portability and continuity of health insurance coverage. When this did not happen, the Department of Health and Human Services (DHHS) stepped in and issued the appropriate regulations (Charters, 2003). The first version of the privacy rule was issued in December 2000 under the Clinton administration, but it was modified by the Bush administration before it was ever implemented (HHS Privacy, 2002). It continues to be modified even as it is being implemented. It behooves managers to be aware of the latest edition of this act.

HIPAA essentially represents two areas for implementation. The first is the *Administrative Simplification plan* and the second area includes the *Privacy Rules*. The Administrative Simplification plan is directed at restructuring the coding of health information to simplify the digital exchange of information among health care providers and to improve the efficiency of health care delivery. The privacy rules are directed at ensuring strong privacy protections for patient without threatening access to care (Erickson & Millar, 2005).

The Privacy Rule applies to three primary covered entities (CE): health plans, health care clearinghouses, and health care providers. It also covers all patient records and other individually identifiable health information used or disclosed by a CE in any form (electronic, paper, or oral) (Maddox, 2002). Although there are many components to HIPAA, key components of the Privacy Rule are that direct treatment providers must make a good faith effort to obtain written acknowledgement of the notice of privacy rights and practices from patients. In addition, health care providers must disclose protected health information to patients requesting their own information or when oversight agencies request the data (HHS Privacy, 2002). Reasonable efforts must be taken, however, to limit the disclosure of personal health information to the minimum information necessary to complete the transaction. There are situations, however, when limiting the information is not required. For example, a minimum of information is not required for treatment purposes, since it is clearly better to have too much information than too little.

The HIPAA Privacy Rule also requires that written authorization is needed before protected health information can be used for marketing purposes, such as selling lists of enrollees to third parties (Charters, 2003). The rule exempts face-to-face encounters or communication offering a promotional gift of nominal value.

Because of the complexity of the HIPAA regulations, it is not expected that a nursing manager would be responsible for compliance alone. Instead, it is most important that the manager work with the administrative team to develop compliance procedures. It is equally important that managers remain cognizant of ongoing changes to the guidelines and are aware of how rules governing these issues may differ in the state in which they are employed. Some provisions of the Privacy Rules mention "reasonable efforts" toward achieving compliance. It is important to realize that being reasonable is provision specific and does not apply to achieving compliance with the entire Privacy Rules. Enforcement of HIPAA falls to the Office of Civil Rights (2003), which states that it is taking a "cooperative" approach in helping covered entities achieve compliance.

Staff nurses are also impacted by HIPAA. Erickson & Millar (2005) say that there are many opportunities for private information to be inadvertently overheard, read, transmitted, or otherwise unintentionally disclosed as nurses go about their daily work. For example, nurses talking in elevators, the hospital gift shop, or in a restaurant for lunch need to be aware of their surroundings and remain alert about not revealing any patient information in a public place.

LEGAL CONSIDERATIONS OF MANAGING A DIVERSE WORKFORCE

Currently, minorities constitute about one quarter of the labor force, with a significant growth in the number of Hispanic, Asian, and African American employees expected over the next two decades. As will be discussed in later chapters, a primary area of diversity is language, including word meanings, accents, or dialects. Problems arising from this could be misunderstanding or reluctance to ask questions. Staff from cultures in which assertiveness is not promoted may find it difficult to disagree with or question others. How the manager handles these manifestations of cultural diversity is of major importance. If the manager's response is seen as discriminatory, the employee may file a complaint with one of the state or federal agencies that oversee civil rights or equal opportunity enforcement. Such things as overt or subtle discrimination are prohibited by Title VII (Civil Rights Act of 1964). Managers have a responsibility to be fair and just. Lack of promotions and unfair assignments may occur with minority employees just because they are different.

In addition, English-only rules in the workplace may be viewed as discriminatory under Title VII. Such rules may not violate Title VII if employers require English only during certain periods of time. Even in these circumstances, the employees must be notified of the rules and how they are to be enforced.

Clearly, managers should be taught how to deal sensitively and appropriately with an increasingly diverse workforce. Enhancing self-awareness and staff awareness of personal cultural biases, developing a comprehensive cultural diversity program, and role modeling cultural sensitivity are some of the ways that managers can effectively avoid many legal problems associated with discriminatory issues. However, it is hoped that future goals for the manager would go beyond compliance with Title VII and move toward understanding of and respect for other cultures.

PROFESSIONAL VERSUS INSTITUTIONAL LICENSURE

In general, a *license* is a legal document that permits a person to offer special skills and knowledge to the public in a particular jurisdiction when such practice would otherwise be unlawful. Licensure establishes standards for entry into practice, defines a scope of practice, and allows for disciplinary action. Currently, licensing for nurses is a responsibility of state boards of nursing or state boards of nurse examiners, which also provide discipline as necessary. The manager, however, is responsible for monitoring that all licensed subordinates have a valid, appropriate, and current license to practice.

Licensure is a privilege and not a right.

All nurses must safeguard the privilege of licensure by knowing the standards of care applicable to their work setting. Deviation from that standard should be undertaken only when nurses are prepared to accept the consequences of their actions, both in terms of liability and loss of licensure.

Nurses who violate specific norms of conduct, such as securing a license by fraud, performing specific actions prohibited by the nurse practice act, exhibiting unprofessional or illegal conduct, performing malpractice, and abusing alcohol or drugs, may have their licenses suspended or revoked by the licensing boards in all states. Frequent causes of license revocation are shown in Display 5.4.

DISPLAY 5.4   Common Causes of Professional Nursing License
Suspension or Revocation

- Professional negligence
- Practicing medicine or nursing without a license
- Obtaining a nursing license by fraud or allowing others to use your license
- Felony conviction for any offense substantially related to the function or duties of an RN
- Participating professionally in criminal abortions
- Not reporting substandard medical or nursing care
- Providing patient care while under the influence of drugs or alcohol
- Giving narcotic drugs without an order
- Falsely holding oneself out to the public or to any health care practitioner as a "nurse practitioner"

Typically, suspension and revocation proceedings are administrative. Following a complaint, the board of nursing completes an investigation. Most of these investigations reveal no grounds for discipline. If the investigation supports the need for discipline, nurses are notified of the charges and are allowed to prepare a defense. At the hearing, which is very similar to a trial, the nurse is allowed to present evidence. Based on the evidence, an administrative law judge makes a recommendation to the state board of nursing, which makes the final decision. The entire process, from complaint to final decision may take up to 2 years.

Some professionals have advocated shifting the burden of licensure, and thus accountability, from individual practitioners to an institution or agency. Proponents for this move believe that *institutional licensure* would provide more effective use of personnel and greater flexibility. Most professional nursing organizations oppose this move strongly because they believe that it has the potential for diluting the quality of nursing care.

An alternative to institutional licensure has been the development of *certification programs* by the ANA. By passing specifically prepared written examinations, nurses are able to qualify for certification in most nurse practice areas. This voluntary testing program represents professional organizational certification. In addition to ANA certification, other specialties, such as cardiac care, offer their own certification examinations. Many nursing leaders today strongly advocate professional certification as a means of enhancing the profession. However, "certification is really only helpful in determining a nurse's continued competence if that nurse is functioning in the areas of his or her certified competence" (Huston, 2006b, p. 360).

INTEGRATING LEADERSHIP ROLES AND MANAGEMENT FUNCTIONS IN LEGAL AND LEGISLATIVE ISSUES

Legislative and legal controls for nursing practice have been established to clarify the boundaries of nursing practice and to protect clients. The leader uses established legal guidelines to role model nursing practice that meets or exceeds accepted standards of care. Leaders also are role models in their efforts to expand expertise in their field and to achieve specialty certification. Perhaps the most important leadership roles in law and legislation are those of vision, risk taking, and energy. The leader is active in professional organizations and groups that define what nursing is and what it should be in the future. This is an internalized responsibility that must be adopted by many more nurses if the profession is to be a recognized and vital force in the political arena.

Management functions in legal and legislative issues are more directive. Managers are responsible for seeing that their practice and the practice of their subordinates are in accord with current legal guidelines. This requires that managers have a working knowledge of current laws and legal doctrines that affect nursing practice. Because laws are not static, this is an active and ongoing function. The manager has a legal obligation to uphold the laws, rules, and regulations affecting the organization, the patient, and nursing practice.

Managers have a responsibility to be fair and nondiscriminatory in dealing with all members of the workforce, including those whose culture differs from their own. The effective leader goes beyond merely preventing discriminatory charges and instead strives to develop sensitivity to the needs of a culturally diverse staff.

The integrated leader–manager reduces the personal risk of legal liability by creating an environment that prioritizes patient needs and welfare. In addition, caring, respect, and honesty as part of nurse–patient relationships are emphasized. If these functions and roles are truly integrated, the risks of patient harm and nursing liability are greatly reduced.

Key Concepts

* *Sources of law* include constitutions, statutes, administrative agencies, and court decisions.
* The burden of proof required to be found guilty and the punishment for the crime varies significantly between *criminal*, civil, and *administrative* courts.
* *Nurse practice acts* define and limit the practice of nursing in each state.
* Professional organizations generally espouse standards of care that are higher than those required by law. These voluntary controls often are forerunners of legal controls.
* Legal doctrines such as *stare decisis* and *res judicata* frequently guide courts in their decision making.
* Currently, licensing for nurses is a responsibility of state boards of nursing or state boards of nurse examiners. These state boards also provide discipline as necessary.
* Some professionals have advocated shifting the burden of licensure, and thus accountability, from individual practitioners to an institution or agency. Many professional nursing organizations oppose this move.
* *Malpractice* or *professional negligence* is the failure of a person with professional training to act in a reasonable and prudent manner. Five components must be present for an individual to be found guilty of malpractice.
* Employers of nurses can now be held liable for an employee's acts under the concept of *vicarious liability*.
* Each person, however, is liable for his or her own tortuous conduct.
* Managers are not automatically held liable for all acts of negligence on the part of those they supervise, but they may be held liable if they were negligent in supervising those employees at the time that they committed the negligent acts.

* While professional negligence is considered to be an unintentional tort, assault, battery, false imprisonment, invasion of privacy, defamation, and slander are intentional torts.
* Consent can be either *informed*, *implied*, or *expressed*. Nurses need to understand the differences between these types of consents and use the appropriate one.
* Although the patient owns the information in a medical record, the actual record belongs to the facility that originally made it and is storing it.
* It has been shown that despite good technical competence, nurses who have difficulty establishing positive interpersonal relationships with clients and their families are at greater risk of being sued.
* Each nurse should be aware how laws such as Good Samaritan immunity or legal access to incident reports are implemented in the state in which they live.
* New legislation pertaining to confidentiality (HIPAA) and patient rights (e.g., PSDA) continue to shape nurse—client interactions in the health care system.

ADDITIONAL LEARNING EXERCISES AND APPLICATIONS

LEARNING EXERCISE 5.7

Where Does Your Responsibility Lie?

Mrs. Shin is a 68-year-old patient with liver cancer. She has been admitted to the oncology unit at Memorial Hospital. Her admitting physician has advised chemotherapy, even though she believes that there is little chance of it working. The patient asks her doctor, in your presence, if there is an alternative treatment to chemotherapy. She replies, "Nothing else has proved to be effective. Everything else is quackery, and you would be wasting your money." After the doctor leaves, the patient and her family ask you if you know anything about alternative treatments. When you indicate that you do have some current literature available, they beg you to share your information with them.

● ASSIGNMENT: What do you do? What is your legal responsibility to your patient, the doctor, and the hospital? Using your knowledge of the legal process, the nurse practice act, patients' rights, and legal precedents (look for the case *Tuma v. Board of Nursing*, 1979), explain what you would do, and defend your decision.

LEARNING EXERCISE 5.8

Legal Ramifications for Exceeding One's Duties

You have been the evening charge nurse in the emergency room at Memorial Hospital for the last 2 years. Besides yourself, you have two LVNs and four RNs working in your department. Your normal staffing is to have two RNs and one LVN on duty Monday through Thursday and one LVN and three RNs on during the weekend.

It has become apparent that one of the LVNs, Maggie, resents the recently imposed limitations of LVN duties because she has had 10 years of experience in nursing, including a tour of duty as a medic in the first Gulf War. The emergency room physicians admire her and are always

(Learning Exercise continues on page 116)

asking her to assist them with any major wound repair. Occasionally, she has exceeded her job description as an LVN in the hospital, although she has done nothing illegal of which you are aware. You have given her satisfactory performance evaluations in the past, even though everyone is aware that she sometimes pretends to be a "junior physician." You also suspect that the physicians sometimes allow her to perform duties outside her licensure, but you have not investigated this or actually seen it yourself.

Tonight, you come back from supper and find Maggie suturing a deep laceration while the physician looks on. They both realize that you are upset, and the physician takes over the suturing. Later, the doctor comes to you and says, "Don't worry! She does a great job, and I'll take the responsibility for her actions." You are not sure what you should do. Maggie is a good employee, and taking any action will result in unit conflict.

● ASSIGNMENT: What are the legal ramifications of this case? Discuss what you should do, if anything. What responsibility and liability exist for the physician, Maggie, and yourself? Use appropriate rationale to support your decision.

LEARNING EXERCISE 5.9

To Float or Not to Float

You have been an obstetrical staff nurse at Memorial Hospital for 25 years. The obstetrical unit census has been abnormally low lately, although the patient census in other areas of the hospital has been extremely high. When you arrive at work today, you are told to float to the thoracic surgery critical care unit. This is a highly specialized unit, and you feel ill prepared to work with the equipment on the unit and the type of critically ill patients who are there. You call the staffing office and ask to be reassigned to a different area. You are told that the entire hospital is critically short staffed, that the thoracic surgery unit is four nurses short, and that you are at least as well equipped to handle that unit as the other three staff who also are being floated. Now your anxiety level is even higher. You will be expected to handle a full RN patient load. You also are aware that more than half the staff on the unit today will have no experience in thoracic surgery. You consider whether to refuse to float. You do not want to place your nursing license in jeopardy, yet you feel conflicting obligations.

● ASSIGNMENT: To whom do you have conflicting obligations? You have little time to make this decision. Outline the steps that you use to reach your final decision. Identify the legal and ethical ramifications that may result from your decision. Are they in conflict?

(Web Links)──────────────────────────────

Managed Care & Patient Privacy
http://www.managedcareandpatientprivacy.com/
Collection of newspaper articles dealing with managed care and patient privacy issues.

Office for Civil Rights—HIPAA
http://www.hhs.gov/ocr/hipaa/
View the Department of Health and Human Services recommendations on the confidentiality of individual identifiable health information.

Nursing & Health Care Directories on: The Nursefriendly Nursing Malpractice Case Studies by Date

http://www.lopez1.com/lopez/clinical.cases/nursing.malpractice.cases.by.date.htm
Provides a summary of precedent cases involving nurses in malpractice cases and includes URL addresses to more comprehensive legal summaries.

University of Cincinnati College of Law—Legal Resources for the Nurse–Paralegal

http://www.law.uc.edu/library/nurse.pdf
Comprehensive bibliography for the nurse–paralegal.

References

Barrett, R. (2005). Quality of informed consent: Measuring understanding among participants in oncology clinical trials. *Oncology Nursing Forum, 32*(4),751–755.

Brooke, P. S. (2006a). Taking heat for an error. *Nursing2006, 36*(3), 10.

Brooke, P. S. (2006b). Signed, sealed, delivered. *Nursing2006, 36*(2), 67.

Brooke, P. S. (2004). Stretching the Good Samaritan law. *Nursing2004, 34*(7), 22.

Bross, W. (2005). Healthcare contracts, organizational responsibility and licensing. *The Alabama Nurse, 33*(3), 3.

Charters, K. G. (2003). HIPAA's latest privacy rule. *Policy, Politics and Nursing Practice, 4*(1), 21–25.

Erickson, J. L., & Millar, S. (2005). Caring for patients while respecting their privacy: Renewing our commitment. *Online Journal of Issues in Nursing, 10*(2), 1–11.

HHS privacy rule's marketing provisions criticized by Kennedy as not strong enough. (2002). *Federal News, 10,* 1115.

Huston, C. J. (2006a). Unlicensed assistive personnel and the registered nurse. In C. J. Huston (Ed.), *Professional issues in nursing* (p. 157). Philadelphia: Lippincott Williams & Wilkins.

Huston, C. J. (2006b). Assuring provider competence through licensure, continuing education and certification. In C. J. Huston (Ed.), *Professional issues in nursing* (p. 360). Philadelphia: Lippincott Williams & Wilkins.

Joint Commission on Accreditation of Healthcare Organizations. (2005). *Health care in the crossroads: Strategies for improv-ing the medical liability system and preventing patient injury.* Oakbrook Terrace, IL: Author.

Klutz, D. L. (2004). Tort reform: An issue for nurse practitioners. *Journal of the American Academy of Nurse Practitioners, 16*(2), 70–75.

Maddox, P. J. (2002). HIPAA: Update on rule revisions and compliance requirements. *Nursing Economics, 20*(2), 88–92.

Murphy, E. K. (2004). Judicial recognition of nursing as a unique profession. *AORN Journal, 80*(5), 924–927.

Nursing malpractice: Understanding the risks. (2003, June). In *Travel nursing 2003:* Supplement to *Nursing2003, 33*(6), 7–12.

Nursing News. (2004). Criminal background checks: It's the law! *Nursing News, 28*(1), 1–5.

Office of Civil Rights (last revised August, 2003). HIPAA. Retrieved January 7, 2004, from *http://www.hhs.gov/ocr/hipaa/*.

Resnick, B. (2004). Documentation: Proactive prevention of litigation. *Nursing Service Organization.* (2004, Fall). Retrieved August 27, 2007, from http://nso.com/newsletters/advisor/2004_fall/documentation.php.

Smith, A. P. (2005). As we lie in the bed we made: The malpractice and regulatory consequences of failing leadership. *Nursing Economics, 23*(2), 97–99.

Salmond, S. W., & David, E. (2005). Attitudes toward advance directives and advance directive completion rates. *Orthopaedic Nursing, 24*(2), 28–34.

White, K. (2005). Medical malpractice: A crisis in cost and access. *Nursing Management, 36*(3), 22–25.

Bibliography

Alley, N. M. (2005). Nurses' promise to safeguard the public: Is it time for nationally mandated background checks? *JONA's Healthcare Law, Ethics and Regulation, 7*(4), 119–124.

Austin, S. (2005). Hold the phone: Are you liable for telephone advice? *Nursing2005, 35*(10), 54–55.

Boliin, J. N. (2005). When nurses are reported to the National Practitioner's Data Bank. *Journal of Nursing Law, 10*(3), 114–148.

Carol, R. (2005, Winter). Overcoming bias in the nursing workplace: Whether it's racist remarks from patients, problems with culturally insensitive co-workers or being passed up for a promotion because of your race or gender, the key is to stay cool and know your rights. *Minority Nurse,* 28–32.

Henson, S. W. (2005). Legal and regulatory education and training needs in the healthcare industry. *JONA's Healthcare Law, Ethics and Regulation, 7*(4), 114–118.

Hogue, E. E. (2005). Liability for failure to provide CSE management services. *Care Management, 11*(5), 27.

Jacobson, J. (2005). AJN reports. When providing care is a moral issue: Is nurses' first priority protecting the patient or their own moral convictions? *American Journal of Nursing, 105*(10), 27–28.

King, T. L. (2005). Is collaborative practice a malpractice risk? Myth versus reality. *Journal of Midwifery and Women's Health, 50*(6), 451–452.

Ryan, B. A. (2005). Advice of counsel. Pregnancy may not merit special treatment. *RN, 68*(11), 70.

Wimberley, P. (2005). Faculty forum. HIPAA and nursing education: How to teach in a paranoid health care environment. *Journal of Nursing Education, 44*(11), 489–492.

Zink, S. (2005). Informed consent. *Progress in Transplantation, 15*(4), 371–378.

6

Patient, Subordinate, and Professional Advocacy

> . . . to see what is right, and not do it, is want of courage, or of principles.
>
> —*Confucius*

> . . . in our imperfect state of conscience and enlightenment, publicity and the collision resulting from publicity are the best guardians of the interest in the sick.
>
> —*Florence Nightingale*

*A*dvocacy—helping others to grow and self-actualize—is a critically important leadership role. Many of the leadership skills that will be described in the following chapters, such as risk taking, vision, self-confidence, ability to articulate needs, and assertiveness, are used in the advocacy role.

Managers, by virtue of their many roles, must be advocates for the profession, subordinates, and patients. The actions of an advocate are to inform others of their rights and to ascertain that they have sufficient information on which to base their decisions. The term *advocacy* can be stated in its simplest form as standing up for what one believes in for both self and others (Corish, 2005).

Foley (2004) defined *nursing advocacy* as representing patients when they are not able to speak for themselves and maintains that nurturing advocacy by nurse administrators may be crucial to nurse retention. The goals of the advocate are to inform, enhance autonomy, and respect the decisions of others.

Advocacy has been recognized as one of the most vital and basic roles of the nursing profession since the time of Florence Nightingale. The role, however, is complex. Nurses may act as advocates by promoting informed decisions, by acting as liaison, or by interceding for another individual (Smith, 2004).

Nurses may act as advocates by either helping others make informed decisions, by acting as an intermediary in the environment, or by directly intervening on the behalf of others.

This chapter will examine the processes through which advocacy is learned as well as the ways in which leader–managers can advocate for their patients, subordinates, and the profession. The role of "whistle-blower" as an advocacy role will be discussed. Specific suggestions for interacting with legislators and the media to influence health policy are included. Leadership roles and management functions essential for advocacy are shown in Display 6.1.

BECOMING AN ADVOCATE

Foley (2004) suggested that although advocacy is assumed to be an inherent part of all nursing curricula and present in all clinical practice settings, the nursing literature contains little descrip-

DISPLAY 6.1 **Leadership Roles and Management Functions Associated With Advocacy**

Leadership Roles

1. Creates a climate where advocacy and its associated risk taking are valued
2. Seeks fairness and justice for individuals who are unable to advocate for themselves
3. Seeks to strengthen patient and subordinate support systems to encourage autonomous, well-informed decision making
4. Influences others by providing information necessary to empower them to act autonomously
5. Assertively advocates on behalf of patients and subordinates when an intermediary is necessary
6. Participates in professional nursing organizations and other groups that seek to advance the profession of nursing
7. Role models proactive involvement in health care policy through both formal and informal interactions with the media and legislative representatives

Management Functions

1. Gives subordinates and patients adequate information to make informed decisions
2. Assures that rights and values of patients supersede those of their health care providers
3. Seeks appropriate consultation when advocacy results in intrapersonal or interpersonal conflict
4. Promotes and protects the workplace safety and health of subordinates and patients
5. Encourages subordinates to bring forth concerns about the employment setting and seeks impunity for whistle blowers
6. Demonstrates the skills needed to interact appropriately with the media and legislators regarding nursing and health care issues
7. Is aware of current legislative efforts affecting nursing practice and organizational and unit management

DISPLAY 6.2   **Nursing Values Central to Advocacy**

1. Each individual has a right to autonomy in deciding what course of action is most appropriate to meet his or her health care goals.
2. Each individual has a right to hold personal values and to use those values in making health care decisions.
3. All individuals should have access to the information they need to make informed decisions and choices.
4. The nurse must act on behalf of patients who are unable to advocate for themselves.
5. Empowerment of patients and subordinates to make decisions and take action on their own is the essence of advocacy.

tion of how nurses learn the advocacy role. However, Corish (2005) feels that often new nurses have not had much practice acting as advocates and that it is up to nurse–leaders to assist staff in developing advocacy skills. She maintains that this can be done by teaching such skills in orientation, identifying senior nurses who can demonstrate the appropriate communication in the advocacy role, and helping staff to understand the difference between assertive and aggressive advocacy.

Regardless of how advocacy is learned, there are nursing values central to advocacy. These values emphasize caring, autonomy, respect, and empowerment (Display 6.2).

LEARNING EXERCISE 6.1

Values and Advocacy
How important a role do you believe advocacy to be in nursing? Do you believe that your willingness to assume this role is a learned value? Were the values of caring and service emphasized in your family and/or community when you were growing up? Have you identified any role models in nursing who actively advocate for patients, subordinates, or the profession? What strategies might you use as a new nurse to impart the need for advocacy to your peers and to the student nurses who work with you?

PATIENT ADVOCACY AND PATIENT RIGHTS

Standard V, Number 3, of the American Nurses Association (ANA) Standards of Professional Performance in Clinical Practice (1998) states that the nurse acts as a patient advocate and assists patients in developing skills so that they can advocate for themselves. This patient advocacy is necessary because disease almost always results in decreased independence, loss of freedom, and interference with the ability to make choices autonomously. Benner (2003) concurs, arguing that being a "good" practitioner means more than just examining patient rights; it requires that we are moved

DISPLAY 6.3   Common Areas Requiring Nurse–Patient Advocacy

1. End of life decisions
2. Technological advances
3. Health care reimbursement
4. Access to health care
5. Provider–patient conflicts regarding expectations and desired outcomes
6. Withholding of information or blatant lying to patients
7. Insurance authorizations, denials, and delays in coverage
8. Medical errors
9. Patient information disclosure (privacy and confidentiality)
10. Patient grievance and appeals processes
11. Cultural and ethnic diversity and sensitivity
12. Respect for patient dignity
13. Inadequate consents
14. Incompetent health care providers
15. Complex social problems including AIDS, teenage pregnancy, violence, poverty
16. Aging population

by the patient's plight and that we respond to the patient as a person. Thus, advocacy becomes the foundation and essence of nursing, and nurses have a responsibility to promote human advocacy.

Managers also must advocate for patients with regard to distribution of resources and the use of technology. The advances in science and limits of financial resources have created new problems and ethical dilemmas. For example, although diagnosis-related groupings may have eased the strain on government fiscal resources, they have created ethical problems, such as patient dumping, premature patient discharge, and inequality of care. Common areas in which nurses must advocate for patients are shown in Display 6.3.

First- and middle-level managers are in the best position to advocate for patients affected by such problems. Benner (2003) states:

> Meeting patients and their families and recognizing their concerns about healthcare comprise the everyday ethical comportment of the practitioner. Patients and families, while encouraged to become empowered and take more responsibility for their health, are often vulnerable due to lack of knowledge of healthcare or due to crisis and reduced capacities. Thus, ethically and legally, healthcare workers are expected to act in the best interests of patients (p. 374).

It is important, however, for the patient advocate to know the difference between controlling patient choices and assisting patients to choose. Nurses must not use paternalism as a means to reduce patient autonomy. A true nurse advocate acts for the patient even when the decisions of the patient differ from those of the nurse (Hickman, 2004; Walsh, 2005).

 It is important for the patient advocate to be able to differentiate between controlling patient choices (domination and dependence) and in assisting patient choices (allowing freedom).

Although Smith (2004) says that the philosophical debate around the role of nurses as patient advocates continues, she maintains that the term *patient advocacy* represents a need that can be described as a commitment to uncompromised professional practice. "The conditions contributing to the need for advocacy include the vulnerability created by illness, the complexity of health information, the complexity of health care systems and the resulting risk for loss of basic human rights through truly informed consent and self-determination" (p. 88).

LEARNING EXERCISE 6.2

Culture and Decisions

You are a staff nurse on a medical unit. One of your patients, Mr. Dau, is a 56-year-old Hmong immigrant to the United States. He has lived in the United States for 4 years and became a citizen 2 years ago. His English is marginal, although he understands more than he can verbalize. He was admitted to the hospital with sepsis resulting from urinary tract infection. His condition is now stable.

Today, Mr. Dau's physician informed him that his CT scan shows a large tumor in his prostrate that is likely cancer. The physician wants to do immediate follow-up testing and surgical resection of the tumor to relieve his symptoms of hesitancy and urinary retention. Although the tumor is probably cancerous, the physician believes that it will respond well to traditional oncology treatments. The expectation is that Mr. Dau should recover fully.

One hour later, when you go in to check on Mr. Dau, you find him sitting on his bed with his suitcase packed, waiting for a ride home. He informs you that he is checking out of the hospital. He states that he believes he can make himself better at home with herbs and through prayers by the Hmong "faith healer." He concludes by telling you, "if I am meant to die, there is little anyone can do." When you reaffirm the hopeful prognosis reported by his physician that morning, Mr. Dau says "The doctor is just trying to give me false hope. I need to go home and prepare for my death."

● ASSIGNMENT: What should you do? How can you best advocate for this patient? Is the problem a lack of information? How does culture play a role in the patient's decision? Does a lack of understanding on this patient's part justify paternalism?

The legislative controls of nursing practice primarily protect the rights of patients. Until the 1960s, patients had few rights; in fact, patients often were denied basic human rights during a time when they were most vulnerable. Since that time, the National League for Nursing (NLN), the American Hospital Association, and many states such as California have passed a bill of rights for patients (Display 6.4).

A *bill of rights* that has become law or state regulation has the most legal authority because it provides the patient with legal recourse. A bill of rights issued by health care organizations and professional associations is not legally binding but may influence federal or state funding and certainly should be considered professionally binding. However, although there has been significant progress in the field of patient rights since 1960, such as HIPAA—the new privacy law (Erickson & Millar, 2005)—there is still no comprehensive federal legislation, except the privacy law, that is directed to the granting and protection of other patient rights.

Today, patients are more assertive and involved in their health care. They have more information to review when looking at treatment options and are demanding to be participants in decisions about their health care. The client's right to information and participation in medical care decisions has led to conflicts in the areas of informed consent and access to medical records. Although the manager has a responsibility to see that all patient rights are met in the unit, the areas that are particularly sensitive involve the right to privacy and personal liberty, both guaranteed by the Constitution.

DISPLAY 6.4 List of Patient Rights in California

In accordance with section 70707 of the California Administrative Code, the hospital and medical staff have adopted the following list of patient rights to:

1. Exercise these rights without regard to sex; cultural, economic, educational, or religious background; or the source of payment for care.
2. Considerate and respectful care.
3. Knowledge of the name of the physician who has primary responsibility for coordinating care and the names and professional relationships of other physicians who will see the patient.
4. Receive information from physician about illness, course of treatment, and prospects for recovery in terms the patient can understand.
5. Receive as much information about any proposed treatment or procedure as the patient may need to give informed consent or to refuse this course of treatment. Except in emergencies, this information shall include a description of the procedure or treatment, the medically significant risks involved in this treatment, alternate course of treatment or nontreatment and the risks involved in each, and the name of the person who will carry out the procedure or treatment.
6. Participate actively in decisions regarding medical care. To the extent permitted by law, this includes the right to refuse treatment.
7. Full consideration of privacy concerning medical care program. Case discussion, consultation, examination, and treatment are confidential and should be conducted discreetly. The patient has the right to be advised of the reason for the presence of any individual.
8. Confidential treatment of all communications and records pertaining to the patient's care and stay in the hospital. Written permission shall be obtained before medical records are made available to anyone not directly concerned with the patient's care.
9. Reasonable responses to any reasonable requests for service.
10. Ability to leave the hospital even against the advice of the physician.
11. Reasonable continuity of care and to know in advance the time and location of appointment and the physician providing care.
12. Be advised if hospital/personal physician proposes to engage in or perform human experimentation affecting care or treatment. The patient has the right to refuse to participate in such research projects.
13. Be informed by the physician or a delegate of the physician of continuing health care requirements following discharge from the hospital.
14. Examine and receive an explanation of the bill, regardless of source of payment.
15. Know which hospital rules and policies apply to the patient's conduct.
16. Have all patient's rights apply to the person who may have legal responsibility to make decisions regarding medical care on behalf of the patient.

Source: Available at *http://www.calpatientguide.org/index.html*.

Subordinate Advocacy

Standard V of the ANA Scope and Standards for Nurse Administrators (2004) suggests that nurse administrators should advocate for subordinates as well as patients. *Subordinate advocacy* is a neglected concept in management theory but is an essential part of the leadership role. In this area of advocacy, the manager must help subordinates to resolve ethical problems and live with the solutions at the unit level.

Smith (2004) suggests that organizations and leaders within organizations have a responsibility to followers in their organization for creating a climate of patient advocacy. For example, leaders must create a work environment for subordinates that promotes empowerment so that they have the courage to speak up for patients. "In its broadest definition, the endpoint of nurse advocacy can be patient advocacy" (p. 90).

The following are suggestions for creating an environment that promotes subordinate advocacy:

- Invite collaborative decision making.
- Listen to staff needs.
- Get to know staff personally.
- Take time to understand the challenges faced by the staff in delivering care.
- Face challenges and solve problems together.
- "Go to bat" for staff when needed.
- Promote shared governance.
- Empower staff.
- Promote nurse autonomy.
- Provide staff with workable systems.

Managers must recognize what subordinates are striving for and the goals and values that subordinates consider appropriate. The leader–manager should be able to guide subordinates toward actualization while defending their right to autonomy. To help nurses deal with ethical dilemmas in their practice, nurse–managers should establish and utilize appropriate support groups, ethics committees, and channels for dealing with ethical problems.

Another critical part of subordinate advocacy is *workplace advocacy*. In this type of advocacy, the manager works to see that the work environment is both safe and conducive to professional and personal growth for subordinates. Occupational health and safety must be assured by interventions such as reducing worker exposure to needle sticks or blood and body fluids. Subordinates should also be able to have the expectation that their work hours and schedules will be reasonable, that staffing ratios will be adequate to support safe patient care, that wages will be fair and equitable, and that nurses will be allowed participation in organizational decision making. When these working conditions do not exist, managers must advocate to higher levels of the administrative hierarchy to correct the problems.

Upper-level managers can advocate for subordinates in a different way. For example, when the health care industry has faced the crisis of inadequate human resources and nursing shortages, many organizations have made quick, poorly thought-out decisions to find short-term solutions to a long-term and severe problem. New workers have been recruited at a phenomenally high cost, yet the problems that caused high worker attrition have not been solved. Upper-level managers must advocate for subordinates in solving problems and making decisions about how best to use limited resources. These decisions must be made carefully, following a thorough examination of the political, social, economic, and ethical costs.

WHISTLE-BLOWING AS ADVOCACY

The public has become much more aware of ethical malfeasance within its institutions and corporate organizations as a result of various scandals that have occurred in the last 50 years. From Watergate to Enron, the American public has been fed a diet of wrongdoing that has led to an increase in moral awareness. Wrongdoing does not stop at large corporations or political activity, it also occurs within health care organizations. When it occurs within a health care institution, nurses must individually or collectively take action. Such action may lead to what is often referred to as whistle-blowing.

Huston (2006a) states that there are basically two types of whistle-blowing. Internal whistle-blowing occurs within an organization, reporting up the chain of command. External whistle-blowing involves reporting outside the organization such as the media or an elected official. An example of whistle-blowing by a nurse might be to report abuse to a patient by one of the physicians. Huston states, "In an era of managed care, declining reimbursements and the ongoing pressure to remain fiscally solvent, the risk of fraud, misrepresentation, and ethical malfeasance in healthcare organizations has never been higher. As a result, the need for whistle-blowing has also likely never been greater " (p. 297). While much of the public wants wrongdoing or corruption to be reported, such behavior is often looked upon with distrust, and whistle-blowing individuals may be considered disloyal. Upper-level managers must be willing to advocate for the so-called whistle-blower.

 Upper-level managers must also be willing to advocate for *whistle-blowers*, who speak out about organizational practices that they believe may be harmful or inappropriate.

Subordinates want the assurance that if they are acting within the scope of their expertise, they will be able to speak up through appropriate channels without fear of retaliation (Huston, 2006a). While whistle-blower protection has been advocated for at the federal level and has passed in some states, many employees are reluctant to report unsafe conditions for fear of retaliation. Nurses should check with their state association to assess the status of whistle-blower protection in their state. At present, there is no universal legal protection for whistle-blowers in the United States. However, the United Kingdom does have legislation that protects employees (Huston, 2006a).

LEARNING EXERCISE 6.3

How Can You Best Advocate?

You are a unit supervisor in a skilled nursing facility. One of your aides, Martha Greenwald, recently reported that she suffered a "back strain" several weeks ago when she was lifting an elderly patient. She did not report the injury at the time because she did not think it was serious. Indeed, she finished the remainder of her shift and has performed all of her normal work duties since that time.

Today, Martha reports that she has just left her physician's office and that he has advised her to take 4 to 6 weeks off from work to fully recover from her injury. He has also prescribed physical therapy and electrical nerve stimulation for the chronic pain. Martha is a relatively new employee, so she has not yet accrued enough sick leave to cover her absence. She asks you to complete the paperwork for her absence and the cost of her treatments to be covered as a work-related injury.

When you contact the workers' compensation case manager for your facility, she states that the claim will be investigated; however, with no written or verbal report of the injury at the time it occurred, there is great likelihood that the claim will be rejected.

● ASSIGNMENT: How best can you advocate for this subordinate?

PROFESSIONAL ADVOCACY

Managers also must be advocates for the nursing profession. This type of advocacy has a long history in nursing. It was nurses who pushed for accountability through state nurse practice acts and state licensing, although this was not accomplished until 1903. Huston (2006b) states that "nurse leaders collaborated on defining the profession, achieving legal recognition of the profession and establishing a culture for professional nursing which has continued to the present time" (p. 464). Advocating for professional nursing is a leadership role.

Joining a profession requires making a personal decision to involve oneself in a system of socially defined roles. Thus, entry into a profession involves a personal and public promise to serve others with the special expertise that a profession can provide and that society legitimately expects it to provide.

Professional issues are always ethical issues. When nurses find a discrepancy between their perceived role and society's expectations, they have a responsibility to advocate for the profession. At times, individual nurses believe that the problems of the profession are too big for them to make a difference; however, their commitment to their profession obligates them to ask question and think about problems that affect the profession. They cannot afford to become powerless or helpless or claim that one person cannot make a difference. Often, one voice is all it takes to raise the consciousness of colleagues within a profession.

> A professional commitment means that people cannot shrink from their duty to question and contemplate problems that face the profession.

If nursing is to advance as a profession, practitioners and managers must broaden their sociopolitical knowledge base to better understand the bureaucracies in which they live. This includes speaking out on consumer issues, continuing and expanding attempts to influence legislation, and increasing membership on governmental health policy-making boards and councils. Only then will nurses be able to influence the tremendous problems facing society today in terms of the homeless, teenage pregnancy, drug and alcohol abuse, inadequate health care for the poor and elderly, and medical errors. These are essential advocacy roles for the profession.

There are many ways that both the profession and individual nurses can advocate to advance social issues. For example, the ANA has advocated for more diversity in nursing. A leadership role would be one that supports and advocates for diversity within an organization. In April 2002, the ANA and more than 60 other partner organizations issued a report entitled *Nursing's Agenda for the Future*, which detailed the complex factors leading to and exacerbating the current nursing shortage.

Other issues that the ANA and its constituent member associations have been working to bring attention to include the impact of the current nursing shortage on the quality of care; staffing ratios; and working conditions for nurses, including mandatory overtime. Indeed, the ANA has created a Center for American Nurses (CAN) that is devoted to workplace advocacy to address workplace issues for all ANA members (Hatmaker, 2004).

Blakeney (2003) suggests that other organizations outside of nursing are also stepping forward to bring these issues to the attention of the public, media, and policy makers. For example, in July 2002, the U.S. Department of Health and Human Services released a report entitled *Projected Supply, Demand, and Shortages of Registered Nurses: 2000–2020*. In August 2002, The Joint Commission released *Health Care at the Crossroads: Strategies for Addressing the Evolving*

Nursing Crisis. In addition, Johnson and Johnson Health Care Systems Inc. launched a $20 million campaign in February 2002 to attract more people to nursing and to increase awareness of the value of the nursing profession in society and America's health care system (Nursing Shortage, 2002).

LEARNING EXERCISE 6.4

Write It Down. What Would You Change?
List five things that you would like to change about nursing or the health care system. Prioritize the changes that you have identified. Write a one-page essay about the change that you believe is most needed. Identify the strategies that you could use individually and collectively as a profession to make the change happen. Be sure that you are realistic about the time, energy, and fiscal resources you have to implement your plan.

Nursing's Advocacy Role in Legislation and Public Policy

A distinctive feature of American society is the manner in which citizens can participate in the political process. People have the right to express their opinions about issues and candidates by voting. People also have relatively easy access to lawmakers and policy makers and can make their individual needs and wants known. Theoretically, then, any one person can influence those in policy-making positions. In reality, this rarely happens; policy decisions are generally focused on group needs or wants.

Much attention has recently been paid to nurses and the importance of the nursing profession and how nurses impact health care delivery. This has been especially true in the areas of patient safety and staff shortages. Both Smith (2004) and Green and Jordan (2004) cite the Institute of Medicine's (IOM) recent report *Keeping Patients Safe: Transforming the Work Environment for Nurses* (2004) as evidence that quality of nursing has an impact on health care and is gaining national attention. Smith suggests that reports such as these may be a boon for clarifying public policy and nursing, and they serve to solidify patient advocacy in the professional practice of nurses. She states that "The imperative for action, the political and popular pressures, and the regulatory obligations have never been so clear" (p. 90).

Nurses in Canada echo the call for active involvement in the political process. Falk-Rafael (2005) maintains that political, social, and economic action is an expression of caring that enacts Nightingale's legacy of political activism. "Nurses, who practice at the intersection of public policy and personal lives are, therefore, ideally situated and morally obligated to include political advocacy and efforts to influence health policy in their practice. The health of the public and the future of the profession may depend upon it" (p. 212).

Using research to influence health care policy is another avenue open to nurses. Examining the Evidence 6.1 shows an example of nursing research that could be used to effect public policy. This is an example of community health nurses recognizing a problem and using evidenced-base practices to demonstrate a need for assistance to low-income families. These families were coping with being health care providers while attempting to remain employed. The research demonstrated an overlooked aspect of welfare reform and showed that public health nurses were uniquely positioned to be policy advocates.

In addition to nurse–leaders and individual nurses, there is a need for collective influence to impact health care policy. The need for organized group efforts by nurses to influence legislative

EXAMINING THE EVIDENCE 6.1

Source: Kneipp, S. M., Castelman, J. B., & Gailor, N. (2004). The informal caregiving burden: An overlooked aspect of the lives and health of women transitioning from welfare to employment. *Public Health Nursing, 21*(1), 24–31.

This study examined the extent of informal caregiver burden in low-income women transitioning off welfare and the relationship between caregiving and continued employment. The random sample was 32 adults. More than 30% of the participants reported having to leave a job within the past year because of caregiving responsibilities. Caregiver burden scores were highest in the time-dependence dimension of caregiving.

The researchers concluded that the public health nurses were uniquely positioned to partner with local welfare-to-work organizations, to educate program staff, and to further develop existing caregiving assessment processes.

policy has long been recognized in this country. In fact, the first state associations were organized expressly for unifying nurses to influence the passage of state licensure laws. *Political action committees* (PACs) of the Congress of Industrial Organizations attempt to persuade legislators to vote in a particular way. Lobbyists of the PAC may be members of a group interested in a particular law or paid agents of the group that wants a specific bill passed or defeated. Nursing must become more actively involved with PACs to influence health care legislation, and PACs provide one opportunity for small donors to feel like they are making a difference.

In addition, professional organizations generally espouse standards of care that are higher than those required by law. Voluntary controls often are forerunners of legal controls. What nursing is and should be depends on nurses taking an active part in their professional organizations.

 Nurses who participate in professional organizations are integral in determining whether voluntary or legal controls represent what nursing is and should be.

Currently, nursing lobbyists in our nation's capital are influencing legislation on quality of care, access to care issues, patient and health-worker safety, health care restructuring, direct reimbursement for advanced practice nurses, and funding for nursing education. Representatives of the ANA regularly attend and provide testimony for meetings of the U.S. Department of Health and Human Services, the Department of Health, the National Institutes of Health, the Occupational Safety and Health Administration (OSHA), and the White House to be sure that the "nursing perspective" is heard in health policy issues (Huston, 2006c).

As a whole, the nursing profession has not yet recognized the full potential of collective political activity. Nurses must exert their collective influence and make their concerns known to policy makers before they can have a major impact on political and legislative outcomes. Because they have been reluctant to become politically involved, nurses have failed to have a strong legislative voice in the past. Legislators and policy makers are more willing to deal with nurses as a group rather than as individuals; thus, joining and supporting professional organizations allows nurses to become active in lobbying for a stronger nurse practice act or for the creation or expansion of advanced nursing roles.

In addition to active participation in national nursing organizations, nurses can influence legislation and health policy in many other ways. Nurses who want to be directly involved can lobby legislators either in person or by letter. This process may seem intimidating to the new nurse; however, there are many books and workshops available that deal with the subject and a common format is used.

Personal letters are more influential than form letters, and the tone should be formal but polite. The letter should also be concise (no more than one page). Be sure to address the legislator properly by title. Establish your credibility early in the letter as both a constituent and as a health care expert. State your reason for writing the letter in the first paragraph, and refer to the specific bill that you are writing about. Then, state your position on the issue, and give personal examples as necessary to support your position. Offer your assistance as a resource person for additional information. Sign the letter, including your name and contact information. Remember to be persistent, and write legislators repeatedly who are undecided on an issue. Display 6.5 displays a format common to letters written to legislators.

DISPLAY 6.5 Sample: A Letter to a Legislator

March 15, 2007

The Honorable John Doe
Member of the Senate
State Capitol, Room ____
City, State, Zip Code

Dear Senator Doe,

I am a registered nurse and member of the American Nurses Association (ANA). I am also a constituent in your district. I am writing in support of SB XXX, which requires the establishment of minimum RN staffing ratios in acute care facilities. As a staff nurse on an oncology unit in our local hospital, I see firsthand the problems that occur when staffing is inadequate to meet the complex needs of acutely ill patients: medical errors, patient and nurse dissatisfaction, workplace injuries, and perhaps most importantly, the inability to spend adequate time with and comfort patients who are dying.

I have enclosed a copy of a recent study conducted by John Smith and published in the January 2007 edition of *Nurses Today*. This article details the positive impact of legislative staffing ratio implementation on patient outcomes as measured by medication errors, patient falls, and nosocomial infection rates.

I strongly encourage you to vote for SB XXX when it is heard by the Senate Business and Professions Committee next week. Thank you for your ongoing concern with nursing and health care issues and for your past support of legislation to improve health care staffing. Please feel free to contact me if you have any questions or would like additional information
Respectfully,

Nurse Nancy

Nurse Nancy, R.N., B.S.N.
Street
City, State, Zip Code
Phone number including area code
Email address

Other nurses may choose to monitor the progress of legislation, count congressional votes, and track a specific legislator's voting intents as well as past voting records. Still other nurses may choose to join *network groups*, where colleagues meet to discuss professional issues and pending legislation.

For nurses interested in a more indirect approach to professional advocacy, their role may be to influence and educate the public about nursing and the nursing agenda to reform health care. This may be done by speaking with professional and community groups about health care and nursing issues and by interacting directly with the media. Never underestimate the influence that a single nurse may have even in writing letters to the editor of local newspapers or by talking about nursing and health care issues with friends, family, neighbors, teachers, clergy, and civic leaders.

LEARNING EXERCISE 6.5

Realistic Advocacy for the Nursing Profession
Do you belong to your state nursing organization or student nursing organization? Why or why not? Make a list of six other things that you could do to advocate for the profession. Be specific. Is your list realistic in terms of your energy and commitment to nursing?

Nursing and the Media

Although nurses have the greatest expertise about nursing issues, too few are willing to interact with the media about vital nursing and health care issues. This is especially unfortunate because both the media and the public place a high trust in nurses and want to hear about health care issues from a nursing perspective. Despite this, there remains many false stereotypes of nurses and nursing in the media, both regarding who they are and what they do. Nurses have some responsibility to correct false assumptions about nurses.

Many nurses avoid media exposure because they believe that they lack the expertise to do so or because they lack self-confidence. The reality is that the responsibility for nursing's image as perceived by the public lies solely upon the shoulders of those who claim nursing as their profession. "Until such time as nurses are able to agree upon the desired collective image and are willing to do what is necessary to both tell and show the public what that image is, little will change" (Huston, 2006d, p. 408).

Nurses should take every opportunity to appear in the media—in newspapers, radio, and television. Trossman (2003) suggests that nurses can ease into the spokesperson role by first presenting information on a current or controversial health care topic in a group setting where they already feel comfortable. Nurses should also complete special training programs to increase their self-confidence in working with journalists and other media representatives. Regardless, the first few media interactions will likely be stressful, just like any new task or learning. Trossman, however, offers the following basic tips to help nurses navigate media waters (Display 6.6):

- Be prepared or at least as prepared as possible given a reporter's deadline. This means researching the topic if there is time, knowing up-to-date information, and knowing three to four facts or figures that can be cited about pertinent issues.
- Stick to three or four key points that will drive home your message, and repeat them during the interview.

DISPLAY 6.6   Tips for Interacting With the Media

1. Be prepared.
2. Meet the reporter's deadlines.
3. Know three to four facts or figures that can be cited about pertinent issues.
4. Stick to three or four clear, concise key points and repeat them during the interview.
5. Stay on track by sticking to predetermined points.
6. Avoid negative language, and focus on solutions or strategies to solve problems.
7. Do not be afraid to say you do not have enough information to answer a question.

Source: Adapted from Trossman, S. (2003). Media relations 101. *American Journal of Nursing, 103*(1), 69–70.

- Make it easy for the media by providing them with clear, concise information and by meeting the reporter's deadlines.
- Stay on track by sticking to predetermined points, using phrases such as "I think the important point is. . . ." Also, avoid repetition of any negative language that a reporter might pick up on and instead focus on solutions or strategies to solve problems.
- Do not be afraid to say that you do not have enough information or expertise to answer a question. Be sure not to guess when factual data is needed.

The bottom line is that "stories about health care are hot" right now and nurses need to be able to respond "when the iron is hot" (Trossman, 2003, p. 69) to advocate both for their profession and for the clients they serve.

LEARNING EXERCISE 6.6

Preparing for a Media Interview

You are the staffing coordinator for a medium-sized community hospital in California. Minimum staffing ratios were implemented in January 2004. While this has represented an even greater challenge in terms of meeting your organization's daily staffing needs, you believe that the impetus behind the legislative mandate was sound. You also are a member of the state nursing association that sponsored this legislation and wrote letters of support for its passage. The hospital that employs you and the state hospital association fought unsuccessfully against the passage of minimum staffing ratios.

The local newspaper contacted you this morning and wants to interview you about staffing ratios in general as well as how these ratios are impacting the local hospital. You approach your chief nursing officer (CNO), and she tells you to go ahead and do the interview if you want but to remember that you are a representative of the hospital.

● ASSIGNMENT: Assume that you have agreed to participate in the interview.
   1. How might you go about preparing for the interview?
   2. Identify three or four factual points that you can state during the interview as your sound bytes. What would be your primary points of emphasis?
   3. Is there a way to reconcile the conflict between your personal feelings about staffing ratios and those of your employer? How would you respond if asked directly by the reporter to comment about whether staffing ratios are a good idea?

INTEGRATING LEADERSHIP ROLES AND MANAGEMENT FUNCTIONS IN ADVOCACY

Nursing leaders and managers recognize that they have an obligation not only to advocate for the needs of their patients, subordinates, and themselves at a particular time but also to be active in furthering the goals of the profession. To accomplish all of these types of advocacy, nurses must value autonomy and empowerment.

However, the leadership roles and management functions to achieve advocacy with patients, subordinates, and for the profession differ greatly. Advocating for patients requires that the manager create a work environment that recognizes patient's needs and goals as paramount. This means creating a work culture where patients are respected, well informed, and empowered. The leadership role required to advocate for patients is often one of risk taking, particularly when advocating for a client may be in direct conflict with a provider or institutional goal. Leaders must also be willing to accept and support patient choices that may be different from their own.

Advocating for subordinates requires that the manager create a safe and equitable work environment where employees feel valued and appreciated. When working conditions are less than favorable, the manager is responsible for relaying these concerns to higher levels of management and advocating for needed changes. The same risk taking that is required in patient advocacy is a leadership role in subordinate advocacy, since subordinate needs and wants may be in conflict with the organization. There is always a risk that the organization will view the advocate as a troublemaker, but this does not provide an excuse for managers to be complacent in this role. Managers also must advocate for subordinates in creating an environment where ethical concerns, needs, and dilemmas can be openly discussed and resolved.

Advocating for the profession requires that the nurse–manager be informed and involved in all legislation affecting the unit, organization, and the profession. The manager also must be an astute handler of public relations and demonstrate skill in working with the media. It is the leader, however, who proactively steps forth to be a role model and active participant in educating the public and improving health care through the political process.

Key Concepts

- *Advocacy* is helping others to grow and self-actualize and is a leadership role.
- Managers, by virtue of their many roles, must be advocates for patients, subordinates, and the profession.
- It is important for the patient advocate to be able to differentiate between controlling patient choices (domination and dependence) and in assisting patient choices (allowing freedom).
- Since the 1960s, the NLN, the American Hospital Association, and many states have passed *bills of rights for patients*. Although these are not legally binding, they can be used to guide professional practice.
- In *workplace advocacy*, the manager works to see that the work environment is both safe and conducive to professional and personal growth for subordinates.
- Professional issues are ethical issues. When nurses find a discrepancy between their perceived role and society's expectations, they have a responsibility to advocate for the profession.
- If nursing is to advance as a profession, practitioners and managers must broaden their sociopolitical knowledge base to better understand the bureaucracies in which they live.

* Because legislators and policy makers are more willing to deal with nurses as a group rather than as individuals, joining and actively supporting professional organizations allow nurses to have a greater voice in health care and professional issues.
* Nurses need to exert their collective influence and make their concerns known to policy makers before they can have a major impact on political and legislative outcomes.
* Nurses have great potential to educate the public and influence policy through the media as a result of the public's high trust in nurses and because the public wants to hear about health care issues from a nursing perspective.

ADDITIONAL LEARNING EXERCISES AND APPLICATIONS

LEARNING EXERCISE 6.7

Ethics and Advocacy

You are a new graduate staff nurse in a home health agency. One of your clients is a 23-year-old male with acute schizophrenia who was just released from the local county, acute-care, behavioral health care facility, following a 72-hour hold. He has no insurance. His family no longer has contact with him, and he is unable to hold a permanent job. He is noncompliant in taking his prescription drugs for schizophrenia. He is homeless and has been sleeping and eating intermittently at the local homeless shelter; however, he was recently asked not to return because he is increasingly agitated and, at times, violent. He calls you today and asks you "to help him with the voices in his head."

You approach the senior RN case manager in the facility for help in identifying options for this individual to get the behavioral health care services that he needs. She suggests that you tell the patient to go to Maxwell's Mini Mart, a local convenience store, at 3 PM today and wait by the counter. Then, she tells you that you should contact the police at 2:55 PM and tell them that Maxwell's Mini Mart is being robbed by your patient so that he will be arrested. She states, "I do this with all of my uninsured mental health patients, since the state Medicaid program offers only limited mental health services and the state penal system provides full mental health services for the incarcerated." She goes on to say that the store owner and the police are aware of what she is doing and support the idea, since it is the only way "patients really have a chance of getting better." She ends the conversation by saying, "I know you are a new nurse and don't understand how the real world works, but the reality is that this is the only way I can advocate for patients like this, and you need to do the same for your patients."

● ASSIGNMENT:
1. Will you follow the advice of the senior RN case manager?
2. If not, how else can you advocate for this patient?

LEARNING EXERCISE 6.8

Letter Writing in Advocacy

Identify three legislative bills affecting nursing that are currently being considered either in committee, the House of Representatives, or the Senate. Select one, and draft a letter to your state assemblyperson, representative, or senator regarding your position on the bill.

LEARNING EXERCISE 6.9

Determining Nursing's Entry Level

Grandfathering is the term used to grant certain people working within the profession for a given period of time or prior to a deadline date the privilege of applying for a license without having to take the licensing examination. Grandfathering clauses have been used to allow licensure for wartime nurses—those with on-the-job training and expertise—even though they did not graduate from an approved school of nursing.

Some professional nursing organizations are once again proposing that the BSN become the entry-level requirement for professional nursing. Some have suggested that as a concession to current ADN and diploma-prepared nurses, all nurses who have passed the state board of registered nursing licensure examination before the new legislation, regardless of educational preparation or experience, would retain the title of professional nurse. Non-baccalaureate nurses after that time would be unable to use the title of professional nurse.

● ASSIGNMENT: Do you believe that the "BSN as entry level" proposal advocates the advancement of the nursing profession? Is grandfathering conducive to meeting this goal? Would you personally support both of these proposals? Does the long-standing internal dissension about making the BSN the entry level into professional nursing reduce nursing's status as a profession? Do lawmakers or the public understand this dilemma or care about it?

LEARNING EXERCISE 6.10

How Would You Proceed?

You are an RN case manager for a large insurance company. Sheila Johannsen is a 34-year-old mother of two small children. She was diagnosed with advanced, metastatic breast cancer 6 months ago. Traditional chemotherapy and radiation seem to have slowed the spread of the cancer, but the prognosis is not good.

Sheila contacted you this morning to report that she has been in contact with a physician at one of the most innovative medical centers in the country. He told her that she might benefit from an experimental gene therapy treatment; however, she is ineligible for participation in the free clinical trials since her cancer is so advanced. The cost for the treatment is approximately $150,000. Sheila states that she does not have the financial resources to pay for the treatment and begs you "to do whatever you can to get the insurance company to pay. Otherwise, she will die."

You know that the cost of experimental treatments is almost always disallowed by your insurance company. You also know that even with the experimental treatment, Sheila's probability of a cure is very small.

● ASSIGNMENT: Decide how you will proceed. How can you best advocate for this patient?

LEARNING EXERCISE 6.11

Conflict of Values

Following is a case study that deals with individual and organizational or professional values and how they may conflict. Read the case, and answer the questions that follow. Use some form of group process in your decision making.

Your next-door neighbor, Joe, is a 75-year-old man with multiple chronic health problems. His history includes four prior myocardial infarctions, implantation of a pacemaker, open-heart surgery, an inoperable abdominal aneurysm, repeated episodes of congestive heart failure, and cardiac arrhythmias. Because of his poor health, he cannot operate the small business he owns or work for any length of time at his gardening or other hobbies. Both Joe and his wife talk about his "impending" death as a relief to his nearly constant discomfort and depression. Although his wife cares very much for him, the constant emotional and physical strain on her is very apparent. Joe is aware of this.

During the 3 years that you have been Joe's neighbor, both he and his wife have called on you as a neighbor, friend, and nurse. Frequently, they request that you auscultate Joe's chest to confirm the recurrence of heart failure. They rely on your judgment as to whether further medical care is needed. You have assisted and taught them about the multiple medications that Joe takes daily. Your nursing assessments confirm the poor prognosis that Joe's doctor has given.

One weekend, as you are leisurely enjoying your lunch, Joe's granddaughter appears at your door, frantically begging you to come quickly because "something is wrong with Grandpa." When you arrive with your stethoscope, you find Joe lying on the floor in his hobby shop; he has no pulse or respirations. He is grossly cyanotic and cool and has a small laceration on his chin that probably occurred when he fell. Joe had been noticeably absent for about 10 to 15 minutes before family members, visiting for the weekend, found him.

Joe's wife and family implore you to do something for him. "Do anything you can. Please help him. Hurry," Joe's wife states. As you begin cardiopulmonary resuscitation (CPR), you realize that many members of the family do not understand what is happening or what you are doing. Joe's wife, although shaken, is fairly calm and rational. She is reassuring her family that something is being done and that Joe's pain and suffering are almost over. After 10 minutes of continuous CPR with no change in Joe's condition, you hear the distant approach of an ambulance. Joe's wife, also hearing the ambulance, places her hand on your back to signal your attention. She says she has had a chance to think now and wants you to stop CPR: "Let Joe be. His pain is over."

You immediately wonder about the legal ramifications of stopping CPR without an order and are reluctant to stop. At the same time, you reflect on the gentleness of this man and the quality of his life during the last few years. As the siren draws nearer (you are still doing CPR), his wife becomes hysterical and begs for you to stop. After repeatedly asking her if she is sure, you stop CPR. A family member meets the ambulance at the driveway to inform the team that their services are not desired. His wife very tenderly takes Joe's head in her lap and says her good-byes.

At that moment, the paramedics enter and tell Joe's wife that the law specifies that they must implement basic life support. They also inform her that once the emergency medical support system is activated, it cannot be canceled, leaving Joe's wife aghast and speechless. Although the paramedics have already restarted CPR, you repeat the patient and spouse's wishes and the patient's medical history. You tell them that the arrest was unwitnessed and that 15 minutes had probably elapsed before CPR was started. You inform them that CPR has just been stopped at the family's insistence. The paramedics make you feel as if you were somehow morally and legally negligent for stopping CPR.

You begin to feel helpless as IV lines are established and drug therapy is initiated. Joe is intubated and defibrillated many times as his family watches this technical display with apparent horror. Joe's wife is quiet with resignation. Joe is transported to the hospital by ambulance, where he is pronounced dead 2 hours after CPR was initiated.

● ASSIGNMENT: In an ideal situation, you would have discussed more clearly with Joe and his wife what his wishes would be in a situation like this, and you could act accordingly. Unfortunately, however, as all too often in real life, this did not happen. This real case happened before the introduction of advanced directives and living wills.

The final decision about whether to start or stop CPR typically reflects one's values. It also requires a determination of whose needs and wants should be paramount in this case: your own, Joe's wife and family, or Joe himself. How would you have responded if you were the neighbor in this situation? Would your actions have been different if Joe were a stranger and the same situation occurred? How could you have advocated for the patient and family as the RN on the ambulance crew? How does a health care professional decide what to do when advocating for a patient or family poses a potential conflict with professional values?

Web Links

ANA—PAC
http://www.nursingworld.org/gova/federal/gfederal.htm
This American Nurses Association web page has a large selection of political action sites to choose from.

ANA—National Awards Program
http://www.nursingworld.org/HomepageCategory/Announcements/NominationsforANANationalAwards.aspx
This American Nurses Association web page details the award criteria and includes nomination forms for the Staff Nurse Advocate of the Year Award. The Staff Nurse Advocacy Award was established in 1998 to recognize excellence in individual staff nurses who provide direct patient care in all practice settings and who have advocated for their patients.

Judge David L. Bazelon Center for Mental Health Law
http://www.bazelon.org/about/index.htm
This center is one of the nation's leading advocates for people with mental disabilities, with precedent-setting litigation outlawing institutional abuse and providing protections against arbitrary confinement.

The Electronic Policy Network
http://movingideas.org/
A source for current public policy issues, including health care policy. Provides search engine for current policy issues.

Foundation for Informed Medical Decision Making
http://www.fimdm.org/
The primary mission of the Foundation for Informed Medical Decision Making (FIMDM) is to strengthen the role that patients play in selecting treatments for their medical conditions. The site includes a bibliography as well as helpful links.

Sigma Theta Tau International: Media Guide to Health Care Experts
http://www.nursingsociety.org/media/ME_intro.html
Source for health care experts from various medical specialties and practices who are willing to interact with the media.

References

American Nurses Association. (1998). *Standards of clinical nursing practice* (2nd ed.). Washington, DC: American Nurses Publishing.

American Nurses Association. (2004). *Scope and standards for nurse administrators* (2nd ed.). Washington, DC: American Nurses Publishing.

Benner, P. (2003). Current controversies in critical care. Enhancing patient advocacy and social ethics. *American Journal of Critical Care, 12*(4), 374–375.

Blakeney, B. (2003, January). Addressing the nursing shortage. *American Journal of Nursing. 103*(suppl), 16.

Corish, C. L. (2005). Advocacy—The power to influence. *Journal of Oncology Nursing, 9*(4), 478.

Erickson, J. L., & Millar, S. (2005). Caring for patients while respecting their privacy: Renewing our commitment. *Online Journal of Nursing Issues, 10*(2), 1–11.

Falk-Rafael, A. (2005). Speaking truth to power: Nursing's legacy and moral imperative. *Advances in Nursing Sciences, 28*(3), 212–223.

Foley, B. J. (2004). Advocacy: A skill that must be nurtured. Retrieved August 10, 2006, from *http://nsweb.nursingspectrum.com/cfforms/GuestLecture/AdvocacySkill.cfm.*

Green, A., & Jordan, C. B. (2004). Common denominators: Shared governance and work place advocacy—Strategies for nurses to gain control over their practice. *Online Journal of Issues in Nursing, 9*(1), 1–7.

Hatmaker, D. (2004, September–October). President's column: A passion for workplace advocacy. *American Nurse, 26*(5), 13.

Retrieved August 19, 2006, from *http://www.Nursing World. org.*

Hickman, S. E. (2004). Honoring resident autonomy in long-term care. *Journal of Psychosocial Nursing, 42*(1),12–16.

Huston, C. (2006a). Whistle-blowing in nursing. In C. Huston (Ed.), *Professional issues in nursing.* Philadelphia: Lippincott Williams & Wilkins.

Huston, C. (2006b). Nursing's professional associations by Marjorie Beyers. In C. Huston (Ed.), *Professional issues in nursing.* Philadelphia: Lippincott Williams & Wilkins.

Huston, C. (2006c). Nursing and public policy: Getting involved. In C. Huston (Ed.), *Professional issues in nursing.* Philadelphia: Lippincott Williams & Wilkins.

Huston, C. (2006d). Professional identity and image. In C. Huston (Ed.), *Professional issues in nursing.* Philadelphia: Lippincott Williams & Wilkins.

Institute of Medicine. (2004). *Keeping patients safe: Transforming the work environment for nurses.* Washington, DC: The National Academies Press.

Nursing shortage: Johnson & Johnson campaign aims to increase awareness, generate interest. (2002). *Nursing Economics, 20*(2), 93–95.

Smith, A. P. (2004). Patient advocacy: Roles for nurses and leaders. *Nursing Economics, 22*(2), 88–90.

Trossman, S. (2003). Media relations 101. *American Journal of Nursing, 103*(1), 69–70.

Walsh, D. (2005). Professional power and maternity care: The many faces of paternalism. *British Journal of Midwifery, 13*(11), 708.

Bibliography

Beu, B. (2004). Health policy issues. Advocacy day preview—Meeting with success. *AORN Journal, 80*(3), 563–565.

Bruhn, J. G. (2005). The lost art of the covenant: Trust as a commodity in health care. *Practice Nurse, 24*(4), 311–319.

Dumpel, H. (2006). Technology and patient advocacy: RNs must exercise independent judgment at all times. *California Nurse, 101*(4), 18–19.

Erlen, J. A. (2004). Functional health illiteracy: Ethical concerns. *Orthopaedic Nursing, 23*(2), 150–153.

Hellquist, K., & Spector, N. (2004). Building a sphere of influence. *Journal of Nursing Administration's Healthcare Law and Regulation, 6*(2), 42–43.

Kim, S. H. (2005). Deferred decision making: Patients' reliance on family and physicians for CPR decisions in critical care. *Nursing Ethics, 12*(5), 493–506.

Meeker, M. A. (2004). Family surrogate decision making at the end of life: Seeing them through with care and respect. *Qualitative Health Research*, *14*(2), 204–225.

Partin, B. (2006). Advocacy in practice. Who, if not you, will determine NP scope of practice? *Nurse Practitioner*, *31*(2), 6.

Pearch, J. (2005). Restraining children for clinical procedures. *Paediatric Nursing*, *17*(9), 36–38.

Roberts, D. (2004). Advocacy through patient teaching. *MEDSURG Nursing*, *13*(6), 363, 382.

Sellman, D. (2005). Towards an understanding of nursing as a response to human vulnerability. *Nursing Philosophy*, *6*(1), 2–10.

Stinson, C. K., Godkin, J., & Robinson, R. (2004). Ethical dilemma: Voluntarily stopping eating and drinking. *Dimensions of Critical Care Nursing*, *23*(1) 38–43.

7

Operational and Strategic Planning

. . . in the absence of clearly defined goals, we are forced to concentrate on activity and ultimately become enslaved by it.

—Chuck Conradt

. . . he who fails to plan, plans to fail.

—Anonymous

Planning is critically important to and precedes all other management functions. Without adequate planning, the management process fails and organizational needs and objectives cannot be met. *Planning* may be defined as deciding in advance what to do; who is to do it; and how, when, and where it is to be done. Therefore, all planning involves choosing among alternatives.

All planning involves choice: A necessity to choose from among alternatives.

This implies that planning is a proactive and deliberate process that reduces risk and uncertainty. It also encourages unity of goals and continuity of energy expenditure (human and fiscal resources) and directs attention to the objectives of the organization. Adequate planning also provides the manager with some means of control and encourages the most appropriate use of resources.

In effective planning, the manager must identify short- and long-term goals and changes needed to ensure that the unit will continue to meet its goals. Identifying such short- and long-term goals requires leadership skills such as vision and creativity, since it is impossible to plan what cannot be dreamed or envisioned. Likewise, planning requires flexibility and energy—two other leadership characteristics. Yet planning also requires management skills such as data gathering, forecasting, and transforming ideas into action.

Unit II focused on several aspects of planning, including strategic and operational planning, planned change, time management, fiscal planning, and career planning. This chapter deals with skills needed by the leader–manager to implement strategic and operational planning. In addition, the leadership roles and management functions involved in developing, implementing, and evaluating the planning hierarchy are discussed (Display 7.1).

DISPLAY 7.1 **Leadership Roles and Management Functions Associated With Operational and Strategic Planning**

Leadership Roles

1. Assesses the organization's internal and external environment in forecasting and identifying driving forces and barriers to strategic planning
2. Demonstrates visionary, innovative, and creative thinking in organizational and unit planning, thus inspiring proactive rather than reactive planning
3. Influences and inspires group members to be actively involved in long-term planning
4. Periodically completes value clarification to increase self-awareness
5. Encourages subordinates toward value clarification by actively listening and providing feedback
6. Communicates and clarifies organizational goals and values to subordinates
7. Encourages subordinates to be involved in policy formation, including developing, implementing, and reviewing unit philosophy, goals, objectives, policies, procedures, and rules
8. Is receptive to new and varied ideas
9. Role models proactive planning methods to subordinates

Management Functions

1. Is knowledgeable regarding legal, political, economic, and social factors affecting health care planning
2. Demonstrates knowledge of and uses appropriate techniques in both personal and organizational planning
3. Provides opportunities for subordinates, peers, competitors, regulatory agencies, and the general public to participate in planning
4. Coordinates unit-level planning to be congruent with organizational goals
5. Periodically assesses unit constraints and assets to determine available resources for planning
6. Develops and articulates a unit philosophy that is congruent with the organization's philosophy
7. Develops and articulates unit goals and objectives that reflect unit philosophy
8. Develops and articulates unit policies, procedures, and rules that put unit objectives into operation
9. Periodically reviews unit philosophy, goals, policies, procedures, and rules and revises them to meet the unit's changing needs
10. Actively participates in organizational strategic planning, defining and operationalizing such strategic plans at the unit level

PROACTIVE PLANNING

Planning has a specific purpose and is one approach to developing strategy. In addition, planning represents specific activities that help to achieve objectives; therefore, planning should be purposeful and proactive. Although there is always some crossover between types of planning within organizations, there is generally an orientation toward one of four planning modes: reactive planning, inactivism, preactivism, or proactive planning.

Reactive planning occurs *after* a problem exists. Because there is dissatisfaction with the current situation, planning efforts are directed at returning the organization to a previous, more comfortable state. Frequently, in reactive planning, problems are dealt with separately without integration with the whole organization. In addition, because it is done in response to a crisis, this type of planning can lead to hasty decisions and mistakes.

Inactivism is another type of conventional planning. Inactivists seek the status quo, and they spend their energy preventing change and maintaining conformity. When changes do occur, they occur slowly and incrementally.

A third planning mode is *preactivisim*. Preactive planners utilize technology to accelerate change and are future oriented. Unsatisfied with the past or present, preactivists do not value experience and believe that the future is always preferable to the present.

The last planning mode is *interactive* or *proactive planning*. Planners who fall into this category consider the past, present, and future and attempt to plan the future of their organization rather than react to it. Because the organizational setting changes often, adaptability is a key requirement for proactive planning.

> Proactive planning is dynamic, and adaptation is considered to be a key requirement since the environment changes so frequently.

Proactive planning occurs, then, in anticipation of changing needs or to promote growth within an organization and is required of all leader–managers so that personal as well as organizational needs and objectives are met.

LEARNING EXERCISE 7.1

What Is Your Planning Style?
Individually write a plan for the current year. How would you describe your planning? Which type of planner are you? Write a brief essay that describes your planning style. Use specific examples and then share your insights in a group.

Forecasting

A mistake common to novice managers is a failure to complete adequate proactive planning. Instead, many managers operate in a crisis mode and fail to use available historical patterns to assist them in planning. Nor do they examine present clues and projected statistics to determine future needs. In other words, they fail to forecast. *Forecasting* involves trying to estimate how a condition will be in the future. Forecasting takes advantage of input from others, gives sequence in activity, and protects an organization against undesirable changes.

With changes in technology, payment structures, and resource availability, the manager who is unwilling or unable to forecast accurately impedes the organization's efficiency and the unit's effectiveness. Increased competition, changes in government reimbursement, and decreased hospital revenues have reduced intuitive managerial decision making. To avoid disastrous outcomes when making future professional and financial plans, managers need to stay well informed about the legal, political, and socioeconomic factors affecting health care.

Managers who are uninformed about the legal, political, economic, and social factors affecting health care make planning errors that may have disastrous implications for their professional development and the financial viability of the organization.

STRATEGIC PLANNING

Planning has many dimensions. Two of these dimensions are time span and complexity or comprehensiveness. Generally, complex organizational plans that involve a long period (usually 3 to 10 years) are referred to as *long-range* or *strategic* plans. However, strategic planning may be done once or twice a year in an organization that changes rapidly. At the unit level, any planning that is at least 6 months in the future may be considered long-range planning.

Strategic planning focuses on purpose, mission, philosophy, and goals related to the external organizational environment.

Strategic planning typically examines an organization's purpose, mission, philosophy, and goals in the context of its external environment.

Strategic planning also forecasts the future success of an organization by matching and aligning an organization's capabilities with its external opportunities. For instance, an organization could develop a strategic plan for dealing with a nursing shortage, preparing succession managers in the organization, developing a marketing plan, redesigning workload, developing partnerships, or simply planning for organizational success.

SWOT Analysis

There are many effective tools that assist in strategic planning. One of the most commonly used in health care organizations is *SWOT analysis* (identification of strengths, weaknesses, opportunities, and threats) (Display 7.2). SWOT analysis, also known as *TOWS analysis*, was developed by Albert Humphrey at Stanford University in the 1960s and 1970s.

DISPLAY 7.2 SWOT Definitions

Strengths are those *internal* attributes that help an organization to achieve its objectives.
Weaknesses are those *internal* attributes that challenge an organization in achieving its objectives.
Opportunities are *external* conditions that promote achievement of organizational objectives.
Threats are *external* conditions that challenge or threaten the achievement of organizational objectives.

The first step in SWOT analysis is to define the desired end state or objective. After the desired objective is defined, the SWOTs are discovered and listed. Decision makers must then decide if the objective can be achieved in view of the SWOTs. If the decision is no, a different objective is selected and the process repeats.

SWOT analysis is a relatively common strategic planning tool. Performed correctly, it allows strategic planners to identify those issues most likely to impact a particular organization or situation in the future and then to develop an appropriate plan for action. *Marketing Teacher* (2000–2006), however, warns that several simple rules must be followed for SWOT analysis to be successful. These are shown in Display 7.3.

Balanced Scorecard

Balanced Scorecard, developed by Robert Kaplan and David Norton in the early 1990s, is another tool that is highly assistive in strategic planning. Indeed, Mindsolve (2006) notes that the *Harvard Business Review* calls Balanced Scorecard "one of the most significant ideas of the last 75 years."

Strategic planners using a Balanced Scorecard, develop metrics (performance measurement indicators), collect data, and analyze that data from four organizational perspectives: financial, customers, internal business processes (or simply processes), and learning and growth. This avoids an overemphasis on financial results as the primary measure of an organization's health and performance (Schwartz, 2005). Clarity Systems (2006) concurs, arguing that "organizations

DISPLAY 7.3 Simple Rules for SWOT Analysis

- Be realistic about the strengths and weaknesses of your organization.
- Be clear about how the present organization differs from what might be possible in the future.
- Be specific about what you want to accomplish.
- Always apply SWOT in relation to your competitors.
- Keep SWOT short and simple.
- Remember that SWOT is subjective.

Source: Adapted from Marketing Teacher. (2000–2006). *SWOT analysis: Lesson.* Retrieved August 26, 2006, from *http://www.marketingteacher.com/Lessons/lesson_swot.htm*.

who embrace the Balanced Scorecard buy into a philosophy where 75% of their organization's value is locked in metrics that are not financial, namely, their customers, their internal business processes and their learning and growth initiatives" (para 4). Instead, all of the measures are considered to be related, and all of the measures are assumed to eventually lead to outcomes. So the scorecard is "balanced" in that outcomes are in balance.

The value of Balanced Scorecards in strategic planning is that they allow organizations to align their strategic activities with the strategic plan and to implement that strategy on a continuous basis (Schwartz, 2005). "This requires communicating strategy to every level within the organization so that corporate strategy is integrated with everyday decision making. The best Balanced Scorecards are not a static set of measurements, but instead remain a work in progress and involve a multi-year progress of testing and tweaking performance measures to reflect better information and changes in business climate" (Clarity Systems, 2006, para 4). Because the Balanced Scorecard is able to translate strategy into action, it is an effective tool for translating an organization's strategic vision into clear and realistic objectives.

Strategic Planning as a Management Process

While SWOT and Balanced Scorecard are different, they are also similar in that they can help organizations assess what they do well and what they need to do to continue to be effective and financially sound. Many other strategic planning tools exist as well, but they are not discussed in this text. Regardless of the tool(s) used, strategic planning as a management process generally includes the following steps:

1. Clearly define the purpose of the organization.
2. Establish realistic goals and objectives consistent with the mission of the organization.
3. Identify the organization's external constituencies or stakeholders and then determine their assessment of the organization's purposes and operations.
4. Clearly communicate the goals and objectives to the organization's constituents.
5. Develop a sense of ownership of the plan.
6. Develop strategies to achieve the goals.
7. Ensure that the most effective use is made of the organization's resources.
8. Provide a base from which progress can be measured.
9. Provide a mechanism for informed change as needed.
10. Build a consensus about where the organization is going.

It should be noted, though, that some critics argue that strategic planning is rarely this linear. Nor is it static. Strategic planning instead involves various actions and reactions that are partially planned and partially unplanned.

 The *dynamic model of strategy* suggests that strategic planning is dynamic and interactive; that is, it involves a complex pattern of actions and reactions.

Who Should Be Involved in Strategic Planning?

Long-range planning for health care organizations historically has been accomplished by top-level managers and the board of directors, with limited input from middle-level managers. To give the strategic plan meaning and to implement it successfully, input from subordinates from all organizational levels may be solicited.

There is increasing recognition, however, of the importance of subordinate input from all levels of the organization to give the strategic plan meaning and to increase the likelihood of its successful implementation.

The first-level manager is generally more involved in long-range planning at the unit level. However, because the organization's strategic plans affect unit planning, managers at all levels must be informed of organizational long-range plans so that all planning is coordinated.

All organizations should establish annual strategic planning conferences, involving all departments and levels of the hierarchy; this action should promote increased effectiveness of nursing staff, better communication between all levels of personnel, a cooperative spirit relative to solving problems, and a pervasive feeling that the departments are unified, goal-directed, and doing their part to help the organization accomplish its mission.

LEARNING EXERCISE 7.2

Making a Long-Term Plan

The human resource manager in the facility where you are a supervisor has just completed a survey of the potential retirement plans of the nursing staff and found that within 5 years, 45% of the staff will probably be retiring. You know that past and present available statistics show that you normally replace 10% to 20% of your staff each year with new hires. You are concerned, as you do not know how you will be able to handle this new increase in your need for staff.

● ASSIGNMENT: Make a 5-year, long-term plan that will increase the likelihood of your being able to meet this new demand. Remember that other units within your facility and other health care organizations in your region may also be facing the same problem.

LOOKING TO THE FUTURE

Due to rapidly changing technology, increasing government involvement in health care, and scientific advances, health care organizations are finding it increasingly difficult to identify long-term needs appropriately and plan accordingly. In fact, most long-term planners find it difficult to plan even 5 years ahead.

Unlike the 20-year strategic plans of the 1960s and 1970s, most long-term planners today find it difficult to look even 5 years in the future.

The health care system is in chaos, as is much of the business world. Traditional management solutions no longer apply, and a lack of strong leadership in the health care system has limited the innovation needed to create solutions to the new and complex problems that the future will bring.

Because change is occurring so rapidly, managers can easily become focused on short-range plans and miss changes that can drastically alter specific long-term plans. Health care facilities are particularly vulnerable to external social, economic, and political forces; long-range planning, then, must address how these forces may change. It is imperative, therefore, that long-range plans be flexible, permitting change as external forces assert their impact on health care facilities. In as far as it is possible, a picture of the future should be used as we formulate long-range planning. One reason for envisioning the future is to study developments that may have an impact on the organization.

 One of the reasons that we attempt to see and understand the future for long-ranging planning is to study potential developments that may affect an organization.

This process of learning about the future allows us to determine what we want to happen. Identifying what may or could happen allows us to avert, encourage, or direct the course of events. "The purpose of learning about the future is not to predict it but to understand the elements that shape it and to envision desirable circumstances, so that progress can be made toward a preferred future rather than a catastrophic one" (Dickenson-Hazard, 2003, p. 4).

There are many factors emerging in the rapidly changing health care system that must be incorporated in planning for a health care organization's future. Some emerging paradigms include:

- There will be a need to build different work relationships because the way we manage systems will change. For example, health care continues to move toward managing populations rather than individuals.
- The health care industry will continue to move away from illness care to wellness care to reduce the demand for expensive, acute-care services.
- The use of *complementary and alternative medicine* (CAM) will likely continue to grow as public acceptance and demand for these services increases.
- The transformation from revenue management to cost management will continue as declining reimbursement forces providers to focus on how to maximize limited resources and provide care at less cost.
- There will be a move to interdependence of professionals rather than professional autonomy. With the movement toward managed care, autonomy has decreased for all health professionals, including managers.
- There will continue to be a shift to patient as consumer of cost and quality information. Historically, many providers assumed that consumers, both payers and patients, had minimal interest in or knowledge about the services that they received. A change in the balance of power among payers, patients, and providers has occurred, and providers will increasingly be held accountable for the quality of outcomes that their patients experience.
- A transition from continuity of provider to continuity of information will occur. Historically, continuity of care was maintained by continuity of provider. In the future, however, the meaning and operationalizing of continuity will become predicated on having complete, accurate, and timely information that moves with the patient. *Electronic health records* (EHR) provide promise for such real-time, point of care information (Huston, 2006).
- Information technology will increasingly provide immediate access to this type of information. Brailer (2005) suggests that through *health care information exchange and interoperability* (HIEI), clinicians everywhere will soon have a longitudinal medical record with full information about each patient.

In addition, Huston (2006) suggests the following factors will influence the future of health care:

- Robotic technology and the use of prototype nurse robots called *nursebots* will increasingly serve as an adjunct to scarce human resources in the provision of health care.
- *Biometrics*, the science of identifying people through physical characteristics such as fingerprints, handprints, retinal scans, voice recognition, and facial structure, will increasingly be used to assure targeted and appropriate access to client records.
- A growing elderly population, medical advances that increase the need for well-educated nurses, consumerism, the increased acuity of hospitalized patients, and a ballooning health care system will continue to increase the demand for RNs.
- An aging workforce, inadequate enrollment in nursing schools to meet projected demand, increased employment of nurses in outpatient or ambulatory care settings, high turnover due to worker dissatisfaction, and inadequate long-term pay incentives will continue to exacerbate the current nursing shortage in acute-care hospitals.
- The Internet and electronic access to health care information will continue to change how providers interact with patients, with consumers increasingly adopting the role of *expert patient.*

Because the paradigm shifts and trends affecting health care are constantly changing and because by the time a trend is recognized, it may be too late to plan proactively for such a change, managers are encouraged to take a broad approach to information gathering in the strategic planning process. Administrators should move toward the visionary and participative strategic planning processes that will be needed for health care agencies to function successfully in the 21st century.

LEARNING EXERCISE 7.3

Forces Affecting Health Care
In small groups, identify six additional forces, beyond those identified in this chapter, affecting today's health care system. You may include legal, political, economic, social, or ethical forces. Try to prioritize these forces in terms of how they will affect you as a manager or RN. For at least one of the six forces you have identified, brainstorm how that force would affect your strategic planning as a unit manager or director of a health care agency.

ORGANIZATIONAL PLANNING: THE PLANNING HIERARCHY

There are many types of planning; in most organizations, these plans form a hierarchy, with the plans at the top influencing all the plans that follow. As depicted in the pyramid in Figure 7.1, the hierarchy broadens at lower levels, representing an increase in the number of planning components. In addition, planning components at the top of the hierarchy are more general, and lower components are more specific.

VISION AND MISSION STATEMENTS

Vision statements are used to describe future goals or aims of an organization. The Alliance for Nonprofit Management (2003–2004) says that if strategic plan is the "blueprint" for an

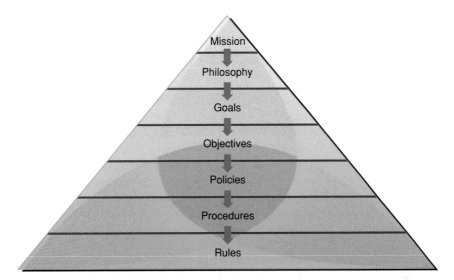

Figure 7.1 The planning hierarchy.

organization's work, then the vision is the "artist's rendering" of the achievement of that plan. It is a description in words that conjures up a picture for all group members of what they want to accomplish together.

Simpson (2005), in describing the value of a vision, says that "Without a vision, any road, even one filled with potholes, will take you there. But what an uncomfortable journey that will be" (p. 100). It is critical, then, that organization leaders recognize that the organization will never be greater than the vision that guides it. "Thus, the vision statement should require all organization members to stretch their expectations, aspirations, and performance" (Alliance for Nonprofit Management, 2003–2004, para 5). An appropriate vision statement for a hospital is shown in Display 7.4.

An organization will never be greater than the vision that guides it.

The purpose or *mission statement* is a brief statement (typically no more than three or four sentences) identifying the reason that an organization exists. The mission statement identifies the organization's constituency and addresses its position regarding ethics, principles, and standards of practice. An example of a mission statement for County Hospital, a teaching hospital, is shown in Display 7.5.

The mission statement is of highest priority in the planning hierarchy because it influences the development of an organization's philosophy, goals, objectives, policies, procedures, and rules.

DISPLAY 7.4 Sample Vision Statement

County Hospital will be the leading center for trauma care in the region.

DISPLAY 7.5   Sample Mission Statement

County Hospital is a tertiary care facility that provides comprehensive, holistic care to all state residents who seek treatment. The purpose of County Hospital is to combine high-quality, holistic health care with the provision of learning opportunities for students in medicine, nursing, and allied health sciences. Research is encouraged to identify new treatment regimens and to promote high-quality health care for generations to come.

Managers employed by County Hospital would have two primary goals to guide their planning: (a) to provide high-quality, holistic care and (b) to provide learning opportunities for students in medicine, nursing, and other allied health sciences. To meet these goals, adequate fiscal and human resources would have to be allocated for preceptorships and clinical research. In addition, an employee's performance appraisal would examine the worker's performance in terms of organizational and unit goals.

Hader (2006) suggests that a mission statement "needs to be a managerial and staff commitment that's developed by an organization's leaders following an exhaustive dialogue between all levels of the organization" (p. 6). BPlans.com (2006) concurs that the best mission statements are developed with input from all members of an organization.

Both Hader and BPlans.com emphasize that an organization must believe and act upon its mission statement.

> An organization must truly believe and act upon its mission statement; otherwise, the statement has little value.

Ingersoll, Witzel, and Smith (2005) concur, arguing that "an organization's mission, vision, and values statements are the guiding force behind the institution's administrative strategic planning" and that "each of these foundational documents assures that their values, beliefs, and intentions are evident in daily work life" (p. 86). Similarly, Luthans and Jensen (2005) state that "given current and projected challenges in the healthcare industry, the need for nurses who are committed to the mission of the organization has never been greater" (p. 304). Bolon (2005), however, in his research comparing mission statements of for-profit and not-for-profit hospitals, found no significant differences in content. This suggests that the hospital industry may be lagging behind other industries in designing thorough and complete mission statements that truly reflect the constituencies being served.

THE ORGANIZATION'S PHILOSOPHY STATEMENT

The *philosophy* flows from the purpose or mission statement and delineates the set of values and beliefs that guide all actions of the organization. It is the basic foundation that directs all further planning toward that mission. A statement of philosophy can usually be found in policy manuals at the institution or is available on request. A philosophy that might be generated from County Hospital's mission statement is shown in Display 7.6.

The *organizational philosophy* provides the basis for developing nursing philosophies at the unit level and for nursing service as a whole. Written in conjunction with the organizational philosophy, the *nursing service philosophy* should address fundamental beliefs about nursing

DISPLAY 7.6   **Sample Philosophy Statement**

The board of directors, medical and nursing staff, and administrators of County Hospital believe that human beings are unique, due to different genetic endowments, personal experiences in social and physical environments, and the ability to adapt to biophysical, psychosocial, and spiritual stressors. Thus, each patient is considered a unique individual with unique needs. Identifying outcomes and goals, setting priorities, prescribing strategy options, and selecting an optimal strategy will be negotiated by the patient, physician, and health care team.

As unique individuals, patients provide medical, nursing, and allied health students invaluable diverse learning opportunities. Because the board of directors, medical and nursing staff, and administrators believe that the quality of health care provided directly reflects the quality of the education of its future health care providers, students are welcomed and encouraged to seek out as many learning opportunities as possible. Because high-quality health care is defined by and depends on technological advances and scientific discovery, County Hospital encourages research as a means of scientific inquiry.

and nursing care; the quality, quantity, and scope of nursing services; and how nursing specifically will meet organizational goals. Frequently, the nursing service philosophy draws on the concepts of holistic care, education, and research. The nursing service philosophy in Display 7.7 builds on County Hospital's mission statement and organizational philosophy.

The *unit philosophy*, adapted from the nursing service philosophy, specifies how nursing care provided on the unit will correspond with nursing service and organizational goals. This congruence in philosophy, goals, and objectives among the organization, nursing service, and unit is shown in Figure 7.2.

DISPLAY 7.7   **Sample Nursing Service Philosophy**

The philosophy of nursing at County Hospital is based on respect for the individual's dignity and worth. We believe that all patients have the right to receive effective nursing care. This care is a personal service that is based on patients' needs and their clinical disease or condition.

Recognizing the obligation of nursing to help restore patients to the best possible state of physical, mental, and emotional health and to maintain patients' sense of spiritual and social well-being, we pledge intelligent cooperation in coordinating nursing service with the medical and allied professional practitioners. Understanding the importance of research and teaching for improving patient care, the nursing department will support, promote, and participate in these activities. Using knowledge of human behavior, we shall strive for mutual trust and understanding between nursing service and nursing employees to provide an atmosphere for developing the fullest possible potential of each member of the nursing team. We believe that nursing personnel are individually accountable to patients and their families for the quality and compassion of the patient care rendered and for upholding the standards of care as delineated by the nursing staff.

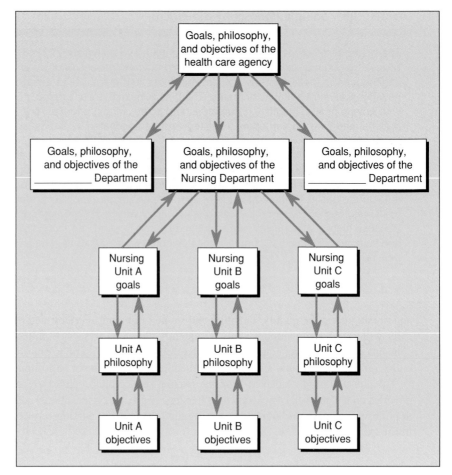

Figure 7.2 Philosophical congruence in the planning hierarchy.

Although unit-level managers have limited opportunity to help develop the organizational philosophy, they are active in determining, implementing, and evaluating the unit philosophy. In formulating this philosophy, the unit manager incorporates knowledge of the unit's internal and external environments and an understanding of the unit's role in meeting organizational goals. The manager must understand the planning hierarchy and be able to articulate ideas both verbally and in writing. Leader–managers also must be visionary, innovative, and creative in identifying unit purposes or goals so that the philosophy not only reflects current practice but also incorporates a view of the future.

Like the mission statement, statements of philosophy in general can be helpful only if they truly direct the work of the organization toward a specific purpose. A department's decisions, priorities, and accomplishments reflect its working philosophy.

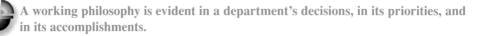

A working philosophy is evident in a department's decisions, in its priorities, and in its accomplishments.

A person should be able to identify exactly how the organization is implementing its stated philosophy by observing members of the staff, reviewing the budgetary priorities, and talking to consumers of health care. The decisions made in an organization make the philosophy visible to all—no matter what is espoused on paper. A philosophy that is not or cannot be implemented is useless.

LEARNING EXERCISE 7.4

Developing a Philosophy Statement
Recover Inc., a fictitious for-profit home health agency, provides complete nursing and supportive services for in-home care. Services include skilled nursing, bathing, shopping, physical therapy, occupational therapy, meal preparation, housekeeping, speech therapy, and social work. The agency provides round-the-clock care, 7 days a week, to a primarily underserved rural area in northern California. The brochure the company publishes says that it is committed to satisfying the needs of the rural community and that it is dedicated to excellence.

● ASSIGNMENT: Based on this limited information, develop a brief philosophy statement that might be appropriate for Recover Inc. Be creative, and embellish information if appropriate.

SOCIETAL PHILOSOPHIES AND VALUES

Societies and organizations have philosophies or sets of beliefs that guide their behavior. These beliefs that guide behavior are called *values*. Values have an intrinsic worth for a society or an individual. Some strongly held American values are individualism, the pursuit of self-interest, and competition. These values have profoundly affected health care policy formation and implementation. The result is a health care system that promotes structured inequalities. Despite spending trillions of dollars on health care annually, millions of American citizens have no health insurance, and millions of others are underinsured.

Although values seem to be of central importance for health care policy development and analysis, public discussion of this crucial variable is often neglected. Instead, health care policy makers tend to focus on technology, cost–benefit analysis, and cost-effectiveness. Although this type of evaluation is important, it does not address the underlying values in this country that have led to unequal access to health care.

LEARNING EXERCISE 7.5

Health Care at What Cost?
Both Canada and Germany have been held up as models in health care reform because they provide health care for all citizens. Although the United States spends more per capita than either Germany or Canada, many citizens do not have access to comprehensive, quality health care. Canadians receive hospitalization, doctor visits, and most dental care free of charge. Germany spends even less and provides a level of service similar to Canada but with a very

(Learning Exercise continues on page 154)

small co-payment for hospitalization. Unlike the emphasis on specialized care in the United States with limited choice of physicians, health care systems in Canada and Germany emphasize primary care, unlimited choice of physicians, free physician visits, and an emphasis on health promotion. With little financial incentive for physician specialization and a nationwide focus on health promotion, there are many more general practitioners per capita in Germany and Canada than in the United States.

At what cost is this health care offered? Canadians and Germans experience longer waits for some high-tech procedures, and the governments of those countries have limitations on the proliferation of technology. However, the United States continues to have a higher incidence of infant mortality and low birth weight than either country and the lowest life expectancy at birth. Despite the highest spending as a percentage of gross domestic product, American consumers had the least number of physician visits and the shortest average hospital stay.

● ASSIGNMENT: In small groups, discuss the following: Do you agree or disagree that the U.S. health care system represents societal values of individualism, the pursuit of self-interests, and competition? Do you believe that the American people are willing to pay the costs required to pursue collectivism, cooperation, and equality in health care? Would you be willing to have fewer choices about your health care if access could be guaranteed to all? Do you believe that the cost of universal coverage should be picked up by the consumer or by the employer? Recognize that both societal and individual values will affect your feelings.

INDIVIDUAL PHILOSOPHIES AND VALUES

As discussed in Chapter 1, values have a tremendous impact on the decisions that people make. For the individual, personal beliefs and values are shaped by that person's experiences.

 Personal philosophies and values are shaped by the socialization processes experienced by that person.

All people should carefully examine their value system and recognize the role that it plays in how they make decisions and resolve conflicts and even how they perceive things. Therefore, the nurse–leader must be self-aware and provide subordinates with learning opportunities or experiences that foster increased self-awareness.

At times, it is difficult to assess whether something is a *true value*. McNally's (1980) classic work identified the following four characteristics that determine a true value:
1. It must be freely chosen from among alternatives only after due reflection.
2. It must be prized and cherished.
3. It is consciously and consistently repeated (part of a pattern).
4. It is positively affirmed and enacted.

If a value does not meet all four criteria, it is a *value indicator*. Most people have many value indicators but few true values. For example, many nurses assert that they value their national nursing organization, yet they do not pay dues or participate in the organization. True values require that the person take action, whereas value indicators do not. Thus, the value ascribed to the national nursing organization is a value indicator for these nurses and not a true value. In addition, because our values change with time, periodic clarification is necessary to determine how our values may have changed. Values clarification includes examining values, assigning priorities to those values, and determining how they influence behavior so that one's lifestyle is consistent with prioritized values. Sometimes, values change as a result of life experiences or newly acquired knowledge. Most of the values we have as children reflect our parents' values. Later, our values are modified by peers and role models. Although they are learned, values cannot be forced on a person because they must be internalized. However, restricted exposure to other viewpoints also limits the number of value choices a person is able to generate. Therefore, becoming more worldly increases our awareness of alternatives from which we select our values.

LEARNING EXERCISE 7.6

Reflecting on Your Values
Using what you have learned about values, value indicators, and value clarifications, answer the following questions. Take time to reflect on your values before answering. This may be used as a writing exercise.
1. List three or four of your basic beliefs about nursing.
2. Knowing what you know now, ask yourself, "Do I value nursing? Was it freely chosen from among alternatives after appropriate reflection? Do I prize and cherish nursing? If I had a choice to do it over, would I still choose nursing as a career?"
3. Are your personal and professional values congruent? Are there any values espoused by the nursing profession that are inconsistent with your personal values? How will you resolve resultant conflicts?

Hader (2006) suggests that "when an organization's mission is in line with staff values, that the base on which to build a winning culture is strong" (p. 6). Occasionally, however, individual values are in conflict with those of the organization. Because the philosophy of an organization determines its priorities in goal selection and distribution of resources, nurses need to understand the organization's philosophy. For example, assume that a nurse is employed by County Hospital, which clearly states in its philosophy that teaching is a primary purpose for the hospital's existence. Consequently, medical students are allowed to practice endotracheal intubation on all people who die in the hospital, allowing the students to gain needed experience in emergency medicine. This practice disturbs the nurse a great deal; it is not consistent with his or her own set of values and thus creates great personal conflict.

Nurses who frequently make decisions that conflict with their personal values may experience confusion and anxiety. This intrapersonal struggle ultimately will lead to job stress and dissatisfaction, especially for the novice nurse who comes to the organization with inadequate values clarification. The choices that nurses make about client care are not merely strategic options; they are moral choices. Internal conflict and burnout may result when personal and organizational values do not mesh.

 When a nurse experiences cognitive dissonance between personal and organizational values, the result may be intrapersonal conflict and burnout.

As part of the leadership role, the manager should encourage all potential employees to read and think about the organization's mission statement or philosophy before accepting the job. The manager should give a copy of the philosophy to the prospective applicant before the hiring interview. The applicant also should be encouraged to speak to employees in various positions within the organization regarding how the philosophy is implemented at their job level. For example, a potential employee may want to determine how the organization feels about cultural diversity and what policies they have in place to ensure that patients from diverse cultures and languages have a mechanism for translation as needed. Finally, new employees should be encouraged to speak to community members about the institution's reputation for care. New employees who understand the organizational philosophy will not only have clearer expectations about the institution's purposes and goals but will also have a better understanding of how they fit into the organization.

Although all nurses should have a philosophy comparable with that of their employer, it is especially important for the new manager to have a value system consistent with that of the organization. Institutional changes that closely align with the value system of the nurse–manager will receive more effort and higher priority than those that are not true values or that conflict with the nurse–manager's value system. Managers who take a position with the idea that they can change the organization's philosophy to more closely agree with their own philosophy are likely to be disappointed.

It is unrealistic for managers to accept a position under the assumption that they can change the organization's philosophy to more closely match their personal philosophy.

Such a change will require extraordinary energy and precipitate inevitable conflict because the organization's philosophy reflects the institution's historical development and the beliefs of those people who were vital in the institution's development. Nursing managers must recognize that closely held values may be challenged by current social and economic constraints and that philosophy statements must be continually reviewed and revised to ensure ongoing accuracy of beliefs.

GOALS AND OBJECTIVES

Goals and objectives are the ends toward which the organization is working. All philosophies must be translated into specific goals and objectives if they are to result in action. Thus, goals and objectives "operationalize" the philosophy.

A *goal* may be defined as the desired result toward which effort is directed; it is the aim of the philosophy. Although institutional goals are usually determined by the organization's highest administrative levels, there is increasing emphasis on including workers in setting organizational goals. Goals, much like philosophies and values, change with time and require periodic reevaluation and prioritization.

Goals, although somewhat global in nature, should be measurable and ambitious but realistic. Goals also should clearly delineate the desired end product. When goals are not clear, simple misunderstandings may compound, and communication may break down. Organizations usually set long- and short-term goals for services rendered; economics; use of resources, including people,

DISPLAY 7.8   Sample Goal Statements

- All nursing staff will recognize the patient's need for independence and right to privacy and will assess the patient's level of readiness to learn in relation to his or her illness.
- The nursing staff will provide effective patient care relative to patient needs insofar as the hospital and community facilities permit through the use of care plans, individual patient care, and discharge planning, including follow-up contact.
- An ongoing effort will be made to create an atmosphere that is conducive to favorable patient and employee morale and that fosters personal growth.
- The performance of all employees in the nursing department will be evaluated in a manner that produces growth in the employee and upgrades nursing standards.
- All nursing units within County Hospital will work cooperatively with other departments within the hospital to further the mission, philosophy, and goals of the institution.

funds, and facilities; innovations; and social responsibilities. Display 7.8 lists sample goal statements.

Although goals may direct and maintain the behavior of an organization, there are several dangers in using goal evaluation as the primary means of assessing organizational effectiveness. The first danger is that goals may be in conflict with each other, creating confusion for employees and consumers. For example, the need for profit maximization in health care facilities today may conflict with some stated patient goals or quality goals. The second danger with the goal approach is that publicly stated goals may not truly reflect organizational goals. In addition, some organizational goals may be developed simply as a conduit for individual or personal goals. The final danger is that because goals are global, it is often difficult to determine whether they have been obtained.

 Although goals may direct and maintain the behavior of an organization, there are several dangers in using goal evaluation as the primary means of assessing organizational effectiveness.

Objectives are similar to goals in that they motivate people to a specific end and are explicit, measurable, observable or retrievable, and obtainable. Objectives, however, are more specific and measurable than goals because they identify how and when the goal is to be accomplished.

Goals usually have multiple objectives that are each accompanied by a targeted completion date. The more specific the objectives for a goal can be, the easier for all involved in goal attainment to understand and carry out specific role behaviors. This is especially important for the nurse–manager to remember when writing job descriptions; if there is little ambiguity in the job description, there will be little role confusion or distortion. Clearly written goals and objectives must be communicated to all those in the organization responsible for their attainment. This is a critical leadership role for the nurse–manager.

Objectives can focus on either the desired process or the desired result. *Process objectives* are written in terms of the method to be used, whereas *result-focused objectives* specify the desired outcome. An example of a process objective might be "100% of staff nurses will orient new patients to the call-light system, within 30 minutes of their admission, by first demonstrating its appropriate use and then asking the patient to repeat said demonstration." An example of a result-focused objective might be "All postoperative patients will perceive a decrease in their pain levels following the administration of parenteral pain medication." Writing good objectives requires time and practice.

For the objectives to be measurable, they should have certain criteria. There should be a specific time frame in which the objectives are to be completed, and the objectives should be stated in behavioral terms, be objectively evaluated, and identify positive rather than negative outcomes.

As a sample objective, one of the goals at Mercy Hospital is that "all RNs will be proficient in the administration of intravenous fluids." Objectives for Mercy Hospital might include the following:

- All RNs will complete Mercy Hospital's course "IV Therapy Certification" within 1 month of beginning employment. The hospital will bear the cost of this program.
- RNs who score less than 70% on a comprehensive examination in "IV Therapy Certification" must attend the remedial 4-hour course "Review of Basic IV Principles" not more than 2 weeks after the completion of "IV Therapy Certification."
- RNs who achieve a score of 70% or better on the comprehensive examination for "IV Therapy Certification" after completing "Review of Basic IV Principles" will be allowed to perform IV therapy on patients. The unit manager will establish individualized plans of remediation for employees who fail to achieve this score on the examination.

The leader–manager clearly must be skilled in determining and documenting goals and objectives. Prudent managers assess the unit's constraints and assets and determine available resources before developing goals and objectives. The leader must then be creative and futuristic in identifying how goals might best be translated into objectives and thus implemented. The willingness to be receptive to new and varied ideas is a critical leadership skill. In addition, well-developed interpersonal skills allow the leader to involve and inspire subordinates in goal setting. The final step in the process involves clearly writing the identified goals and objectives, communicating changes to subordinates, and periodically evaluating and revising goals and objectives as needed.

LEARNING EXERCISE 7.7

Writing Goals and Objectives
Practice writing goals and objectives for County Hospital based on the mission and philosophy statements in this chapter. Identify three goals and three objectives to operationalize each of these goals.

POLICIES AND PROCEDURES

Policies are plans reduced to statements or instructions that direct organizations in their decision making. A policy is a statement of expectations that sets boundaries for action taking and decision making (Paige, 2003). These comprehensive statements, derived from the organization's philosophy, goals, and objectives, explain how goals will be met and guide the general course and scope of organizational activities. Thus, policies direct individual behavior toward the organization's mission and define broad limits and desired outcomes of commonly recurring situations while leaving some discretion and initiative to those who must carry out that policy. Although some policies are required by accrediting agencies, many policies are specific to the individual institution, thus providing management with a means of internal control.

Policies also can be implied or expressed. *Implied policies*, neither written nor expressed verbally, have usually developed over time and follow a precedent. For example, a hospital may have an implied policy that employees should be encouraged and supported in their activity in community, regional, and national health care organizations. Another example might be that nurses who limit their maternity leave to 3 months can return to their former jobs and shifts with no status change.

Expressed policies are delineated verbally or in writing. Most organizations have many written policies that are readily available to all people and promote consistency of action. Expressed policies may include a formal dress code, policy for sick leave or vacation time, and disciplinary procedures. Paige (2003) implies that organizations can be held liable for failing to develop facility wide polices and procedures that are followed. She suggests forming a committee of key players to address the policy and procedure process within an institution. Unfortunately, in most health care organizations, *nursing policy and procedure committees* (NPPCs) are centralized with one person, or small group, managing this ongoing task (Hudson, 2006). Involving more individuals in the process should increase the quality of the end product and the likelihood that procedures will be implemented as desired. Such a shared governance approach to policy and procedure management can also improve patient care and worker satisfaction (Hudson, 2006). See Examining the Evidence 7.1.

Although top-level management is more involved in setting organizational policies (usually by policy committees), unit managers must determine how those policies will be implemented on their units. Input from subordinates in forming, implementing, and reviewing policy allows the leader–manager to develop guidelines that all employees will support and follow. Even if

 EXAMINING THE EVIDENCE 7.1

Source: Hudson, K. (2006). Policy and procedure management: A job that's never done. *Nursing Management, 37*(6), 34–38.

This article provided anecdotal evidence of the benefits of transitioning from a centralized nursing policy and procedure committee (NPPC) to a shared governance model. Forming a shared governance NPPC required obtaining a diverse cadre of nurse representatives from each clinical area, articulating the new committee's mission, writing objectives, creating a framework for subcommittee task teams, and developing a formal meeting protocol. The work of this new committee was accountable to and reported to the nursing executive team.

Benefits of the shared governance NPPC model included more comprehensive and current policies and procedures, better patient care as a result of increased awareness of policies and procedures by staff, and greater collaboration between disciplines and units. In addition, staff reported enhanced commitment to progressive nursing practice and less reliance on education and administrative support for improvements in practice. Personal rewards for NPPC members included improved skill in writing and speaking, literature critiquing, project management, and interpersonal communication.

unit-level employees are not directly involved in policy setting, their feedback is crucial to its successful implementation. Having uniform policies and procedures developed through collaboration is critical.

After policy has been formulated, the leadership role of managers includes the responsibility for communicating that policy to all who may be affected by it. This information should be transmitted in writing and verbally. A policy's perceived value often depends on how it is communicated.

 The relative value of a policy is often perceived in relation to how it is communicated.

Procedures are plans that establish customary or acceptable ways of accomplishing a specific task and delineate a sequence of steps of required action. Established procedures save staff time, facilitate delegation, reduce cost, increase productivity, and provide a means of control. Procedures identify the process or steps needed to implement a policy and are generally found in manuals at the unit level of the organization. Procedures may have some variation in the steps as long as the same outcome is obtained (Paige, 2003).

The manager also has a responsibility to review and revise policies and procedure statements to ensure currency and applicability. Given the current explosion of evidence-based research as well as new regulations, technology, and drugs, keeping policies and procedures current and relevant is a tremendous management challenge. In addition, because most units are in constant flux, the needs of the unit and the most appropriate means of meeting those needs constantly change. For example, the unit manager is responsible for seeing that a clearly written policy regarding holiday and vacation time exists and that it is communicated to all those it affects. The unit manager also must provide a clearly written procedural statement regarding how to request vacation or holiday time on that specific unit. The unit manager would assess any long-term change in patient census or availability of human resources and revise the policy and procedural statements accordingly.

Because procedural instructions involve elements of organizing, some textbooks place the development of procedures in the organizing phase of the management process. Regardless of where procedural development is formulated, there must be a close relationship with planning—the foundation for all procedures.

RULES

Rules and regulations are plans that define specific action or nonaction. Generally included as part of policy and procedure statements, *rules* describe situations that allow only one choice of action. Rules are fairly inflexible, so the fewer rules, the better.

 Because rules are the least flexible type of planning in the planning hierarchy, there should be as few rules as possible in the organization.

Existing rules, however, should be enforced to keep morale from breaking down and to allow organizational structure. Chapter 25, on discipline, includes a more detailed discussion of rules and regulations.

OVERCOMING BARRIERS TO PLANNING

Benefits of effective planning include timely accomplishment of higher-quality work and the best possible use of capital and human resources. Because planning is essential, managers must be able to overcome barriers that impede planning. For successful organizational planning, the manager must remember several points:

- The organization can be more effective if movement within it is directed at specified goals and objectives. Unfortunately, the novice manager frequently omits establishing a goal or objective. Setting a goal for a plan keeps managers focused on the bigger picture and saves them from getting lost in the minute details of planning. Just as the nursing care plan establishes patient care goals before delineating problems and interventions, managers must establish goals for their planning strategies that are congruent with goals established at higher levels.

- Because a plan is a guide to reach a goal, it must be flexible and allow for readjustment as unexpected events occur. This flexibility is a necessary attribute for the manager in all planning phases and the management process.

- The manager should include in the planning process all people and units that could be affected by a plan. Although time-consuming, employee involvement in how things are done and by whom increases commitment to goal achievement. Although not everyone will want to contribute to unit or organizational planning, all should be invited. The manager also needs to communicate clearly the goals and specific individual responsibilities to all those responsible for carrying out the plans so that work is coordinated.

- Plans should be specific, simple, and realistic. A vague plan is impossible to implement. A plan that is too global or unrealistic discourages rather than motivates employees. If a plan is unclear, the nurse–leader must restate the plan in another manner or use group process to clarify common goals.

- Know when to plan and when not to plan. It is possible to overplan and underplan. For example, one who overplans may devote excessive time to arranging details that might be better left to those who will carry out the plan. Underplanning occurs when the manager erroneously assumes that people and events will naturally fall into some desired and efficient method of production.

- Good plans have built-in evaluation checkpoints so that there can be a midcourse correction if unexpected events occur. A final evaluation should always occur at the end of the plan. If goals were not met, the plan should be examined to determine why it failed. This evaluation process assists the manager in future planning.

INTEGRATING LEADERSHIP ROLES AND MANAGEMENT FUNCTIONS IN PLANNING

Planning requires managerial expertise in health care economics, human resource management, political and legislative issues affecting health care, and planning theory. Planning also requires the leadership skills of being sensitive to the environment, being able to appraise accurately the social and political climate, and being willing to take risks. Hader (2006) suggests that it is organizational leaders who make the mission "come alive through active participation in its formation, role modeling appropriate behaviors, and holding staff accountable to the highest care standards" (p. 6).

Clearly, the leader–manager must be skilled in determining, implementing, documenting, and evaluating all types of planning in the hierarchy because an organization's leaders are integral to realizing the mission of the organization. Managers then must draw on the philosophy and goals established at the organizational and nursing service levels in implementing planning at the unit level. Initially, managers must assess the unit's constraints and assets and determine its resources available for planning. The manager then draws on his or her leadership skills in creativity, innovation, and futuristic thinking to problem solve how philosophies can be translated into goals, goals into objectives, and so on down the planning hierarchy. The wise manager will develop the interpersonal leadership skills needed to inspire and involve subordinates in this planning hierarchy. The manager also must demonstrate the leadership skill of being receptive to new and varied ideas.

The final step in the process involves articulating identified goals and objectives clearly; this learned management skill is critical to the success of the planning. If the unit manager lacks management or leadership skills, the planning hierarchy fails.

Key Concepts

* The planning phase of the management process is critical and precedes all other functions.
* Planning is a proactive function required of all nurses.
* Plans should be specific, simple, and realistic.
* A plan is a guide for action in reaching a goal and must be flexible.
* Organizations and planners tend to use one of four planning modes: *reactive*, *inactivism*, *preactivism*, or *proactive*. A proactive planning style is always the goal.
* All people and organizational units affected by a plan should be included in the planning.
* Plans have a time for evaluation built into them so that there can be a midcourse correction if necessary.
* Strategic planning tools such as *SWOT* and *Balanced Scorecard* help planners to identify those issues most likely to impact a particular organization or situation in the future and then to develop an appropriate plan for action.
* A philosophy that is not or cannot be implemented is useless.
* To avoid ongoing intrapersonal values conflicts, employees should have a philosophy compatible with that of their employer.
* All planning must include an evaluation step and requires periodic reevaluation and prioritization.
* All planning in the hierarchy must flow from and be congruent with planning done at higher levels in the hierarchy.
* Due to rapidly changing technology, increasing government involvement in health care, changing population demographics, and reduced provider autonomy, health care organizations are finding it increasingly difficult to appropriately identify long-term needs and plan accordingly.

ADDITIONAL LEARNING EXERCISES
AND APPLICATIONS

LEARNING EXERCISE 7.8

Exploring the Impact of Philosophy on Management Action

Susan is the supervisor of the 22-bed oncology unit at Memorial Hospital, a 150-bed hospital. Unit morale and job satisfaction are high, despite a unit occupancy rate of less than 50% in the last 6 months. Patient satisfaction on this unit is as high as or higher than that of any other unit in the hospital.

Susan's personal philosophy is that oncology patients have physical, social, and spiritual needs that are different from other patients. Both the unit and nursing service philosophy reflect this belief. Thus, nurses working in the oncology unit receive additional education, orientation, and socialization regarding their unique roles and responsibilities in working with oncology patients.

At this morning's regularly scheduled department head meeting, the chief executive nursing officer suggests that because of extreme budget shortfalls and continuing low census, the oncology unit should be closed and its patients merged with the general medical–surgical patient population. The oncology nursing staff would be reassigned to the medical–surgical unit, with Susan as the unit's co-supervisor.

The idea receives immediate support from the medical–surgical supervisor because of the current staffing shortage on her unit. Susan, startled by the proposal, immediately voices her disapproval and asks for 2 weeks to prepare her argument. Her request is granted.

● ASSIGNMENT: What values or beliefs are guiding Susan, the chief executive nursing officer, and the medical–surgical unit supervisor? Determine an appropriate plan of action for Susan. What impact does a unit or nursing service philosophy have on the actions of management and employees?

LEARNING EXERCISE 7.9

Incremental Goal Setting

Assume that your career goal is to become a nurse–lawyer. You are currently an RN in an acute-care facility in a large, metropolitan city. You have your BSN degree but will need to take at least 12 units of prerequisite classes for acceptance into law school. A law school within commuting distance of your home offers evening classes that would allow you to continue your current day job at least part-time. Quitting your job entirely would be financially unfeasible.

● ASSIGNMENT: Identify at least four objectives that you need to set to achieve your career goal. Be sure that these objectives are explicit, measurable, observable or retrievable, and obtainable. Then identify at least three actions for each objective that delineate how you will achieve them.

LEARNING EXERCISE 7.10

Current Events and Planning

You are a manager in a public health agency. In reading the morning paper before going to work today, you pursue an article about the influx of Hmong families in your county. There has been an increase of 10% in this population in the last year, and it is expected to continue to rise. You ponder how this will affect your client population and your agency.

You decide to gather your staff together and develop a strategic plan for dealing with the problems and opportunities that this change in client demographics presents.

● ASSIGNMENT: In examining the 10 steps listed in development of strategic plans, what are things that you can personally influence, and what other individuals in the organization should be involved with the strategic plan? Make a list of 10 to 12 strategies that will assist you in planning for this new client population. What other statistics will you need to help you plan? What are some other future developments in your county that could have a positive or negative influence on your plan?

(Web Links)

Basics of Developing Mission, Vision and Values Statements
http://www.managementhelp.org/plan_dec/str_plan/stmnts.htm
Learn how to develop mission, vision, and values statements.

Strategic Planning (in Nonprofit or For-Profit Organizations)
http://www.managementhelp.org/plan_dec/str_plan/str_plan.htm
Identifies basics of strategic planning in both nonprofit and for-profit organizations.

University of Iowa Hospitals & Clinics: Nursing Services and Patient Care
http://www.uihealthcare.com/depts/nursing/about/mission.html
Find out the philosophy and goals of this health care organization.

Balanced Scorecard Collaborative
http://www.bscol.com/
The Balance Scorecard Collaborative portal helps organizations throughout the world to build and implement the Balanced Scorecard to drive strategic change.

References

Alliance for Nonprofit Management. (2003–2004) *Frequently asked questions. What's in a vision statement?* Retrieved August 13, 2006, from *http://www.allianceonline. org/FAQ/strategic_planning/what_s_in_vision_statement.faq.*

Bolon, D. S. (2005). Comparing mission statement content in for-profit and not-for-profit hospitals: Does mission really matter? *Hospital Topics, 83*(4), 2–9.

BPlans.com. (2006). *Writing a mission statement.* Retrieved August 13, 2006, from *http://www.bplans.com/dp/ missionstatement.cfm/?CMP=KNC-google&gclid= CObs5OvU34YCFRYmWAodZg3O3A.*

Brailer, D. J. (2005, January 19). Interoperability: The key to the future health care system. *Health Affairs.* Retrieved August 28, 2006, from *http://content.healthaffairs.org/cgi/content/ full/hlthaff.w5.19/DC1.*

Clarity Systems. (2006). *Management methodologies. Balanced scorecard.* Retrieved August 26, 2006, from *http://www.claritysystems.com/default.asp?item= managementmethodologies.*

Dickenson-Hazard, N. (2003). Future study or the magic 8 ball? *Reflections on Nursing Leadership, 29*(4), 4.

Hader, R. (2006). More than words: Provide a clear and concise mission statement. *Nursing Management, 37*(7), 6.

Hudson, K. (2006). Policy and procedure management. A job that's never done. *Nursing Management, 37*(6), 34–38.

Huston, C. (2006). *Professional issues in nursing.* Philadelphia: Lippincott Williams & Wilkins.

Ingersoll, G. L., Witzel, P. A., & Smith, T. C. (2005). Using organizational mission, vision, and values to guide professional practice model development and measurement of nurse performance. *Journal of Nursing Administration, 35*(2), 86–93.

Luthans, K. W., & Jensen, S. M. (2005). The linkage between psychological capital and commitment to organizational mission. *Journal of Nursing Administration, 35*(6), 304–310.

Marketing Teacher. (2000–2006). *SWOT analysis: Lesson.* Retrieved August 26, 2006, from *http://www.marketing teacher.com/Lessons/lesson_swot.htm.*

McNally, M. (1980). Values. Part 1. *Supervisor Nurse, 11,* 27–30.

Mindsolve. (2006). Strategic alignment. Executing strategy from the top desk to every desktop. *The Balanced Scorecard.* Retrieved August 26, 2006, from *http://www.mindsolve.com/ site/landing/BalancedScorecard.aspx.*

Paige, J. B. (2003). Solve the policy and procedure puzzle. *Nursing Management, 34*(3),45–48.

Schwartz, J. (2005). The Balanced Scorecard versus Total Quality Management: Which is better for your organization? *Military Medicine, 170*(10), 855–858.

Simpson, R. L. (2005). Patient and nurse safety. How information technology makes a difference. *Nursing Administration Quarterly, 29*(1), 97–101.

Bibliography

Balanced scorecard helps CMs focus on improvement: Charts show trends in LOS, charges, readmissions. (2006). *Hospital Case Management, 14*(5), 72–73.

Bolon, D. S. (2005). Comparing mission statement content in for-profit and not-for-profit hospitals: Does mission really matter? *Hospital Topics, 83*(4), 2–9.

Brunke, L. (2006). On reflection. Developing a strategic plan. *Nursing BC, 38*(2), 37.

Huang, S., Chen, P., Yang, M., Change, W., & Lee, H. (2004). Using a balanced scorecard to improve the performance of an emergency department. *Nursing Economics, 22*(3), 140–146.

Jeffs, L., Merkley, J., Heffrey, J., Ferris, E., Dusek, J., & Hunter, C. (2006). Case study: Reconciling the quality and safety gap through strategic planning. *Canadian Journal of Nursing Leadership, 19*(2), 32–40.

Jones, D. L. (2006). Balanced scorecards: Improving your outcomes measures. *ACSM's Health and Fitness Journal, 10*(2), 28–31.

Kane-Urrabazo, C. (2006). Management's role in shaping organizational culture. *Journal of Nursing Management, 14*(3), 188–194.

Kreitzer, M. J., Zhang, L., Trotter, M. J. (2006). Transformative professional development: Outcomes of the inner life renewal program. *Complementary Health Practice Review, 11*(1), 57–62.

McAndrew, F., & Taylor, R. (2006). Consultation. How all voices are heard for strategic planning. *Journal of Dementia Care, 14*(3), 22–24.

McKernan, J. (2006). Management forum. Nurses involved with strategic planning. *Dermatology Nursing, 18*(1), 63.

Sharma, M. (2005). Health education in India: A strengths, weaknesses, opportunities, and threats (SWOT) analysis. *International Electronic Journal of Health Education, 16*(5), 80–85.

Smalley, J. (2005). Notes from the field. What's your nursing philosophy? *Nursing Management, 36*(12), 59–61.

To chapter leaders: Reconnect to core values. (2006). *AACN News, 23*(7), 9.

Write your personal mission statement. (2006). *Explorer, 32*(1), 3.

Zager, L. R., & Walker, E. C. (2005). One vision, one voice: Transforming caregiving in nursing. *Orthopaedic Nursing, 24*(2), 130–133.

8

Planned Change

> *. . . managing and innovation did not always fit comfortably together. That's not surprising. Managers are people who like order. They like forecasts to come out as planned. In fact, managers are often judged on how much order they produce. Innovation, on the other hand, is often a disorderly process. Many times, perhaps most times, innovation does not turn out as planned. As a result, there is tension between managers and innovation.*
>
> *——Lewis Lehro (about the first years at Minnesota Mining and Manufacturing)*

> *. . . I can't understand why people are frightened of new ideas. I'm frightened of old ones.*
>
> *——John Cage*

Many forces are driving change in contemporary health care, including rising health care costs, declining reimbursement, workforce shortages, increasing technology, information availability, and a growing elderly population. Burritt (2005) suggests that these dynamic forces have led to a progressive destabilization in some health care organizations to such an extent that they threaten viability. The reality then is that today's health care agencies are continually instituting change to upgrade their structure, promote greater quality, and keep their workers.

Today, most health care organizations find themselves undergoing continual change directed at organizational restructuring, quality improvement, and employee retention. In most cases, these changes are planned. *Planned change*, in contrast to accidental change or *change by drift*, results from a well-thought-out and deliberate effort to make something happen. Planned change is the deliberate application of knowledge and skills by a leader to bring about a change.

One key role, then, of health care leaders today is "facilitating changes in the workplace to continually improve care and meet fiscal realities" (Cummings & McLennan, 2005, p. 61).

Successful leader–managers must be well grounded in change theories and be able to apply such theories appropriately.

> Today, most health care organizations find themselves undergoing continual change directed at organizational restructuring, quality improvement, and employee retention.

Still, change is not easy. Regardless of the type of change, all major change brings feelings of achievement and pride as well as loss and stress. Porter-O'Grady (2003) stresses that the skills necessary to move reticent groups cannot be understated. The leader must use developmental, political, and relational expertise to ensure that needed change is not sabotaged. Burritt (2005) agrees, suggesting that "putting an organization on a positive, healthier course is about leadership that focuses on re-energizing and empowering a workforce. It is about restoring people's confidence in themselves and inspiring them to embrace and initiate change" (p. 482).

What often differentiates a successful change effort from an unsuccessful one is the ability of the *change agent*—a person skilled in the theory and implementation of planned change—to deal appropriately with these very real human emotions and to connect and balance all aspects of the organization that will be affected by that change. In organizational planned change, the manager is often the change agent.

In some large organizations today, however, multidisciplinary teams of individuals, representing all key stakeholders in the organization, are assigned the responsibility for managing the change process. In such organizations, this team manages the communication between the people leading the change effort and those who are expected to implement the new strategies. In addition, this team manages the organizational context in which change occurs and the emotional connections essential for any transformation.

It becomes clear that initiating and coordinating change requires well-developed leadership and management skills. It also requires vision and expert planning skills because a vision is not the same as a plan. The failure to reassess goals proactively and to initiate these changes results in misdirected and poorly used fiscal and human resources. Leader–managers must be visionary in identifying where change is needed in the organization. And they must be flexible in adapting to change that they directly initiated as well as change that has indirectly affected them. Display 8.1 delineates selected leadership roles and management functions necessary for leader–managers acting either in the change agent role or as a coordinator of the planned change team.

THE DEVELOPMENT OF CHANGE THEORY: KURT LEWIN

Most of the current research on change builds on the classic change theories developed by Kurt Lewin in the mid-20th century. Lewin (1951) identified three phases through which the change agent must proceed before a planned change becomes part of the system: unfreezing, movement, and refreezing.

Unfreezing occurs when the change agent convinces members of the group to change or when guilt, anxiety, or concern can be elicited. Thus, people become discontented and aware of a need to change. Kerfoot (2006) says that "change that is sustained does not happen in organizations with top-down edicts" (p. 208). That is because before any change can occur, people must believe

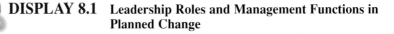

DISPLAY 8.1 Leadership Roles and Management Functions in Planned Change

Leadership Roles

1. Is visionary in identifying areas of needed change in the organization and the health care system
2. Demonstrates risk taking in assuming the role of change agent
3. Demonstrates flexibility in goal setting in a rapidly changing health care system
4. Anticipates, recognizes, and creatively problem solves resistance to change
5. Serves as a role model to subordinates during planned change by viewing change as a challenge and opportunity for growth
6. Role models high-level interpersonal communication skills in providing support for followers undergoing rapid or difficult change
7. Demonstrates creativity in identifying alternatives to problems
8. Demonstrates sensitivity to timing in proposing planned change
9. Takes steps to prevent aging in the organization and to keep nursing current with the new realities of nursing practice

Management Functions

1. Forecasts unit needs with an understanding of the organization and unit's legal, political, economic, social, and legislative climate
2. Recognizes the need for planned change and identifies the options and resources available to implement that change
3. Appropriately assesses the driving and restraining forces when planning for change
4. Identifies and implements appropriate strategies to minimize or overcome resistance to change
5. Seeks subordinates' input in planned change and provides them with adequate information during the change process to give them some feeling of control
6. Supports and reinforces the individual efforts of subordinates during the change process
7. Identifies and uses appropriate change strategies to modify the behavior of subordinates as needed
8. Periodically assesses the unit/department for signs of organizational aging and plans renewal strategies

the change is needed. Palfrey (2006) concurs, arguing, "that to implement change, the team has to be signed up to the vision" (para 2). Similarly, Cummings and McLennan (2005) assert that it is necessary in a planned change "to understand the perspectives of each stakeholder and align the changes to be meaningful to them" (p. 65). For effective change to occur, the change agent needs to have made a thorough and accurate assessment of the extent of and interest in change, the nature and depth of motivation, and the environment in which the change will occur.

Because human beings have little control over many changes in their lives, the change agent must remember that people need a balance between stability and change in the workplace. Change for change's sake subjects employees to unnecessary stress and manipulation.

Change should be implemented only for good reasons.

LEARNING EXERCISE 8.1

Unnecessary Change
Try to remember a situation in your own life that involved unnecessary change. Why do you think the change was unnecessary? What types of turmoil did it cause? Were there things a change agent could have done that would have increased unfreezing in this situation?

The second phase of planned change is *movement*. In movement, the change agent identifies, plans, and implements appropriate strategies, ensuring that driving forces exceed restraining forces. Because change is such a complex process, it requires a great deal of planning and intricate timing. Recognizing, addressing, and overcoming resistance may be a lengthy process. Any change of human behavior, or the perceptions, attitudes, and values underlying that behavior, takes time. Therefore, any change must allow enough time for those involved to be fully assimilated in that change.

 Whenever possible, change should be implemented gradually.

The last phase is *refreezing*. During the refreezing phase, the change agent assists in stabilizing the system change so that it becomes integrated into the status quo. If refreezing is incomplete, the change will be ineffective and the prechange behaviors will be resumed. For refreezing to occur, the change agent must be supportive and reinforce the individual adaptive efforts of those affected by the change. Because change needs at least 3 to 6 months before it will be accepted as part of the system, the change agent must be sure that he or she will be on hand until the change is completed.

Change should never be attempted unless the change agent can make a commitment to be available until the change is complete.

It is important to remember though, that refreezing does not eliminate the possibility of further improvements to the change. Indeed, measuring the impact of change should always be a part of refreezing, for "without measurement, the capacity to achieve administrative and clinical outcomes remains an intuitive undertaking" (Smith et al., 2005, p. 67). Display 8.2 illustrates the change agent's responsibilities during the various stages of planned change.

A CONTEMPORARY ADAPTATION OF LEWIN'S MODEL

Building on Lewin's model, Cummings and McLennan (2005) outlined five steps in their successful planned change to integrate the advanced practice nurse role into an acute-care setting. The first step was to use a change model to guide the process. The second step was to assign a champion (*change agent*) to support, coordinate, and market the change at all levels of the organization (*unfreezing*). In the second step, the planned change and desired outcomes were clearly outlined and communicated to those affected by the change. In the third step, a forum was created to facilitate open communication between all affected by the change during the actual

DISPLAY 8.2 **Stages of Change and Responsibilities of the Change Agent**

Stage 1—Unfreezing

1. Gather data.
2. Accurately diagnose the problem.
3. Decide if change is needed.
4. Make others aware of the need for change; often involves deliberate tactics to raise the group's discontent level; do not proceed to Stage 2 until the status quo has been disrupted and the need for change is perceived by the others.

Stage 2—Movement

1. Develop a plan.
2. Set goals and objectives.
3. Identify areas of support and resistance.
4. Include everyone who will be affected by the change in its planning.
5. Set target dates.
6. Develop appropriate strategies.
7. Implement the change.
8. Be available to support others and offer encouragement through the change.
9. Use strategies for overcoming resistance to change.
10. Evaluate the change.
11. Modify the change, if necessary.

Stage 3—Refreezing

Support others so that the change remains.

change process (*movement*). The final step was to attend to support staff during the transition period (*refreezing*).

Cummings and McLennan concluded that because complex change takes time and innovation to achieve the desired outcome, the change agent must be patient and open to new opportunities during refreezing.

 Change agents must be patient and open to new opportunities during refreezing, as complex change takes time and several different attempts may be needed before desired outcomes are achieved.

Additionally, they emphasized the importance of the change agent knowing whether similar changes were attempted in the past, understanding why the change attempts failed, and articulating the difference in the current change effort (Cummings & McLennan, 2005).

LEWIN'S DRIVING AND RESTRAINING FORCES

Lewin also theorized that people maintain a state of status quo or equilibrium by the simultaneous occurrence of both *driving forces* (facilitators) and *restraining forces* (barriers) operating within any field. Driving forces advance a system toward change; restraining forces impede change.

> The forces that push the system toward change are *driving forces*, whereas the forces that pull the system away from change are called *restraining forces*.

Lewin's model maintained that for change to occur, the balance of driving and restraining forces must be altered. The driving forces must be increased or the restraining forces decreased.

Driving forces may include a desire to please one's boss, to eliminate a problem that is undermining productivity, to get a pay raise, or to receive recognition. Restraining forces include conformity to norms, an unwillingness to take risks, and a fear of the unknown. In Figure 8.1, the person wishing to return to school must reduce the restraining forces or increase the driving forces to alter the present state of equilibrium. There will be no change or action until this occurs. Therefore, creating an imbalance within the system by increasing the driving forces or decreasing the restraining forces is one of the tasks required for a change agent.

Numerous factors affect successful implementation of planned change. Many good ideas are never realized because of poor timing or a lack of power on the part of the change agent. For example, both organizations and individuals tend to reject outsiders as change agents because they are perceived as having inadequate knowledge or expertise about the current status, and their motives often are not trusted. Therefore, there is more widespread resistance if the change agent is an insider. The outside change agent, however, tends to be more objective in his or her assessment, whereas the inside change agent is often influenced by a personal bias regarding how the organization functions.

Likewise, some greatly needed changes are never implemented because the change agent lacks sensitivity to timing. If the organization or the people within that organization have recently undergone a great deal of change or stress, any other change should wait until group resistance decreases.

LEARNING EXERCISE 8.2

Making Change Possible
Identify a change that you would like to make in your personal life (such as losing weight, exercising daily, or stopping smoking). List the restraining forces keeping you from making this change. List the driving forces that make you want to change. Determine how you might be able to change the status quo and make the change possible.

ORGANIZATIONAL CHANGE ASSOCIATED WITH NONLINEAR DYNAMICS

Most organizations frequently experience stability followed by intense transformation. Some later organizational theorists feel that Lewin's refreezing to establish equilibrium should not be the focus of contemporary organizational change since change is unforeseeable and ever present. This is particularly true in health care organizations, where long-term outcomes are almost always unpredictable.

GOAL: RETURN TO SCHOOL

Forces driving to reach goal	Forces restraining from reaching goal
Opportunity for advancement	Low energy level
Status—Social gratification	Limited financial resources
Enhanced self-esteem	Unreliable transportation
Family supportive of efforts	Time with family already limited

Figure 8.1   Driving and restraining forces.

In the past, organizations looked at change and organizational dynamics as linear, occurring both in steps and sequentially. More contemporary theorists maintain that the world is so unpredictable that such dynamics are truly nonlinear. As a result, nonlinear change theories such as *complex adaptive systems theory* and *chaos theory* now influence the thinking of many organizational leaders.

Complexity and Complex Adaptive Systems Change Theory

"*Complexity science* is the latest generation of systems thinking that investigates patterns and has emerged from the exploration of the subatomic world and quantum physics" (Holden, 2005, p. 651). Complexity science argues that the world is complex as are the individuals who operate within it. Thus, control and order are emergent rather than predetermined, and mechanistic formulas do not provide the flexibility needed to predict what actions will result in what outcomes. Benson (2005) agrees, suggesting that the principles of complexity science state that the whole of the system of process is greater than the sum of its parts and that systems are self-organizing and highly adaptive because of these constantly interacting components and feedback loops. Brown (2006) echoes a similar assertion in his statement that complexity theory "reiterates that many contemporary problems are a consequence of highly interactive contexts and agents and cannot be reduced to a single cause-and-effect analysis" (p. 592).

Complex adaptive system theory, an outgrowth of complexity theory, suggests that the relationship between elements or agents within any system is nonlinear and that these elements are the key players in changing settings or outcomes.

 Complex adaptive system theory, which grew out of complexity theory, suggests that the relationship between elements or agents within any system is nonlinear and that these elements are constantly in play to change the environment or outcome.

For example, while an individual may have behaved one way in the past, complex adaptive system theory suggests that future behavior may not always be the same (not always predictable). This is because that individuals' prior experience and past learning may change her or his future choices. In addition, the rules or parameters of each situation are different, even if

DISPLAY 8.3   **Main Features of Olson and Eoyang's (2001) Complex Adaptive Systems Approach to Change**

- Change should be achieved through connections among change agents instead of from the top down.
- There should be adaptation to uncertainty during the change instead of trying to predict stages of development.
- Goals, plans, and structures should be allowed to emerge instead of depending on clear, detailed plans and goals.
- Value differences should be amplified and explored instead of focusing on consensus in change efforts.
- Patterns in one part of the organization are often repeated in another part. Thus, change does not need to begin at the top of an organization to be successful. The goal instead is self-similarity rather than differences in how change is implemented in different parts of the organization.
- Successful change fits with the current organizational environment instead of with an ideal. This is what makes it sustainable.

these differences are subtle; even small variations can dramatically alter choice of action. Complex adaptive systems theory also suggests that the actions of any agent within the system affect all other agents in the system; that is, that context and action are interconnected. Finally, complex adaptive system theory suggests that there are always hidden or unanticipated elements in systems that make linear thinking almost impossible.

In their theory of *complex adaptive systems* (CAS), Olson and Eoyang (2001) suggest that the self-organizing nature of human interactions in a complex organization leads to surprising effects. Rather than focusing on the macro level of the organization system, complexity theory suggests that most powerful change processes occur at the micro level, where relationships, interactions, and simple rules shape emerging patterns. The main features of the CAS approach are shown in Display 8.3.

In applying complex adaptive system theory to planned change, it becomes clear that the multidimensionality of health care organizations, and the individuals who work within them, results in significant challenges for the change agent. Change agents then must carefully examine and focus on the relationships between the elements and be careful not to look at any one element in isolation from the others. It also suggests that time and attention must be given to trying to understand these relationships and interactions even before unfreezing is attempted and that continual monitoring and adaptation will likely be needed for movement and refreezing to be successful.

Chaos Theory

The roots of *chaos theory*, considered by Holden (2005) to be a subset of complexity science, likely emerged from the early work of meteorologist Edward Lorenz in the 1960s to improve weather forecasting techniques (Benson, 2005). Lorenz discovered that even tiny changes in variables often dramatically affected outcomes. Lorenz also discovered that even though these chaotic changes appeared to be random, they were not. Instead, he found that there were "deterministic sequences and certain physical laws, which prevail in nature, even among structures or situations that seem highly irregular or disorganized" (Benson 2005, p. 4). This is why Rae (n.d.) argues that chaos theory is really about finding order in what appears to be random data.

> **Chaos theory is really about finding the underlying order in apparently random data.**

Determining this underlying order, however, is challenging, and the order itself is constantly changing. This chaos makes it difficult to predict the future. In addition, chaos theory suggests that even small changes in conditions can drastically alter a system's long-term behavior (commonly known as the *butterfly effect*). Thus, changes in outcomes are not proportional to the degree of change in the initial condition. As a result of this sensitivity, the behavior of a system exhibiting chaos appears to be random, even though the system is deterministic in the sense that it is well defined and contains no random parameters. Benson (2005) argues that chaos and complexity theories have great application within the social sciences, particularly in regard to organizational development and leadership. For example, in the health care arena, Benson argues that chaos theory could be used to impart insight to issues of quality patient care and patient safety. For example, annual quality plans with sharply delivered strategies and targets are rarely effective. Instead, Benson suggests that general goals and boundaries for improvement should be developed and that measurement approaches must be created that continually look for hidden variables.

The use of nonlinear theories to explain organizational functioning and change are expected to increase in the 21st century. Such theories offer "fresh ways to think about challenges facing healthcare, not just within organizations, but also across the healthcare continuum. Many of the principles and concepts within these new sciences make intuitive sense, but applying them will require new competencies on the part of leaders and their organizations" (Benson, 2005, p. 9). Rae (n.d.) agrees, arguing that:

> Chaos has already had a lasting effect on science, yet there is much still . . . to be discovered. Many scientists believe that twentieth century science will be known for only three theories: relativity, quantum mechanics, and chaos. Aspects of chaos show up everywhere around the world, from the currents of the ocean and the flow of blood through fractal blood vessels to the branches of trees and the effects of turbulence. Chaos has inescapably become part of modern science. As chaos changed from a little-known theory to a full science of its own, it has received widespread publicity. Chaos theory has changed the direction of science: in the eyes of the general public, physics is no longer simply the study of subatomic particles in a billion-dollar particle accelerator, but the study of chaotic systems and how they work (para 33).

CLASSIC CHANGE STRATEGIES

Three classic strategies for effecting change in others were described by Bennis, Benne, and Chinn (1969), with the most appropriate strategy for any situation depending on the power of the change agent and the amount of resistance expected from the subordinates. One of these strategies is to give current research as evidence to support the change. This group of strategies is often referred to as *rational–empirical* strategies. The change agent using this set of strategies assumes that resistance to change comes from a lack of knowledge and that humans are rational beings who will change when given factual information documenting the need for change. This type of strategy is used when there is little anticipated resistance to the change or when the change is perceived as reasonable. Cummings and McLennan (2005) argue, however, that evidence alone is rarely sufficient to induce change, since changing thinking and culture often involves values and beliefs.

Because peer pressure is often used to effect change, another group of strategies exists which use group process and these are called *normative–re-educative* strategies. These strategies use group norms and peer pressure to socialize and influence people so that change will occur. The change agent assumes that humans are social animals, more easily influenced by others than by facts. This strategy does not require the change agent to have a legitimate power base. Instead, the change agent gains power by skill in interpersonal relationships. He or she focuses on noncognitive determinants of behavior, such as people's roles and relationships, perceptual orientations, attitudes, and feelings, to increase acceptance of change.

The third group of strategies, *power–coercive* strategies, features the application of power by legitimate authority, economic sanctions, or political clout of the change agent. These strategies include influencing the enactment of new laws and using group power for strikes or sit-ins. Using authority inherent in an individual position to effect change is another example of a power–coercive strategy. These strategies assume that people often are set in their ways and will change only when rewarded for the change or when they are forced by some other power–coercive method. Resistance is handled by authority measures; the individual must accept it or leave.

Often, the change agent uses strategies from each of these three groups. An example may be reflected in the change agent who wants someone to stop smoking. The change agent might present the person with the latest research on cancer and smoking (the rational–empirical approach); at the same time, the change agent might have friends and family encourage the person socially (normative–re-educative approach). The change agent also might refuse to ride in the smoker's car if the person smokes while driving (power–coercive approach). By selecting from each set of strategies, the change agent increases the chance of successful change.

LEARNING EXERCISE 8.3

Using Change Strategies to Increase Sam's Compliance

You are a staff nurse in a home health agency. One of your patients, Sam Little, is a 38-year-old man with type 1 diabetes. He has developed some loss of vision and had to have two toes amputated as consequences of his disease process. Sam's compliance with four-times-daily blood glucose monitoring and sliding-scale insulin administration has never been particularly good, but he has been worse than usual lately. However, he does seem willing to follow a prescribed diabetic diet and has kept his weight to a desired level.

Sam's wife called you at the agency yesterday and asked you to work with her in developing a plan to increase Sam's compliance with his blood glucose monitoring and insulin administration. She said that Sam, while believing it "probably won't help," has agreed to meet with you to discuss such a plan.

● ASSIGNMENT: What change strategy or combination thereof (rational–empirical, normative–re-educative, power–coercive) do you believe has the greatest likelihood of increasing Sam's compliance? How could you use this strategy? Who would be involved in this change effort? What efforts might you undertake to increase the unfreezing so that Sam is more willing to actively participate in such a planned change effort?

RESISTANCE: THE EXPECTED RESPONSE TO CHANGE

Resistance almost always accompanies change because change alters the balance of a group.

> **Because change disrupts the homeostasis or balance of the group, resistance should always be expected.**

The level of resistance generally depends on the type of change proposed. Technological changes encounter less resistance than changes that are perceived as social or that are contrary to established customs or norms. For example, nursing staff are more willing to accept a change in the type of IV pump to be used than a change regarding who is able to administer certain types of IV therapy. Nursing leaders also must recognize that subordinates' values, educational levels, cultural and social backgrounds, and experiences with change (positive or negative) will have a tremendous impact on the degree of resistance. It also is much easier to change a person's behavior than it is to change an entire group's behavior. Likewise, it is easier to change knowledge levels than attitudes. But all major change takes time (Burritt, 2005).

In an effort to eliminate resistance to change in the workplace, managers historically used an autocratic leadership style with specific guidelines for work, an excessive number of rules, and a coercive approach to discipline. The resistance, which occurred anyway, was both covert (such as delaying tactics or passive–aggressive behavior) and overt (openly refusing to follow a direct command). The result was wasted managerial energy and time and a high level of frustration.

Today, resistance is recognized as a natural and expected response to change. Contemporary managers immerse themselves in identifying and implementing strategies to minimize or manage this resistance to change. One such strategy is to encourage subordinates to speak openly so that options can be identified to overcome objections. Likewise, workers are encouraged to talk about their perceptions of the forces driving the planned change so that the manager can accurately assess change support and resources. In addition, managers should be sure to plan for and create *short-term wins* so that followers can recognize and celebrate progressive change along the way (Burritt, 2005).

> Today, resistance is recognized as a natural and expected response to change.

Still, there are individual variations in terms of risk taking and willingness to accept change. Pesut (2000) classifies individuals as either crusaders or tradition bearers in response to their propensity to seek change. *Crusaders* are change agents who see problems in the present and want to make things better for the future. *Tradition bearers* are the preservers of what is best from the past and the present.

Similarly, Kerfoot (2006) suggests that "just as Johnny Appleseed carried and planted apple seeds that sprouted throughout the Northwest Territory, there are seed carriers in every organization with the seeds of positive change or a negative reaction to change" (p. 208). When there are enough positive seed carriers, their effect "can be felt for days, months, and even years as the seeds take root in the organization, re-seed themselves, and flourish" (p. 208).

Early in the planned change, managers should assess which workers will promote or resist a specific change, both by observation and direct communication. Then, the manager can collaborate with change promoters on how best to convert those individuals more resistant to change.

Jones and Moss (2006) suggest that "the employment of 'early adopters' and those initially more hesitant and resistant to change as champions, will exponentially increase the number of acceptors, or at least those willing to comply" (p. 138).

LEARNING EXERCISE 8.4

What Is Your Attitude Toward Change?
How do you typically respond to change? Do you embrace it? Seek it out? Accept it reluctantly? Avoid it at all cost? Is this behavioral pattern similar to your friends' and that of your family? Has your behavior always fit this pattern, or has the pattern changed throughout your life? If so, what life events have altered how you view and respond to change?

Perhaps the greatest factor contributing to the resistance encountered with change is a lack of trust between the employee and the manager or the employee and the organization. Workers want security and predictability. That is why trust erodes when the ground rules change, as the assumed "contract" between the worker and the organization is altered. Subordinates' confidence in the change agent's ability to manage change depends on whether they believe they have sufficient resources to cope with it. In addition, the leader–manager must remember that subordinates in an organization will generally focus more on how a specific change will affect their personal lives and status than on how it will affect the organization.

PLANNED CHANGE AS A COLLABORATIVE PROCESS

Oftentimes, the change process begins with a few people who meet to discuss their dissatisfaction with the status quo, and an inadequate effort is made to talk with anyone else in the organization. This approach virtually guarantees that the change effort will fail. People abhor "information vacuums," and when there is no ongoing conversation about the change process, gossip usually fills the void. These rumors are generally much more negative than anything that is actually happening.

As a rule, anyone who will be affected by a change should be included in planning it.

 Whenever possible, all those who may be affected by a change should be involved in planning for that change.

When change agents fail to communicate with the rest of the organization, they prevent people from understanding the principles that guided the change, what has been learned from prior experience, and why compromises have been made. Likewise, subordinates affected by the change should thoroughly understand the change and how it affects them as individuals. Good, open communication throughout the process can reduce resistance. Leaders must ensure that group members share perceptions about what change is to be undertaken, who is to be involved and in what role, and how the change will directly and indirectly affect each person in the organization. This was especially apparent in Gradwell's (2004) research, which examined the impact

EXAMINING THE EVIDENCE 8.1

Source: Gradwell, S. S. (2004, June). *Communicating planned change: A case study of leadership credibility.* Drexel University (doctoral dissertation). Retrieved October 1, 2006, from *http://dspace.library.drexel.edu/retrieve/2651/gradwell_thesis.pdf.*

This research study used a qualitative approach with phenomenological interviewing of 25 participants to investigate how the executive (i.e., CEO, COO, CIO) leaders of a Midwest financial organization increased their credibility during a planned organizational change. Specifically, this research focused on the relationship between the leaders' communication of a planned change and the leadership teams' credibility. Three themes emerged from analysis of the data: (a) the change, (b) the leaders, and (c) the communication.

This study suggested that leadership credibility in a planned change exists when the three themes are present and inextricably linked together. In addition, leadership was perceived as a unified team that communicates planned change in a meaningful and consistent manner, using well-structured and well-planned multiple methods to communicate the planned change.

of the leader's communication of a planned change on the leadership team's credibility to carry out that change (Examining the Evidence 8.1).

The easiest way for the manager to ensure that subordinates share this perception is to involve them in the change process. When information and decision making are shared, subordinates feel that they have played a valuable role in the change. Palfrey (2006) suggests that to encourage and maintain motivation within the team, staff must feel empowered to develop their own initiatives. Change agents and the elements of the system—the people or groups within it—must openly develop goals and strategies together. All must have the opportunity to define their interest in the change, their expectation of its outcome, and their ideas on strategies for achieving change.

It is not always easy to attain grassroots involvement in planning efforts. Even when managers communicate that change is needed and that subordinate feedback is wanted, the message often goes unheeded. Some people in the organization may need to hear a message repeatedly before they listen, understand, and believe the message. If the message is one that they do not want to hear, it may take even longer for them to come to terms with the anticipated change.

THE LEADER–MANAGER AS A ROLE MODEL DURING PLANNED CHANGE

Leader–managers must act as role models to subordinates during the change process. The leader–manager must attempt to view change positively and to impart this view to subordinates.

It is critical that managers not view change as a threat.

Rather than viewing change as a threat, managers should embrace it as a challenge and the chance or opportunity to do something new and innovative. Porter-O'Grady (2003) suggests that these dramatically changing times in the practice of nursing have given leaders a more demanding role in health care and that the manager's behavior is the single most important factor in how people in the organization accept change. Burritt (2005) agrees, arguing that the nurse executive's skill in managing change is absolutely pivotal in an organization's ability to change as necessary to meet new demands.

The leader has two responsibilities in facilitating change in nursing practice. First, leader–managers must be actively engaged in change in their own work and model this behavior to staff. Secondly, leaders must be able to assist staff members in making the needed change requirements in their work. Kerfoot (2006) suggests that in every work unit, there are "natural networkers who carry information and culture within their units and others" (p. 209). Since these individuals may have little formal power, the unit manager must mentor and support these individuals so that "they will carry important messages forward to craft and support the organizational changes in process" (p. 209). This is because for a change to become part of the organization, staff must internalize it. One way to assist staff with this internalization is to show a relationship between the process of change and outcome. When this can be measured, then the evidence to support the change is convincing (Porter-O'Grady, 2003).

Managers must believe that they can make a difference. This feeling of control is probably the most important trait for thriving in a changing environment. Friends, family, and colleagues should be used as a support network for managers during change. Likewise, managers should learn to recognize their own stress signals during change and take appropriate steps when the stress level rises too high.

ORGANIZATIONAL AGING: CHANGE AS A MEANS OF RENEWAL

Organizations progress through developmental stages, just as people do—birth, youth, maturity, and aging. As organizations age, structure increases to provide greater control and coordination. The young organization is characterized by high energy, movement, and virtually constant change and adaptation. Aged organizations have established "turf boundaries," function in an orderly and predictable fashion, and are focused on rules and regulations. Change is limited.

It is clear that organizations must find a balance between stagnation and chaos, between birth and death. In the process of maturing, workers within the organization can become prisoners of procedures, forget their original purposes, and allow means to become the ends. Without change, the organization may stagnate and die. Organizations need to keep foremost what they are going to do, not what they have done.

LEARNING EXERCISE 8.5

Young or Old Organization?
Reflect on the organization in which you work or the nursing school you attend. Do you believe that this organization has more characteristics of a young or aged organization? Diagram on a continuum from birth to death where you feel that this organization would fall. What efforts has this organization taken to be dynamic and innovative? What further efforts could be made? Do you agree or disagree that most organizations change unpredictably? Can you support your conclusions with examples?

IS THE NURSING PROFESSION IN NEED OF RENEWAL?

This is a time of changing nursing practice, a change that often creates crisis when nurses try to defend existing models of practice instead of embracing change. Porter-O'Grady (2003) posits that the profession must examine and adapt to the changing context of nursing practice. The traditional realities are:

- Institutionally based care
- Process oriented
- Procedurally driven
- Based on mechanical and manual intervention
- Provider driven
- Treatment based
- Reflective of late-stage intervention
- Based on vertical clinical relationships

According to Porter-O'Grady (2003), the emerging realities of nursing practice for this century will be:

- Mobility based or multisettings
- Outcome driven
- Best-practice oriented
- Emphasized by technology and minimally invasive intervention
- User driven
- Health based
- Geared for early intervention
- Based on horizontal clinical relationships

Perhaps there is no greater need for the leader, at this point in the changing profession, than to be the catalyst for change. Many people attracted to the profession now find that their values and traditional expectations no longer fit as they once did. It is the leader's role to help the staff turn around and confront the opportunities and challenges of the realties of emerging nursing practice; to create enthusiasm and passion for renewing the profession; to embrace the change of locus of control, which now belongs to the health care consumer; and to engage a new social context for nursing practice.

INTEGRATING LEADERSHIP ROLES AND MANAGEMENT FUNCTIONS IN PLANNED CHANGE

It should be clear that leadership and management skills are necessary for successful planned change to occur. The manager must understand the planning process and planning standards and be able to apply both to the work situation. The manager is also cognizant of the specific driving and restraining forces within a particular environment for change and is able to provide the tools or resources necessary to implement that change. The manager, then, is the mechanic who implements the planned change.

The leader, however, is the inventor or creator. Leaders today are forced to plan in a chaotic health care system that is changing at a frenetic pace. Out of this chaos, leaders must identify trends and changes that may affect their organizations and units and proactively prepare for these changes. Thus, the leader must retain a big-picture focus while dealing with each part of the system. In the inventor or creator role, the leader displays such traits as flexibility, confidence, tenacity, and the ability to articulate vision through insights and versatile thinking. The leader also must constantly look for and attempt to adapt to the changing and unpredictable interactions between agents and environmental factors as outlined by the complexity science theorists.

Both leadership and management skills are necessary in planned change. The change agent fulfills a management function when identifying situations where change is necessary and appropriate and when assessing the driving and restraining forces affecting the plan for change. The leader is the role model in planned change. He or she is open and receptive to change and views change as a challenge and an opportunity for growth. Perhaps the most critical elements in successful planned change are the change agent's leadership skills—interpersonal communication, group management, and problem-solving abilities.

 Key Concepts

* Change should not be viewed as a threat but as a challenge and a chance to do something new and innovative.
* Change should be implemented only for good reason.
* Because change disrupts the homeostasis or balance of the group, *resistance* should be expected as a natural part of the change process.
* The level of resistance to change generally depends on the type of change proposed. Technological changes encounter less resistance than changes that are perceived as social or that are contrary to established customs or norms.
* Perhaps the greatest factor contributing to the resistance encountered with change is a lack of trust between the employee and the manager or the employee and the organization.
* It is much easier to change a person's behavior than it is to change an entire group's behavior. It also is easier to change knowledge levels than attitudes.
* Change should be planned and thus implemented gradually, not sporadically or suddenly.
* Those who may be affected by a change should be involved in planning for it. Likewise, workers should thoroughly understand the change and its effect on them.
* The feeling of control is critical to thriving in a changing environment.
* Friends, family, and colleagues should be used as a network of support during change.
* The change agent has the leadership skills of problem solving and decision making and has good interpersonal skills.
* In contrast to *planned change*, *change by drift* is unplanned or accidental.
* Historically, many of the changes that have occurred in nursing or have affected the profession are the results of change by drift.
* People maintain status quo or equilibrium when both *driving* and *restraining forces* operating within any field simultaneously occur. For change to happen, this balance of driving and restraining forces must be altered.
* Organizations are preserved by change and constant renewal. Without change, the organization may stagnate and die.
* Emerging theories such as *complexity science* suggest that change is unpredictable, occurs at random and is dependent upon rapidly changing relationships between agents and factors in the system and that even small changes can effect an entire organization.

ADDITIONAL LEARNING EXERCISES AND APPLICATIONS

LEARNING EXERCISE 8.6

Implementing Planned Change in a Family Planning Clinic

You are a Hispanic RN who has recently received a 2-year grant to establish a family planning clinic in an impoverished, primarily Hispanic area of a large city. The project will be evaluated at the end of the grant to determine whether continued funding is warranted. As project director, you have the funds to choose and hire three health care workers. You will essentially be able to manage the clinic as you see fit.

The average age of your patients will be 14 years, and many come from single-parent homes. In addition, the population with which you will be working has high unemployment, high crime and truancy levels, and great suspicion and mistrust of authority figures. You are aware that many restraining forces exist that will challenge you, but you feel strongly committed to the cause. You believe that the high teenage pregnancy rate and maternal and infant morbidity can be reduced.

● ASSIGNMENT:
1. Identify the restraining and driving forces in this situation.
2. Identify realistic short- and long-term goals for implementing such a change. What can realistically be accomplished in 2 years?
3. How might the project director use hiring authority to increase the driving forces in this situation?
4. Is refreezing of the planned change possible so that changes will continue if the grant is not funded again in 2 years?

LEARNING EXERCISE 8.7

Retain the Status Quo or Implement Change?

Assume that morale and productivity are low on the unit where you are the new manager. In an effort to identify the root of the problem, you have been meeting informally with staff to discuss their perceptions of unit functioning and to identify sources of unrest on the unit. You believe that one of the greatest factors leading to unrest is the limited advancement opportunity for your staff nurses. You have a fixed charge nurse on each shift. This is how the unit has been managed for as long as everyone can remember. You would like to rotate the charge nurse position but are unsure of your staff's feelings about the change.

● ASSIGNMENT: Using the phases of change identified by Lewin (1951), identify the actions you could take in unfreezing, movement, and refreezing. What are the greatest barriers to this change? What are the strongest driving forces?

LEARNING EXERCISE 8.8

How Would You Handle This Response to Change?

You are the unit manager of a cardiovascular surgical unit. The work station on the unit is small, dated, and disorganized. The unit clerks have complained for some time that the chart racks on the counter above their desk are difficult to reach, that staff frequently impinge on the clerks' work space to discuss patients or to chart, that the call-light system is antiquated, and that supplies and forms need to be relocated. You ask all eight of your shift unit clerks to make a "wish list" of how they would like the work station to be redesigned for optimum efficiency and effectiveness.

Construction is completed several months later. You are pleased that the new work station incorporates what each unit clerk included in his or her top three priorities for change. There is a new revolving chart rack in the center of the work station, with enhanced accessibility to both staff and unit clerks. A new state-of-the-art, call-light system has been installed. A small, quiet room has been created for nurses to chart and conference, and new cubbyholes and filing drawers now put forms within arm's reach of the charge nurse and unit clerk.

Almost immediately, you begin to be barraged with complaints about the changes. Several of the unit clerks find the new call-light system's computerized response system overwhelming and complain that patient lights are now going unanswered. Others complain that with the chart rack out of their immediate work area, charts can no longer be monitored and are being removed from the unit by physicians or left in the charting room by nurses. One unit clerk has filed a complaint that she was injured by a staff member who carelessly and rapidly turned the chart rack. She refuses to work again until the old chart racks are returned. The regular day-shift unit clerk complains that all the forms are filed backward for left-handed people and that after 20 years, she should have the right to put them the way that she likes it. Several of the nurses are complaining that the work station is "now the domain of the unit clerk" and that access to the telephones and desk supplies is limited by the unit clerks. There have been some rumblings that several staff members believe that you favored the requests of some employees over others.

Today, when you make rounds at change of shift, you find the day-shift unit clerk and charge nurse involved in a heated conversation with the evening-shift unit clerk and charge nurse. Each evening, the charge nurse and unit clerk reorganize the work station in the manner that they believe is most effective, and each morning, the charge nurse and unit clerk put things back the way they had been the prior day. Both believe that the other shift is undermining their efforts to "fix" the work station organization and that their method of organization is the best. Both groups of workers turn to you and demand that you "make the other shift stop sabotaging our efforts to change things for the better."

● ASSIGNMENT: Despite your intent to include subordinate input into this planned change, resistance is high and worker morale is plummeting. Is the level of resistance a normal and anticipated response to planned change? If so, would you intervene in this conflict? How? Was it possible to have reduced the likelihood of such a high degree of resistance?

LEARNING EXERCISE 8.9

Old and New Roles of Nursing Practice

Examine the old and new realities of nursing practice as identified by Porter-O'Grady (2003) under the heading "Is the Nursing Profession in Need of Renewal?"

● ASSIGNMENT: In a small group, discuss the old and new roles of nursing practice. In your observations, based on your nursing school clinical experiences, theory-based classes, and watching other nurses in their roles, what type of nursing practice do you see being implemented? Give specific examples. Are the practice models in the evidence provider driven or user driven? Is the nursing practice process oriented or outcome driven? As an organization, do you believe that nursing would be classified as (a) an aging organization, (b) in constant motion and ever renewing, or (c) a closed system that does not respond well to change?

Web Links

Kurt Lewin
http://muskingum.edu/%7Epsychology/psycweb/history/lewin.htm
Biography, overview of planned change theory, timeline of his theoretical developments, and bibliography.

The New Science of Leadership: An Interview with Margaret Wheatley
http://www.scottlondon.com/interviews/wheatley.html
An interview excerpt with best-selling author Margaret Wheatley about organizational change, chaos theory, and complex adaptive change.

Employee Resistance to Organizational Change
http://search.mywebsearch.com/mywebsearch/AJmain.jhtml?t=&st=kwd&ptnrS=zuzeb004
YYUS&searchfor=resistance+to+change
This updated 2005 literature review by Albert F. Bolognese presents different theoretical approaches to understanding employee resistance to change.

References

Bennis, W., Benne, K., & Chinn, R. (1969). *The planning of change* (2nd ed.). New York: Holt, Rinehart, & Winston.

Benson, H. (2005). Chaos and complexity: Applications for healthcare quality and patient safety. *Journal for Healthcare Quality: Promoting Excellence in Healthcare, 27*(5), 4–10.

Brown, C. A. (2006). The application of complex adaptive systems theory to clinical practice in rehabilitation. *Disability and Rehabilitation, 28*(9), 587–593.

Burritt, J. E. (2005). Organizational turnaround. The role of the nurse executive. *Journal of Nursing Administration, 35*(11), 482–489.

Cummings, G., & McLennan, M. (2005). Advanced practice nursing. Leadership to effect policy change. *Journal of Nursing Administration, 35*(2), 61–66.

Gradwell, S. S. (2004, June). *Communicating planned change: A case study of leadership credibility.* Drexel University (doctoral dissertation). Retrieved October 1, 2006, from *http://dspace. library.drexel.edu/retrieve/2651/gradwell_thesis.pdf.*

Holden, L. M. (2005). Complex adaptive systems: Concept analysis. *Journal of Advanced Nursing, 52*(6), 651–657.

Jones, S., & Moss, J. (2006). Computerized provider order entry. *Journal of Nursing Administration, 36*(3), 136–139.

Kerfoot, K. (2006). On leadership. The Johnny Appleseeds of organizational change. *Dermatology Nursing, 18*(2), 208–210.

Lewin, K. (1951). *Field theory in social sciences.* New York: Harper & Row.

Olson, E. E., & Eoyang, G. H. (2001). *Facilitating organization change: Lessons from complexity science.* San Francisco: Jossey-Boss/Pfeiffer.

Palfrey, G. (2006). Reflections of a nurse partner. Managing change. *Practice Nurse, 31*(5), 66.

Pesut, D. (2000). Crusaders and tradition bearers. *Nursing Outlook, 48*(6), 262.

Porter-O'Grady, T. (2003). A different age for leadership part 2: New rules, new roles. *Journal of Nursing Administration, 33*(3), 173–178.

Rae, G. (n.d.). *Chaos theory: A brief introduction.* Retrieved September 13, 2006, from *http://www.imho.com/grae/chaos/chaos.html.*

Smith, C. E., Rebeck, S., Schaag, H., Kleinbeck, S., Moore, J. J., & Bleich, M. R. (2005). A model for evaluating systemic change. Measuring outcomes of hospital discharge education redesign. *Journal of Nursing Administration, 35*(2), 67–73.

Bibliography

Brown, H. (2006). Too much change in our working environment? *Geriatric Medicine, 36*(3), 11.

Buck, K., & McPherson, B. (2006). Co-creating the space for change: Through dialogue, ministry leaders will find confidence to move into the future. *Health Progress, 87*(3), 62–65.

Doutrich, D., & Storey, M. (2006). Cultural competence and organizational change: Lasting results of an institutional linkage. *Home Health Care Management and Practice, 18*(5), 356–360.

Grimes, P. (2006). Cycle of perpetual change adversely affects care. *Nursing Standard, 20*(19), 38–39.

Hadden, K. (2004, February 23). *Strategies for planned change.* Retrieved September 11, 2006, from *http://portfolio.educ.kent.edu/haddenk/Strategies/categories.htm.*

Hernandez, N. (2006). Organizational culture and organizational change. *AMT Events, 23*(2), 66–67, 75–77.

Kaplan, S. A., Calman, N. S., Golub, M., Ruddock, C., & Billings, J. (2006). Fostering organizational change through a community-based initiative. *Health Promotion Practice, 7*(3)(suppl), 181S–190S.

Kuokkanen, L., Suominen, T., Rankinen, S., Kukkurainen, M.L., Savikko, N. and Doran, D. (2007, July). Organizational change and work-related empowerment. Nursing Management, *15*(5), 500–507.

Lindstrom-Forneri, W., Tuokko, H., & Rhodes, R.E. (2007, August). "Getting around town": A preliminary investigation of the theory of planned behavior and intent to change driving behaviors among older adults. *Journal of Applied Gerontology, 26*(4), 385–398.

Nagelkerk, J. (2006). Psychosocial work environment and mental health: Job-strain and effort-reward imbalance models in a context of a major organizational changes. *Clinical Nurse Specialist: The Journal for Advanced Nursing Practice, 20*(2), 93–94.

Penprase, B., & Norris, D. (2005). What nurse leaders should know about complex adaptive systems theory. *Nursing Leadership Forum, 9*(3), 127–132.

9

Time Management

. . . nothing is particularly hard if you divide it into small jobs.

—*Henry Ford*

. . . things which matter most must never be at the mercy of things that matter least.

—*Johann Wolfgang von Goethe*

Another part of the planning process is short-term planning. This operational planning focuses on achieving specific tasks. Short-term plans involve a period of 1 hour to 3 years and are usually less complex than strategic or long-range plans. Short-term planning may be done annually, bimonthly, weekly, daily, or even hourly.

Previous chapters examined the need for prudent planning of resources, such as money, equipment, supplies, and labor. Time is an equally important resource. If managers are to direct employees effectively and maximize other resources, they must first be able to find the time to do so. *Time management* is making optimal use of available time. Because time is a finite and valuable resource, learning to use it wisely requires both leadership skills and management functions. The leader–manager must initiate an analysis of time management on the unit level, involve team members and gain their cooperation in maximizing time use, and guide work to its conclusion and successful implementation.

There is a close relationship between time management and stress. Managing time appropriately is one way to reduce stress and increase productivity. The current status of health care, the nursing shortage, and decreasing reimbursements, have resulted in many health care organizations trying to do more with less. The effective use of time-management tools, therefore, becomes even more important to enable managers to meet personal and professional goals. Managing time well allows an individual more time to spend on priority issues.

 Good time-management skills allow an individual to spend time on things that matter.

Unfortunately, some individuals lack self-awareness about what is important or how they currently spend their time. The first step then to making better use of time, is to examine how you currently spend it and to consider "how much of your time goes to waste every day because of

DISPLAY 9.1 Leadership Roles and Management Functions in Time Management

Leadership Roles

1. Is self-aware regarding personal blocks and barriers to efficient time management as well as how one's own value system influences his/her use of time and the expectations of followers
2. Functions as a role model, supporter, and resource person to subordinates in setting priorities
3. Assists followers in working cooperatively to maximize time use
4. Prevents and/or filters interruptions that prevent effective time management
5. Role models flexibility in working cooperatively with other people whose primary time management style is different
6. Presents a calm and reassuring demeanor during periods of high unit activity

Management Functions

1. Appropriately prioritizes day-to-day planning to meet short-term and long-term unit goals
2. Builds time for planning into the work schedule
3. Analyzes how time is managed on the unit level by using job analysis and time-and-motion studies
4. Eliminates environmental barriers to effective time management for unit staff
5. Handles paperwork promptly and efficiently and maintains a neat work area
6. Breaks down large tasks into smaller ones that can more easily be accomplished by unit members
7. Utilizes appropriate technology to facilitate timely communication and documentation
8. Discriminates between inadequate staffing and inefficient use of time when time resources are inadequate to complete assigned tasks

unscheduled developments, frequent interruptions, tardiness, bad planning, and crisis management" (Where Does the Time Go?, 2006, para 2). Leadership roles and management functions needed for effective time management are included in Display 9.1.

THREE BASIC STEPS TO TIME MANAGEMENT

There are three basic steps to time management (Fig. 9.1). The first step requires that time be set aside for planning and establishing priorities. The second step entails completing the highest-priority task (as determined in step 1) whenever possible and finishing one task before beginning another. In the final step, the person must reprioritize what tasks will be accomplished based on new information received. Because this is a cyclic process, all three steps must be accomplished sequentially. Managers who are new to time management may underestimate the importance of regular planning and fail to allot enough time for it.

 Unfortunately, two mistakes common to novice managers are underestimating the importance of a daily plan and not allowing adequate time for planning.

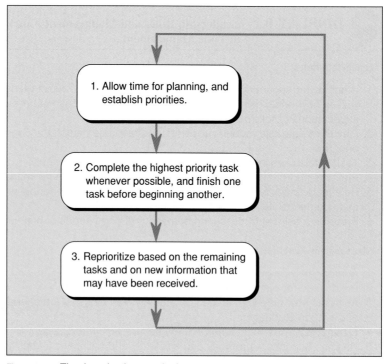

Figure 9.1   The three basic steps in time management.

Taking Time to Plan

Daily planning is essential if the manager is to manage by efficiency rather than by crisis. The old adage "fail to plan—plan to fail" is timeless. Managers may believe they are unproductive if they sit at their desk designing the plan for the day, rather than accomplishing a specific task. Without adequate planning, however, the manager finds it difficult to get started and begins to manage by crisis. In addition, there can be no sense of achievement at day's end if the goals for the day are not clearly delineated.

LEARNING EXERCISE 9.1

Targeting Personal Procrastination
Spend a few moments reflecting on the last 2 weeks of your life. What are the things you put off doing? Do these things form a pattern? For instance, do you always put off writing a school paper until the last minute? Do you wait to do certain tasks at work until you cannot avoid the task any longer? What things do you do when you really do not want to do something? Do you eat? Play video games? Watch TV? Read?

● ASSIGNMENT: Write a one-page essay on at least two things that you procrastinate and then develop two strategies for breaking each of these habits.

Planning takes time; it requires the ability to think, analyze data, envision alternatives, and make decisions. Setting aside time at the beginning of each day to plan the day allows the manager to spend time on high-priority tasks. During this planning time, the manager should review short-term, intermediate, and long-term goals and determine what progress will be made toward these goals. Sometimes, the manager does allow time for planning but has problems accurately predicting the length of time it will take to complete an activity.

Priority Setting and Procrastination

Because managers are inundated with many requests for their time and energy, the next step in time management is prioritizing, which may well be the key to good time management.

> Priority setting is perhaps the most critical skill in good time management, because all actions we take have some type of relative importance.

Vacarro (2001) suggests that there are five priority-setting traps (Display 9.2). The first is "whatever hits first." This trap occurs when an individual simply responds to things as they happen rather than thinking first and then acting. The second trap is the "path of least resistance." In this trap, the individual makes an erroneous assumption that it is always easier to do a task personally and fails to delegate appropriately. The third trap is the "squeaky wheel." In this trap, the individual falls prey to those who are most vocal about their urgent requests. Compounding the trap is that the individual often feels a need to respond to the time frame imposed by the "squeaky wheel," rather than his or her own. The fourth trap is called "managing by default." In this trap, the individual feels obligated to take on tasks that no one else has come forward to do. To keep this from happening, the individual must determine whether the undone job is truly his or her responsibility and whether it serves to accomplish his or her stated goals. The last trap is "waiting for inspiration." In this trap, individuals wait until they become "inspired" to accomplish a task. Some necessary tasks will never be inspiring, and the wise manager recognizes that the only thing that will complete these tasks is hard work and appropriate attention to the matter.

One simple means of prioritizing what needs to be accomplished is to divide all requests into three categories: "don't do," "do later," and "do now" (Display 9.3). The "don't do" items probably reflect problems that will take care of themselves, are already outdated, or are better accomplished by someone else. The manager either throws away the unnecessary information or passes it on to the appropriate person in a timely fashion. In either case, the manager removes unneeded clutter from his or her work area.

DISPLAY 9.2 Five Priority-Setting Traps

1. Whatever hits first
2. Path of least resistance
3. Squeaky wheel
4. Managing by default
5. Waiting for inspiration

DISPLAY 9.3   **Three Categories of Prioritization**

1. "Don't do"
2. "Do later"
3. "Do now"

Some "do later" items reflect trivial problems or those that do not have immediate deadlines; thus, they may be procrastinated. To *procrastinate* means to put off something until a future time, to postpone, or to delay needlessly. Procrastination is a difficult problem to solve because it rarely results from a single cause and can involve a combination of dysfunctional attitudes, rationalizations, and resentment.

Blunt and Pychyl (2005) suggest that procrastination is closely related to personality and temperament. They suggest that people tend to be either action oriented or state oriented (more likely to procrastinate) and that changing this orientation is very difficult (Examining the Evidence 9.1)

Marano (2006) is quick to point out, however, that procrastination does not mean lazy. Instead, it is "an active mental process of diverting yourself from doing high-priority things in the delusion that tomorrow will be better—because you'll know more, you'll have more time, or the sun will shine differently" (p. 41).

 Procrastination is not the same as laziness.

Although managers should selectively procrastinate, they should not avoid a task because it is overwhelming or unpleasant. Before setting "do later" items aside, the manager must be

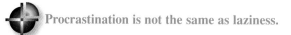

EXAMINING THE EVIDENCE 9.1

Source: Blunt, A., & Pychyl, T. A. (2005). Project systems of procrastinators: A personal project-analytic and action control perspective. *Personality and Individual Differences, 38*(8), 1771–1780.

As part of research completed with the Ottawa Carleton University Procrastination Research Group, Blunt and Pychyl suggest that there are two basic ways of functioning in the world. There are the state-oriented souls, who have a lot of inertia—and are most likely to procrastinate, and action-oriented people, who move easily from task to task.

State-oriented people rate tasks more negatively; they experience greater uncertainty, boredom, frustration, and guilt than do their action-oriented peers. What helps them is priming the pump or shifting from one action to the next.

The authors suggest that state-oriented individuals "follow a 10-minute rule" whereby they do the task they do not want to do for 10 minutes and then decide whether to continue. This is because many tasks are easier to continue once they have been started. The authors also conclude that succeeding at a task does not require that you like doing it.

sure that large projects have been broken down into smaller projects and that a specific time line and plan for implementation are in place. The plan should include short-term, intermediate, and final deadlines. Likewise, a manager cannot ignore items without immediate time limits forever and must make a definite time commitment in the near future to address these requests.

The "do now" requests most commonly reflect a unit's day-to-day operational needs. These requests may include daily staffing needs, dealing with equipment shortages, meeting schedules, conducting hiring interviews, and giving performance appraisals. "Do now" requests also may represent items that had been put off earlier.

In prioritizing all the "do now" items, the manager may find preparing a written list helpful. Remember, however, that a list is a plan, not a product, and that the creation of the list is not the final goal. The list is a planning tool. Although the manager may use monthly or weekly lists, a list also can assist in coordinating daily operations. This daily list, however, should not be longer than what can be realistically accomplished in 1 day; otherwise, it demotivates instead of assists the manager. In addition, although the manager must be cognizant of and plan for routine tasks, it is not always necessary to place them on the list because they may only distract attention from other priority tasks. Lists should allow adequate time for each task and have blocks of time built in for the unexpected.

In addition, individuals who use lists to help them organize their day must be careful not to confuse importance and urgency. Not all important things are urgent, and not all urgent things are important. This is especially true when the urgency is coming from an external source.

In addition, the manager should periodically review lists from previous days to see what was not accomplished or completed. If a task appears on a list for several successive days, the manager must re-examine it and assess why it was not accomplished. Some projects need to be removed from the list. A project may remain unaccomplished if it is not divided into steps or tasks that can be completed.

 Some projects are not accomplished because they are not broken down into manageable tasks.

For example, many well-meaning people begin thinking about completing their tax returns in early January but feel overwhelmed by a project that cannot be accomplished in 1 day. If preparing a tax return is not broken down into several smaller tasks with intermediate deadlines, it may be almost perpetually procrastinated.

LEARNING EXERCISE 9.2

Making Big Projects Manageable
Masikiewicz (2000) states that the best way to get big projects done is to break them down, with mini-deadlines that you set yourself. Think of the last major paper you wrote for a class. Did you set short-term and intermediate deadlines? Did you break the task down into smaller tasks to eliminate a last-minute crisis? What short-term and intermediate deadlines have you set to accomplish major projects that have been assigned to you this quarter or semester?

The manager must remember that because the list is a planning tool, there must be some flexibility in its implementation. In fact, the last step in time management is reprioritizing. Often, the manager's priorities or list will change during a day, week, or longer because new information is received. If the manager does not take time to reprioritize after each major task is accomplished, other priorities set earlier may no longer be accurate. In addition, despite outstanding planning, an occasional crisis may erupt.

No amount of planning can prevent an occasional crisis.

If a crisis does occur, the individual may need to set aside the original priorities for the day and reorganize, communicate, and delegate a new plan reflecting the new priorities associated with the unexpected event causing the crisis.

LEARNING EXERCISE 9.3

Creating Planning Lists
Do you make a daily plan to organize what needs to be done? Mentally or on paper, develop a list of five items that must be accomplished today. Prioritize that list. Now make a list of five items that must be done this week. Prioritize that list as well.

MANAGING TIME AT WORK

Being overwhelmed by work and time constraints leads to increased errors, the omission of important tasks, and general feelings of stress and ineffectiveness. Although some people seem to be "naturals" with time management, the skill is learned and improves with practice.

All workers need to allow time for daily planning to appropriately manage time at work. Examples of the types of plans a charge nurse might make in day-to-day planning include staffing schedules, patient care assignments, coordination of lunch- and work-break schedules, and interdisciplinary coordination of patient care. Examples of an acute-care staff nurse's day-to-day planning might include determining how reports will be given and received; the timing and method used for initial patient assessments; the coordination of medication administration, treatments, and procedures; and the organization of documentation of the day's activities.

Some staff nurses appear disorganized in their efforts to care for patients. Usually, this disorganization results from poor planning. Planning occurs first in the management process because the ability to be organized develops from good planning. During planning, there should be time to think about how plans will be translated into action. The planner must pause and decide how people, activities, and materials are going to be put together to carry out the objectives. The following suggestions using industrial engineering principles may assist the staff nurse in planning work activities:

• *Gather all the supplies and equipment that will be needed before starting an activity.*
   Breaking a job down mentally into parts before beginning the activity may help the

staff nurse identify what supplies and equipment will be needed to complete the activity.

- *Group activities that are in the same location.* If you have walked a long distance down a hallway, attempt to do several things there before going back to the nurses' station. If you are a home health nurse, group patient visits geographically when possible to minimize travel time and maximize time with patients.
- *Use time estimates.* For example, if you know an intermittent intravenous medication (IV piggyback) will take 30 minutes to complete, then use that time estimate for planning some other activity that can be completed in that 30-minute window of time.
- *Document your nursing interventions as soon as possible after an activity is completed.* Waiting until the end of the workday to complete necessary documentation increases the risk of inaccuracies and incomplete documentation.
- *Always strive to end the workday on time.* Although this is not always possible, delegating appropriately to others and making sure that the workload goal for any given day is reasonable are two strategies that will accomplish this goal.

Like staff nurses, unit managers need to coordinate how their duties will be carried out and devise methods to make work simpler and more efficient. Often, this includes simple tasks such as organizing how supplies are stored or determining the most efficient lunch and break schedules for staff. The goal in planning work and activities is to facilitate greater productivity and satisfaction. Daily planning actions that may help the unit manager identify and utilize time as a resource most efficiently might include:

- At the start of each workday, identify key priorities to be accomplished that day. Identify what specific actions need to be taken to accomplish those priorities and in what order they should be done. Also identify specific actions that should be taken to meet ongoing, long-term goals.
- Determine the level of achievement that you expect for each prioritized task. Is a maximizing or "satisficing" approach more appropriate or more reasonable for each of the goals you have identified?
- Assess the staff assigned to work with you. Assign work that must be delegated to staff members who are both capable and willing to accomplish the priority task that you have identified. Be sure that you have clearly expressed any expectations you may have about how and when a delegated task must be completed. (Delegation is discussed further in Chapter 20.)
- Review the short- and long-term plans of the unit regularly. Include colleagues and subordinates in identifying unit problems or concerns so that they can be fully involved in planning for needed change.
- Plan ahead for meetings. Prepare and distribute agendas in advance.
- Allow time at several points throughout the day and at the end of the day to assess progress in meeting established daily goals and to determine if unanticipated events have occurred or if new information has been received that may have altered your original plan. Ongoing realities for the unit manager include work situations that are constantly changing, and with them, setting new priorities and adjusting older ones.

 Setting new priorities or adjusting priorities to reflect ever-changing work situations is an ongoing reality for the unit manager.

LEARNING EXERCISE 9.4

Setting Daily Priorities

Assume that you are the RN leader of a team with one LVN and one nursing assistant on the 7 AM to 3 PM shift at an acute-care hospital. The three of you are responsible for providing total care to 10 patients. Prioritize the following list of 10 things that you need to accomplish this morning. Use a "1" for the first thing you will do and a "10" for the last. Be prepared to provide rationale for your priorities.

___ Check medication cards/sheets against the rand or Kardex.

___ Listen to night shift report 0700–0720.

___ Take brief walking rounds to assess the night shift report and to introduce yourself to patients.

___ Hang four 0900 IV medications.

___ Set up the schedule for breaks and lunch among your team members.

___ Give 0845 preop on patient going to surgery at 0900.

___ Pass 0830 breakfast trays.

___ Meet with team members to plan the schedule for the day and to clarify roles.

___ Read charts of patients who are new to you.

___ Check 0600 blood sugar lab results for 0730 insulin administration.

Taking Breaks

Planning for periodic breaks from work during the workday is an integral part of an individual's time and task management. Taking regularly scheduled breaks from work is important, as breaks allow the worker to refresh both physically and mentally. Hatcher and colleagues (2006) suggest that having time off, whether it be for vacation or for on-the-job breaks, provides time for renewal as well as reflection. In addition, it reduces stress; minimizes shoulder, neck, and low back pain; and reduces eyestrain. This is especially true for the older nurse.

Kriegel (2002) says that when individuals are overworked, they must recognize that longer hours on the job do not necessarily produce the desired outcomes. Most people's knee-jerk response to pressure is to run harder and faster, but Kriegel maintains that working longer at a rushed pace not only increases the potential for stress and burnout but also results in more mistakes. Taking a 15-minute daily time-out to think creatively about how to achieve work objectives is recommended.

Dealing with Interruptions

All managers experience interruptions, but lower-level managers experience the most. This occurs in part because first- and middle-level managers are more involved in daily planning than higher-level managers and thus directly interact with a greater number of subordinates. In addition, many lower-level managers do not have a quiet work space or clerical help to filter interruptions. Frequent work interruptions result in situational stress and lowered job satisfaction. Managers need to develop skill in preventing interruptions that threaten effective time management.

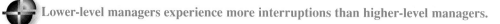 **Lower-level managers experience more interruptions than higher-level managers.**

Time Wasters

Four time wasters warrant special attention here. The first of these surprisingly is technology. Marano (2006) suggests that what differentiates procrastination today from a century ago is the variety of distractions and diversion available, including the Internet, chat rooms, online card games, and X box. Belkin (2005) echoes a similar theme in her assertion that technology provides endless ways to waste time. A joint poll released in 2005 by AOL and Salary.com found that "the average worker wastes two hours every day (not including lunch), and that nearly 45 percent of respondents name the computer as their primary distraction" (para 5).

A second time waster is socializing. The AOL and Salary.com poll also showed that 23 percent of respondents reported socializing with colleagues during their workday as well as making personal phone calls (probably the primary time guzzler before the computer came along) and running errands (Belkin, 2005).

Although socializing can help workers meet relationship needs or build power, it can tremendously deter productivity. This is especially true for managers with an open door policy. Subordinates can be discouraged from taking up a manager's time with idle chatter in several ways:

- *Do not make yourself overly accessible.* Make it easy for people to ignore you. Try not to "work" at the nursing station, if this is possible. If charting is to be done, sit with your back to others. If you have an office, close the door. Have people make appointments to see you. All these behaviors will discourage casual socializers.
- *Interrupt.* When someone is rambling on without getting to the point, break in and say gently, "Excuse me. Somehow I'm not getting your message. What exactly are you saying?"
- *Avoid promoting socialization.* Having several comfortable chairs in your office, a full candy dish, and posters on your walls that invite comments encourage socializing in your office.
- *Be brief.* Watch your own long-winded comments, and stand up when you are finished. This will signal an end to the conversation.
- *Schedule long-winded pests.* If someone has a pattern of lengthy chatter and manages to corner you on rounds or at the nurse's station, say, "I can't speak with you now, but I'm going to have some free time at 11 AM. Why don't you see me then?" Unless the meeting is important, the person who just wishes to chat will not bother to make a formal appointment.

If you would like to chat and have the time to do so, use coffee breaks and lunch hours for socializing.

The other external time wasters that a manager must conquer are paperwork overload and a poor filing system. Managers are generally inundated with paper clutter, including organizational memos, staffing requests, quality assurance reports, incident reports, and patient evaluations. Because paperwork is often redundant or unnecessary, the manager needs to become an expert at handling it. Whenever possible, incoming correspondence should be handled the day it arrives; it should either be thrown away or filed according to the date to be completed. Try to address each piece of correspondence only once.

An adequate filing system also is invaluable to handling paper overload. Keeping correspondence organized in easily retrievable files rather than disorganized stacks saves time when the manager needs to find specific information. The manager also may want to consider increased use of computerization and email to reduce the paper use and to increase response time in time-sensitive communication.

Personal Time Management

Personal time management refers in part to self-knowledge. Self-awareness is a leadership skill. For people who are not certain of their own short- to long-term goals, time management in general poses difficulties.

> Managing time is difficult if a person is unsure of his or her priorities for time management, including personal short-term, intermediate, and long-term goals.

These goals give structure to what should be accomplished today, tomorrow, and in the future. However, goals alone are not enough; a concrete plan with time lines is needed. Plans outlined in manageable steps are clearer, more realistic, and attainable. By being self-aware and setting goals accordingly, people determine how their time will be spent. If goals are not set, others often end up deciding how a person should spend his or her time.

Think for a moment about last week. Did you accomplish all that you wanted to accomplish? How much time did you or others waste? In your clinical practice, did you spend your time hunting for supplies and medicines instead of teaching your patient about his or her diabetes? Too often, irrelevant decisions and insignificant activities take priority over real purposes. Clearly, work redesign, clarification of job descriptions, or a change in the type of care delivery system may alleviate some of these problems. However, the same general principle holds: Professional nurses who are self-aware and have clearly identified personal goals and priorities have greater control over how they expend their energy and what they accomplish. In addition, organized individuals "experience less stress, are healthier, and perform better on the job than their disorganized peers" (Cohen, 2006, p. 128).

Cohen (2006) suggests that using a planner or appointment book to organize your day can help make a day feel less chaotic. It can also help you to identify pockets of spare time that you could use for breaks. Computer-savvy individuals might choose to use one of the newer personal digital assistants (PDAs) such as a Palm Pilot or an electronic calendar associated with an email system to help organize their day.

In addition to being self-aware regarding the values that influence how people prioritize the use of their time, people must be self-aware regarding their general tendency to complete tasks in isolation or in combination. Some people prefer to do one thing at a time, whereas others typically do two or more things simultaneously. Some individuals begin and finish projects on time, have clean and organized desks because of handling each piece of paperwork only once, and are highly structured. Others tend to change plans, borrow and lend things frequently, emphasize relationships rather than tasks, and build longer-term relationships. It is important to recognize one's own preferred time-management style and to be self-aware about how this orientation may affect your interaction with others in the workplace.

Finally, each individual should be cognizant of how he or she values the time of others. For example, being punctual goes beyond common courtesy. Kennedy (2006) suggests that "being punctual gives you the right—the positioning—to expect and demand that others treat your time with utmost respect" (p. 243). Likewise, tardiness reflects some disregard for the value of other people's time.

> A lack of punctuality suggests that you do not value other people's time.

Kennedy also suggests that it is imperative to be where you are supposed to be when you are supposed to be there if you want to win friends and influence people. He cautions latecomers to remember that not being punctual is almost certain to result in being negatively judged by those very people you are trying to impress.

Personal Time Wasters

A significant part of personal time management depends on self-awareness about how and when a person is most productive. Everyone has ways to waste time or steer clear of certain activities.

 Everyone avoids certain types of work or has methods of wasting time.

Likewise, each person works better at certain times of the day or for certain lengths of time. Self-aware people schedule complex or difficult tasks during the periods when they are most productive and simpler or routine tasks during less productive times.

Using a Time Inventory

Because most people have an inaccurate perception of the time they spend on a particular task or the total amount of time they are productive during the day, a time inventory may provide insight. A time inventory is shown in Display 9.4. A time inventory allows you to compare what you planned to do, as outlined by your appointments and "to do" entries, with what you actually did. "It will reveal how much you are letting situations, events and other people control your time instead of you being in command of your schedule" (Where Does the Time Go?, 2006, para 4).

Because the greatest benefit from a time inventory is being able to objectively identify patterns of behavior, it may be necessary to maintain the time inventory for several days or even several weeks. It also may be helpful to repeat the time inventory annually to see if long-term behavior changes have been noted. Remember, there is no way to beg, borrow, or steal more hours in the day. If time is habitually used ineffectively, being a manager will be very stressful.

LEARNING EXERCISE 9.5

Writing a Personal Time Inventory
Use the time inventory shown in Display 9.4 to identify your activities for a 24-hour period. Record your activities on the time inventory on a regular basis. Be specific. Do not trust your memory. Star the periods of time when you were most productive. Circle periods of time when you were least productive. Do not include sleep time. Was this a typical day for you? Could you have modified your activity during your least productive time periods? If so, how?

INTEGRATING LEADERSHIP ROLES AND MANAGEMENT FUNCTIONS IN TIME MANAGEMENT

The leadership skills needed to manage time resources draw heavily on interpersonal communication skills. The leader is a resource and role model to subordinates in how to manage

DISPLAY 9.4 Time Inventory

5:00 AM	_____
6:00 AM	_____
6:30 AM	_____
7:00 AM	_____
7:30 AM	_____
8:00 AM	_____
8:30 AM	_____
9:00 AM	_____
9:30 AM	_____
10:00 AM	_____
10:30 AM	_____
11:00 AM	_____
11:30 AM	_____
12:00 PM	_____
12:30 PM	_____
1:00 PM	_____
1:30 PM	_____
2:00 PM	_____
2:30 PM	_____
3:00 PM	_____
3:30 PM	_____
4:00 PM	_____
4:30 PM	_____
5:00 PM	_____
5:30 PM	_____
6:00 PM	_____
6:30 PM	_____
7:00 PM	_____
7:30 PM	_____
8:00 PM	_____
8:30 PM	_____
9:00 PM	_____
9:30 PM	_____
10:00 PM	_____
11:00 PM	_____
12:00 PM	_____
1:00 AM	_____
2:00 AM	_____
3:00 AM	_____
4:00 AM	_____

time. As has been stressed in other phases of the management process, the leadership skill of self-awareness also is necessary in time management. Leaders must understand their own value system, which influences how they use time and how they expect subordinates to use time.

The management functions inherent in using time resources wisely are more related to productivity. The manager must be able to prioritize activities of unit functioning to meet short- and long-term unit needs.

Successful leader–managers are able to integrate leadership skills and management functions; they accomplish unit goals in a timely and efficient manner in a concerted effort with subordinates. They also recognize time as a valuable unit resource and share responsibility for the use of that resource with subordinates. Perhaps most importantly, the integrated leader–manager with well-developed, time-management skills can maintain greater control over time and energy constraints in his or her personal and professional life.

 Key Concepts

* Because time is a finite and valuable resource, learning to use it wisely is essential for effective management.
* *Time management* can be reduced to three cyclic steps: (a) allow time for planning, and establish priorities; (b) complete the highest priority task, and whenever possible, finish one task before beginning another; and (c) reprioritize based on remaining tasks and new information that may have been received.
* Setting aside time at the beginning of each day to plan the day allows the manager to spend appropriate time on high-priority tasks.
* Making lists is an appropriate tool to manage daily tasks. This list should not be any longer than what can realistically be accomplished in a day and must include adequate time to accomplish each item on the list and time for the unexpected.
* A common cause of *procrastination* is failure to break large tasks down into smaller ones so that the manager can set short-term, intermediate, and long-term goals.
* Lower-level managers have more interruptions in their work than higher-level managers. This results in situational stress and lowered job satisfaction.
* Managers must learn strategies to cope with interruptions from socializing.
* Because so much paperwork is redundant or unnecessary, the manager needs to develop expertise at prioritizing it and eliminating unnecessary clutter at the work site.
* An efficient filing system is invaluable to handling paper overload.
* *Personal time management* refers to "the knowing of self." Managing time is difficult if a person is unsure of his or her priorities, including personal short-term, intermediate, and long-term goals.
* Being punctual implies that you value other people's time and creates an imperative for them to value your time as well.
* Using a *time inventory* is one way to gain insight into how and when a person is most productive. It also assists in identifying internal time wasters.

ADDITIONAL LEARNING EXERCISES AND APPLICATIONS

LEARNING EXERCISE 9.6

A Busy Day at the Public Health Agency

You work in a public health agency. It is the agency's policy that at least one public health nurse is available in the office every day. Today is your turn to remain in the office. From 1 PM to 5 PM, you will be the public health nurse at the scheduled immunization clinic; you hope to be able to spend some time finishing your end-of-month reports, which are due at 5 PM. The office stays open during lunch; you have a luncheon meeting with a Cancer Society group from noon to 1 PM today. The RN in the office is to serve as a resource to the receptionist and handle patient phone calls and drop-ins. In addition to the receptionist, you may delegate appropriately to a clerical worker. However, the clerical worker also serves the other clinic nurses and usually is fairly busy. While you are in the office today trying to finish your reports, the following interruptions occur:

8:30 AM: Your supervisor, Anne, comes in and requests a count of the diabetic and hypertensive patients seen in the last month.

9:00 AM: An upset patient is waiting to see you about her daughter who just found out that she is pregnant.

9:00 AM: Three drop-in patients are waiting to be interviewed for possible referral to the chest clinic.

9:30 AM: The public health physician calls you and needs someone to contact a family about a child's immunization.

9:30 AM: The dental department drops off 20 referrals and needs you to pull charts of these patients.

10:00 AM: A confused patient calls to find out what to do about the bills that he has received.

10:45 AM: Six families have been waiting since 8:30 AM to sign up for food vouchers.

11:45 AM: A patient calls about her drug use; she doesn't know what to do. She has heard about Narcotics Anonymous and wants more information now.

● ASSIGNMENT: How would you handle each interruption? Justify your decisions. Do not forget lunch for yourself and the two office workers. *Note:* Attempt your own solution before reading the possible solution presented in the back of this book.

LEARNING EXERCISE 9.7

Realistic Prioritizing

You are an RN providing total patient care to four patients on an orthopedic unit during the 7 AM to 3 PM shift. Given the following patient information, prioritize your activities for the shift in eight 1-hour blocks of time. Be sure to include time for reports, planning your day's activities, breaks, and lunch. Be realistic about what you can accomplish. What activities will you delegate to the next shift? What overall goals have guided your time management? What personal values or priorities were factors in setting your goals?

Room 101 A	Ms. Jones	84 years old. Fractured left hip, secondary to fall at home. Disoriented since admission, especially at night. Soft restraints in use. Moans frequently. Being given IV pain medication every 2 hours prn. Vital signs and checks for circulation, feeling, and movement in toes ordered every 2 hours. Scheduled for surgery at 1030. Preoperative medications scheduled for 0930 and 1000. Consent yet to be signed. Family members will be here at 0800 and have expressed questions about the surgery and recovery period. Patient to return from surgery at approximately 1430. Will require postoperative vital signs every 15 minutes.
Room 101 B	Ms. Wilkins	26 years old. Compound fracture of the femur with postoperative fat emboli, now resolved. 10-lb Buck's traction. Has been in the hospital 3 weeks. Very bored and frustrated with prolonged hospitalization. Upset about roommate who calls out all night and keeps her from sleeping. Wants to be moved to new room. Has also requested to have hair washed during bath today. Has IV medication running at 100 mL/h. IV antibiotic piggybacks at 0800 and 1200. Oral medications at 0800, 0900, and 1200.
Room 102 A	Mr. Jenkins	47 years old. T-6 quadriplegic due to diving accident 14 years ago. Two days postoperative above-knee amputation due to osteomyelitis. Cultures show methicillin-resistant *Staphylococcus aureus* (MRSA). Strict wound isolation. Has been hospitalized for 2 weeks. Expressing great deal of anger and frustration to anyone who enters room. IV site red and puffy. IV needs to be restarted. Dressing change of operative site ordered daily. Heat lamp treatments ordered b.i.d. to small pressure sores on coccyx. IV antibiotic piggybacks at 0800, 1000, 1200, and 1400. Main IV bag to run out at 1000. 0600 lab work results to be called to physician this morning. Needs total assistance in performing activities of daily living, such as bathing and feeding self.
Room 103 A	Mr. Novak	19 years old. Severe tear of rotator cuff in left shoulder while playing football. One-day postoperative rotator cuff repair. Very quiet and withdrawn. Refusing pain medication, which has been ordered every 2 hours prn. Says he can handle pain and does not want to "mess up his body with drugs." He wants to be recruited into professional football after this semester. Nonverbal signs of grimacing, moaning, and inability to sleep suggest that moderate pain is present. Physician states that likelihood of Mr. Novak ever playing football again is very low but has not yet told patient. Girlfriend frequently in room at patient's bedside. IV infusing at 150 mL/h. IV antibiotics at 0800 and 1400. Has not had a bath since admission 2 days ago.

LEARNING EXERCISE 9.8

Creating a Shift Time Inventory

You are a 3 PM to 11 PM shift coordinator for a skilled-nursing facility. You are the only RN on your unit this shift. All the other personnel assigned to work with you this evening are unlicensed. The unit census is 21. As the shift coordinator, your responsibility is to make shift assignments, provide needed patient treatments, administer IV medications, and coordinate the work of team members. This evening, you will need to administer treatments and/or medications to the following patients:

Room 101 A	Gina Adams	88 years old. Senile dementia. Resident for 6 years. Confused—strikes out at staff. Soft wrist restraints bilaterally. Has small grade 2 pressure ulcer on coccyx, which requires evaluation and dressing change each shift.
Room 102 B	Gus Taylor	64 years old. Diabetes. New resident. Bilateral AK amputee. Right amputation 2 weeks ago. Left amputation performed 8 years ago. Needs stump dressing on right amputation site this shift. Has developed MRSA in wound site. Wound isolation ordered. IV antibiotics due at 4 PM and 10 PM tonight. Blood glucose monitoring due at 4:30 PM and 9:00 PM with sliding-scale coverage.
Room 106 A	Marvin Young	26 years old. Closed head injury 5 years ago. Resident since that time. Decerebrate posturing only. Does not follow commands. PEG feeding tube site red and inflamed; MD has not yet been notified. Needs feeding solution bag change this PM.
Room 107 A	Sheila Abood	93 years old. Functional decline. Refusing to eat. Physician has written an order not to resuscitate in the event of cardiac or respiratory failure but wants an IV line begun this PM to minimize patient dehydration. Family will also be here this PM and wants to talk about their mother's status.
Room 109 C	Tina Crowden	89 years old. Admit from local hospital, 2 weeks postop left hip replacement. Anticipated length of stay—2 weeks. Arrives by ambulance at 3:30 PM. Needs to have admission assessment and paperwork completed and care plan started.

Oral Medications Schedule
    Room 101 A—4 PM, 8 PM
    Room 101 B—4 PM, 8 PM
    Room 102 A—5 PM, 9 PM
    Room 103 B—4 PM, 10 PM
    Room 104 C—5 PM, 6 PM, 9 PM
    Room 106 B—6 PM, 9 PM
    Room 108 C—9 PM
    Room 109 C—5 PM, 6 PM, 8 PM, 9 PM

● ASSIGNMENT: Create a time inventory from 3:00 PM to 11:30 PM by using 1-hour blocks of time. Plan what activities you will do during each 1-hour block. Be sure that you start with the activities you have prioritized for the shift. Also, remember that you will be in shift report from

3:00 to 3:30 PM and from 11:00 to 11:30 PM and that you need to schedule a dinner break for yourself. Allow adequate time for planning and dealing with the unexpected. Compare the inventory that you created with other students in your class. Did you identify the same priorities? Were you more focused on professional, technical, or amenity care? Will your plan require multitasking? Was the time inventory that you created realistic? Is this a workload that you believe you could handle?

LEARNING EXERCISE 9.9

Plan Your Day

It is October of your second year as coordinator of nursing management for the surgical department. A copy of your appointment calendar for Monday, October 27, follows.

You will review your unfinished business from the preceding Friday and look at the new items of business that have arrived on your desk this morning. (The new items follow the appointment calendar.) The unit ward clerk is usually free in the afternoon to provide you with 1 hour of clerical assistance, and you have a charge nurse on each shift to whom you may delegate.

1. Assign a priority to each item, with "1" being the most important and "5" being the least important.
2. Decide when you will deal with each item, being careful not to use more time than you have open on your calendar.
3. If the problem is to be handled immediately, explain how you will do this (e.g., delegated, phone call).
4. Explain the rationale for your decisions.

Monday, October 27

8:00 AM	Arrive at work
8:15 AM	Daily rounds with each head nurse in your area
8:30 AM	Continuation of daily rounds with head nurses
9:00 AM	Open
9:30 AM	Open
10:00 AM	Department Head meeting
10:30 AM	United Givers committee
11:00 AM	United Givers committee continued
11:30 AM	Open
Noon	Lunch
12:30 PM	Lunch
1:00 PM	Weekly meeting with administrator—budget and annual report due
1:30 PM	Open
2:00 PM	Infection control meeting
2:30 PM	Infection control meeting continued
3:00 PM	Fire drill and critique of drill
3:30 PM	Fire drill and critique of drill continued
4:00 PM	Open
4:30 PM	Open
5:00 PM	Off duty

(Learning Exercise continues on page 204)

Correspondence

Item 1
From the desk of M. Jones, personnel manager
October 24
Dear Joan:

I am sending you the names of two new graduate nurses who are interested in working in your area. I have processed their applications; they seem well qualified. Could you manage to see them as early as possible in the week? I would hate to lose these prospective employees, and they are anxious to obtain definite confirmation of employment.

Item 2
From the desk of John Brown, purchasing agent
October 23
Joan:

We really must get together this week and devise a method to control supplies. Your area has used three times the amount of thermometer covers as any other area. Are you taking that many more temperatures? This is just one of the supplies your area uses excessively. I'm open to suggestions.

Item 3
Roger Johnson, MD, chief of surgical department
October 24
Ms. Kerr:

I know you have your budget ready to submit, but I just remembered this week that I forgot to include an arterial pressure monitor. Is there another item that we can leave out? I'll drop by Monday morning, and we'll figure something out.

Item 4
October 23
Ms. Kerr:

The following personnel are due for merit raises, and I must have their completed and signed evaluations by Tuesday afternoon: Mary Rocas, Jim Newman, Marge Newfield.
M. Jones, personnel manager

Item 5
Roger Johnson, MD, chief of surgical department
October 23
Ms Kerr:

The physicians are complaining about the availability of nurses to accompany them on rounds. I believe you and I need to sit down with the doctors and head nurses to discuss this recurring problem. I have some free time Monday afternoon.

Item 6
5 AM
Joan:

Sally Knight (your regular night RN) requested a leave of absence due to her mother's illness. I told her it would be OK to take the next three nights off. She is flying out of town on the 9 AM commuter flight to San Francisco, so phone her right away if you don't want her to go. I felt I had no choice but to say yes.
Nancy Peters, night supervisor P.S. You'll need to find a replacement for her for the next three nights.

Item 7
To: Ms Kerr
From: Administrator
Re: Patient complaint
Date: October 23

Please investigate the following patient complaint. I would like a report on this matter this afternoon.
Dear Sir:

My mother, Gertrude Boswich, was a patient in your hospital, and I just want to tell you that no member of my family will ever go there again.

She had an operation on Monday, and no one gave her a bath for 3 days. Besides that, she didn't get anything to eat for 2 days, not even water. What kind of a hospital do you run anyway?
Elmo Boswich

Item 8
To: Joan Kerr
From: Nancy Newton, RN, head nurse
Re: Problems with x-ray department
Date: October 23

We have been having problems getting diagnostic x-ray procedures scheduled for patients. Many times, patients have had to stay an extra day to get x-ray tests done. I have talked to the radiology chief several times, but the situation hasn't improved. Can you do something about this?

Item 9
To: All department heads
From: Store room
Re: Supplies
Date: October 23

The storeroom is out of the following items: Toilet tissue, paper clips, disposable diapers, and pencils. We are expecting a shipment next week.

Telephone Messages
Item 10

Sam Surefoot, Superior Surgical Supplies, Inc., returned your call at 7:50 AM on October 27. He will be at the hospital this afternoon to talk about problems with defective equipment received.

Item 11

Donald Drinkley, Channel 32-TV, called at 8:10 AM on October 27 to say he will be here at 11:30 AM to do a feature story on the open-heart unit.

Item 12

Lila Green, director of nurses at St. Joan's Hospital, called at 8:05 AM on October 24 about a phone reference on Jane Jones, RN. Ms. Jones has applied for a job there. Isn't that the one we fired last year?

Item 13

Betty Brownie, Bluebird Troop 35, called at 8 AM on October 27 about the Bluebird troop visit to patients on Halloween with trick-or-treat candy. She will call again.

LEARNING EXERCISE 9.10

Avoiding Crises

Some people always seem to manage by crisis. The following scenarios depict situations that likely could have been avoided with better planning. Write down what could have been done to prevent the crisis. Then outline at least three alternatives to deal with the problem, as it already exists.

- It is the end of your 8-hour shift. Your team members are ready to go home. You have not yet begun to chart on any of your six patients. Neither have you completed your intake/output totals or given patients the medications that were due 1 hour ago. The arriving shift asks you to give a report now.
- You need to use the home computer to write your midterm essay, which is due tomorrow, but your mother is online doing the family's taxes, which must be mailed by midnight. The taxes will likely take several additional hours.
- Your computer hard drive crashes when you try to print your term paper, which is due tomorrow.
- An elderly, frail patient pulls out her IV line. You make six attempts, over a 1-hour period, to restart the line but are unsuccessful. You have missed your lunch break and now must choose between taking time for lunch and finishing your shift on time.

Web Links

Time Management Strategies for Improving Academic Performance
http://www.ucc.vt.edu/lynch/TimeManagement.htm
This site, produced by Virginia Tech, includes information on time management and priority setting for students as well as tools for assessing personal time-management behaviors.

Organizational Skills: Are You Ready for a Change?
http://www.womensmedia.com/organize-goals-0200.htm
A women's resource for organizational skills.

Personal Time Management for Busy Managers
http://www.ee.ed.ac.uk/~gerard/Management/art2.html
This article looks at the basics of personal time management and describes how the manager can assume control of this basic resource.

Center for Learning and Teaching
http://www.clt.cornell.edu/campus/learn/SSWorkshops/SKResources.html
Includes a variety of links to time-management strategies, including weekly planners, making lists, time estimates, and tips for overcoming procrastination

References

Belkin, L. (2005, July 17). *On the job, the pauses that refresh.* New York Times Job Market. Retrieved October 10, 2006, from *http://www.nytimes.com/2005/07/17/jobs/17wcol.html?ex= 1279252800&en=0821af5c57da032d&ei=5090&partner= rssuserland&emc=rss.*

Blunt, A., & Pychyl, T. A. (2005). Project systems of procrastinators: A personal project-analytic and action control perspective. *Personality and Individual Differences, 38*(8), 1771–1780.

Cohen, A. (2006). Me time. Mission: control. *Health, 20*(2), 127–128, 130.

Hatcher, B. J., Bleich, M. R., Connolly, C., Davis, K., O'Neill Hewlett, P., & Stokley Hill, K. (2006, June). *Wisdom at work. The importance of the older and experienced nurse in the workplace.* Robert Wood Johnson Foundation. Retrieved October 10, 2006, from *http://www.rwjf.org/files/ publications/other/wisdomatwork.pdf.*

Kennedy, D. (2006). The magic of punctuality. *Podiatry Management, 25*(3), 243–246.

Kriegel, R. (2002). *How to succeed in business without working so damn hard: Rethinking the rules, reinventing the game.* New York: Warner Books.

Marano, H. E. (2006). Getting out from under: How to stop procrastinating—now! *Psychology Today, 39*(2), 41–42.

Masikiewicz, M. (2000). Get ready, get set, get organized. *Career World, 29*(1), 6–11.

Vacarro, P. J. (2001). Five priority-setting traps. *Family Practice Management, 8*(4), 60.

Where does the time go? (2006). Day-Timer. Retrieved October 10, 2006, from *http://www.daytimer.com/ Time-Management-Resources/Where-Does-the-Time-Go/684AC8ECEE8C465FA5F8AA4624E940DA/False.*

Bibliography

Bryan-Brown, C. W., & Dracup, K. (2004). Procrastination is the thief of time: Surviving guidelines. *American Journal of Critical Care, 13*(4), 287–289.

Cox, S. (2006). Better time management: A matter of perspective. *Nursing, 36*(3), 43.

Fink-Samnick, E. (2006). Self and balance amid chaos. *Case Manager, 17*(1), 69–71.

Fry, M. (2005). An educational framework for triage nursing based on gatekeeping, timekeeping and decision-making processes. *Accident and Emergency Nursing, 13*(4), 214–219.

Hedrick, L. H. (2006). *15 ways to save time.* Day-Timer. Retrieved October 10, 2006, from *http://www.daytimer.com/ Time-Management-Resources/15-Ways-to-Save-Time/684AC8ECEE8C465FA5F8AA4624E940DA/False.*

Kamienski, M. C., & Zimmerman, P. G. (2006). Managers forum. Dealing with interruptions of nurse managers during office time. *Journal of Emergency Nursing, 32*(3), 272–273.

Lehmkuhl, D. (2006). *15 principles for organizing your business life.* Day-Timer. Retrieved October 10, 2006, from

http://www.daytimer.com/Time-Management-Resources/ 15-Principles-for-Organizing-Your-Business-Life/684AC8ECEE8C465FA5F8AA4624E940DA/False.

McConnell, C. R. (2006). From the editor. The ultimate unrenewable resource: Time. *Health Care Manager, 25*(1), 1–3.

O'Regan H., & Fawcett, T. (2006). Learning to nurse: Reflections on bathing a patient. *Nursing Standard, 20*, 46, 60–64.

Palfrey, G. (2006, April 7). Reflections of a nurse partner. Work/life balance = living. *Practice Nurse, 31*(7), 54.

Taigman, M., Shost, D. A., & DuGray, R. (2003). Time savers: 3 experts tackle a real-life management problem. *EMS Manager and Supervisor, 5*(4), 1r–2r.

Watson, D. (2006). *Timesaving tips for e-mail.* Day-Timer. Retrieved October 10, 2006, from *http://www.daytimer.com/ Time-Management-Resources/Timesaving-Tips-for-E-mail/684AC8ECEE8C465FA5F8AA4624E940DA/False.*

Weinstein, L. B. (2006, March 13). Guarding a nonrenewable resource . . . "A life of a nurse: A simple time-management tool," by Tamela Garcia, RN. *Nursing Spectrum—Florida Edition, 16*(13), 4.

10

Fiscal Planning

. . . nurses are practicing caring in an environment where the economics and costs of health care permeate discussions and impact decisions.

—*Marian C. Turkel*

. . . the trouble with a budget is that it's hard to fill up one hole without digging another.

—*Dan Bennett*

O'Kane (2006) states that "hospitals and health systems throughout the United States are trying to maintain their balance against buffeting financial pressures, with one eye on rising clinical costs and the other on shrinking payments. Chief financial officers (CFOs) and other leaders live daily with the "on the ground" realities of those pressures, while the larger health care policy debate continues to focus on big picture issues, such as financing mechanisms, infrastructure, quality, and access" (para 1). Scarce resources and soaring health care costs are a reality of all contemporary health care delivery systems. There has never been a time more than now when health care organizations need to operate more efficiently or be more aware of cost containment.

Historically, nursing management played a limited role in determining and monitoring resource allocation in health care institutions. Nurse–managers were often given budgets with little rationale and were allowed only limited input in fiscal decision making. Because nursing was generally classified as a "nonincome-producing service," nursing input was undervalued. During the last 2 to 3 decades, however, health care organizations have come to recognize the importance of nursing input in fiscal planning, and nurse leader–managers in the 21st century are expected to be expert financial managers. The reality is that nursing budgets generally account for the greatest share of the total expenses in health care institutions, and participation in fiscal planning has become a fundamental and powerful tool for nursing.

Many managers perceive fiscal planning to be the most difficult type of planning. Some managers encounter difficulty with forecasting costs based on current and projected needs. This may occur if the manager has had little formal education or training on budget preparation. It is important to remember that fiscal planning is an acquired skill that improves with use.

Fiscal planning is not intuitive; it is a learned skill that improves with practice.

Fiscal planning also requires vision, creativity, and a thorough knowledge of the political, social, and economic forces that shape health care. Fiscal planning, then, must be included in nursing program curricula and in management preparation programs. This chapter discusses the leader–manager's role in fiscal planning, identifies types of budgets, and delineates the budgetary process. Learners will also examine health care reimbursement concepts with specific attention given to the impact of managed care on contemporary health care organizations. The leadership roles and management functions involved in fiscal planning are outlined in Display 10.1.

DISPLAY 10.1 **Leadership Roles and Management Functions in Fiscal Planning**

Leadership Roles

1. Is visionary in identifying or forecasting short- and long-term unit needs, thus inspiring proactive rather than reactive fiscal planning
2. Is knowledgeable about political, social, and economic factors that shape fiscal planning in health care today
3. Demonstrates flexibility in fiscal goal setting in a rapidly changing system
4. Anticipates, recognizes, and creatively solves budgetary constraints
5. Influences and inspires group members to become active in short- and long-range fiscal planning
6. Recognizes when fiscal constraints have resulted in an inability to meet organizational or unit goals and communicates this insight effectively, following the chain of command
7. Ensures that patient safety is not jeopardized by cost containment

Management Functions

1. Identifies the importance of and develops short- and long-range fiscal plans that reflect unit needs
2. Articulates and documents unit needs effectively to higher administrative levels
3. Assesses the internal and external environment of the organization in forecasting to identify driving forces and barriers to fiscal planning
4. Demonstrates knowledge of budgeting and uses appropriate techniques to budget effectively
5. Provides opportunities for subordinates to participate in relevant fiscal planning
6. Coordinates unit-level fiscal planning to be congruent with organizational goals and objectives
7. Accurately assesses personnel needs by using predetermined standards or an established patient classification system
8. Coordinates the monitoring aspects of budget control
9. Ensures that documentation of patient's need for services and services rendered is clear and complete to facilitate organizational reimbursement

BALANCING COSTS AND QUALITY

Complicating fiscal planning in health care organizations today are the dual goals of cost containment and quality care, which do not always have a linear relationship. *Cost containment* refers to effective and efficient delivery of services while generating needed revenues for continued organizational productivity. Cost containment is the responsibility of every health care provider, and the viability of most health care organizations today depends on their ability to use their fiscal resources wisely.

Being *cost-effective*, however, is not the same as being inexpensive; a dictionary definition of *cost-effective* incorporates the concept of being economical in terms of the goods or services received for the money spent, meaning that the product is worth the price (American Heritage Dictionary of the English Language, 2005). Cost-effectiveness takes into account factors such as anticipated length of service, need for such a service, and availability of other alternatives.

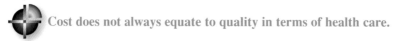 Cost does not always equate to quality in terms of health care.

In terms of health care, cost and quality do not mean the same thing. O'Kane (2006) suggests that "higher spending does not buy higher quality care. In fact, what higher spending often buys is unnecessary care, which not only has no value, but also exposes patients to risk and wastes time, resources, and money, all of which could be put to better use" (para 4). O'Kane goes on to say that "the current incentives, perverse and firmly embedded in the payment structure for generations, reward physicians and hospitals for providing units of care regardless of the quality of that care. For example, there are more than 100 diagnosis-related groups that actually pay more when a patient gets a hospital-acquired, preventable staph infection" (para 22).

RESPONSIBILITY ACCOUNTING AND FORECASTING

An essential feature of fiscal planning is *responsibility accounting*, which means that each of an organization's revenues, expenses, assets, and liabilities is someone's responsibility. As a corollary, the person with the most direct control or influence on any of these financial elements should be held accountable for them. At the unit level, this accountability generally falls to the manager. The manager, then, should be an active participant in unit budgeting, have a high degree of control over what is included in the unit budget, receive regular data reports that compare actual expenses with budgeted expenses, and be held accountable for the financial results of the operating unit.

Because unit managers are involved in daily operations and see firsthand their unit's functioning, they often have expertise in forecasting patient census trends as well as supply and equipment needs for their units. *Forecasting* involves making an educated budget estimate by using historical data.

The unit manager also can best monitor and evaluate all aspects of a unit's budget control. Like other types of planning, the unit manager has a responsibility to communicate budgetary planning goals to staff. The more the staff understands the budgetary goals and the plans to carry out those goals, the more likely goal attainment is. Sadly, many nurses have little knowledge of the nursing budget model used by their hospital system.

BASICS OF BUDGETS

A *budget* is a financial plan that estimates expenditures and revenues by an agent for a stated future period (About, Inc., 2006). In other words, it includes estimated expenses as well as income for a period of time. Accuracy dictates the worth of a budget; the more accurate the budget blueprint, the better the institution can plan the most efficient use of its resources.

The budget's value is directly related to its accuracy.

Because a budget is at best a prediction, a plan, and not a rule, fiscal planning requires flexibility, ongoing evaluation, and revision. Indeed, Barr (2005) suggests that budgeting must be treated as a continuous process rather than an annual exercise because the process is so dynamic. In the budget, expenses are classified as fixed or variable and either controllable or noncontrollable. *Fixed* expenses do not vary with volume, whereas *variable* expenses do. Examples of fixed expenses might be a building's mortgage payment or a manager's salary; variable expenses might include the payroll of hourly wage employees and the cost of supplies.

Controllable expenses can be controlled or varied by the manager, whereas *noncontrollable* expenses cannot. For example, the unit manager can control the number of personnel working on a certain shift and the staffing mix; he or she cannot, however, control equipment depreciation, the number and type of supplies needed by patients, or overtime that occurs in response to an emergency. A list of the fiscal terminology that a manager needs to know is shown in Display 10.2.

LEARNING EXERCISE 10.1

Would You Accept This Gift?
One of the oncologists on your unit (Dr. Sam Jones) has offered to give you his old photocopier because his office is purchasing a new one. As a condition of acceptance, he requires that all the oncologists and radiologists be allowed to use the copier free of charge.

● ASSIGNMENT:
    1. Justify acceptance or rejection of the gift. What influenced your choice?
    2. What are the fixed and variable costs?
    3. What are the controllable and noncontrollable costs?
    4. How much control will you, as a unit manager, have over the use of the copier?

STEPS IN THE BUDGETARY PROCESS

The nursing process provides a model for the steps in budget planning:
    1. The first step is to assess what needs to be covered in the budget. Generally, this determination should reflect input from all levels of the organizational hierarchy, since budgeting is most effective when all personnel using the resources are involved in the process. A composite of unit needs in terms of labor, equipment, and operating expenses can then be compiled to determine the organizational budget.

DISPLAY 10.2 Fiscal Terminology

Acuity index—Weighted statistical measurement that refers to severity of illness of patients for a given time. Patients are classified according to acuity of illness, usually in one of four categories. The acuity index is determined by taking a total of acuities and then dividing by the number of patients.

Assets—Financial resources that a health care organization receives, such as accounts receivable.

Baseline data—Historical information on dollars spent, acuity level, patient census, resources needed, hours of care, and so forth. This information is used as basis on which future needs can be projected.

Break-even point—Point at which revenue covers costs. Most health care facilities have high fixed costs. Because per-unit fixed costs in a noncapitated model decrease with volume, health care facilities under this model need to maintain a high volume to decrease unit costs.

Capitation—A prospective payment system that pays health plans or providers a fixed amount per enrollee per month for a defined set of health services, regardless of how many (if any) services are used.

Case mix—Type of patients served by an institution. A hospital's case mix is usually defined in such patient-related variables as diagnosis, personal characteristics, and patterns of treatment.

Cash flow—Rate at which dollars are received and dispersed.

Controllable costs—Costs that can be controlled or that vary. An example would be the number of personnel employed, the level of skill required, wage levels, and quality of materials.

Cost–benefit ratio—Numerical relationship between the value of an activity or procedure in terms of benefits and the value of the activity's or procedure's cost. The cost–benefit ratio is expressed as a fraction.

Cost center—Smallest functional unit for which cost control and accountability can be assigned. A nursing unit is usually considered a cost center, but there may be other cost centers within a unit (orthopedics is a cost center, but often the cast room is considered a separate cost center within orthopedics).

Diagnosis-related groups (DRGs)—Rate-setting prospective payment system used by Medicare to determine payment rates for an inpatient hospital stay based on admission diagnosis. Each DRG represents a particular case type for which Medicare provides a flat dollar amount of reimbursement. This set rate may, in actuality, be higher or lower than the cost of treating the patient in a particular hospital.

Direct costs—Costs that can be attributed to a specific source, such as medications and treatments. Costs that are clearly identifiable with goods or service.

Fee-for-service (FFS) system—A reimbursement system under which insurance companies reimburse health care providers after the needed services are delivered.

Fixed budget—Style of budgeting that is based on a fixed, annual level of volume, such as number of patient-days or tests performed, to arrive at an annual budget total. These totals are then divided by 12 to arrive at the monthly average. The fixed budget does not make provisions for monthly or seasonal variations.

Fixed costs—Costs that do not vary according to volume. Examples of fixed costs are mortgage or loan payments.

For-profit organization—Organization in which the providers of funds have an ownership interest in the organization. These providers own stocks in the for-profit organization and earn dividends based on what is left when the cost of goods and of carrying on the business is subtracted from the amount of money taken in.

Full costs—Total of all direct and indirect costs.

Full-time equivalent (FTE)— Number of hours of work for which a full-time employee is scheduled for a weekly period. For example, 1.0 FTE = five 8-hour days of staffing, which equals 40 hours of staffing per week. One FTE can be divided in different ways. For example, two part-time employees, each working 20 hours per week, would equal 1 FTE. If a position requires coverage for more than 5 days or 40 hours per week, the FTE will be greater than 1.0 for that position. Assume a position requires 7-day coverage, or 56 hours; then the position requires 1.4 FTE coverage (56 divided by 40 = 1.4). This means that more than one person is needed to fill the FTE positions for a 7-day period.

Health maintenance organization (HMO)—Historically, a prepaid organization that provided health care to voluntarily enrolled members in return for a preset amount of money on a per-person, per-month basis. Often referred to as a managed care organization (MCO).

Hours per patient-day (HPPD)—Hours of nursing care provided per patient per day by various levels of nursing personnel. HPPD are determined by dividing total production hours by the number of patients.

Indirect costs—Costs that cannot be directly attributed to a specific area. These are hidden costs and are usually spread among different departments. Housekeeping services are considered indirect costs.

Managed care—Term used to describe a variety of health care plans designed to contain the cost of health care services delivered to members while maintaining the quality of care.

Medicaid—Federally assisted and state-administered program to pay for medical services on behalf of certain groups of low-income individuals. Generally, these people are not covered by Social Security. Certain groups of people (e.g, the elderly, blind, disabled, members of families with dependent children, and certain other children and pregnant women) also qualify for coverage if their incomes and resources are sufficiently low.

Medicare—Nationwide health insurance program authorized under Title 18 of the Social Security Act that provides benefits to people 65 years of age or older. Medicare coverage also is available to certain groups of people with catastrophic or chronic illness, such as patients with renal failure requiring hemodialysis, regardless of age.

Noncontrollable costs—Indirect expenses that cannot usually be controlled or varied. Examples might be rent, lighting, and depreciation of equipment.

Not-for-profit organization—This type of organization is financed by funds that come from several sources, but the providers of these funds do not have an ownership interest. Profits generated in the not-for-profit organization are frequently funneled back into the organization for expansion or capital acquisition.

Operating expenses—Daily costs required to maintain a hospital or health care institution.

Patient classification system—Method of classifying patients. Different criteria are used for different systems. In nursing, patients are usually classified according to acuity.

Preferred provider organization (PPO)—Health care financing and delivery program with a group of providers, such as physicians and hospitals, who contract to give services on a fee-for-service basis. This provides financial incentives to consumers to use a select group of preferred providers and pay less for services. Insurance companies usually promise the PPO a certain volume of patients and prompt payment in exchange for fee discounts.

Production hours—Total amount of regular time, overtime, and temporary time. This also may be referred to as actual hours.

Prospective payment system (PPS)—A hospital payment system with predetermined reimbursement ratio for services given.

Revenue—Source of income or the reward for providing a service to a patient.

Staffing mix—Ratio of RNs, LVNs/LPNs, and unlicensed workers (e.g., a shift on one unit might have 40 percent RNs, 40 percent LPNs/LVNs, and 20 percent other). Hospitals vary on their staffing mix policies.

Third-party payment system—A system of health care financing in which providers deliver services to patients, and a third party, or intermediary, usually an insurance company or a government agency, pays the bill.

Turnover ratio—Rate at which employees leave their jobs for reasons other than death or retirement. The rate is calculated by dividing the number of employees leaving by the number of workers employed in the unit during the year and then multiplying by 100.

Variable costs—Costs that vary with the volume. Payroll costs are an example.

Workload units—In nursing, workloads are usually the same as patient-days. For some areas, however, workload units might refer to the number of procedures, tests, patient visits, injections, and so forth.

2. The second step is to develop a plan. The budget plan may be developed in many ways. A budgeting cycle that is set for 12 months is called a *fiscal-year budget*. This fiscal year, which may or may not coincide with the calendar year, is then usually broken down into quarters or subdivided into monthly or semiannual periods. Most budgets are developed for a 1-year period, but a *perpetual budget* may be done on a continual basis each month so that 12 months of future budget data are always available.

Selecting the optimal time frame for budgeting also is important. Errors are more likely if the budget is projected too far in advance. If the budget is shortsighted, compensating for unexpected major expenses or purchasing capital equipment may be difficult.

A budget that is predicted too far in advance has greater probability for error.

3. The third step is implementation. In this step, ongoing monitoring and analysis occur to avoid inadequate or excess funds at the end of the fiscal year. In most health care institutions, monthly statements outline each department's projected budget and deviations from that budget. Some managers artificially inflate their department budgets as a cushion against budget cuts from a higher level of administration. If several departments partake in this unsound practice, the entire institutional budget may be ineffective. If a major change in the budget is indicated, the entire budgeting process must be repeated. Top-level managers must watch for and correct unrealistic budget projections before they are implemented.

4. The last step is evaluation. The budget must be reviewed periodically and modified as needed throughout the fiscal year. Each unit manager is accountable for budget deviations in his or her unit. Most units can expect some change from the anticipated budget, but large deviations must be examined for possible causes and remedial action taken if necessary.

TYPES OF BUDGETS

Three major types of budgets that the unit manager is directly involved in with fiscal planning are personnel, operating, and capital budgets.

The Personnel Budget

The largest of the budget expenditures is the *workforce* or *personnel budget* because health care is *labor intensive*. To handle fluctuating patient census and acuity, managers need to use historical data about unit census fluctuations in forecasting short- and long-term personnel needs. Likewise, a manager must monitor the personnel budget closely to prevent understaffing or overstaffing. As patient days or volume decreases, managers must decrease personnel costs in relation to the decrease in volume.

In addition to numbers of staff, the manager must be cognizant of the *staffing mix*. Staffing mix refers to the mix (percentages) of licensed (RN, LVN) and unlicensed (CNA, UAP) staff working at a given time. The manager also must be aware of the patient acuity so that the most economical level of nursing care that will meet patient needs can be provided.

Although Unit V discusses staffing, it is necessary to briefly discuss here how staffing needs are expressed in the personnel budget. Most staffing is based on a predetermined *standard*. This standard may be addressed in hours per patient day (medical units), visits per month (home health agencies), or minutes per case (the operating room). Because the patient census, number of visits, or cases per day never remains constant, the manager must be ready to alter staffing when volume increases or decreases. Sometimes, the population and type of cases change so that the established standard is no longer appropriate. For example, an operating room that begins to perform open-heart surgery would involve more nursing time per case; therefore, the standard (number of nursing minutes per case) would need to be adjusted. Normally, the standard is adjusted upward or downward once a year, but staffing is adjusted daily depending on the volume.

The standard formula for calculating *nursing care hours (NCH) per patient-day (PPD)* is shown in Figure 10.1. A unit manager in an acute-care facility might use this formula to calculate daily staffing needs. For example, assume that your budgeted nursing care hours are 6 NCH/PPD. You are calculating the NCH/PPD for today, January 31; at midnight, it will be February 1. The patient census at midnight is 25 patients. In checking staffing, you find the following information:

Shift	Staff on Duty	Hours Worked
11 PM (1/30) to 7 AM (1/31)	2 RNs	8 hours each
(last night)	1 LVN	8 hours
	1 CNA	8 hours
7 AM to 3 PM	3 RNs	8 hours each
	2 LVNs	8 hours each
	1 CNA	8 hours
	1 ward clerk	8 hours
3 PM to 11 PM	2 RNs	8 hours each
	2 LVNs	8 hours each
	1 CNA	8 hours
	1 ward clerk	8 hours
11 PM (1/31) to 7 AM (2/1)	2 RNs	8 hours each
(last night)	2 LVNs	8 hours each
	1 CNA	8 hours

Ideally, you would use 12 midnight to 12 midnight to compute the NCH/PPD for January 31, but most staffing calculations based on traditional 8-hour shifts are made beginning at 11 PM and ending at 11 PM the following night. Therefore, in this case, it would be acceptable to figure the NCH/PPD for January 31 by using numerical data from the 11 PM to 7 AM shift last night and the 7 AM to 3 PM and 3 PM to 11 PM shifts today. The first step in this calculation requires a computation of total nursing care hours worked in 24 hours (including the ward clerk's hours). This can be calculated by multiplying the total number of staff on duty each shift by the hours each worked in their shift. Each shift total then is added together to get the total number of nursing hours worked in all three shifts or 24 hours:

Last night:	11 PM to 7 AM, 4 staff @ 8 hours each	= 32 hours
Today:	7 AM to 3 PM, 7 staff @ 8 hours each	= 56 hours
Today:	3 PM to 11 PM, 6 staff @ 8 hours each	= 48 hours
		= 136 hours

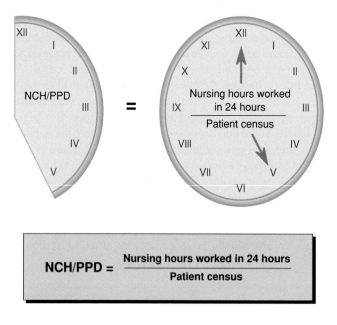

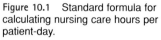

$$NCH/PPD = \frac{\text{Nursing hours worked in 24 hours}}{\text{Patient census}}$$

Figure 10.1   Standard formula for calculating nursing care hours per patient-day.

The nursing hours worked in 24 hours are 136 hours.

The second step in solving NCH/PPD requires that you divide the nursing hours worked in 24 hours by the patient census. The patient census in this case is 25. Therefore, 136 divided by 25 = 5.44.

The NCH/PPD for January 31 was 5.44, which is less than your budgeted NCH/PPD of 6.0. It would be possible to add up to 14 additional hours of nursing care in the next 24 hours and still maintain the budgeted nursing care hours standard. However, the unit manager must remember that the standard is flexible and that patient acuity and staffing mix may suggest the need for even more staff for Feb. 1 than the budgeted NCH/PPD.

The personnel budget includes actual *worked time* (also called *productive time* or *salary expense*) and time that the organization pays the employee for not working (*nonproductive* or *benefit time*). Nonproductive time includes the cost of benefits, new employee orientation, employee turnover, sick and holiday time, and education time. For example, the average 8.5-hour shift includes a 30-minute lunch break and two 15-minute breaks. Thus, this employee would work 7.5 productive hours and have 1.0 hours of nonproductive time.

LEARNING EXERCISE 10.2

Calculating NCH/PPD
Calculate the NCH/PPD if the midnight census remained the same as on page 215, but use the following as the number of hours worked:

12 midnight to 12 noon	2 RNs	12 hours each
	2 LVNs	12 hours each
	1 CNA	12 hours
	1 ward clerk	5 hours

12 noon to 12 midnight	3 RNs	12 hours each
	2 LVNs	12 hours each
	1 CNA	12 hours
	1 ward clerk	12 hours

Now, calculate the NCH/PPD if the following staff were working:

12 midnight to 12 noon	3 RNs	12 hours each
	1 LVN	12 hours
12 noon to 12 midnight	2 RNs	12 hours each
	1 LVN	12 hours
	1 ward clerk	4 hours

The Operating Budget

The *operating budget* is the second area of expenditure that involves all managers. The operating budget reflects expenses that change in response to the volume of service, such as the cost of electricity, repairs and maintenance, and supplies. While personnel costs lead the hospital budget, the cost of supplies runs a close second.

 Next to personnel costs, *supplies* are the second most significant component in the hospital budget.

Effective unit managers should be alert to the types and quantities of supplies used in their unit. They also should understand the relationship between supply use and patient mix, occupancy rate, technology requirements, and types of procedures performed on the unit. Saving unused supplies from packs or trays, reducing obsolete and slow-moving inventory, eliminating pilferage, and monitoring the uncontrolled usage of supplies and giveaways all represent potential cost savings. Other ways to cut supply costs might be in rental versus facility-owned equipment, stocking products on consignment, and just-in-time stockless inventory. *Just-in-time ordering* is a process whereby inventory is delivered to the organization by suppliers only when it is needed and immediately before it is to be used.

LEARNING EXERCISE 10.3

Missing Supplies
You are a unit manager in an acute-care hospital. You are aware that staff occasionally leave at the end of the shift with forgotten hospital supplies in their pockets. You remember how often as a staff nurse you would unintentionally take home rolls of adhesive tape, syringes, penlights, and bottles of lotion. Usually, you remembered to return the items, but other times you did not.

Recently, however, your budget has shown a dramatic and unprecedented increase in missing supplies, including gauze wraps, blood pressure cuffs, stethoscopes, surgical instruments, and personal hygiene kits. Although this increase represents only a fraction of your total operating budget, you believe that it is necessary to identify the source of their use. An audit of patient charts and charges reveals that these items were not used in patient care.

(Learning Exercise continues on page 218)

When you ask your charge nurses for an explanation, they reveal that a few employees have openly expressed that taking a few small supplies is, in effect, an expected and minor fringe benefit of employment. Your charge nurses do not believe that the problem is widespread, and they cannot objectively document which employees are involved in pilfering supplies. The charge nurses suggest that you ask all employees to document in writing when they see other employees taking supplies and then turn in the information to you anonymously for follow-up.

● ASSIGNMENT: Because supplies are such a major part of the operating budget, you believe that some action is indicated. You must determine what that action should be. Analyze your actions in terms of the desirable and undesirable effects on the employees involved in taking the supplies and those who are not. Is the amount of the fiscal debit in this situation a critical factor? Is it worth the time and energy that would be required to truly eliminate this problem?

The Capital Budget

The third type of budget used by managers is the *capital budget*. Capital budgets plan for the purchase of buildings or major equipment, which include equipment that has a long life (usually greater than 5 to 7 years), is not used in daily operations, and is more expensive than operating supplies. Capital budgets are composed of long-term planning, or a major acquisitions component, and a short-term budgeting component. The long-term major acquisitions component outlines future replacement and organizational expansion that will exceed 1 year. Examples of these types of capital expenditures might include the acquisition of a positron emission tomography imager or the renovation of a major wing in a hospital. The short-term component of the capital budget includes equipment purchases within the annual budget cycle, such as call-light systems, hospital beds, and medication carts.

Often, the designation of capital equipment requires that the value of the equipment exceed a certain dollar amount. That dollar amount will vary from institution to institution, but $1,000 to $5,000 is common. Managers are usually required to complete specific capital equipment request forms either annually or semiannually and to justify their request.

Barr (2005) warns that many health care institutions underestimate the cost of capital equipment, as they examine only the original purchase price and not the cost of implementation, installation, upkeep, and necessary technological updates. These and other "budget busters" are noted in Display 10.3.

DISPLAY 10.3 Budget Busters

- Going through the difficult process of completing a budget estimate for the coming year but never using it.
- Relying on the current year's budget numbers as a starting point for the next year's budget.
- Neglecting or underestimating costs related to capital expenditures.
- Ignoring declining patient volumes in the hope that the trend will be temporary.
- Failing to set aside enough money for unexpected capital expenses.

Source: Adapted from Barr, P. (2005). Flexing your budget: Experts urge hospitals, systems to trade in their traditional budgeting process for a more dynamic and versatile model. *Modern Healthcare, 35*(37), 24, 26.

BUDGETING METHODS

Budgeting is frequently classified according to how often it occurs and the base on which budgeting takes place. Four of the most common budgeting methods are incremental budgeting (also called flat-percentage increase budgeting), zero-based budgeting, flexible budgeting, and new performance budgeting.

Incremental Budgeting

Incremental or the *flat-percentage increase method* is the simplest method for budgeting. By multiplying current-year expenses by a certain figure, usually the inflation rate or consumer price index, the budget for the coming year may be projected. Although this method is simple and quick and requires little budgeting expertise on the part of the manager, it is generally inefficient fiscally because there is no motivation to contain costs and no need to prioritize programs and services. Wilkes, a health care management and economic consultant suggests that most (hospital) budgets use "history plus" to determine their budget needs, meaning department heads simply look at last year's budget and add a fixed percentage to the figures (Barr, 2005).

Zero-Based Budgeting

In comparison, managers who use *zero-based budgeting* must rejustify their program or needs every budgeting cycle. This method does not automatically assume that because a program has been funded in the past, it should continue to be funded. Thus, this budgeting process is labor intensive for nurse–managers. The use of a *decision package* to set funding priorities is a key feature of zero-based budgeting. Key components of decision packages are shown in Display 10.4.

The following is an *example* of a decision package for implementing a mandatory hepatitis B vaccination program at a nursing school.

Objective: All nursing students will complete a hepatitis B vaccination series.

Driving forces: Hepatitis B is a severely disabling disease that carries significant mortality. The Occupational Safety and Health Association (OSHA) requires that hepatitis B vaccine be offered to health care workers (which includes student nurses) who have a reasonable expectation of being exposed to blood on the job. Vaccination will greatly reduce the risk for contracting this disease. The current vaccination series has proved to have few serious side effects. The nursing school risks liability if it does not follow recommendations to have all high-risk groups vaccinated.

Restraining forces: The vaccination series costs $175 per student. Some students do not want to have the vaccinations and believe that requiring them to do so is a violation of free choice. It is unclear whether the school is liable if a student experiences a damaging side effect from the vaccinations.

DISPLAY 10.4 **Key Components of Decision Packages in Zero-Based Budgeting**

1. Listing of all current and proposed objectives or activities in the department
2. Alternative plans for carrying out these activities
3. Costs for each alternative
4. Advantages and disadvantages of continuing or discontinuing an activity

Alternative 1: Require the vaccinations. Because the school of nursing cannot afford to pay for the cost of the series, require that the students pay for it.

Advantage: No cost to the school. All students receive the vaccinations.
Disadvantage: Many students cannot afford the cost of the vaccination and believe that requiring it infringes on their right to control choices about their bodies.

Alternative 2: Do not require the vaccination series.

Advantage: No cost to anyone. Students have choice regarding whether to have the vaccinations and assume the responsibility of protecting their health themselves.
Disadvantage: Some nursing students will be unprotected against hepatitis B while working in a high-risk clinical setting.

Alternative 3: Require the vaccination series but share the cost between the student and the school.

Advantage: Decreased cost to students. All students would be vaccinated.
Disadvantage: Costs and limited choice.

Decision packages and zero-based budgeting are advantageous because they force managers to set priorities and to use resources most efficiently. This rather lengthy and complex method also encourages participative management because information from peers and subordinates is needed to analyze adequately and prioritize the activities of each unit.

LEARNING EXERCISE 10.4

Developing a Decision Package
Given the following objective, develop a decision package to aid you in fiscal priority setting.
   Objective: To have reliable, economic, and convenient transportation when you enter nursing school in 3 months.
   Additional information: You currently have no car and rely on public transportation, which is inexpensive and reliable but not very convenient. Your current financial resources are limited, although you could probably qualify for a car loan if your parents were willing to cosign the loan. Your nursing school's policy states that you must have a car available to commute to clinical agencies outside the immediate area. You know that this policy is not enforced and that some students do carpool to clinical assignments.

● ASSIGNMENT: Identify at least three alternatives that will meet your objective. Choose the best alternative based on the advantages and disadvantages that you identify. You may embellish information presented in the case to help your problem solving.

Flexible Budgeting

Flexible budgets are budgets that adjust automatically over the course of the year depending on variables such as volume, labor costs, and capital expenditures (Barr, 2005). A flexible budget automatically calculates what expenses should be, given the volume that is occurring. Thus, costs can be allocated on a volume basis. Barr suggests that while "not a new concept, flexible budgets have gained greater adoption in the past 10 years" (para 7). This is because most health care institutions face rapidly changing census and manpower needs that are difficult to predict, despite historical forecasting tools. The flexible budget "can be designed to quickly identify where such variations occur and create a better picture of current finances as well as a more realistic outlook" (para 15).

New Performance Budgeting

The fourth method of budgeting, *new performance budgeting*, emphasizes outcomes and results instead of activities or outputs. Thus, the manager would budget as needed to achieve specific outcomes and would evaluate budgetary success accordingly. For example, a home health agency would set and then measure a specific outcome in a group, such as diabetic patients, as a means of establishing and justifying a budget.

CRITICAL PATHWAYS

Critical pathways (also called *clinical pathways* and *care pathways*) are one method of planning, assessing, implementing, and evaluating the cost-effectiveness of patient care. They are relatively standardized predictions of patients' progress for a specific diagnosis or procedure. For example, a critical pathway for a specific diagnosis might suggest an average length of stay (ALOS) of 4 days, with certain interventions completed by certain points on the pathway (much like a PERT diagram; see page 24). Patient progress that differs from the critical pathway prompts a *variance analysis*.

> **Critical pathways are predetermined courses of progress that patients should make after admission for a specific diagnosis or after a specific surgery.**

First developed in the 1980s as a tool to reduce length of stay, with an emphasis on nursing care (Goldszer et al., 2004), critical pathways also provide a useful tool for monitoring quality of care. Once the cost of a pathway is known, analyzing the cost-effectiveness of the pathway as well as the associated cost variances is possible. By using clinical and cost variance data, decisions on changing the pathway can be made with both clinical and financial outcome projections.

The advantage of critical pathways is that they do provide some means of standardizing medical care for patients with similar diagnoses. Their weakness, however, is the difficulties that they pose in accounting for and accepting what are often justifiable differentiations between unique patients who have deviated from their pathway. Critical pathway documentation also poses one more paperwork and utilization review function in a system that is already burdened with administrative costs. The challenges and lessons learned in implementing clinical pathways at a Boston hospital are discussed in Examining the Evidence 10.1.

HEALTH CARE REIMBURSEMENT

Historically, health care institutions used incremental budgeting and placed little or no emphasis on budgeting. Because insurance carriers reimbursed fully on virtually a limitless basis, there was little motivation to save costs and organizations found it unnecessary to justify charges.

EXAMINING THE EVIDENCE 10.1

Source: Goldszer, R. C., Rutherford, A., Banks, P., Zou, K. H., Curley, M. Brita Rossi, P., et al. (2004, March). Implementing clinical pathways for patients admitted to a medical service: Lessons learned. *Critical Pathways in Cardiology, 3*(1), 35–41. Retrieved October 18, 2006, from *http://www.brighamandwomens.org/gms/News/GoldzerEtAl.pdf*.

This article details the implementation of two pathways for patients admitted to medical service at Brigham and Women's Hospital in Boston, Massachusetts, beginning in 2003; one was a clinical care plan (CCP) for use with all patients, and the other was a Pancreatitis Pathway (PP) for patients admitted with acute pancreatitis. The pathways, developed by teams including attending physicians (general internists and gastroenterologists), medicine house officers, nurses, and care coordinators provided printed standards of care and a mechanism for daily multidisciplinary documentation.

Many physicians and nurses provided feedback following implementation of the pathways. Many were critical and raised concerns. The project leaders, the steering committee, and the nurse-managers discussed these concerns and made changes to the pathways based on this feedback. Their expectation, however, is to continue to use CCPs throughout the hospital for all patients. Lessons learned from the experience included:

1. Senior leadership support is essential.
2. There must be physician and nurse champions.
3. All stakeholders must be involved in developing the pathways.
4. Nursing documentation improved as a result of pathway use.
5. Physicians need ongoing encouragement and education about the value of pathways.
6. There is considerable work involved for unit coordinators in using pathways on a medical–surgical unit.
7. There must be ongoing feedback to users.
8. Edits and continuous input from users improve the product.

Reimbursement was based on costs incurred to provide the service plus profit (*fee-for-service* [*FFS*]), with no ceiling placed on the total amount that could be charged. Indeed, under FFS, the more services provided, the greater the amount that can be billed. Therefore, FFS reimbursement encourages overtreatment of clients.

The end result of uncontrolled FFS reimbursement was skyrocketing health care costs with health care increasingly assuming a greater percentage of gross domestic product (GDP) each year. Currently, the United States spends more of its GDP on medical care than any other nation (Cowen, 2006)—15 percent compared with 8 percent for other highly developed countries. U.S. health expenditure is $7,129 per capita, twice that of the average industrialized nation. In addition, a new *Commonwealth Fund* report notes that U.S. health administration costs are high, with 31 cents of each patient care dollar going for administration, much of which is profit (Whitney, 2006).

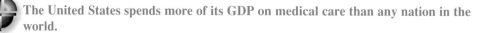

The United States spends more of its GDP on medical care than any nation in the world.

MEDICARE AND MEDICAID

The U.S. federal government became a major insurer of health care with the advent of Medicare and Medicaid in the mid-1960s. *Medicare* is a federally sponsored health insurance program for the elderly (over age 65) and for certain groups of people with catastrophic or chronic illness, regardless of age. Medicare currently provides coverage for items and services for over 43 million beneficiaries (Centers for Medicare and Medicaid Services [CMMS], 2006a). Part A Medicare is the hospital insurance program. Part B is the supplementary medical insurance program that pays for outpatient care (including laboratory and x-ray services) and physician (or other primary care provider) services. Part C (now called Medicare Advantage) allows patients more choices for participating in managed care plans. And the newest, Medicare Part D, which became effective January 1, 2006, allows Medicare patients to purchase prescription drug coverage.

Medicaid is a federal–state cooperative health insurance plan directed primarily for the financially indigent. Medicaid now covers 59 million Americans—one in six—according to the National Association of State Budget Officers. It pays for 37 percent of all U.S. births, helps to pay for more than 60 percent of all patients in nursing homes, and accounts for 22 percent of state spending (Supersize Me, 2006). Both programs are coordinated by CMMS.

With the advent of Medicare and Medicaid and FFS reimbursement, health care costs skyrocketed. As a result, the government began establishing regulations requiring organizations to justify the need for services and to monitor the quality of services. Health care providers were forced for the first time to submit budgets and justify costs. This new surveillance and existence of external controls had a tremendous effect on the health care industry.

THE PROSPECTIVE PAYMENT SYSTEM

The advent of *diagnosis-related groups* (DRGs) in the early 1980s added to the need for monitoring cost containment. DRGs were predetermined payment schedules that reflected historical costs for treatment of specific patient conditions. The first version of DRGs included 383 categories. Approximately 550 DRGs, or "product lines," currently exist.

With DRGs, hospitals join the *prospective payment system* (PPS), whereby they receive a specified amount for each Medicare patient's admission, regardless of the actual cost of care. Exceptions to this occur when providers can demonstrate that a patient's case is an *outlier*, meaning that the cost of providing care for that patient justifies extra payment. PPS and consequent cost-containment efforts lead to decreased length of stays for most patients.

 As a result of the PPS and the need to contain costs, the length of stay for most hospital admissions has decreased greatly.

Many argue that quality standards have been lowered and that patients are being discharged before they are ready. It is the nurse–leader's responsibility to recognize when cost containment is impinging on patient safety and to take appropriate action to guarantee at least a minimum standard of care. Chapter 23 further discusses the PPS and its impact on quality control.

The government again deeply affected health care administration in the United States in 1997 with the passage of the *Balanced Budget Act* (BBA). This act contained numerous cost-containment measures, including reductions in provider payments for traditional FFS Medicare program partici-pants. The bulk of the savings resulted from limiting the growth rates for hospital and physician pay-ments. A second major source of savings derived from restructuring the payment methods for reha-bilitation hospitals, home health agencies, skilled nursing facilities, and outpatient services. The BBA also, for the first time, authorized payments to nurse practitioners for Medicare-provided serv-ices at 85 percent of the physician-fee schedule.

The ever-increasing impact of the federal government on how health care is delivered in the United States must be recognized. Accompanying this funding is an increase in regulations for facilities treating these patients and a system that rewards cost containment. Health care providers are encountering financial crises as they attempt to meet unlimited health care needs and services with limited fiscal reimbursement. Competition has intensified, reimbursement lev-els have declined, and utilization controls have increased. In addition, rapidly changing federal and state reimbursement policies make long-range budgeting and planning very difficult for health care facilities.

THE MANAGED CARE MOVEMENT

"Since around 1990, managed care has been the single most dominant force in the fundamental transformation of health care delivery in the United States" (Shi & Singh, 2005, p. 197.) Almost 100 million Americans were participating in some type of managed care early this century. "In 2002, 95% of Americans receiving employer-provided health benefits were enrolled in managed care plans, compared to only 27% in 1988" (p. 202).

Broadly defined, *managed care* is a system that attempts to integrate efficiency of care, access, and cost of care. Shi and Singh suggest that it is a "mechanism of providing healthcare services in which a single organization takes on the management of financing, insurance, deliv-ery and payment" (p. 198). Common denominators of managed care include the use of primary care providers as "*gatekeepers*," a focus on prevention, a decreased emphasis on inpatient hos-pital care, the use of clinical practice guidelines for providers, and *selective contracting* (whereby providers agree to lower reimbursement levels in exchange for patient population con-tracts). Managed care typically uses formularies to manage pharmacy care and focuses on con-tinuous quality monitoring and improvement.

Utilization review is another common component of managed care. *Utilization review* is "the determination of medical necessity for medical and surgical in-hospital, outpatient, and alterna-tive setting treatments for acute and rehabilitation care" (Alabama Department of Industrial Relations, 2006, para 3). It includes pre-certification or pre-authorization for elective treatments, concurrent review and, if necessary, retrospective review for emergency cases (Alabama Depart-ment of Industrial Relations, 2006).

Another frequent hallmark of managed care is *capitation*, whereby providers receive a fixed monthly payment regardless of services used by that patient during the month. If the cost to pro-vide care to someone is less than the capitated amount, the provider profits. If the cost is greater than the capitated amount, the provider suffers a loss. The goal, then, for capitated providers is to see that patients receive the essential services to stay healthy or to keep from becoming ill but to eliminate unnecessary use of health care services. Critics of capitation argue that this reim-bursement strategy leads to undertreatment of patients. A summary of managed care character-istics is found in Display 10.5.

DISPLAY 10.5   Managed Care at a Glance

- Represents a wide range of financing alternatives that focus on managing the cost and quality of health care by:
    - Using panels of selectively contracted providers
    - Limiting benefits to subscribers who use noncontracted providers
    - Implementing some type of authorization system
    - Focusing on primary care rather than specialists and inpatient services
    - Emphasizing preventive health care
    - Relying on clinical practice guidelines for providers
    - Regularly reviewing the use of health care resources
    - Continuously monitoring and improving the quality of health services
- Patients have less choice about the providers they can see and services they can access, in exchange for small co-payments and no deductibles.
- Managed care organizations often use primary care *gatekeepers* to:
    - Be sure that the provider-ordered services are needed and appropriate
    - See that patients are cared for in outpatient settings whenever possible
    - Ration care by queuing and wait times for authorizations
    - Encourage providers to follow more standardized care pathways and clinical guidelines for treatment
- Managed care is based on the concept of *capitation*, whereby providers prospectively receive a fixed monthly payment, regardless of what services are used by that patient during the month. This encourages providers to treat less, because their potential profits decline as treatment increases.

Types of Managed Care Organizations

One of the most common types of managed care organizations (MCO) is the *health maintenance organization* (HMO). An HMO is a corporate body funded by insurance premiums. The HMO's physicians and other professionals practice medicine within certain financial, geographic, and professional limits to individuals and families who have enrolled in the HMO.

The *Health Maintenance Organization Act of 1973* authorized spending $375 million over 5 years to set up and evaluate HMOs in communities across the country. Although HMOs originated as an alternative to traditional health insurance plans, some of the largest private insurers, including Blue Cross & Blue Shield and Aetna, have created HMOs within their organization while maintaining their traditional indemnity plans.

In discussing HMOs, it is important to remember that there are different types of HMOs as well as different types of plans within HMOs to which members may subscribe. Several types of HMOs include (a) *staff*, (b) *independent practice association* (IPA), (c) *group*, and (d) *network*. In *staff HMOs*, physician providers are salaried by the HMO and under direct control of the HMO. In *IPA HMOs*, the HMO contracts with a group of physicians through an intermediary to provide services for members of the HMO. In a *group HMO*, the HMO contracts directly with one independent physician group. In *network HMOs*, the HMO contracts with multiple independent physician group practices.

The types of plans available within HMOs typically vary according to the degree of provider choice available to enrollees. Two such plans include *point-of-service* (POS) and *exclusive provider organization* (EPO) options. In POS plans, the patient has the option, at the time of service, to select a provider outside the network but pays a higher premium as well as a *co-payment* (amount of money enrollees pay out of their pocket at the time a service is provided) for the flexibility to do so. In the EPO option, enrollees must seek care from the designated HMO provider or pay all of the cost out of pocket.

Another common type of MCO is the *preferred provider organization* (PPO). PPOs render services on a fee-for-service basis but provide financial incentives to consumers (they pay less) when the preferred provider is used. Providers are motivated to become part of a PPO because it ensures them an adequate population of patients.

Medicare and Medicaid Managed Care

Although Medicare and Medicaid patients historically were excluded from managed care under the *free choice of physician rule*, these restrictions were lifted in the 1970s and 1980s. As a result, these patients could participate in private HMOs and other types of managed care programs through *Medicare Part C* (formerly the Medicare + Choice program, and now known as Medicare Advantage). To join a Medicare Advantage Plan, patients must have both Medicare Part A and Part B. The payment system for these programs (effective 1982) was to be prospective, and the HMO was at risk for providing all benefits in return for the capitated payment.

MCOs receive reimbursement for Medicare-eligible patients based on a formula established by the CMMS, which looks at age, gender, geographic region, and the average cost per patient at a given age. Then, the government gives itself a 5-percent discount and gives the rest to the MCO.

The *BBA of 1997* expanded the role of private plans under Medicare + Choice to include PPOs, *provider-sponsored organizations* (PSOs), *private fee-for service* (PFFS) plans, and *medical savings accounts* (MSAs), coupled with high-deductible insurance plans. Private plan options were offered primarily at the county level (Henry J. Kaiser Family Foundation, 2005). The CMMS is now the largest managed care buyer in the United States.

 The Centers for Medicare and Medicaid Services is now the largest purchaser of managed care in the country.

Of the total Medicaid enrollment in the United States in 2004, approximately 60 percent of participants are receiving Medicaid benefits through managed care (CMMS, 2006b.) In addition, all states except Alaska, New Hampshire, and Wyoming have all or a portion of their Medicaid population enrolled in an MCO. A report, prepared by the University of California comparing fee-for-service with managed care for Medi-Cal (California's program for Medicaid) patients, suggests that managed care is a better system to improve access and health outcomes (California HealthCare Foundation, 2004).

PROPONENTS AND CRITICS OF MANAGED CARE SPEAK UP

Proponents of managed care argue that prepaid health care plans, such as those offered by HMOs, decrease health care costs, provide broader benefits for patients than under the traditional FFS model, appropriately shift care from inpatient to outpatient settings, result in higher physician productivity, and have high enrollee satisfaction levels. This was certainly the case in a study by Deb, Li, Trivedi, and Zimmer (2006), which suggested that an individual enrolled in an HMO plan has 2 more visits to a doctor and 0.1 more visits to the emergency room per year than would the same individual enrolled in a nonmanaged care plan.

Critics, however, suggest that participation in MCOs may result in a loss of existing physician–patient relationships, a limited choice of physicians for consumers, a lower level of continuity of care, reduced physician autonomy, longer wait times for care, and consumer confusion about the many rules to be followed. A common complaint heard from managed care subscribers is that services must be preapproved or preauthorized by a gatekeeper or that second opinions must be obtained before surgery. Although this loss of autonomy is difficult for consumers accustomed to an FFS system with few limits on choice and access, such utilization constraints are necessary due to *moral hazard*, which is the risk that the insured will overuse services just because the insurance will pay the costs. Because the co-payment is typically small for patients in managed care programs, the risk of moral hazard rises.

 Moral hazard refers to the propensity of insured patients to use more medical services than necessary because their insurance covers so much of the cost.

Another aspect complicating health care reimbursement through the PPS, an HMO, or a PPO is that clear and comprehensive documentation of the need for services and actual services provided is mandatory. Provision of service no longer guarantees reimbursement. Thus, the fiscal accountability of nurses goes beyond planning and implementing; it includes responsible recording and communication of activities.

Provision of service no longer guarantees reimbursement.

Perhaps the most serious concern about the advancement of managed care in this country is the change in relationships among insurers, physicians, nurses, and patients. The full impact on clinical judgment of tying physician and nursing salaries to bonuses, incentives, and penalties designed to reduce utilization of services and resources and increase profit is unknown. As a result, a need for self-awareness regarding the values that guide individual professional nursing practice has never been greater.

LEARNING EXERCISE 10.5

Providing Care With Limited Reimbursement

You are the manager at a home health agency. One of your elderly patients has insulin-dependent diabetes. He has no family support. He speaks limited English and has little understanding of his disease. He lives alone. Your reimbursement from a government agency pays $90 per visit. Because this gentleman needs so much care, you find that the actual cost to your agency is $130 for each visit to him. What will be the impact to your agency if this patient is seen twice a week for 3 months? How can you recover the lost revenue? How can you make each visit less costly and still meet the needs of the patient?

THE FUTURE OF MANAGED CARE

Managed care continues to change the face of health care in the United States. Abbott and Keller (2006) suggest that managed care contracts account for 30 percent to 70 percent of a hospital's revenues. Because most hospitals contract with multiple payers and every payer has contracts for each of its products, the terms and rates for reimbursement vary tremendously. Hospitals can have 50 to 150 individual active contracts at any point in time (Abbott & Keller, 2006).

This contractual complexity and the use of prospective payment makes it much more difficult for providers to anticipate potential revenues and then to bill for and collect reimbursement for services provided. Indeed, some critics of managed care suggest that health care practitioners and institutions now bear much more of the financial risk for the cost of care than insurers. D'Cruz and Welter (2005) suggest that auditing commercial payments will be the single most important job for many hospitals in the short-term future since 8 percent to 14 percent of commercial revenue goes uncollected (underpayments from a provider's perspective). Although managed care is a major component in health care, recent trends suggest that participation is declining.

Recent trends suggest that participation in managed care plans (both by consumers and providers) is actually declining, although it continues to be a major force impacting contemporary health care.

This decline has occurred in part because managed care plans are no longer significantly less expensive for consumers to purchase or for insurers to provide. In addition, providers have grown increasingly frustrated with limited and delayed reimbursement for services provided as well as the need to justify need for services ordered. This phenomenon has been referred to as the *managed care backlash*. The Center for Studying Health System Change, based on phone interviews with more than 6,000 physicians, found that the percentage of U.S. physicians who do not participate in any managed care plans rose to 11.5 percent in 2004–2005, up from 9.2 percent in 2000–2002 (Managed by Whom?, 2006).

Managed care is not going to go away—at least not any time soon. It will, however, continue to change. "According to some, managed care and its strategies are evolving. According to others, managed care is dying" (American Psychiatric Association, 2003, p. 1). In any case, most agree that managed care and the delivery of health care in the United States will look very different in the future. Certainly, in reviewing the health care reimbursement milestones of the past 75 years (Display 10.6), one can see that health care reimbursement has changed dramatically in a relatively short time and that managed care is just one more reimbursement schema that has changed the face of health care in the United States.

To provide care and appropriately advocate for patients in the 21st century, all nurses need at least a basic understanding of health care costs. They also need to know how reimbursement strategies directly and indirectly affect their practice. Only then can nurses be active participants in the proactive and visionary fiscal planning required to survive in the current health care marketplace.

DISPLAY 10.6   U.S. Health Care Milestones: 75 Years of Reimbursement

1929 First HMO, the Ross-Loos Clinic, established in Los Angeles.

1929 Origins of Blue Cross, when Baylor University Hospital agreed to provide 1500 schoolteachers up to 21 days of hospital care for $6.00 per year.

1935 Passage of Social Security Act. This act originally included compulsory health insurance for states that voluntarily chose to participate, but the American Medical Association fought it and the health insurance provisions were omitted from the act.

1942 First nationwide hospital insurance bill introduced into Congress, but it failed to pass.

1946 Hill Burton Act promoted hospital development and renovation after World War II. Authorized $75 million yearly for 5 years to aid in hospital construction.

1965 Passage of Medicare and Medicaid as part of Lyndon B. Johnson's Great Society. Resulted in 50-percent increase in the number of medical schools in the United States.

1972 Professional Standards Review Organizations (PSROs) established by Congress to prevent excess hospitalization and utilization by Medicare and Medicaid patients.

1973 The Health Maintenance Act authorized the spending of $375 million over 5 years to set up and evaluate HMOs in communities across the country.

1974 The National Planning Act created a system of state and local health planning agencies largely supported by federal funds. This created Health Systems Agencies (HSAs) to inventory each community's health care resources and to issue Certificates of Need.

1974 The Employment Retirement Income and Security Act (ERISA) passed, generally preempting state regulation of self-insuring employee benefit plans.

1983 DRGs established, which changed the structure of Medicare payments from a retrospectively adjusted cost-reimbursement system to a prospective, risk-based one.

1986 COBRA Act of 1986 passed. Allowed terminated employees or those who lose coverage because of reduced work hours to buy group coverage for themselves and their families for limited periods of time (up to 60 days to decide).

1988 Medicare Catastrophic Coverage Act (MCCA) enacted, which expanded Medicare benefits greatly to include a portion of out-of-pocket drug and physician expenses.

1989 Medicare system of paying physician charges was changed to a resource-based relative value scale (RBRVS) to be phased in starting in 1992.

1993 President William J. Clinton introduced the Health Security Act, legislation assuring universal access to all Americans. The act failed to pass.

1996 Health Insurance Portability and Accountability Act passed. Created MSAs and required the Department of Health and Human Services to establish national standards for electronic health care transactions and national identifiers for providers, health plans, and employers. It also addressed the security and privacy of health data.

1997 Approximately one quarter of Americans enrolled in HMOs. Almost 6 million Medicare beneficiaries enrolled in HMOs. Balanced Budget Act gives states the authority to implement managed care programs without federal waivers.

1999 Health care spending comprises approximately 15 percent of the GDP of the United States, exceeding $1 trillion in annual health care expenditures. Approximately 37 million Americans are uninsured and between 50 and 70 million are inadequately insured.

2001 People in the United States make over 1 billion visits to physician offices, have hundreds of millions of contacts with other health caregivers, and spend over 170 million days in acute-care hospitals (Bodenheimer & Grumbach, 2005). Over 1.5 million elderly

(continued)

DISPLAY 10.6   U.S. Health Care Milestones: 75 Years of Reimbursement (continued)

Medicare HMO patients forced to find new insurance arrangements as their HMOs pulled out of the Medicare program after losing money on Medicare enrollees. Increasing disenchantment noted with managed care.

2003 The Medicare Prescription Drug, Improvement, and Modernization Act of 2003 passes, providing a voluntary program for prescription drug coverage under the Medicare program. Included a provision that Americans can have tax-free health savings accounts (Shi & Singh, 2005).

2005 There are "187.4 million Americans with private health insurance coverage, 35.2 million Medicare beneficiaries, and 31.5 million Medicaid recipients. Health insurance can be purchased from approximately 1000 health insurance companies and 70 Blue Cross & Blue Shield plans. The managed care sector includes approximately 540 licensed HMOs and 925 preferred provider organizations (PPOs)" (Shi & Singh, 2005, p. 3).

INTEGRATING LEADERSHIP ROLES AND MANAGEMENT FUNCTIONS IN FISCAL PLANNING

Managers must understand fiscal planning, be aware of their budgetary responsibilities, and be cost-effective in meeting organizational goals. The ability to forecast unit fiscal needs with sensitivity to the organization's economic, social, and legislative climate is a high-level management function. Managers also must be able to articulate unit needs through budgeting to ensure adequate nursing staff, supplies, and equipment. Finally, managers must be skillful in the monitoring aspects of budget control.

Leadership skills allow the manager to involve all appropriate stakeholders in developing the budget. Other leadership skills required in fiscal planning include flexibility, creativity, and vision regarding future needs. The skilled leader is able to anticipate budget constraints and act proactively. In contrast, many managers allow budget constraints to dictate alternatives. In an age of inadequate fiscal resources, the leader is creative in identifying alternatives to meet patient needs. The skilled leader, however, also ensures that cost containment does not jeopardize patient safety. As well, leaders are assertive, articulate people who ensure that their department's budgeting receives a fair hearing. Because leaders can delineate unit budgetary needs in an assertive, professional, and proactive manner, they generally obtain a fair distribution of resources for their unit.

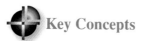 **Key Concepts**

* *Fiscal planning*, as in all types of planning, is a learned skill that improves with practice.

* Historically, nursing management played a limited role in determining resource allocation in health care institutions.
* The *personnel–workforce budget* often accounts for the majority of health care organization's expenses because health care is *labor intensive*.
* Personnel budgets include actual worked time (*productive time* or *salary expense*) and time that the organization pays the employee for not working (*nonproductive* or *benefit time*).
* A *budget* is at best a forecast or prediction; it is a plan and not a rule. Therefore, a budget must be flexible and open to ongoing evaluation and revision.
* A budget that is predicted too far in advance is open to greater error. If the budget is shortsighted, compensating for unexpected major expenses or capital equipment purchases may be difficult.
* The desired outcome of budgeting is maximal use of resources to meet organizational short- and long-term needs. Its value to the institution is directly related to its accuracy.
* The *operating budget* reflects expenses that flex up or down in a predetermined manner to reflect variation in volume of service provided.
* *Capital budgets* plan for the purchase of buildings or major equipment. This includes equipment that has a long life (usually greater than 5 years), is not used daily, and is more expensive than operating supplies.
* Managers must rejustify their program or needs every budgeting cycle in *zero-based budgeting*. Using a *decision package* to set funding priorities is a key feature of zero-based budgeting.
* With the advent of state and federal reimbursement for health care in the 1960s, providers were forced to submit budgets and costs to payers that more accurately reflected their actual cost to provide these services.
* With *diagnosis-related groups* (DRGs), hospitals join the *prospective payment system* (PPS), whereby they receive a specified amount for each Medicare patient's admission, regardless of the actual cost of care. Exceptions occur when the provider can demonstrate that a patient's case is an *outlier*, meaning that the cost of providing care for that patient justifies extra payment.
* Key principles of managed care include the use of primary care providers as *gatekeepers*, a focus on prevention, a decreased emphasis on inpatient hospital care, the use of clinical practice guidelines for providers, selective contracting, capitation, utilization review, the use of formularies to manage pharmacy care, and continuous quality monitoring and improvement.
* The types of plans available within HMOs typically vary according to the degree of provider choice available to enrollees.
* Managed care has altered the relationships among insurers, physicians, nurses, and patients, with providers today often having to assume a role as agent for the patient as well as agent of resource allocation for an insurance carrier, hospital, or particular practice plan.
* Provision of service no longer guarantees reimbursement. Clear and comprehensive documentation of the need for services and actual services provided is needed for reimbursement.

ADDITIONAL LEARNING EXERCISES AND APPLICATIONS

LEARNING EXERCISE 10.6

How Does Policy Influence Your Decision?

You are the evening house supervisor of a small, private, rural hospital. In your role as house supervisor, you are responsible for staffing the upcoming shift and for troubleshooting any and all problems that cannot be handled at the unit level.

Because of legislative changes and reductions in federal monies being reimbursed to your facility over the last few years, the hospital has developed a policy that says that emergency care will be provided to indigent patients (patients who cannot pay for services) only when the patient needs immediate medical intervention and would not tolerate a transfer to county facilities, which are approximately 30 minutes away.

Tonight, you receive a call to come to the emergency room to handle a "patient complaint." When you arrive, you find a Hispanic woman in her mid-20s arguing vehemently with the emergency room charge nurse and physician. When you intercede, the patient introduces herself as Teresa Garcia and states, "There is something wrong with my father, and they won't help him because we can't pay. They say we must go to the county hospital, and the care he would get there will not be as good. If we had money, you would be willing to do something." The charge nurse intercedes by saying, "Teresa's father began vomiting about 2 hours ago and blacked out approximately 45 minutes ago, following a 14-hour drinking binge." The ER physician added, "Mr. Garcia's blood alcohol level is 0.25 (two and one-half times the level required to be declared legally intoxicated), and my baseline physical examination would indicate nothing other than he is drunk and needs to sleep it off. Besides, I have seen Mr. Garcia in the ER before, and it's always for the same thing. If he wants further treatment, it should be provided at the county facility."

Teresa persists in her pleas to you that "there is something different this time" and that she believes this hospital should evaluate her father further. She intuitively feels that something terrible will happen to her father if he is not cared for immediately. The ER physician becomes even angrier after this comment and states to you, "I am not going to waste my time and energy on someone who is just drunk, and I refuse to order any more expensive lab tests or x-rays on this patient. If you want something else done, you will have to find someone else to order it." With that, he walks off and returns to the examination room, where other patients are waiting to be seen. The ER nurse turns to look at you and is waiting for further directions.

● ASSIGNMENT: How will you handle this situation? Would your decision be any easier if there were no limitations in resource allocation? Are your values to act as an agent for the patient or for the agency more strongly developed?

LEARNING EXERCISE 10.7

Weighing Choices in Budget Spending

One of your goals as the unit manager of a critical care unit is to prepare all your nurses to be certified in advanced cardiac life support. You currently have five staff nurses who need this certification. You can hire someone to teach this class locally and rent a facility for $800; however, the cost will be taken out of the travel and education budget for the unit, and this will leave you short for the rest of the fiscal year. It also will be a time-consuming effort because you must coordinate the preparation and reproduction of educational materials needed for the course and make arrangements for the rental facility. A certification class also will be provided in the near future in a large city approximately 150 miles from the hospital. The cost per participant will be $200. In addition, there would be travel and lodging expenses.

● ASSIGNMENT: You have several decisions to make. Should the class be held locally? If so, how will you organize it? Are you going to require your staff to have this certification or merely highly recommend that they do so? If it is required, will the unit pay the costs of the certification? Will you pay the staff nurses their regular hourly wage for attending the class on regularly scheduled work hours? Can this certification be cost-effective? Use group process in some way to make your decision.

LEARNING EXERCISE 10.8

How Will You Meet New Budget Restrictions?

You are the director of the local agency that cares for ill and well elderly patients. You are funded by a private corporation grant, which requires matching of city and state funds. You received a letter in the mail today from the state that says state funding will be cut by $35,000, effective in 2 weeks, when the state's budget year begins. This means that your private funding also will be cut $35,000, for a total revenue loss of $70,000. It is impossible at this time to seek alternative funding sources.

In reviewing your agency budget, you note that, as in many health care agencies, your budget is labor intensive. More than 80 percent of your budget is attributable to personnel costs, and you believe that the cuts must come from within the personnel budget. You may reduce the patient population that you serve, although you do not really want to do so. You briefly discuss this communication with your staff; no one is willing to reduce his or her hours voluntarily, and no one is planning to terminate his or her employment at any time in the near future.

● ASSIGNMENT: Given the following brief description of your position and each of your five employees, decide how you will meet the new budget restrictions. What is the rationale for your choice? Which decision do you believe will result in the least disruption of the agency and of the employees in the agency? Should group decision making be involved in fiscal decisions such as this one? Can fiscal decisions such as this be made without value judgments?

Your position is project director. As the project director, you coordinate all the day-to-day activities in the agency. You also are involved in long-term planning, and a major portion of your time is allotted to securing future funding for the agency to continue. As the project director, you have the authority to hire and fire employees. You are in your early 30s and have a master's degree in nursing and health administration. You enjoy your job and believe that you have done well in this position since you started 4 years ago. Your yearly salary as a full-time employee is $80,000.

Employee #1 is Mrs. Potter. Mrs. Potter has worked at the agency since it started 7 years ago. She is an RN with 30 years' experience working with the geriatric population in public health nursing, care facilities, and private duty. She plans to retire in 7 years and travel with her independently wealthy husband. Mrs. Potter has a great deal of expertise that she can share

(Learning Exercise continues on page 234)

with your staff, although at times you believe she overshadows your authority because of her experience and your young age. Her yearly salary as a full-time employee is $65,000.

Employee #2 is Mr. Boone. Mr. Boone has BS degrees in both nursing and dietetics and food management. As an RN and Registered Dietician (RD), he brings a unique expertise to your staff, which is highly needed when dealing with a chronically ill and improperly nourished elderly population. In the 6 months since he joined your agency, he has proven to be a dependable, well-liked, and highly respected member of your staff. His yearly salary as a full-time employee is $55,000.

Employee #3 is Miss Barns. Miss Barns is the receptionist–secretary in the agency. In addition to all the traditional secretarial duties, such as typing, filing, and transcription of dictation, she screens incoming telephone calls and directs people who come to the agency for information. Her efficiency is a tremendous attribute to the agency. Her full-time yearly salary is $26,000.

Employee #4 is Ms. Lake. Ms. Lake is an LPN/LVN with 15 years of work experience in a variety of health care agencies. She is especially attuned to patient needs. Although her technical nursing skills are also good, her caseload frequently is more focused around elderly patients who need companionship and emotional support. She does well at patient teaching because of her outstanding listening and communication skills. Many of your patients request her by name. She is a single mother, supporting six children, and you are aware that she has great difficulty in meeting her personal financial obligations. Her full-time yearly salary is $48,000.

Employee #5 is Mrs. Long. Mrs. Long is an "elderly help aide." She has completed nurse aide training, although her primary role in the agency is to assist well elderly with bathing, meal preparation, driving, and shopping. The time that Mrs. Long spends in performing basic care has decreased the average visit time for each member of your staff by 30 percent. She is widowed and uses this job to meet her social and self-esteem needs. Financially, her resources are adequate, and the money she earns is not a motivator for working. Mrs. Long works 3 days a week, and her yearly salary is $23,000.

LEARNING EXERCISE 10.9

Identifying, Prioritizing, and Choosing Program Goals

Jane is the supervisor of a small cardiac rehabilitation program. The program includes inpatient cardiac teaching and an outpatient exercise rehabilitation program. Because of limited reimbursement by third-party insurance payers for patient education, there has been no direct charge for inpatient education. Outpatient program participants pay $180 per month to attend three 1-hour sessions per week, although the revenue generated from the outpatient program still leaves an overall budget deficit for the program of approximately $4,800 per month.

Today, Jane is summoned to the associate administrator's office to discuss her budget for the upcoming year. At this meeting, the administrator states that the hospital is experiencing extreme financial difficulties due to DRGs and the prospective payment system. He states that the program must become self-supporting in the next fiscal year; otherwise, services must be cut. On returning to her office, Jane decided to make a list of several alternatives for problem solving and to analyze each for driving and restraining factors. These alternatives include the following:

1. *Implement a charge for inpatient education*. This would eliminate the budget deficit, but the cost would probably have to be borne by the patient. (*Implication:* Only patients with adequate fiscal resources would elect to receive vital education.)
2. *Reduce department staffing*. There are currently three staff members in the department, and it would be impossible to maintain the same level or quality of services if staffing were reduced.
3. *Reduce or limit services*. The inpatient education program or educational programs associated with the outpatient program could be eliminated. These are both considered to be valuable aspects of the program.
4. The fee for the outpatient program could be increased. This could easily result in a decrease in program participation, because many outpatient program participants do not have insurance coverage for their participation.

● ASSIGNMENT: Identify at least five program goals, and prioritize them as you would if you were Jane. Based on the priorities that you have established, which alternative would you select? Explain your choice.

LEARNING EXERCISE 10.10

Addressing Conflicting Values

You are a single parent of two children younger than 5 years old and are currently employed as a pediatric office nurse. You enjoy your job, but your long-term career goal is to become a pediatric nurse practitioner, and you have been taking courses part-time preparing to enter graduate school in the fall. Your application for admission has been accepted, and the next cycle for admissions will not be for another 3 years. Your recent divorce and assignment of sole custody of the children have resulted in a need for you to reconsider your plan.

Restraining Forces: You had originally planned to reduce your work hours to part-time to allow time for classes and studying, but this will be fiscally impossible now. You also recognize that tuition and educational expenses will place a strain on your budget even if you continue to work full-time. You have not looked into the availability of scholarships or loans and have missed the deadline for the upcoming fall. In addition, you have not yet overcome your anxiety and guilt about leaving your small children for even more time than you do now.

Driving Forces: You also recognize, however, that gaining certification as a pediatric nurse practitioner should result in a large salary increase over what you are able to make as an office nurse and that it would allow you to provide resources for your children in the future that you otherwise may be unable to do. As well, you recognize that although you are not dissatisfied with your current job, you have a great deal of ability that has gone untapped and that your potential for long-term job satisfaction is low.

● ASSIGNMENT: Fiscal planning always requires priority setting, and often this priority setting is determined by personal values. Priority setting is made even more difficult when there are conflicting values. Identify the values involved in this case. Develop a plan that addresses these value conflicts and has the most desirable outcomes.

LEARNING EXERCISE 10.11

How Would You Change This Budget?

Today is April 1, and you have received the following budget printout. Your charge nurses are requesting an additional RN on each shift since the acuity has increased dramatically over the last 2 years. Dr. Robb has requested two new continuous limb movement machines for the postoperative orthopedic patients on your unit at a cost of $3,000 each. In addition, you would like to attend a national orthopedics conference in New York in August at a projected cost of $1,500. The registration fee is $350 and is due now.

	Annual Budget	Expended in March	Expended Year to Date[*]	Amount Remaining
Personnel	300,000	25,000	175,000	125,000
Overtime	50,000	3,800	50,000	0
Supplies	18,000	1,500	13,500	4,500
Travel (personal)	2,200	0	1,700	500
Equipment	5,000	0	5,000	0
Staff development (personal)	1,000	200	800	200

*Fiscal year begins July 1.

● ASSIGNMENT: How will you deal with these requests based on the budget printout? What expenses can and should be deferred to the new fiscal year? In what budgeting area were your previous projections most accurate? Most inaccurate? What factors may have contributed to these inaccuracies? Were they controllable or predictable?

Web Links

Centers for Medicaid and Medicare Services (CMMS)
http://www.cms.hhs.gov/
Introduces Medicare, Medicaid, and SCHIP and provides information about all programs administered by the CMMS.

United States Department of Health and Human Services (USDHHS)
http://www.os.dhhs.gov
The U.S. government's principal agency for protecting the health of all Americans and providing essential human services.

Managed Care Magazine
http://www.managedcaremag.com
A guide for managed care executives and physicians covering capitation, compensation, and disease management.

Health Insurance—Understanding Your Health Plan's Rules
http://familydoctor.org/734.xml

References

Abbott, K. A., & Keller, H. (2006, September). Retrospective review: The good, the bad, and the ugly: Rigorous retrospective review of managed care accounts should be mandatory for hospitals. *Healthcare Financial Management*. Retrieved October 17, 2006, from *http://www.findarticles.com/ p/articles/mi_m3257/is_9_60/ai_n16728111*.

About, Inc. (2006). *Definition of budget*. Business and Finance—Economics. Retrieved October 15, 2006, from *http://economics.about.com/cs/economicsglossary/g/ budget.htm*.

Alabama Department of Industrial Relations. (2006). *Utilization management and bill screening*. Retrieved October 23, 2006, from *http://dir.alabama.gov/wc/umbs.aspx*.

American Heritage Dictionary of the English Language. (2005). *Definition—Cost-effective*. Houghton-Mifflin Company. Retrieved October 20, 2006, from *http://iwon.ask.com/ reference/dictionary/ahdict/18780/cost-effective*.

American Psychiatric Association (2003, December). *Alternatives to managed care. Resource document*. Retrieved October 23, 2006, from *http://www.psych.org/edu/other_res/ lib_archives/archives/200403.pdf*.

Barr, P. (2005). Flexing your budget: Experts urge hospitals, systems to trade in their traditional budgeting process for a more dynamic and versatile model. *Modern Healthcare, 35*(37), 24, 26.

Bodenheimer, T. S., & Grumbach, K. (2005). *Understanding health policy*. Fourth Edition. New York: Lange Medical Books/McGraw Hill.

California HealthCare Foundation. (2004). *Preventing unnecessary hospitalizations in Medi-Cal: Comparing fee-for-service with managed care*. Retrieved October 15, 2006, from *http://www.chcf.org/topics/medi-cal*.

Centers for Medicare and Medicaid Services (2006a). *Medicare coverage—General information*. Retrieved October 21, 2006, from *http://www.cms.hhs.gov/CoverageGenInfo/*.

Centers for Medicare and Medicaid Services (2006b). *Medicaid managed care*. Retrieved October 22, 2006, from *http://www.cms.hhs.gov/MedicaidManagCare/*.

Cowen, T. (2006, October 5). *Poor U.S. scores in health care don't measure Nobels and innovation*. Retrieved October 23, 2006, from *http://www.nytimes.com/2006/10/05/business/ 05scene.html?ex=1317700800&en=5889b4819eaf787a&ei=5 090&partner=rssuserland&emc=rss*.

D'Cruz, M., & Welter, T. (2005, December). No small change: Payment trends call for big preparation for 2006. *Healthcare Financial Management, 59*(12), 50–56, 58, 60.

Deb, P., Li, C., Trivedi, P. K., & Zimmer, D. M. (2006). The effect of managed care on use of health care services: Results from two contemporaneous household surveys. *Health Economics, 15*(7), 743–760.

Goldszer, R. C., Rutherford, A., Banks, P., Zou, K. H., Curley, M., Brita Rossi, P., et al. (2004, March). Implementing clinical pathways for patients admitted to a medical service: Lessons learned. *Critical Pathways in Cardiology, 3*(1), 35–41. Retrieved October 18, 2006, from *http://www.brighamand-womens.org/gms/News/GoldzerEtAl.pdf*.

Henry J. Kaiser Family Foundation. (2005, April). *Medicare. Medicare advantage*. Retrieved May 25, 2005, from *http://www.kff.org/medicare/loader.cfm?url=/commonspot/ security/getfile.cfm&PageID=52979*.

Managed by whom? (2006, September). *Healthcare Financial Management*. Retrieved October 18, 2006, from *http://www. findarticles.com/p/articles/mi_m3257/is_9_60/ai_n16728086*.

O'Kane, M. (2006, August). Redefining value in health care: A new imperative: Does spending more mean better care? Not necessarily. *Healthcare Financial Management*. Retrieved October 16, 2006 from *http://www.findarticles.com/p/ articles/mi_m3257/is_8_60/ai_n16752984*.

Shi, L., & Singh, D. (2005). *Essentials of the U.S. health care system*. Sudbury, MA: Jones and Bartlett Publishers.

Supersize me. (2006, September). *Healthcare Financial Management*. FindArticles.com. Retrieved October 17, 2006, from *http:// www.findarticles.com/p/articles/mi_m3257/is_9_60/ai_n16728093*.

Whitney, W. T. Jr. (2006, October 12). *U.S. health care falls short*. Retrieved October 23, 2006, from *http://www.pww.org/article/articleview/9989/1/343*.

Bibliography

Barry, P. (2006, May). Perspectives on private practice. Handling the finances: HMO versus private pay. *Perspectives in Psychiatric Care, 42*(2), 133–136.

Beaty, L. (2005). A primer for understanding diagnosis-related groups and inpatient hospital reimbursement with nursing implications. *Critical Care Nursing Quarterly, 28*(4), 360–369.

Bowman, J., Rousseau, A., Silk, D., & Harrison, C. (2006). Access to cancer drugs in Medicare Part D: Formulary placement and beneficiary cost sharing in 2006: Medicare Part D beneficiaries have access to many more cancer drugs than ever before, with low cost sharing. *Health Affairs, 25*(5), 1240–1248.

CMS proposes sweeping changes in hospital payment structure: New rule would require more attention to documentation. (2006). *Hospital Case Management, 14*(8), 113, 123.

CMS to revamp DRGs to eliminate 'bias'. (2006). *OR Manager, 22*(6), 11.

Cooper, P. F., Simon, K. I., & Vistnes, J. (2006). A closer look at the managed care backlash. *Medical Care, 44*(5)(Suppl), I4–I11.

Fine, A. (2006). Medicare evaluates pay-for-performance. *Managed Care Quarterly, 14*(1), 22–23.

Gee, P. (2006). DRG do-over: The need for a service-line strategy. *Healthcare Financial Management, 60*(8), 52–55.

Goodman, R. M. (2006). Relationship between primary care physician financial risk and member emergency department use in a commercial HMO population. *American Journal of Managed Care, 12*(6), 329–340.

Gosden, T. (2005). *Capitation, salary, fee-for-service and mixed systems of payment: Effects on the behaviour of primary care physicians.* The Cochrane Library, n.1 (software—research, systematic review). CINAHL AN: 2005005020.

Hurst, S. A., & Danis, M. (2006). Perspectives. Indecent coverage? Protecting the goals of health insurance from the impact of co-payments. *Cambridge Quarterly of Healthcare Ethics, 15*(1), 107–113.

Johnston, C. (2006, April). Up to the job? Auditing to assess the adequacy of an established ICP. *Journal of Integrated Care Pathways, 10*(1), 13–16.

Lindrooth, R. C., Bazzoli, G. J., Needleman, J., & Hasnain-Wynia, R. (2006). The effect of changes in hospital reimbursement on nurse staffing decisions at safety net and nonsafety net hospitals. *Health Services Research, 41*(3), 701–720.

Physician-case manager team cuts LOS, denials: Collaborative effort focuses on top 10 DRGs. (2006, January). *Hospital Case Management, 14*(1), 4–5.

Rice, M., Broome, M. E., Habermann, B., Kang, D., & Davis, L. L. (2006). Implementing the research budget. *Western Journal of Nursing Research, 28*(2), 234–241.

Rizk, E. (2006, August). Finding opportunity where business models meet. *Managed Care Magazine.* Retrieved October 15, 2006, from *http://www.managedcaremag.com/archives/0608/0608.align.html.*

Russo, M. (2006). Putting the copayment before the horse. *Biotechnology Healthcare, 3*(3), 3.

Specialists track core measure, documentation, DRGs: RNs work on team with case managers, social workers. (2006). *Hospital Case Management, 14*(9), 135–137.

Tseng, C. W., Brook, R. H., Keeler, E., Steers, W. N., Waitzfelder, B. E., & Mangione, C. M. (2006). Effect of generic-only drug benefits on seniors' medication use and financial burden. *American Journal of Managed Care, 12*(9), 525–532.

U.S. health-care system scores a D for quality. (2006, September 20). *Health Day.* Retrieved October 15, 2006, from *http:// www.nlm.nih.gov/medlineplus/news/fullstory_38924.html.*

Watson, J., Hockley, J., & Dewar, B. (2006). Barriers to implementing an integrated care pathway for the last days of life in nursing homes. *International Journal of Palliative Nursing, 12*(5), 234–240.

Welton, J. M., & Halloran, E. J. (2005). Nursing diagnoses, diagnosis-related group, and hospital outcomes. *Journal of Nursing Administration, 35*(12), 541–549.

11

Career Development: From New Graduate to Retirement

. . . every individual you hire for a leadership role should have the capability to grow into that role.

—Carolyn Hope Smeltzer

. . . career plans are about where you are today and, more importantly, where you're going tomorrow.

—Phil McPeck

To be a fully engaged professional requires commitment to career development. *Career development* is intentional career planning and should be viewed as a critical and deliberate life process involving both the individual and the employer. It provides individuals with choices about career outcomes rather than leaving it to chance. Thus, career planning is about career exploration, opportunities, and change. Before the 1970s, organizations did little to help employees plan and develop their careers. Now, subordinate career development is essential to organizational success, and most organizations accept at least some responsibility for assisting employees with this function.

Career development begins with an assessment of self as well as one's work environment, job analysis, education, training, job search and acquisition, and work experience. This is known as *career planning*. Career planning includes evaluating one's strengths and weaknesses, setting goals, examining career opportunities, preparing for potential opportunities, and using appropriate developmental activities.

Career planning in nursing often begins with an individual's decision about educational entry level for practice but quickly expands to developing advanced skills in an area of nursing practice. Even for the entry-level nurse, career planning should include, at minimum, a commitment to the use of evidence-based practice, learning new skills or bettering practice by using role models and mentors, staying aware of and being involved in professional issues, and furthering one's education. At best, it should include long-term career goals as well as a specific, detailed plan to achieve those goals. For the most part, organizational career development efforts have centered on management development rather than activities that promote growth in nonmanagement

DISPLAY 11.1 **Leadership Roles and Management Functions Associated With Career Development**

Leadership Roles

1. Is self-aware of personal values influencing career development
2. Encourages employees to take responsibility for their own career planning
3. Identifies, encourages, and develops future leaders
4. Shows a genuine interest in the career planning and career development of all employees
5. Encourages and supports the development of career paths within and outside the organization
6. Supports employees' personal career decisions based on each employee's needs and values
7. Is a role model for continued professional development via specialty certification, continuing education, and portfolio development
8. Emphasizes the need for employees to develop the skill set necessary for evidence-based practice

Management Functions

1. Develops fair policies on promotions and transfers and communicates them clearly to subordinates
2. Uses organizational transfers appropriately
3. Uses a planned system of short- and long-term coaching for career development and documents all coaching efforts
4. Disseminates career information
5. Posts job openings
6. Works cooperatively with other departments in arranging for the release of employees to take other positions within the organization
7. Provides resources for subordinate training and education

employees. Given that more than 80 percent of an organization's employees are typically non-management, this is a neglected part of career development.

This chapter examines organizational justifications for employee career development, career stages, and career coaching; the use of competency assessment and professional certification as part of career management; appropriate use of lateral, downward, and accommodating transfers; identifying and selecting employees for promotion; management development programs; and the development of professional résumés, résumé cover letters, and portfolios. The leadership roles and management functions for career development are shown in Display 11.1. A comparison of the organization and individual's responsibilities for career development can be seen in Display 11.2.

JUSTIFICATIONS FOR CAREER DEVELOPMENT

For many, nursing is just a job rather than a career. This viewpoint limits opportunities for professional advancement and personal growth, since what cannot be imagined rarely becomes a

DISPLAY 11.2 **The Components of Career Development**

Career Planning (Individual)	**Career Management (Organizational)**
• Self-assess interests, skills, strengths, weaknesses, and values	• Integrate individual employee needs with organizational needs
• Determine goals	• Establish, design, communicate, and implement career paths
• Assess the organization for opportunities	• Disseminate career information
• Assess opportunities outside the organization	• Post and communicate all job openings
• Develop strategies	• Assess employees' career needs
• Implement plans	• Provide work experience for development
• Evaluate plans	• Give support and encouragement
• Reassess and make new plans as necessary, at least biannually	• Develop new personnel policies as necessary
	• Provide training and education

reality. Organizations that employ nurses and nurses themselves then must recognize the benefits of career development. The following, summarized in Display 11.3, is a list of justifications for career development programs:

• *Reduced employee attrition.* Career development can reduce the turnover of ambitious employees who would otherwise be frustrated and seek other jobs because of a lack of job advancement.

• *Equal employment opportunity.* Minorities and other underserved groups will have a better opportunity to move up in an organization if they are identified and developed early in their careers.

• *Improved use of personnel.* When employees are kept in jobs that they have outgrown, their productivity is often reduced. People perform better when they are placed in jobs that fit them and provide new challenges.

• *Improved quality of work life.* Nurses increasingly desire to control their own careers. They are less willing to settle for just any role or position that comes their way. They want greater job satisfaction and more career options.

• *Improved competitiveness of the organization.* Highly educated professionals often prefer organizations that have a good track record of career development. During nursing shortages, a recognized program of career development can be the deciding factor for professionals selecting a position.

• *Obsolescence avoided and new skills acquired.* Because of the rapid changes in health care, especially in the areas of consumer demands and technology, employees may find that their skills have become obsolete. A successful career development program begins to retrain employees proactively, providing them with the necessary skills to remain current in their field and, therefore, valuable to the organization. Some of the most basic career development programs, such as financial planning and general equivalency diploma (GED) programs, can be the most rewarding programs for the staff.

DISPLAY 11.3 Justifications for Career Development

1. Reduces employee attrition
2. Provides equal employment opportunity
3. Improves use of personnel
4. Improves quality of work life
5. Improves competitiveness of the organization
6. Avoids obsolescence and builds new skills
7. Promotes evidence-based practice

• *Evidence-based practice promoted.* Evidence-based practice is now the gold standard for nursing practice. According to Springer, Corbett, and Davis (2006), "many nurses practicing at the bedside are not prepared with the skills needed to base their practice on evidence" (p. 534). The astute manager can recognize this knowledge deficit and use career planning and goal setting to allow these nurses the time and resources needed to acquire these skills.

Before managers can plan a successful career development program, they need to understand the normal career stages of individuals. McNeese-Smith (2000) suggests that there are three different job stages among nurses: entry, mastery, and disengagement. *Entry* is the process of involvement, skill development, and increasing congruity between an individual's self-concept and his or her role in the job. Group membership follows a period of training, orientation, and supervision. If an employee is socialized appropriately, he or she begins to become an "insider."

Mastery begins with the new member having advanced beginner skills; possessing some job esteem; and moving toward seniority, expertise, and high esteem. This is a time of accomplishment, challenge, and a sense of purpose, and the individual often achieves a high enough level of expertise to be a role model to others. However, as the member gains experience and skills, his or her ideal concept of the position begins to decrease.

The last stage, *disengagement*, commences if the congruency and relationship between self-identity and job identity begin to decline. The focus of identity shifts to something else, and the job no longer provides growth and a relevant sense of identity. Thus, the employee may become bored and indifferent to the job. Friends leave or are promoted, the system changes, and the future suggests increasing frustration as the employee can become confined at a level where performance and behavior steadily decline. Clearly, boredom and job indifference leading to disengagement increase with time in the same job. Thus, managers must offer support for a continuous, challenging career program for employees that includes support for advanced degrees and certification as well as specialty skills and job transfer.

Finally, an argument might be made that another career stage exists in nursing—that of *re-entry.* Concurrent with the nursing shortage, many nurses who no longer work in the profession, but who possess the necessary training and experience to do so, are considering re-entering the work setting. McIntosh, Palumbo, and Rambur (2006) studied this "shadow workforce" and found that the factors cited as most important in their decision to return were the accessibility of re-entry programs, flexible work schedules, free or affordable re-entry programs, and an orientation program. In addition, this group placed a high value on development opportunities, educational conference reimbursement, tuition reimbursement, and workshop days. Given that

80 percent of Americans in a 2002 American Association of Retired Persons (AARP) study stated their intent to work at least part-time after retirement, greater attention must be directed at helping shadow workforce nurses identify and succeed at postretirement employment alternatives (McIntosh et al., 2006).

LEARNING EXERCISE 11.1

Exploring Career Stages
In a group, discuss the job stages described by McNeese-Smith. What stage most closely reflects your present situation? In what stages of their careers are nurses who you know (colleagues, managers, your nursing instructors)? Do you believe that male and female nurses have similar or dissimilar career stages?

THE ORGANIZATION'S RESPONSIBILITY FOR CAREER DEVELOPMENT

One of the organization's responsibilities for career development is the creation of career paths and advancement ladders for employees. It also must attempt to match position openings with appropriate people. This includes accurately assessing employees' performance and potential in order to offer the most appropriate career guidance, education, and training. Other organizational responsibilities include:

- *Integrating needs.* The human resources department, nursing division, nursing units, and education department must work and plan together to match job openings with the skills and talents of present employees.
- *Establishing career paths.* Career paths must not only be developed but also communicated to the staff and implemented consistently. When designing career paths, each successive job in each path should contain additional responsibilities and duties that are greater than the previous jobs in that path. Each successive job also must be related to and use previous skills. Once career paths are established, they must be communicated effectively to all concerned staff. What employees must do to advance in a particular path should be very clear. Although various forms of career ladders have existed for some time, they are still not widely used. This problem is not unique to nursing. Even when health care organizations design and use a career structure, the system often breaks down once the nurse leaves that organization. For example, nurses at the level of Clinical Nurse 3 in one hospital will usually lose that status when they leave the organization for another position.
- *Disseminating career information.* The education department, human resources department, and unit manager are all responsible for sharing career information; however, employees should not be encouraged to pursue unrealistic goals.
- *Posting job openings.* Although this is usually the responsibility of the human resources department, the manager should communicate this information, even when it means that one of the unit staff may transfer to another area. Effective managers know who needs to

be encouraged to apply for openings and who is ready for more responsibility and challenges.

• *Assessing employees.* One of the benefits of a good appraisal system is the important information that it gives the manager on the performance, potential, and abilities of all staff members. The use of short- and long-term coaching will give managers insight into their employees' needs and wants so that appropriate career counseling can proceed.

• *Providing challenging assignments.* Planned work experience is one of the most powerful career development tools. This includes jobs that temporarily stretch employees to their maximum skill, temporary projects, assignment to committees, shift rotation, assignment to different units, or shift charge duties.

• *Giving support and encouragement.* Because excellent subordinates make managers' jobs easier, managers are often reluctant to encourage these subordinates to move up the corporate ladder or to seek more challenging experiences outside the manager's span of control. Thus, many managers hoard their talent. A leadership role requires that managers look beyond their immediate unit or department and consider the needs of the entire organization. Leaders recognize and share talent.

• *Developing personnel policies.* An active career development program often results in the recognition that certain personnel policies and procedures are impeding the success of the program. When this occurs, the organization should re-examine these policies and make necessary changes.

• *Providing education and training.* The impact of education and training on career development and retention of subordinate staff is discussed more fully in Chapter 16. The need for organizations to develop leaders and managers is presented later in this chapter.

CAREER COACHING

Organizations also have a responsibility to provide career coaching to employees. This is a role often adopted by the unit manager. *Career coaching* involves helping others to identify professional goals and career options and then designing a career plan to achieve those goals. The Executive Coaching Network (n.d.) suggests that career coaches serve as "facilitators, motivators, consultants and sounding boards dealing with business goals, people interaction and self-management issues. While behavior change will often be a key focus, the coach's role is not that of a therapist. It is not about unraveling personalities, but often involves people doing things differently in the workplace" (para. 4). Raffals (n.d.) suggests that career coaching involves "enabling others to see fresh perspectives, make new decisions, take new actions, and move forward 'growthfully' and productively from these freshly exposed perspectives and choices" (para 15). Career coaching typically has three steps:

1. *Gathering data.* One of the best ways to gather data about employees is to observe their behavior. When managers spend time observing employees, they are able to determine who has good communication skills, who is well organized, who uses effective negotiating skills, and who works collaboratively. Managers also should seek information about the employee's past work experience, performance appraisals, and educational experiences. Data also should include academic qualifications and credentials. Most of this

information is retrievable in the employee's personnel file. Finally, employees themselves are an excellent source of information about career needs and wants.

2. *Asking what is possible*. As part of career planning, the manager should assess the department for possible changes in the future, openings or transfers, and potential challenges and opportunities. The manager should anticipate what type of needs lie ahead, what projects are planned, and what staffing and budget changes will occur. After carefully assessing the employee's profile and future opportunities, managers should consider each staff member and ask the following questions: How can this employee be helped so that he or she is better prepared to take advantage of the future? Who needs to be encouraged to return to school, to become credentialed, or to take a special course? Which employees need to be encouraged to transfer to a more challenging position, given more responsibility on their present unit, or moved to another shift? Managers can create a stimulating environment for career development by being aware of the uniqueness of their employees.

3. *Conducting the coaching session*. The goals of career coaching include helping employees increase their effectiveness; identifying potential opportunities in the organization; and advancing their knowledge, skills, and experience. It is important not to intimidate employees when questioning them about their future and their goals. Although there is no standard procedure for career coaching, the main emphasis should be on employee growth and development. The manager can assist the employee in exploring future options. Coaching sessions give the manager a chance to discover potential future managers—employees who should then begin to be groomed for a future managerial role in subsequent coaching sessions.

Career coaching, then, can be either short or long term. In *short-term career coaching*, the manager regularly asks the employees questions or challenges them to refocus their perspective or improve their performance (Hange-Kukuk, 2006). Thus, it is a means to routinely develop and motivate employees and should be a spontaneous part of the experienced manager's repertoire.

Long-term career coaching, on the other hand, is a planned management action that occurs over the duration of employment. Because this type of coaching may cover a long time, it is frequently neglected unless the manager uses a systematic scheduling plan and a form for documentation. Because employees and managers move frequently within an organization, the lack of record keeping regarding employees' career needs has deterred nursing career development. In the present climate of organizational restructuring and downsizing, a manager's staff is even more in need of career coaching, and documentation of the career coaching takes on an even more important role. Display 11.4 is an example of a long-term coaching form.

Long-term coaching, however, is a major step in building an effective team and an excellent strategy to increase productivity and retention. The effective manager should have at least one coaching session with each employee annually, in addition to any coaching that may occur during the appraisal interview. Although some coaching should occur during the performance appraisal interview, additional coaching should be planned at a less stressful time. Coaching provides opportunities to assist employees in the growth and development necessary for expanded roles and responsibilities. A major leadership role is the development of subordinate staff. This interest in the future of individual employees plays a vital role in retention and productivity.

DISPLAY 11.4   Sample Long-Term Coaching Form

Name of employee _____

Name of supervisor _____

Date _____ Date of last coaching interview _____

1. What new challenges and responsibilities could be given to this employee that would utilize his or her special talents?
   _____
   _____

2. What events happening in the organization do you foresee affecting this employee? (Examples would be plans to go to an all-RN staff, changing the mode of patient care delivery, increasing emphasis on credentialing by the new CEO of the nursing division, changing the medication system, and changing the ratio of nonprofessionals to professionals for nurse staffing.)
   _____
   _____

3. How should the employee be preparing to meet new or changing expectations?
   _____
   _____

4. What specific suggestions and guidance for the future can you give this employee? (Examples would be taking specific courses to prepare for change, urging them to pursue an advanced degree, considering changing shifts, urging them to seek challenges outside of your unit, and suggesting that they apply for the next management opening.)
   _____
   _____

5. What specific organizational resources can you offer the employee?
   _____
   _____

6. What new information regarding this employee's long-term plans, aspirations, and potential have the perusal of the personnel record, your observations, and this interview given you?
   _____
   _____

7. Do the organizational and professional career plans held by the individual match your vision of his or her future? If not, how do they differ?
   _____
   _____

8. What developmental and professional growth has taken place since the last coaching session?
   _____
   _____

9. Date of next coaching interview _____

COMPETENCY ASSESSMENT AS PART OF CAREER DEVELOPMENT

Competency assessment and professional specialty certification are also a part of career management. Competencies are defined as the "knowledge, skills, or attitudes that enable one to effectively perform the activities of a given occupation or function to the standards expected in employment" (Carliner et al., 2006, p. 4). Yet Carliner also points out that "competencies can be considered along a spectrum, from the basic competencies needed to survive in the workforce to a range of advanced competencies needed to sustain employability and advance in one's career" (p. 29).

Managers should appraise each employee's competency level as part of not only performance appraisal but also as part of career development. This appraisal should lead to the development of a plan that outlines what the employee must do to achieve desired competencies in both current and future positions. For example, because of the rapid explosion of information and constant changes in organizations, Carliner and associates (2006) suggest that workers are increasingly taking on new roles as coaches or mentors and that the skills associated with being a good coach or mentor must be intentionally developed.

Often, however, competency assessment focuses only on whether the employee has achieved required minimal competency levels to meet current federal, state, or organizational standards and not on how to exceed these competency levels. Thus, competency assessment and goal setting in career planning is proactive, with the employee identifying areas of potential future growth and the manager assisting in identifying strategies that would help the employee achieve that goal.

 Competency assessment and goal setting in career planning should help the employee identify how to exceed these levels of competency.

In addition, Carliner and colleagues (2006) suggest that further research is needed to better understand how core competencies should be used in assessing not only work performance but career development learning needs. Carliner suggests that future research is needed to address these questions:
- Do core competencies improve performance in the workplace?
- What are the benefits of developing workers' core competencies?
- How can we assess core competencies?
- What are the core competencies required to function in the changing workplace?

- Do core competencies contribute to building a learning organization?
- What core competencies are required to function in a knowledge society?
- Do core competencies improve quality of work experience?
- Do jobs match the competencies identified for them?
- Do core competencies improve workers self-efficacy and self-esteem in the workplace?
- Do core competencies acquired for one occupation transfer to other occupations?

PROFESSIONAL SPECIALTY CERTIFICATION

Professional specialty certification is one way an employee can demonstrate advanced achievement of competencies. *Certification*, as defined by the American Board of Nursing Specialties (ABNS) (2000), is "the formal recognition of the specialized knowledge, skills, and experience demonstrated by the achievement of standards identified by a nursing specialty to promote optimal health outcomes" (para 1). Professional associations such as ABNS grant specialty certification as a formal but voluntary process of demonstrating expertise in a particular area of nursing.

For example, the American Nurses Association (ANA) established the ANA Certification Program in 1973 to provide tangible recognition of professional achievement in a defined functional or clinical area of nursing. The American Nurses Credentialing Center (ANCC), a subsidiary of ANA, became its own corporation in 1991 and since then has certified more than 150,000 nurses throughout the United States and its territories in more than 40 specialty and advanced practice areas of nursing (ANCC, 2006). A few of the other organizations offering specialty certifications for nurses are the American Association of Critical Care Nursing, the American Association of Nurse Anesthetists, the American College of Nurse Midwives, the Board of Certification for Emergency Nursing, and the Rehabilitation Nursing Certification Board. Some of the personal benefits associated with professional certification are shown in Display 11.5. In addition, the value of certification to employers and the impact on a nurse's professional practice are discussed in Examining the Evidence 11.1.

DISPLAY 11.5   **Personal Benefits of Professional Certification**

Professional certification:
- Enhances and validates your nursing specialty knowledge and competence
- Builds confidence in you as a professional, demonstrating that you meet nationally recognized standards in your specialty
- Serves as a testimonial to your dedication to nursing, bringing a greater accountability to the profession
- Recognizes you as a resource and leader to your colleagues in your specialty
- Promotes increased patient and family satisfaction and confidence in their care
- Provides a valuable credential for your professional curriculum vitae, résumé, or portfolio

Source: Massachusetts General Hospital. (n.d.) *Professional certification in nursing.* Retrieved December 1, 2006, from *http://www.mgh.harvard.edu/pcs/CCPD/cpd_Professional_Cert.asp.*

EXAMINING THE EVIDENCE 11.1

Source: American Board of Nursing Specialties (ABNS). (2005, October). *Value of certification survey. Executive summary.* Retrieved December 1, 2006, from *http://www.nursingcertification.org/pdf/executive_summary.pdf.*

In summer 2004, ABNS member organizations undertook a study to validate nurses' perceptions, values, and behaviors related to certification. In particular, the study sought to address perceptions of managers on the value of certification, challenges and barriers to certification, benefits and rewards to nurses for being certified, the impact of certification on lost workdays, and the impact of certification on nurse retention.

Twenty (83 percent) of ABNS's member organizations participated in the survey, which began in 2005. The total sample size for the ABNS Value of Certification Survey was 94,768 nurses, which included certified and noncertified nurses and a subset of nurse–managers.

The study found that certification is greatly valued among nurses; yet, nurses continue to face challenges and barriers in obtaining and maintaining certification. In addition, the study found that certification continues to be a valuable method for nurses to differentiate themselves in the workplace and that health care organizations continue to offer certification incentives to attract and retain professional, certified nurses.

The study findings suggested that health care organizations can support nurses by implementing strategies to overcome barriers to certification and by offering appropriate incentives and rewards for certification. The study also suggested that certified nurses be asked to serve as role models and partner with professional nursing organizations, specialty nursing certification boards, and their health care employers to advocate for meaningful incentives and rewards that foster certification.

EMPLOYEE TRANSFERS

A *transfer* may be defined as a reassignment to another job within the organization. In a strict business sense, a transfer usually implies similar pay, status, and responsibility. Because of the variety of positions available for nurses in any health care organization, coupled with the lack of sufficient higher-level positions available, two additional terms have come into use: lateral transfer and downward transfer.

Appropriate Transfers

A *lateral transfer* describes one staff person moving to another unit, to a position with a similar scope of responsibilities, within the same organization. A *downward transfer* occurs when someone takes a position within the organization that is below his or her previous level. This frequently happens in health care. An example would be the charge nurse who decides to learn another nursing specialty (e.g., a nurse steps down from a charge position on a medical–surgical unit to a staff position in labor and delivery). It may be in a nurse's interest to consider a downward transfer because it often increases the chances of long-term career success.

For example, a nurse's long-term career goal might be to hold a position in cardiac rehabilitation. The nurse determines that most of the cardiac rehabilitation staff are hired out of the hospital's critical care unit (CCU). Although this nurse has had previous experience in a cardiac care unit, he or she has not held that position in this organization. The nurse requests a downward transfer from an evening charge position on a surgical unit to day-shift staff nurse in the CCU. This transfer will provide the nurse with current experience in CCU and more exposure to the manager of the cardiac rehabilitation unit. In this example, a downward transfer increases the likelihood that the nurse's long-term goal will be realized.

Downward transfers also should be considered when nurses are experiencing periods of stress or role overload. Self-aware nurses often request such transfers. In some circumstances, the manager may need to intervene and use a downward transfer to alleviate temporarily a nurse's overwhelming stress. Another type of downward transfer may accommodate employees in the later stages of their career. In many cases, valued employees who wish to reduce their career roles may be accommodated by a manager's assistance with locating a suitable position for their talent and stature in the profession.

 Managers often assist valuable employees who desire a reduced role in their careers to locate a position that will use their talents and still allow them a degree of status.

These *accommodating transfers* generally allow someone to receive a similar salary but with a reduction in energy expenditure. For example, a long-time employee might be given a position as ombudsman to use his or her expertise and knowledge of the organization and at the same time assume a status position that is less physically demanding.

Inappropriate Transfers

One deterrent to successful career development is the *inappropriate transfer*. Some managers solve unit personnel problems by transferring problem employees to another unsuspecting department. Such transfers are harmful in many ways. They contribute to decreased productivity, are demotivating for all employees, and are especially destructive for the employee who is transferred.

This is not to say that employees who do not "fit" in one department will not do well in a different environment. Before such transfers, however, both the manager and the employee must speak candidly regarding the employee's capabilities and the manager's expectations. All types of transfers should be individually evaluated for appropriateness.

 It is not uncommon for an employee to struggle in one department yet improve his or her performance in a new department or unit.

LEARNING EXERCISE 11.3

How Would You Handle This Transfer Request?
You are the manager of a surgical unit. Many novice nurses apply to your unit to perfect their basic skills before transferring to a specialty unit. Although this is somewhat frustrating to you, you recognize that you can do little about it. The hospital policy dictates that nurses requesting another position must fill out a "request for transfer" form when they apply for the new position. This form, which is completed by the nurses' current manager, contains information

regarding when they can be released from their present position for the new position and a current appraisal of their work performance.

Today, you find another "request for transfer" form on your desk. However, when you read the name on the form, you feel a sense of relief rather than despair. The nurse requesting the transfer is one of your more difficult employees. Scott Powell is a very qualified nurse, but he is frequently absent from work, is very critical of the other nurses' work performance, and is generally unpleasant to be around. During the 2 years that he has worked on this unit, you have tried many different approaches in an effort to improve Scott's absenteeism and attitude. There would frequently be temporary improvements only.

Scott has requested a transfer to the emergency room. His career goal is to be part of the flight rescue team. He certainly has the skills and intelligence to be part of this highly skilled group. However, you believe that if you include all the negative aspects of Scott's perform- ance, he may not be selected for the position. On one hand, you believe this job could be a turning point for Scott. It might be what he needs to overcome some of his work problems. On the other hand, the relief that you feel at the possibility of transferring Scott off your unit indi- cates that there are some ethical issues present in this situation.

● ASSIGNMENT: Decide what you should do about Scott's request to transfer to the emer- gency room. Outline your plan. Be specific about the alternatives open to you and what course of action you will take.

PROMOTIONS

Promotions are reassignments to a position of higher rank. It is normal for promotions to include a pay raise. Most promotions include increased status, title changes, more authority, and greater responsibility. Because of the importance that U.S. society places on promotions, certain guide- lines must accompany promotion selection to ensure that the process is fair and equitable. When position openings occur, they are often posted and filled quickly with little thought of long-term organizational or employee goals. This frequently results in negative personnel outcomes. To avoid this, the following elements should be determined in advance:

• *Whether recruitment will be internal or external.* There are obvious advantages and disad- vantages to recruiting for promotions from both inside and outside the organization.

 Recruiting from within can help to develop employees to fill higher-level positions as they become vacant. It can also serve as a powerful motivation and recognition tool.

External candidates often cost more in terms of salary than internal ones. Whitehouse (2006) suggests that companies often have to pay 20 to 30 percent more for external can- didates than they do for internal candidates. This is because external candidates "who pre- sumably already have good jobs, need a financial incentive to leave their current positions for something else. External candidates are also more likely to require employment con- tracts and severance pay" (para 9). Whitehouse argues that poor succession planning has been targeted as one of the main contributing factors to excessive pay for executive level hiring in recent years and that this could be ameliorated if organizations consciously develop an adequate pool of strong internal candidates.

There are advantages to recruiting from outside the organization, however. When promotions are filled with people outside the organization, the organization is infused with people with new ideas. This prevents the stagnation that often occurs when all promotions are internal. Regardless of what the organization decides, the policy should be consistently followed and communicated to all employees. Some companies recruit from within first and recruit from outside the organization only if they are unable to find qualified people from among their own employees.

- *What the promotion and selection criteria will be.* Employees should know in advance what the criteria for *promotion* are and what selection method is to be used. Some organizations use an interview panel as a selection method to promote all employees beyond the level of charge nurse. Decisions regarding the selection method and promotion criteria should be justified with rationale. Additionally, employees need to know what place seniority will have in the selection criteria.
- *The pool of candidates that exists.* When promotions are planned, as in succession management, there will always be an adequate pool of candidates identified and prepared to seek higher-level positions. A word of caution must be given regarding the zeal with which managers urge subordinates to seek promotions. The leader's role is to identify and prepare such a pool. It is not the manager's role to urge the employee to seek a position in a manner that would lead the employee to think that he or she was guaranteed the job or to unduly influence him or her in the decision to seek such a job.

When employees actively seek promotions, they are making a commitment to do well in the new position. When they are pushed into such positions, the commitment to expend the energy to do the job well may be lacking. In addition, for many reasons, the employee may not feel ready, either due to personal commitments or because he or she feels inadequately educated or experienced. Indeed, it is possible to promote an individual beyond his or her level of capability (known as the *Peter Principle*).

 The Peter Principle suggests that individuals often rise "to the level of their incompetence."

- *Handling rejected candidates.* All promotion candidates who are rejected must be notified before the selected candidate is notified. This is common courtesy. They should be thanked for applying and, when appropriate, encouraged to apply for future position openings. Sometimes, managers should tell employees which deficiencies kept them from getting the position. For instance, employees should be told if they lack some educational component or work experience that would make them a stronger competitor for future promotions. This can be an effective way of encouraging career development.
- *How employee releases are to be handled.* Knowledge that the best candidate for the position currently holds a critical job or difficult position to fill should not influence decisions regarding promotions. Managers frequently find it difficult to release employees to another position within the organization. Policies regarding the length of time that a manager can delay releasing an employee should be written and communicated. On the other hand, some managers are so good at developing their employees that they frequently become frustrated because their success at career development results in constantly losing their staff to other departments. In such cases, higher-level management should reward such leaders and set release policies that are workable and realistic.

LEARNING EXERCISE 11.4

Why Won't Beth Apply for the Position?

You have been the evening charge nurse of a large surgical unit for the last 4 years. Each year, you perform a career development conference with all your licensed staff. These sessions are held separately from the performance appraisal interviews. You have been extremely pleased with the results of these conferences. Two of your LVNs/LPNs are now enrolled in an RN program. Several of the RNs from your unit have obtained advanced clinical positions, and many have returned to school. As a result of your encouragement and support, several of the nurses have taken charge positions on other units. You are proud of your ability to recognize talent and to perform successful career counseling.

This is the last time that you will be performing career counseling, because you have resigned your position to return to graduate school. You have encouraged several of the staff to apply for your position but think that one particular nurse—Beth, a 34-year-old woman—would be exceptional. She is extremely capable clinically, very mature, well respected by everyone, and has excellent interpersonal skills. Beth only works 4 days a week but has been invaluable to you in the 4 years since you have been charge nurse. However, Beth is one of the few nurses who has never acted on any of your suggestions at previous career-coaching interviews.

Last week, you had another coaching interview with Beth and told her of your plans. You urged her to apply for your position and told her that you would recommend her to your supervisor, although you would not be making the final selection. Beth told you that she would think about it, and today she told you that she does not wish to apply for the position. You are very disappointed and believe that perhaps you have failed in some way.

● ASSIGNMENT: Examine this scenario carefully. Make a list of the possible reasons that Beth declined the promotion. Be creative. Were the coaching sessions valuable or a waste of your time? Compare your findings with others in the group. After comparison, determine what influence, if any, values had on the development of the lists.

MANAGEMENT DEVELOPMENT

Management development is a planned system of training and developing people so that they acquire the skills, insights, and attitudes needed to manage people and their work effectively within the organization. Management development is often referred to as *succession planning*. Freed and Dawson (2006) suggest that movement to management positions is seen by most nurses as a pathway to career advancement, although many nurses feel uncertain that they have the essential skills for management.

 Many nurses feel that they lack the knowledge and experience necessary to become a manager.

Scott (2006) argues, however, that the same critical thinking skills that staff nurses use in their clinical practice apply to management—they are just applied differently. She also suggests that the world of nursing management can be daunting but that it can also come with great rewards. Clearly, most management roles do "increase the nurse's scope of responsibility and require a greater variety of skills and knowledge" (Freed & Dawson, 2006, p. 43). With the flattening of organizational hierarchies, an expected increase in nursing management vacancies due to retirement, and a continued increase in managerial responsibilities, new leader–managers will likely need the formal education and training that are a part of a management development program. The program must include a means of developing appropriate attitudes through social learning theory as well as adequate content on management theory.

Support for management development programs by the organization should occur in two ways. First, top-level management must do more than bear the cost of management development classes. They must create an organizational structure that allows managers to apply their new knowledge. Therefore, for such programs to be effective, the organization must be willing to practice a management style that incorporates sound management principles.

Second, training outcomes improve if nursing executives are active in planning and developing a systematic and integrated program. Whenever possible, nursing administrators should teach some of the classes and, at the very least, make sure that the program supports top-management philosophy. Just as nurses are required to be certified in critical care before they accept a position in a CCU, so too should nurses be required to take part in a management development program before their appointment to a management position. This requires early identification and grooming of potential management candidates.

The first step in the process would be an appraisal of the present management team and an analysis of possible future needs. The second step would be the establishment of a training and development program. This would require decisions such as the following: How often should the formal management course be offered? Should outside educators be involved, or should in-house staff teach it? Who should be involved in teaching the didactic portion? Should there be two levels of classes, one for first-level and one for middle-level managers? Should the management development courses be open to all, or should people be recommended by someone from management? In addition to formal course content, what other methods should be used to develop managers? Should other methods be used, such as job rotation through an understudy system of pairing selected people with a manager and management coaching?

The inclusion of *social learning activities* also is a valuable part of management development. Management development will not be successful unless learners have ample chance to try out new skills. Providing potential managers with didactic management theory alone inadequately prepares them for the attitudes, skills, and insights necessary for effective management. Case studies, management games, transactional analysis, and sensitivity training also are effective in changing attitudes and increasing self-awareness. All of these techniques appropriately use social learning theory strategies.

RÉSUMÉ PREPARATION

Despite the best efforts of organizations to help subordinates identify career needs, wants, and opportunities, it is how employees represent themselves that often determines whether desired career opportunities become a reality. Creating a positive image often depends on having well-developed interviewing skills (Chapter 15) and a well-prepared résumé. The résumé is an important career-planning tool. It is also a screening tool used by employers to select applicants and make promotion decisions; therefore, maintaining a current, professional résumé is a career-planning necessity for health care professionals and should not be undertaken lightly. According to human resource professionals, nearly 95 percent of résumés in circulation (either on paper or in cyberspace) are poorly written (The Resume Center, 2005–2006).

Résumé Structure

Matias (2005–2006) suggests that how a résumé is structured, organized, and written reflects one's personal characteristics. Résumés should concentrate on what applicants like to do and what they do well. They must also be believable. "If an employer has any inkling you are being deceitful, your résumé will go into the trash. And even if you are able to get through the résumé review and interview process with half-truths, be warned: once hired, you will be expected to deliver" (para 13). Candidates then should always focus on what they have to offer and not attempt to represent themselves as something they are not, regardless of what the agency says they want.

Various acceptable styles and formats of résumés exist. However, because the résumé represents the professionalism of the applicant and recruiters use it to summarize an applicant's qualifications, it must be professionally prepared, make an impression, and quickly capture the reader's attention. The following are general guidelines for résumé preparation:

- The résumé should be typed in a single font format that is easy to read.
- The résumé should maximize strong points and minimize weakness.
- The style should reflect good grammar, correct punctuation, and proper sentence structure. Typographic errors suggest that the candidate may not be serious about the job application or that the quality of his or her work will be substandard.
- High-quality (24 pound with watermark), white, or off-white paper should be used to print the résumé (Vaughan, 2005–2006).

Fox (2005–2006) and Hackett (2005–2006) suggest additional general strategies for résumé preparation:

- Strive to be concise and clear. The purpose of the résumé is to get an interview, not a job, so it is not necessary to go into detail about each accomplishment.
- Use bulleted sentences rather than lengthy paragraphs. A résumé is typically reviewed in just 15 to 30 seconds. Bullets make it easier for someone to quickly scan a résumé and still absorb it.
- Use action words such as *developed*, *created*, or *supervised*.
- Lead with your strengths. Put those strong points first where they are more likely to be read.
- Leave white space. Use a font size no smaller than 10 point. Limit the length of your résumé to one or two pages.

Vaughan (2005–2006) warns, however, not to get so wrapped up in the way the résumé is supposed to look that you forget to include what it is supposed to say. Most résumés begin with a professional objective(s). They also should include educational history, work experience, awards or honors, professional publications or presentations, memberships in professional organizations, community service, and license information, if appropriate. Typically, personal information (age, gender, race, church affiliation, or personal interests) should not be included, as it provides potential objectionable information to an employer (The Resume Center, Inc., 2005–2006). A sample résumé is shown in Figure 11.1.

The Résumé Cover Letter

Cover letters (whether by mail or email) should always be used when submitting a résumé. The purpose of the cover letter is to introduce the applicant, briefly highlight key points of the

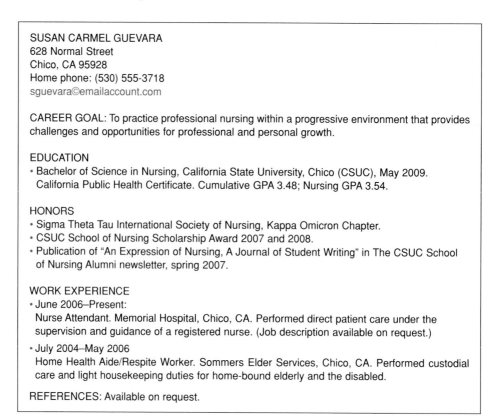

SUSAN CARMEL GUEVARA
628 Normal Street
Chico, CA 95928
Home phone: (530) 555-3718
sguevara©emailaccount.com

CAREER GOAL: To practice professional nursing within a progressive environment that provides challenges and opportunities for professional and personal growth.

EDUCATION
• Bachelor of Science in Nursing, California State University, Chico (CSUC), May 2009. California Public Health Certificate. Cumulative GPA 3.48; Nursing GPA 3.54.

HONORS
• Sigma Theta Tau International Society of Nursing, Kappa Omicron Chapter.
• CSUC School of Nursing Scholarship Award 2007 and 2008.
• Publication of "An Expression of Nursing, A Journal of Student Writing" in The CSUC School of Nursing Alumni newsletter, spring 2007.

WORK EXPERIENCE
• June 2006–Present:
Nurse Attendant. Memorial Hospital, Chico, CA. Performed direct patient care under the supervision and guidance of a registered nurse. (Job description available on request.)
• July 2004–May 2006
Home Health Aide/Respite Worker. Sommers Elder Services, Chico, CA. Performed custodial care and light housekeeping duties for home-bound elderly and the disabled.

REFERENCES: Available on request.

Figure 11.1   Sample nursing résumé.

résumé, and make a positive first impression. Whenever possible, the cover letter should be addressed to a specific individual.

Newfield (2005–2006) suggests that cover letters should begin with the specific job being sought as well as the reason the applicant is interested in working for that particular organization. If possible, the applicant should mention a particular unit or department or comment on the philosophy or reputation of the employer to show that the applicant has done some homework. This also reinforces the idea that the cover letter is not generic or mass produced. In addition, applicants should include two to three reasons why their experience makes a good fit and a brief outline of career highlights (Newfield, 2005–2006).

PREPARING A PROFESSIONAL PORTFOLIO

A professional portfolio, which all nurses should maintain, can be described as a collection of materials that document a nurse's competencies and illustrate the expertise of the nurse.

Oermann (2002) states that there are two types of professional portfolios: best work and growth and development. Best-work portfolios are used for documentation for career ladder promotions, job applications, performance reviews, and other situations where others will review the portfolio.

All nurses should maintain a portfolio to reflect their professional growth throughout their career.

Growth and development portfolios are designed for nurses to monitor their progress in meeting their own individual goals for professional and personal growth. This later portfolio is a working document to be used only by the individual nurse; however, should the nurse choose to do so, selected material can be used from the portfolio to be placed in the best-work portfolio that is shown to others (Oermann, 2002). The individual needs to be selective in collecting best-work documentation and only include those materials that illustrate competency and highlight achievement. Separate files for the following would be helpful:

- Formal education documentation, including a curriculum vitae or résumé; copies of diplomas and state license numbers, and certification of any specialty should be included.
- Continuing education documentation, including programs attended and credits earned, as well as learning outcomes of such programs.
- Performance documentation, including evaluations, position descriptions, reference letters, awards, or commendations.
- Community service documentation, including committee or organizational membership.
- Professional nursing activities documentation, especially offices held or other types of participation.

Maintaining a professional portfolio avoids lost opportunities to save documents. Professional nurses should always have documentation readily available to pursue a promotion, consider a new position, or to apply for another position in their present employment.

INTEGRATING LEADERSHIP ROLES AND MANAGEMENT FUNCTIONS IN CAREER DEVELOPMENT

It is clear that appropriate career management should foster positive career development, alleviate burnout, reduce attrition, and promote productivity. Management functions in career development include disseminating career information and posting job openings. The manager should have a well-developed, planned system for career development for all employees; this system should include long-term coaching, the appropriate use of transfers, and how promotions are to be handled. These policies should be fair and communicated effectively to all employees.

With the integration of leadership, managers become more aware of how their own values shape personal career decisions. Additionally, the leader–manager shows genuine interest in the career development of all employees. Career planning is encouraged, and potential leaders are identified and developed. Present leaders are rewarded when they see those, whom they have helped to develop, advance in their careers and in turn develop leadership and management skills in others.

Effective managers recognize that in all career decisions, the employee must decide when he or she is ready to pursue promotions, return to school, or take on greater responsibility. Leaders are aware that every person perceives success differently. Although career development programs benefit all employees and the organization, there is an added bonus for the professional nurse. When professional nurses have the opportunity to experience a well-planned career development program, a greater viability for and increased commitment to the profession are often evident.

Key Concepts

* There are many outcomes of a *career development* program that justify its implementation.
* Career job sequencing should assist the manager in career management.
* Career development programs consist of a set of personal responsibilities called *career planning* and a set of management responsibilities called *career management*.
* Employees often need to be encouraged to make more formalized long-term career plans.
* Career planning should include, at minimum, a commitment to the use of evidence-based practice, learning new skills or bettering practice through the use of role models and mentors, staying aware of and being involved in professional issues, and furthering one's education.
* Designing *career paths* is an important part of organizational career management.
* Managers should plan specific interventions that promote growth and development in each of their subordinates.
* Most individuals progress through normal and predictable career stages.
* *Career coaching* involves helping others to identify professional goals and career options and designing a career plan to achieve those goals. This coaching should be both short and long term.
* *Competency assessment* and goal setting in career planning should help the employee identify how to exceed the minimum levels of competency required by federal, state, or organizational standards.
* *Professional specialty certification* is one way that an employee can demonstrate advanced achievement of competencies.
* The *transfer*, when used appropriately, may be an effective way to provide career development.
* Because of the importance that American society places on promotions, certain guidelines must accompany promotion selection to ensure that the process is fair and equitable.
* Policies regarding promotion should be in writing and communicated to all employees.
* Recruitment from within has been shown to have a positive effect on employee satisfaction, whereas recruitment from outside the organization allows for new ideas and prevents stagnation.
* To be successful, *management development* must be planned and supported by top-level management. This type of planned program is called *succession management*.
* If appropriate management attitudes and insight are goals of a management development program, *social learning* techniques need to be part of the teaching strategies used.
* It is possible to promote individuals beyond their level of capability. The *Peter Principle*, as it is known, suggests that individuals often rise "to the level of their incompetence."
* Maintaining a current, professional résumé is a career-planning necessity for the health care professional and should not be undertaken lightly.
* Cover letters (whether by mail or email) should always be used when submitting a résumé. Their purpose is to introduce the applicant, briefly highlight key points of the résumé, and make a positive first impression.
* All nurses should maintain a *professional portfolio* (a collection of materials that document a nurse's competencies and illustrate the expertise of the nurse) to reflect their professional growth over their career.

ADDITIONAL LEARNING EXERCISES
AND APPLICATIONS

LEARNING EXERCISE 11.5

Developing a Realistic Twenty-Year Career Plan
Develop a 20-year career plan, taking into account the constraints of family responsibilities such as marriage, children, and aging parents. Have your career plan critiqued to determine whether it is feasible and whether the time lines and goals are realistic.

LEARNING EXERCISE 11.6

Listing Policies Relating to Promotions
You have been appointed to a committee of staff nurses in your home health agency to assist in developing a set of policies regarding how future promotions are to be handled. Lately, there has been some unhappiness about how employees have been selected for promotions. Your committee is to focus on how shift and day charge nurses are to be selected.

● ASSIGNMENT: Develop a list of five to seven policies regarding such promotions. Be able to justify your promotion criteria and policies.

LEARNING EXERCISE 11.7

Preparing a Résumé
The medical center where you have applied for a position has requested that you submit a résumé along with your application. Prepare a professional résumé, using your actual experience and education. You may use any style and format that you desire. The résumé will be critiqued on its professional appearance and appropriateness of included content.

LEARNING EXERCISE 11.8

Constructing a Management Development Program
You are serving on an *ad hoc* committee to construct a management development program. Your organization has requested that the charge nurses work with staff development and plan a 1-week training and education program that would be required of all new charge nurses before their appointment. Because the organization will be bearing the cost of the program (i.e., paying for the educators and employee time), you are required to select appropriate content and educational methods that will not exceed 40 hours, including actual orientation time by a charge nurse.

● ASSIGNMENT: Develop and write up such a plan, and share it with the class. Your plan should depict hours, content, and educational methods.

LEARNING EXERCISE 11.9

Career Mapping

Career planning is often made easier when a career map is created to assist in developing a long-term master plan. Use the career guide shown in Figure 11.2, along with the steps in career planning outlined in Display 11.2, to assist with developing the personal plan described in Learning Exercise 11.5.

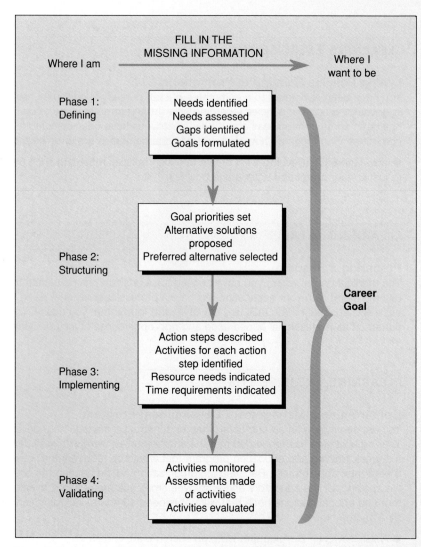

Figure 11.2   A career-planning guide for a professional nurse.

Web Links

American Nurses Credentialing Center (ANCC)
http://www.nursingworld.org/ancc/
Provides a general overview of the ANCC as well as the more than 40 specialty and advanced practice areas of specialty certification/recertification offered.

National Student Nurses' Association Career Center
http://www.nsna.org/career/ultimate_adventure.asp
Includes resources for senior nursing students, new graduates, and RNs, with direct links to hospitals with positions for new graduates. Includes electronic articles on choosing the right first job, tips on getting the job you want, preparing for licensure as an RN, specialty nursing, and more.

Tips on Taking the NCLEX Exam
http://www.nsna.org/career/nclexlink.pdf
This article, by Beulah Hall, includes tips for preparing to take the NCLEX.

National Student Nurses' Association Career Center Specialty Opportunities
http://www.nsna.org/career/career_plan_spnurse.asp
Provides links to articles from NSNA's Imprint magazine to help readers explore specialty options such as community health nursing, critical care nursing, emergency nursing, midwifery, perioperative nursing, school nursing, uniformed services, and more.

HRH Global Resource Center—Succession Planning, Training and Development of Health Leaders
http://www.hrhresourcecenter.org/taxonomy_menu/1/68/84
This is a collection of resources dedicated to succession planning and health leadership development programs in and for developing countries.

University of Sheffield Careers Service—Careers in Nursing and Midwifery, Career Planning—Why Now?
http://www.shef.ac.uk/careers/students/nursing/planning.html
Includes job search strategies, the application process, interviewing, useful contacts, and other pertinent topics.

Template for Writing Résumé Cover Letters
http://jobsearchtech.about.com/od/coverletters/Covers_Letters.htm
Provides a template for writing cover letters to accompany résumés.

References

American Board of Nursing Specialties. (2000). *Homepage.* Retrieved December 1, 2006, from *http://www. nursingcertification.org/.*

American Nurses Credentialing Center. (2006). *American Nurses Credentialing Center—Certified nursing excellence.* Retrieved October 28, 2006, from *http://www.nursingworld.org/ancc/ inside.html.*

Carliner, S., Ally, M., Zhao, N., Bairstow, L., Khoury, S., & Johnston, L. (2006, June). *A review of the state of the field of workplace learning: What we know and what we need to know about competencies, diversity, e-learning, and human performance improvement.* Canadian Society for Training and Development. Retrieved December 1, 2006, from *http://www.cstd.ca/networks/FldRev_WLP_0606.pdf.*

Executive Coaching Network. (n.d.). *What is executive coaching? Retrieved December 1, 2006, from *http://www.execcoachnetwork.com.au/whatis.html.*

Fox, F. (2005–2006). *Resume writing—"Straight talk about your resume."* Media, Inc. Retrieved December 1, 2007, from *http://www.resume-resource.com/article6.html.*

Freed, P. E., & Dawson, S. (2006, October). Is nursing management in your future? *Nursing Management, 37*(10), 43–48.

Hackett, A. (2005–2006). *15 tips for writing winning resumes.* Media, Inc. Retrieved December 1, 2006, from *http://www.resume-resource.com/article59.html.*

Hange-Kukuk, C. (2006). *Coaching increases productivity and morale.* SouthCoast Today. Retrieved December 1, 2006, from *http://www.s-t.com/daily/09-00/09-17-00/d06bu143.htm.*

Matias, L. (2005–2006). *Resume writing help—Your resume should have character.* Media, Inc. Retrieved December 1, 2006, from *http://www.resume-resource.com/article26.html.*

McIntosh, B., Palumbo, M. V., & Rambur, B. (2006, September-October). Does a 'shadow workforce' of inactive nurses exist? *Nursing Economics, 24*(5), 231–238.

McNeese-Smith, D. K. (2000). Job stages of entry, mastery, and disengagement among nurses. *Journal of Nursing Administration, 30*(3), 140–147.

Newfield, P. (2005–2006). *Cover letter article—"Winning cover letters."* Media, Inc. Retrieved December 1, 2006, from *http://www.resume-resource.com/article5.html.*

Oermann, M. H. (2002). Developing a professional portfolio in nursing. *Orthopaedic Nursing, 21*(2), 73–79.

Raffals, R. (n.d.) *What is coaching?* Retrieved December 1, 2006, from *http://www.awakenthemagic.com/coach/whatis.html.*

Resume Center, Inc. (2005–2006). *Resume writing—"Mistakes to avoid on your resume."* Media, Inc. Retrieved December 1, 2006, from *http://www.resume-resource.com/article8.html.*

Scott, D. E. (2006). Is management right for me? *Advance for Nurses. Northern California and Reno, Nevada, 3*(23), 20, 24.

Springer, P. J., Corbett, C., & Davis, N. (2006). Enhancing evidence-based practice through collaboration. *Journal of Nursing Administration, 36*(11), 534–537.

Vaughan, C. (2005–2006). *Resume mistakes: Do not let this happen to you.* Media, Inc. Retrieved December 1, 2006, from *http://www.resume-resource.com/article31.html.*

Whitehouse, K. (2006). *Executive hiring goes on a budget in new succession planning.* CareerJournal.com. Retrieved October 29, 2006, from *http://www.careerjournal.com/salaryhiring/hotissues/20060109-whitehouse.html.*

Bibliography

Baehr, C. (2005–2006). *Graduating with a plan of action—To jumpstart your career.* Media, Inc. Retrieved December 1, 2006, from *http://www.resume-resource.com/article25.html.*

Beyers, M. (2006). Nurse executives' perspectives on succession planning. *Journal of Nursing Administration, 36*(6), 304–312.

Blouin, A. S., McDonagh, K. J., Neistadt, A. M., & Helfand, B. (2006). Leading tomorrow's healthcare organizations: Strategies and tactics for effective succession planning. *Journal of Nursing Administration, 36*(6), 325–330.

Bonczek, M.E., & Woodard, E.K. (2006). Who'll replace you when you're gone? *Nursing Management, 37*(8), 30–35.

Cadmus, E. (2006). Succession planning: Multilevel organizational strategies for the new workforce. *Journal of Nursing Administration, 36*(6), 298–303.

Canadian Nurses Association. (2003). *Succession planning for nursing leadership.* Retrieved October 28, 2006, from *http://www.cna-nurses.ca/CNA/documents/pdf/publications/succession_planning_e.pdf.*

Chapman, M. (2006, September 6–12). Following nurses' career progressions is good reading . . . 'Just a minute' . . . (careers August 30). *Nursing Standard, 20*(52), 33.

Clancy, D., & Oyefeso, A. (2005). Profiling stress among addiction practitioners across career stages: Focus on addiction nurses. *Substance Abuse, 26*(2), 51.

Clark, D. E. (2006). Degrees of success: Student voices. From welder to nurse. *Minority Nurse,* Winter: 62–64.

Dion, K. W. (2006). Nursing portfolios: Drivers, challenges, and benefits. *Dean's Notes, 27*(4), 1–3.

Ferguson-Paré, M. (2006). Sabbatical journey of discovery: Recruitment, retention and quality of work life. *Canadian Journal of Nursing Leadership, 19*(3), 18–20.

Fowlie, P. (2006). Readers speak. Careertalk interest . . . "The mid-career nurse" (May). *Canadian Nurse, 102*(7), 6.

Goacher, A. (2006). Careers. Being prepared for redeployment. *Nursing Times, 102*(34), 20–21.

Hilton, L. (2006). So you want to be a manager? Nurse recruiters look for more than just clinical knowledge. *Nursing Spectrum—Philadelphia Tri-State Edition, 15*(12), 16.

Johnston, S. (2006). See one, do one, teach one: Developing professionalism across the generations. *Clinical Orthopaedics and Related Research, 449,* 186–192.

Krueger, C., Barnard, N. P., & Malone, M. P. (2006). Avoid hiring woes: Keep your good employees: Provide educational opportunities, safe environment. *Hospital Home Health, 23*(11), 123–127.

Kuypers, A. (2006). Developing a portfolio for today's nurse. *ACORN, 19*(2), 15.

Linney, A. (2006). Changing career . . . emergency nurse (May). *Emergency Nurse, 14*(3), 7.

Mathieu, J. (2006). Getting that first job: Search and resume tips. *Journal of the American Dietetic Association, 106*(9), 1338, 1340, 1342–1345.

Matias, L. (2005–2006). *Write resume—There's no need to pad your resume.* Media, Inc. Retrieved December 1, 2006, from *http://www.resume-resource.com/article27.html.*

Percival, J. (2006). Careers. Successful goal-setting. *Nursing Times, 102*(38), 22–23.

Pierce, P. A., & Snyder, J. F. (2006). Résumés for health/fitness students and professionals. *ACSM's Health and Fitness Journal, 10*(2), 19–27.

Resume Center, Inc. (2005–2006). *Cover letter writing—"How to write a winning cover letter."* Media, Inc. Retrieved December 1, 2006, from *http://www.resume-resource.com/article7.html.*

Rose, T. (2005–2006). *Career change—Throw your career a change up in mid-stride.* Media, Inc. Retrieved December 1, 2006, from *http://www.resume-resource.com/article38.html.*

Shirey, M. R. (2005). Celebrating certification in nursing: Forces of magnetism in action. *Nursing Administration Quarterly, 29*(3), 245–253.

Taylor, J. S., & Cantrell, E. J. (2006). Peacock or plum? Reflections on academic research career pathways. *Nurse Education Today, 26*(6), 449–456.

Van der Heijde, C. M., & Van der Heijden, B. I. (2006). A competence-based and multidimensional operationalization and measurement of employability. *Human Resource Management, 45*(3), 449–476.

Walker, D. (2005–2006). *The warning signs of career disaster.* Media, Inc. Retrieved December 1, 2006, from *http://www.resume-resource.com/article18.html.*

Wicker, T. (2006). Do you need a professional portfolio? *Arizona Nurse, 59*(5), 12.

Yang, C., Gau, M., Shiau, S., & Hu, W. (2004). Professional career development for male nurses. *Journal of Advanced Nursing, 48*(6), 642–550.

12

Organizational Structure

> . . . *society, community, family are all conserving institutions. They try to maintain stability, and to prevent, or at least to slow down, change. But the organization of the post-capitalist society of organizations is a destabilizer. Because its function is to put knowledge to work—on tools, processes, and products; on work; on knowledge itself—it must be organized for constant change.*
>
> —*Peter Drucker*

> . . . *in a changing world, organizations must change as surely as individuals must change. Recent years have seen an increase in organizational "flattening," the tendency to shrink the organizational structure through the removal of layers of hierarchy.*
>
> — *Charles R. McConnell*

Unit III provided a background in planning, the first phase of the management process. Organizing follows planning as the second phase of the management process and is explored in this unit. In the organizing phase, relationships are defined, procedures are outlined, equipment is readied, and tasks are assigned. Organizing also involves establishing a formal structure that provides the best possible coordination or use of resources to accomplish unit objectives. This chapter looks at how the structure of an organization facilitates or impedes communication, flexibility, and job satisfaction. Chapter 13 examines the role of authority and power in organizations and how power may be used to meet individual, unit, and organizational goals. Chapter 14 looks at how human resources can be organized to accomplish patient care.

Fayol (1949) suggested that an organization is formed when the number of workers is large enough to require a supervisor. Organizations are necessary because they accomplish more work than can be done by individual effort. Because people spend most of their lives in social, personal, and professional organizations, they need to understand how organizations are structured—their formation, methods of communication, channels of authority, and decision-making processes.

Organizational structure refers to the way in which a group is formed, its lines of communication, and its means for channeling authority and making decisions.

Each organization has a formal and an informal organizational structure. The formal structure is generally highly planned and visible, whereas the informal structure is unplanned and often hidden. *Formal structure*, through departmentalization and work division, provides a framework for defining managerial authority, responsibility, and accountability. In a well-defined formal structure, roles and functions are defined and systematically arranged, different people have differing roles, and rank and hierarchy are evident.

Informal structure is generally social, with blurred or shifting lines of authority and accountability. People need to be aware that informal authority and lines of communication exist in every group, even when they are never formally acknowledged. The primary emphasis of this chapter, however, is the identification of components of organizational structure, the leadership roles and management functions associated with formal organizational structure, and the proper utilization of committees to accomplish organizational objectives (Display 12.1).

ORGANIZATIONAL THEORY

Max Weber, a German social scientist, is known as the father of organizational theory. Generally acknowledged to have developed the most comprehensive classic formulation on the characteristics of *bureaucracy*, Weber wrote from the vantage point of a manager instead of that of a scholar. During the 1920s, Weber saw the growth of the large-scale organization and correctly predicted that this growth required a more formalized set of procedures for administrators. His statement on bureaucracy, published after his death, is still the most influential statement on the subject.

Weber postulated three "ideal types" of authority or reasons why people throughout history have obeyed their rulers. One of these, *legal-rational authority*, was based on a belief in the legitimacy of the pattern of normative rules and the rights of those elevated to authority under such rules to issue commands. Obedience, then, was owed to the legally established impersonal set of rules rather than to a personal ruler. It is this type of authority that is the basis for Weber's concept of bureaucracy.

Weber argued that the great virtue of bureaucracy—indeed, perhaps its defining characteristic—was that it was an institutional method for applying general rules to specific cases, thereby making the actions of management fair and predictable. Other characteristics of bureaucracies as identified by Weber include the following:

• There must be a clear division of labor (i.e., all work must be divided into units that can be undertaken by individuals or groups of individuals competent to perform those tasks).

DISPLAY 12.1 Leadership Roles and Management Functions Associated With Organizational Structure

Leadership Roles

1. Evaluates the organizational structure frequently to determine if management positions can be eliminated to reduce the chain of command
2. Encourages and guides employees to follow the chain of command and counsels employees who do not follow chain of command
3. Supports personnel in advisory (staff) positions
4. Models responsibility and accountability for subordinates
5. Assists staff to see how their roles are congruent with and complement the organization's mission, vision, and goals
6. Facilitates constructive informal group structure
7. Encourages upward communication
8. Fosters a positive organizational culture between work groups and subcultures that facilitates shared values and goals
9. Promotes participatory decision making and shared governance to empower subordinates
10. Uses committees to facilitate group goals, not to delay decisions
11. Teaches group members how to avoid groupthink

Management Functions

1. Continually identifies and analyzes stakeholder interests in the organization
2. Is knowledgeable about the organization's internal structure, including personal and department authority and responsibilities within that structure
3. Provides the staff with an accurate unit organization chart and assists with interpretation
4. When possible, maintains unity of command
5. Clarifies unity of command when there is confusion
6. Follows appropriate subordinate complaints upward through chain of command
7. Establishes an appropriate span of control
8. Is knowledgeable about the organization's culture
9. Uses the informal organization to meet organizational goals
10. Uses committee structure to increase the quality and quantity of work accomplished
11. Works, as appropriate, to achieve a level of operational excellence appropriate to magnet status

- A well-defined hierarchy of authority must exist in which superiors are separated from subordinates; on the basis of this hierarchy, remuneration for work is dispensed, authority is recognized, privileges are allotted, and promotions are awarded.
- There must be impersonal rules and impersonality of interpersonal relationships. In other words, bureaucrats are not free to act in any way they please. Bureaucratic rules provide superiors systematic control over subordinates, thus limiting the opportunities for arbitrary behavior and personal favoritism.
- A system of procedures for dealing with work situations (i.e., regular activities to get a job done) must exist.

• A system of rules covering the rights and duties of each position must be in place.

• Selection for employment and promotion is based on technical competence.

Bureaucracy was the ideal tool to harness and routinize the energy and prolific production of the Industrial Revolution. Weber's work did not, however, consider the complexity of managing organizations in the 21st century. Weber wrote during an era when worker motivation was taken for granted, and his simplification of management and employee roles did not examine the bilateral relationships between employee and management prevalent in most organizations today. Since Weber's research, management theorists have learned much about human behavior, and most organizations have modified their structures and created alternative organizational designs that reduce rigidity and impersonality. For example, a structure that supports autonomy and empowers nurses is likely to benefit effective patient care (Kramer & Schmalenberg, 2005).

 Current research supports the thesis that changing an organization's structure in a manner that increases autonomy and work empowerment for nurses will also lead to more effective patient care.

In fact, Campbell, Fowles, and Weber (2004) found a significant relationship between organizational structure and job satisfaction (Examining the Evidence 12.1). Yet, almost 100 years after Weber's findings, components of bureaucratic structure continue to be found in the design of most large organizations.

COMPONENTS OF ORGANIZATIONAL STRUCTURE

Weber also is credited with the development of the *organization chart* to depict an organization's structure. Because the organization chart (Fig. 12.1) is a picture of an organization, the knowledgeable manager can derive much information from reading the chart. An organization chart can help identify roles and their expectations. By observing elements, such as which departments report directly to the chief executive officer (CEO), the novice manager can make some inferences about the organization. For instance, having the top-level nursing manager reporting to an assistant executive officer rather than to the CEO might indicate the amount of value the organization places on nursing. Managers who understand an organization's structure and relationships will be able to expedite decisions and have a greater understanding of the organizational environment.

 EXAMINING THE EVIDENCE 12.1

Source: Campbell, S. L., Fowles, E. R., & Weber, B. J. (2004). Organizational structure and job satisfaction in public health nursing. *Public Health Nursing*, *21*(6), 564–571.

This descriptive study found a significant relationship between organizational structure variables and job satisfaction in local health departments in a community in Illinois.

The findings suggest that work environments in which supervisors and subordinates consult together concerning job tasks and decisions, as well as in which individuals are involved with peers in decision making and task definition, are positively related to job satisfaction.

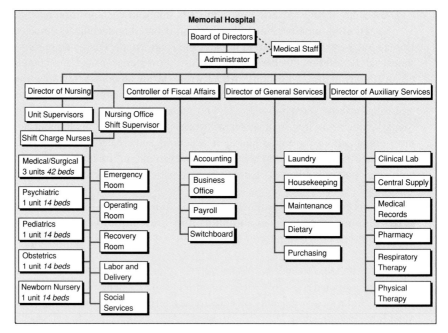

Figure 12.1   Sample organizational chart.

Relationships and Chain of Command

The organization chart defines formal relationships within the institution. Formal relationships, lines of communication, and authority are depicted on a chart by unbroken (solid) lines. These *line* positions can be shown by solid horizontal or vertical lines. Solid horizontal lines represent communication between people with similar spheres of responsibility and power but different functions. Solid vertical lines between positions denote the official *chain of command*, the formal paths of communication and authority. Those having the greatest decision-making authority are located at the top; those with the least are at the bottom. The level of position on the chart also signifies status and power.

Dotted or broken lines on the organization chart represent *staff* positions. Because these positions are advisory, a staff member provides information and assistance to the manager but has limited organizational authority. Used to increase his or her sphere of influence, staff positions enable a manager to handle more activities and interactions than would otherwise be possible. These positions also provide for specialization that would be impossible for any one manager to achieve alone. Although staff positions can make line personnel more effective, organizations can function without them.

Advisory (staff) positions do not have inherent legitimate authority. Clinical specialists and in-service directors in staff positions often lack the authority that accompanies a line relationship. Accomplishing the role expectations in a staff position is therefore more difficult because typically little authority accompanies it. Because only line positions have authority for decision making, staff positions may result in an ineffective use of support services unless job descriptions and responsibilities for these positions are clearly spelled out.

Unity of command is indicated by the vertical solid line between positions on the organizational chart. This concept is best described as one person/one boss in which employees have one manager to whom they report and to whom they are responsible. This greatly simplifies the manager–employee relationship because the employee needs to maintain only a minimum number of relationships and accept the influence of only one person as his or her immediate supervisor.

 Unity of command is difficult to maintain in some large health care organizations because the nature of health care requires a multidisciplinary approach.

Nurses frequently feel as though they have many bosses because health care typically involves a multidisciplinary approach. Additional possible bosses may include the immediate supervisor, the patient, the patient's family, central administration, and the physician. All have some input in directing a nurse's work. Weber was correct when he determined that a lack of unity of command results in some conflict and lost productivity. This is demonstrated frequently when health care workers become confused about unity of command.

LEARNING EXERCISE 12.1

Who's the Boss?
In groups or individually, analyze the following, and give an oral or written report.
1. Have you ever worked in an organization in which the lines of authority were unclear? Have you been a member of a social organization in which this happened? How did this interfere with the organization's functioning?
2. Do you believe that the "one boss/one person" rule is a good idea? Don't hospital clerical workers frequently have many bosses? If you have worked in a situation in which you had more than one boss, what was the result?

Span of Control

Span of control also can be determined from the organization chart. The number of people directly reporting to any one manager represents that manager's span of control and determines the number of interactions expected of him or her. Theorists are divided regarding the optimal span of control for any one manager. Quantitative formulas for determining the optimal span of control have been attempted; suggested ranges are from 3 to 50 employees. When determining an optimal span of control in an organization, the manager's abilities, the employees' maturity, task complexity, geographic location, and level in the organization at which the work occurs must all be considered. The number of people directly reporting to any one supervisor must be the number that maximizes productivity and worker satisfaction.

 Too many people reporting to a single manager delays decision making, whereas too few results in an inefficient, top-heavy organization.

Until the last decade, the principle of narrow spans of control at top levels of management, with slightly wider spans at other levels, was widely accepted. Now, with increased financial pressures on health care organizations to remain fiscally solvent and electronic communication technology advances, many have increased their spans of control and reduced the number of administrative levels in the organization. This reduction in numbers of administrative levels is often termed *flattening the organization* (McConnell, 2005).

Managerial Levels

In large organizations, several levels of managers often exist. *Top-level managers* look at the organization as a whole, coordinating internal and external influences, and generally make decisions with few guidelines or structures. Examples of top-level managers include the organization's chief operating officer (COO) or CEO and the highest-level nursing administrator. Current nomenclature for top-level nurse–managers varies; they might be called vice-president of nursing or patient care services, nurse administrator, director of nursing, chief nurse, assistant administrator of patient care services, or chief nurse officer (CNO).

Some top-level nurse–managers may be responsible for non-nursing departments. For example, a top-level nurse–manager might oversee the respiratory, physical, and occupational therapy departments in addition to all nursing departments. Likewise, the CEO might have various titles, such as president or director. It is necessary to remember only that the CEO is the organization's highest-ranking person, and the top-level nurse–manager is its highest-ranking nurse. Responsibilities common to top-level managers include determining the organizational philosophy, setting policy, and creating goals and priorities for resource allocation. Top-level managers have a greater need for leadership skills and are not as involved in routine daily operations as are lower-level managers.

Middle-level managers coordinate the efforts of lower levels of the hierarchy and are the conduit between lower and top-level managers. Middle-level managers carry out day-to-day operations but are still involved in some long-term planning and in establishing unit policies. Examples of middle-level managers include nursing supervisors, nurse–managers, head nurses, and unit managers.

Currently, there are many health facility mergers and acquisitions, and reduced levels of administration are frequently apparent within these consolidated organizations. This often results in middle-level managers having increased responsibilities and role expansion (McConnell, 2005). Consequently, many health care facilities have renamed middle-level managers using the title of "director" as a way to indicate new roles. The old term *director of nursing,* still used in many small facilities to denote the CNO, is now used in many health care organizations to denote a middle-level manager. The proliferation of titles among health care administrators has made it imperative that individuals understand what roles and responsibilities go with each position.

First-level managers are concerned with their specific unit's work flow. They deal with immediate problems in the unit's daily operations, with organizational needs, and with personal needs of employees. The effectiveness of first-level managers tremendously affects the organization. First-level managers need good management skills. Because they work so closely with patients and health care teams, first-level managers also have an excellent opportunity to practice leadership roles that will greatly influence productivity and subordinates' satisfaction. Examples of first-level managers include primary care nurses, team leaders, case managers, and charge nurses. In many organizations, every RN is considered a first-level manager. All nurses in every situation must manage themselves and those under their care. A composite look at top-, middle-, and first-level managers is shown in Table 12.1.

TABLE 12.1   Levels of Managers

	Top Level	Middle Level	First Level
Examples	Chief nursing officer Chief executive officer Chief financial officer	Unit supervisor Department head Director	Charge nurse Team leader Primary nurse
Scope of responsibility	Look at organization as a whole as well as external influences	Focus is on integrating unit level day-to-day needs with organizational needs	Focus primarily on day-to-day needs at unit level
Primary planning focus	Strategic planning	Combination of long- and short-range planning	Short-range, operational planning
Communication flow	More often top down but receives subordinate feedback both directly and via middle-level managers	Upward and downward with great centrality	More often upward; generally relies on middle-level managers to transmit communication to top-level managers

One of the leadership responsibilities of organizing is to periodically examine the number of people in the chain of command. Organizations frequently add levels until there are too many managers. Therefore, the nursing manager should carefully weigh the advantages and disadvantages of adding a management level. For example, does having a charge nurse on each shift aid or hinder decision making? Does having this position solve or create problems?

Centrality

Centrality, or where a position falls on the organizational chart, is determined by organizational distance. Employees with relatively small organizational distance can receive more information than those who are more peripherally located. This is why the middle manager often has a broader view of the organization than other levels of management. A middle manager has a large degree of centrality because this manager receives information upward, downward, and horizontally.

 Centrality refers to the location of a position on an organization chart where frequent and various types of communication occur.

Because all communication involves a sender and a receiver, messages may not be received clearly because of the sender's hierarchical position. Similarly, status and power often influence the receiver's ability to hear information accurately. An example of the effect of status on communication is found in the "principal syndrome." Most people can recall panic, when they were school-age, at being summoned to the principal's office. Thoughts of "what did I do?" travel through one's mind. Even adults find discomfort in communicating with certain people who hold high status. This may be fear or awe, but both interfere with clear communication. The difficulties with upward and downward communication are more fully discussed in Chapter 19.

LEARNING EXERCISE 12.2

Change Is Coming

This learning exercise refers to the organization chart in Figure 12.1. Because Memorial Hospital is expanding, the Board of Directors has made several changes that require modification of the organization chart. The directors have just announced the following changes:

- The name of the hospital has been changed to Memorial General Hospital and Medical Center.
- State approval has been granted for open-heart surgery.
- One of the existing medical–surgical units will be remodeled and will become two critical care units (one six-bed coronary and open-heart unit and one six-bed trauma and surgical unit).
- A part-time medical director will be responsible for medical care on each critical care unit.
- The hospital administrator's title has been changed to executive director.
- An associate hospital administrator has been hired.
- A new hospitalwide educational department has been created.
- The old pediatric unit will be remodeled into a seven-bed pediatric wing and a seven-bed rehabilitation unit.
- The director of nursing's new title is vice-president of patient care services.

● ASSIGNMENT: If the hospital is viewed as a large, open system, it is possible to visualize areas where problems might occur. In particular, it is necessary to identify changes anticipated in the nursing department and how these changes will affect the organization as a whole. Depict all of these changes on the old organization chart, delineating both staff and line positions. Give the rationale for your decisions. Why did you place the education department where you did? What was the reasoning in your division of authority? Where do you believe there might be potential conflict in the new organization chart? Why?

It is important, then, to be aware of how the formal structure affects overall relationships and communication. This is especially true because organizations change their structure frequently, resulting in new communication lines and reporting relationships. Unless one understands how to interpret a formal organization chart, confusion and anxiety will result when organizations are restructured.

LEARNING EXERCISE 12.3

Cultures and Hierarchies

Having been with the county health department for 6 months, you are very impressed with the physician who is the county health administrator. She seems to have a genuine concern for patient welfare. She has a tea for new employees each month to discuss the department's philosophy and her own management style. She says that she has an open-door policy, so employees are always welcome to visit her.

Since you have been assigned to the evening immunization clinic as charge nurse, you have become concerned with a persistent problem. The housekeeping staff often spends part of the evening sleeping on duty or socializing for long periods. You have reported your concerns to your health department supervisor twice. Last evening, you found the housekeeping staff having another get-together. This mainly upsets you because the clinic is chronically in need of cleaning. Sometimes, the public bathrooms get so untidy that they embarrass you and your staff. You frequently remind the housekeepers to empty overflowing waste paper baskets. You believe that this environment is demeaning to patients. This also upsets you because you and your staff work hard all evening and rarely have a chance to sit down. You believe it is unfair to everyone that the housekeeping staff is not doing its share.

On your way to the parking lot this evening, the health administrator stops to chat and asks you how things are going. Should you tell her about the problem with the housekeeping staff? Is this following an appropriate chain of command? Do you believe that there is a conflict between the housekeeping unit's culture and the nursing unit's culture? What should you do? List choices and alternatives. Decide what you should do, and explain your rationale.

Note: Attempt to solve this problem before referring to a possible solution posted in the Appendix.

Is it ever appropriate to go outside the chain of command? Of course, there are isolated circumstances when the chain of command must be breached. However, those rare conditions usually involve a question of ethics. In most instances, those being bypassed in a chain of command should be forewarned. Remember that unity of command provides the organization with a workable system for procedural directives and orders so that productivity is increased and conflict is minimized.

TYPES OF ORGANIZATIONAL STRUCTURES

Traditionally, nursing departments have used one of the following structural patterns: bureaucratic, ad hoc, matrix, flat, or various combinations of these. The type of structure used in any health care facility affects communication patterns, relationships, and authority.

Line Structures

Bureaucratic organizational designs are commonly called *line structures* or *line organizations*. Those with staff authority may be referred to as *staff organizations*. Both of these types of organizational structures are found frequently in large health care facilities and usually resemble Weber's original design for effective organizations. Because of most people's familiarity with these structures, there is little stress associated with orienting people to these organizations. In these structures, authority and responsibility are clearly defined, which leads to efficiency and simplicity of relationships. The organization chart in Figure 12.1 is a line-and-staff structure.

These formal designs have some disadvantages. They often produce monotony, alienate workers, and make adjusting rapidly to altered circumstances difficult. Another problem with line and line-and-staff structures is their adherence to chain of command communication, which restricts upward communication. Good leaders encourage upward communication to compensate for this disadvantage. However, when line positions are clearly defined, going outside the chain of command for upward communication is usually inappropriate.

Ad Hoc Design

The *ad hoc design* is a modification of the bureaucratic structure and is sometimes used on a temporary basis to facilitate completion of a project within a formal line organization. The ad hoc structure is a means of overcoming the inflexibility of line structure and serves as a way for professionals to handle the increasingly large amounts of available information. Ad hoc structures use a project team or task approach and are usually disbanded after a project is completed. This structure's disadvantages are decreased strength in the formal chain of command and decreased employee loyalty to the parent organization.

Matrix Structure

A *matrix organization* structure is designed to focus on both product and function. Function is described as all the tasks required to produce the product, and the product is the end result of the function. For example, good patient outcomes are the product, and staff education and adequate staffing may be the functions necessary to produce the outcome.

The matrix organization structure has a formal vertical and horizontal chain of command. Figure 12.2 depicts a matrix organizational structure and shows that the director of maternal child care could report both to a vice president for maternal and women's services (product manager) and a vice president for nursing services (functional manager). Although there are less

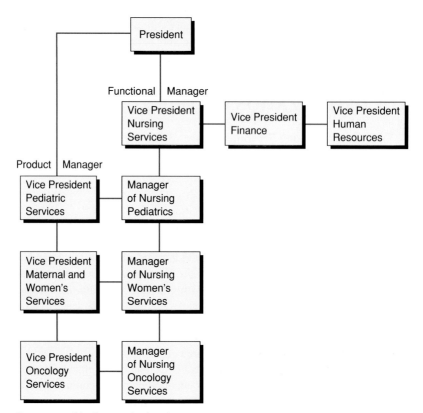

Figure 12.2   Matrix organizational structure.

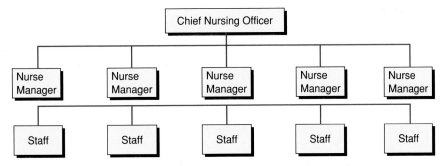

Figure 12.3   Flattened organizational structure.

formal rules and fewer levels of the hierarchy, a matrix structure is not without disadvantages. For example, in this structure, decision making can be slow because of the necessity of information sharing, and it can produce confusion and frustration for workers because of its dual-authority hierarchical design. The primary advantage of centralizing expertise is frequently outweighed by the complexity of the communication required in the design.

Service Line Organization

Similar to the matrix design is service line organization, which can be used in some large institutions to address the shortcomings that are endemic to traditional large bureaucratic organizations. *Service lines*, sometimes called *care-centered organizations*, are smaller in scale than a large bureaucratic system. For example, in this organizational design, the overall goals would be determined by the larger organization, but the service line would decide on the processes to be used to achieve the goals.

Flat Designs

Flat organizational designs are an effort to remove hierarchical layers by flattening the chain of command and decentralizing the organization. In good times, when organizations are financially well off, it is easy to add layers to the organization in order to get the work done, but when the organization begins to feel a financial pinch, they often look at their hierarchy to see where they can cut positions. While there are advantages to a flattened organization, many managers resist such change as it means their work load is greatly increased (McConnell, 2005).

In *flattened organizations*, there continues to be line authority, but because the organizational structure is flattened, more authority and decision making can occur where the work is being carried out. Figure 12.3 shows a flattened organizational structure. Many managers have difficulty letting go of control, and even very flattened types of structure organizations often retain many characteristics of a bureaucracy.

DECISION MAKING WITHIN THE ORGANIZATIONAL HIERARCHY

The decision-making hierarchy, or pyramid, is often referred to as *a scalar chain*. By reviewing the organization chart in Figure 12.1, it is possible to determine where decisions are made within the management hierarchy. Although every manager has some decision-making authority, its type and level are determined by the manager's position on the chart.

In organizations with *centralized decision making*, a few managers at the top of the hierarchy make the decisions. *Decentralized decision making* diffuses decision making throughout the organization and allows problems to be solved by the lowest practical managerial level. Often, this means that problems can be solved at the level at which they occur, which has the potential to improve quality care outcomes and increase organizational efficiency (Caramanica, 2004). As a rule, larger organizations benefit from decentralized decision making.

 In general, the larger the organization, the greater the need to decentralize decision making.

Decision making needs to be decentralized in large organizations because the complex questions that must be answered can best be addressed by a variety of people with distinct areas of expertise. Leaving such decisions in a large organization to a few managers burdens those managers tremendously and could result in devastating delays in decision making.

STAKEHOLDERS

Stakeholders are those entities in an organization's environment that play a role in the organization's health and performance or that are affected by the organization. Stakeholders may be both internal and external, they may include individuals and large groups, and they may have shared goals or diverse goals. *Internal stakeholders,* for example, may include the nurse in a hospital or the dietitian in a nursing home. Examples of *external stakeholders* for an acute-care hospital might be the local school of nursing, home health agencies, and managed care providers who contract with consumers in the area. Even the Chamber of Commerce in a city could be considered a stakeholder for a health care organization.

 Every organization should be viewed as being part of a greater community of stakeholders.

Stakeholders have interests in what the organization does but may or may not have the power to influence the organization to protect their interests. Stakeholders' interests are varied, however, and their interests may coincide on some issues and not others. Organizations do not choose their own stakeholders; rather, the stakeholders choose to have a stake in the organizations' decisions. Stakeholders may have a supportive or threatening influence on organizational decision making. For many decisions an organization makes, it may face a diverse set of stakeholders with varied and conflicting interest and goals.

As a part of planned change, discussed in Chapter 8, and decision making, discussed in Chapter 1, a *stakeholder analysis* is an important aspect of the management process. Such an analysis should be performed when there is a need to clarify the consequences of decisions and changes. In addition to identifying stakeholders who will be impacted by a change, it is necessary to prioritize them and determine their influence. Waymack (2005) maintains that identifying stakeholders is a critical step in organizational change because it helps organizations develop a communication plan to meet the needs of each group of stakeholders. Astute leaders

DISPLAY 12.2 **Examples of Stakeholders in a Community Hospital**

External Stakeholders	Internal Stakeholders
Local businesses	Hospital employees
Area colleges and universities	Physicians
Insurance companies and HMOs	Patients
Community leaders	Patients' families
Unions	Union shop stewards
Professional organizations	Board of directors

and managers, then, must always be cognizant of who their stakeholders are, how they may be connected, and the opportunities for positive collaboration to achieve the organization's mission (Lockyer, 2005). A depiction of some possible stakeholders for a local community hospital appears in Display 12.2.

LIMITATIONS OF ORGANIZATION CHARTS

Because organization charts show only formal relationships, what they can reveal about an institution is limited. The chart does not show the informal structure of the organization. Every institution has in place a dynamic informal structure that can be powerful and motivating. Knowledgeable leaders never underestimate its importance because the informal structure includes employees' interpersonal relationships, the formation of primary and secondary groups, and the identification of group leaders without formal authority. The informal structure, known as the *grapevine*, also has groups, leaders, and channels.

 The informal structure also has its own leaders. In addition, it also has its own communication channels, often referred to as the *grapevine*.

These groups are important in organizations because they provide workers with a feeling of belonging. They also have a great deal of power in an organization; they can either facilitate or sabotage planned change. Their ability to determine a unit's norms and acceptable behavior has a great deal to do with the socialization of new employees. Informal leaders are frequently found among long-term employees or people in select *gatekeeping positions*, such as the CNO's secretary. Frequently, the informal organization evolves from social activities or from relationships that develop outside the work environment.

Organization charts also are limited in their ability to depict each line position's degree of authority. Equating status with authority frequently causes confusion. The distance from the top of the organizational hierarchy usually determines the degree of status: the closer to the top, the higher the status. Status also is influenced by skill, education, specialization, level of responsibility, autonomy, and salary accorded a position. People frequently have status with little accompanying authority.

Because organizations are dynamic environments, an organization chart becomes obsolete very quickly. It also is possible that the organization chart may depict how things are supposed

DISPLAY 12.3   Advantages and Limitations of the Organization Chart

Advantages

1. Maps lines of decision-making authority
2. Helps people understand their assignments and those of their coworkers
3. Reveals to managers and new personnel how they fit into the organization
4. Contributes to sound organizational structure
5. Shows formal lines of communication

Limitations

1. Shows only formal relationships
2. Does not indicate degree of authority
3. May show things as they are supposed to be or used to be rather than as they are
4. Possibility exists of confusing authority with status

to be, when in reality, the organization is still functioning under an old structure because employees have not yet accepted new lines of authority. Another limitation of the organization chart is that although it defines authority, it does not define responsibility and accountability. The manager should understand the interrelationships and differences among these three terms.

Authority is defined as the official power to act. It is power given by the organization to direct the work of others. A manager may have the authority to hire, fire, or discipline others. Because the use of authority, power building, and political awareness are so important to functioning effectively in any structure, Chapter 13 discusses these organizational components in depth.

A *responsibility* is a duty or an assignment. It is the implementation of a job. For example, a responsibility common to many charge nurses is establishing the unit's daily patient care assignment. Managers should always be assigned responsibilities with concomitant authority. If authority is not commensurate to the responsibility, role confusion occurs for everyone involved. For example, supervisors may have the responsibility of maintaining high professional care standards among their staff. If the manager is not given the authority to discipline employees as needed, however, this responsibility is virtually impossible to implement.

Accountability is similar to responsibility, but it is internalized. Thus, to be accountable means that individuals agree to be morally responsible for the consequences of their actions. Therefore, one individual cannot be accountable for another. Society holds us accountable for our assigned responsibilities, and people are expected to accept the consequences of their actions. A nurse who reports a medication error is being accountable for the responsibilities inherent in the position. Display 12.3 discusses the advantages and limitations of an organization chart.

ORGANIZATIONAL CULTURE

Organizational culture is the total of an organization's values, language, traditions, customs, and sacred cows—those few things present in an institution that are not open to discussion or change. For example, the hospital logo that had been designed by the original board of trustees is an item that may not be considered for updating or change.

Organizational culture is a system of symbols and interactions unique to each organization. It is the ways of thinking, behaving, and believing that members of a unit have in common.

Similarly, Waters (2004) defines organizational culture as "the source of motivated and coordinated activities within organizations, activities that serve as a foundation for practices and behaviors that endure because they're meaningful, have a history of working well, and are likely to continue working in the future" (p. 36). Both of these definitions impart a sense of the complexity and importance of organizational culture. It is the "operating system" of an organization and drives the organization and its actions (Waters, 2004).

Organizational culture is often confused with *organizational climate*—how employees perceive an organization. For example, an employee might perceive an organization as fair, friendly, and informal or as formal and very structured. The perception may be accurate or inaccurate, and people in the same organization may have different perceptions about the same organization. Therefore, since the organizational climate is the view of the organization by individuals, the organization's climate and its culture may differ.

Although assessing unit culture is a management function, building a constructive culture, particularly if a negative culture is in place, requires the interpersonal and communication skills of a leader. Wooten and Crane (2003) state that "healthcare organizations have lagged behind trends evident in corporate America that demonstrate how investments in organizational culture translate into high performance" (p. 275). Way (2006) states that it is imperative for health care organizations to support a "nurse friendly" culture where nurses are able to perform their roles.

The leader must take an active role in creating the kind of organizational culture that will ensure success. The more entrenched the culture and pattern of actions, the more challenging the change process is for the leader. Given such entrenchment of culture, success in building a new culture often requires new leadership and/or assistance by the use of outside analysis.

Kane-Urrabazo (2006) maintains that there are four critical cultural components that a leader–manager can influence. She identifies these as trust and trustworthiness, empowerment, consistency, and mentorship. These components exist as managerial traits at all times, regardless of the overall culture present in the organization, and therefore, managers have a special role in shaping organizational culture for their staff.

Organizations, if large enough, also have many different and competing value systems that create subcultures. These subcultures shape perceptions, attitudes, and beliefs and influence how their members approach and execute their particular roles and responsibilities. A critical challenge then for the nurse leader–manager is to recognize these subcultures and to do whatever is necessary to create shared norms and priorities. "Defining a collective mission is a critical first step in creating the team efforts that drive collaborative and productive work and communication" (Wooten & Crane, 2003, p. 275).

Managers must be able to assess their unit's culture and choose management strategies that encourage a shared culture. Such transformation requires both management assessment and leadership direction. Indeed, Wooten and Crane (2003) argue that nursing leaders should take on the responsibility of culture gatekeeper. Pinkerton (2006) relates how managers and leaders can assist with creating a shared culture by storytelling; using narratives about the organization in orientation, meetings, and performance review. These shared stories not only bind groups together but act as motivators.

Much of an organization's culture is not available to staff in a retrievable source and must be related by others. For example, feelings about collective bargaining, nursing education levels, nursing autonomy, and nurse–physician relationships differ from one organization to another. These beliefs and values, however, are rarely written down or appear in a philosophy. Therefore, in addition to creating a constructive culture, a major leadership role is to assist subordinates in understanding the organization's culture. Display 12.4 identifies questions that leaders and followers should ask when assessing organizational culture.

SHARED GOVERNANCE: ORGANIZATIONAL DESIGN FOR THE 21ST CENTURY?

Shared governance, one of the most innovative and idealistic of organization structures, was developed in the mid-1980s as an alternative to the traditional bureaucratic organizational structure. A flat type of organizational structure is often used to describe shared governance but differs somewhat, as shown in Figure 12.4. In shared governance, the organization's governance is shared among board members, nurses, physicians, and management. Thus, decision-making and communication channels are altered. Group structures, in the form of *joint practice committees*, are developed to assume the power and accountability for decision making, and professional communication takes on an egalitarian structure.

In health care organizations, shared governance empowers decision makers, and this empowerment is directed at increasing nurses' authority and control over nursing practice. Shared governance thus gives nurses more control over their nursing practice by being an accountability-based governance system for professional workers.

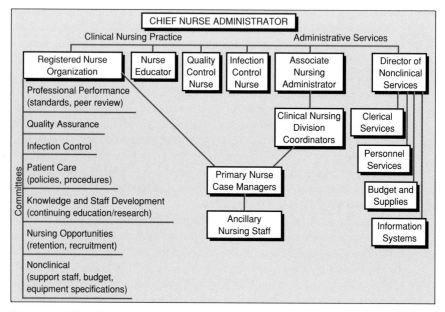

Figure 12.4   Shared governance model.

DISPLAY 12.4 Assessing the Organizational Culture

What Is the Organization's Physical Environment?

1. Is the environment attractive?
2. Does it appear that there is adequate maintenance?
3. Are nursing stations crowded or noisy?
4. Is there an appropriate-size lobby? Are there quiet areas?
5. Is there sufficient seating for families in the dining room?
6. Are there enough conference rooms?

What Is the Organization's Social Environment?

1. Are many friendships maintained beyond the workplace?
2. Is there an annual picnic or holiday party that is well attended by the employees?
3. Do employees seem to generally like each other?
4. Do all shifts and all departments get along fairly well?
5. Are certain departments disliked or resented?
6. Are employees on a first-name basis with co-workers, doctors, charge nurses, and supervisors?

How Supportive Is the Organization?

1. Is educational reimbursement available?
2. Are good, low-cost meals available to employees?
3. Are there adequate employee lounges?
4. Are funds available to send employees to workshops?
5. Are employees recognized for extra effort?
6. Does the organization help pay for the holiday party or other social functions?

What Is the Organizational Power Structure?

1. Who holds the most power in the organization?
2. Which departments are viewed as powerful? Which are viewed as powerless?
3. Who gets free meals? Who gets special parking places?
4. Who carries beepers? Who wears lab coats? Who has overhead pages?
5. Who has the biggest office?
6. Who is never called by his or her first name?

How Safe Is the Organization?

1. Is there a well-lighted parking place for employees arriving or departing when it is dark?
2. Is there an active and involved safety committee?
3. Are security guards needed?

What Is the Communicative Environment?

1. Is upward communication usually written or verbal?
2. Is there much informal communication?
3. Is there an active grapevine? Is it reliable?

(continued)

DISPLAY 12.4   **Assessing the Organizational Culture** (continued)

4. Where is important information exchanged—in the parking lot? the doctors' surgical dressing room? the nurses' station? the coffee shop? during surgery or during the delivery room?

What Are the Organizational Taboos? Who Are the Heroes?

1. Are there special rules and policies that can never be broken?
2. Are certain subjects or ideas forbidden?
3. Are there relationships that cannot be threatened?

> The stated aim of shared governance is the empowerment of employees within the decision-making system.

Although participatory management lays the foundation for shared governance, they are not the same. *Participatory management* implies that others are allowed to participate in decision making over which someone has control. Thus, the act of "allowing" participation identifies the real and final authority for the participant.

There is no single model of shared governance, although all models emphasize the empowerment of staff nurses. Generally, issues related to nursing practice are the responsibility of nurses, not managers, and nursing councils are used to organize governance. These nursing councils, elected at the organization and unit levels, use a congressional format organized like a representative form of government, with a president and cabinet.

A sample operational framework of an organization using shared governance is shown in Figure 12.5. In this model, from Wake Forest University's Baptist Medical Center (n.d.), there are four governance councils and a coordinating council. The governance councils are the Practice

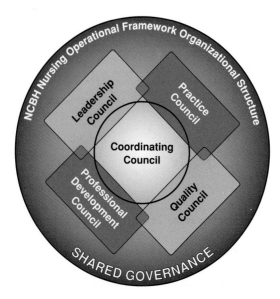

Figure 12.5   Sample nursing councils in a shared governance model. (Source: North Carolina Baptist Hospital, Wake Forest University Medical Center. (n.d.). *Shared governance.* Retrieved November 20, 2003, from *http://www.wfubmc.edu/Nursing/ Shared+Governance*)

Council, Professional Development Council, Quality Council, and Leadership Council. The councils participate in decision making and coordination of the department of nursing and provide input through the shared governance process in all other areas where nursing care is delivered.

Black (2003) describes another shared governance model, called the Professional Nurse Practice Model (PNPM). This model was implemented at Central Iowa Health System and involves staff nurses in making decisions about nursing practice via participation in a committee structure. Issues include nursing quality, nursing policy and procedure, nursing research, resource utilization, and professional growth. Some of the accomplishments of the PNPM over the first year included the development of a model for evidence-based practice, a clinical advancement program that recognizes clinical excellence at the bedside, and nursing grand rounds.

The number of health care organizations using shared governance models has been revitalized due to the current nurse shortage (Hess, 2004). Hospitals using a shared governance model report that shared governance improve staff nurses' perceptions of their job and practice environment (Caramanica, 2004). Additionally, recent research examining shared governance models in hospitals revealed that using a shared governance model results in lessening nursing shortages (Huston, 2006).

However, a major impediment to the implementation of shared governance has been the reluctance of managers to change their roles. The nurse–manager's role becomes one of consulting, teaching, collaborating, and creating an environment with the structures and resources needed for the practice of nursing and shared decision making between nurses and the organization. This new role is foreign to many managers and difficult to accept. In addition, consensus decision making takes more time than autocratic decision making, and not all nurses want to share decisions and accountability. Although many positive outcomes have been attributed to implementation of shared governance, the expense of introducing and maintaining this model also must be considered because it calls for a conscientious commitment both on the part of the workers and the organization.

> Shared governance requires a substantial and long-term commitment on the part of the workers and the organization.

ORGANIZATIONS AND MAGNET STATUS

During the early 1980s, the American Academy of Nursing (AAN) first began identifying hospitals that maintained well-qualified nurse executives in a decentralized environment, with organizational structures that emphasized open, participatory management (Upenieks, 2003). These *magnet hospitals,* as they came to be called, also offered autonomous, self-managing, self-governing climates that allowed nurses to fully practice their clinical expertise, flexible staffing, adequate staffing ratios, and clinical career opportunities (Upenieks, 2003).

Becoming a magnet hospital is not easy. First, the hospital must create and promote a professional practice culture in all aspects of nursing care (Bumgarner & Beard, 2003). Then, the hospital must apply to the American Nurses Credentialing Center (ANCC), submit comprehensive documentation that demonstrates its compliance with standards in the American Nurses Association's (ANA) Scope and Standards for Nurse Administrators, and undergo a multiday onsite evaluation to verify the information in the documentation submitted and to assess the presence of the

DISPLAY 12.5 The Fourteen Forces of Magnetism for Magnet Hospital Status

1. Quality of nursing leadership
2. Organizational structure
3. Management style
4. Personnel policies and programs
5. Professional models of care
6. Quality of care
7. Quality improvement
8. Consultation and resources
9. Autonomy
10. Community and the hospital
11. Nurses as teachers
12. Image of nursing
13. Interdisciplinary relationships
14. Professional development

14 "forces of magnetism" (Display 12.5) within the organization (American Nurses Credentialing Center [ANCC], 2006a). This process may take up to 2 years (Bumgarner & Beard, 2003). Magnet status is awarded for a 4-year period, after which the organization must reapply. As of September 29, 2006, there were 209 magnet-designated organizations in 42 states and one in Australia (ANCC, 2006b). While nurses fare better in magnet hospitals, patients fare better as well with improved outcomes, including lower morality rates (Drenkard, 2005; Huston, 2006; Kramer & Schmalenberg, 2004).

 RNs employed in magnet hospitals experience better staffing, lower use of agency nurses, lower levels of burnout, and higher levels of job satisfaction.

LEARNING EXERCISE 12.4

Why Work for Them?
A list of current magnet hospitals and their contact information can be found at the ANCC website: *http://www.nursecredentialing.org/magnet/facilities.html*.

● ASSIGNMENT: Select one of the current magnet hospitals, and prepare a one-page written report about how that particular hospital demonstrates the excellence exemplified by magnet status. Speak to at least five of the "forces of magnetism." Would you want to work for this particular hospital?

COMMITTEE STRUCTURE IN AN ORGANIZATION

Managers also are responsible for designing and implementing appropriate committee structures. Poorly structured committees can be nonproductive for the organization and frustrating for committee members. However, there are many benefits to and justifications for well-structured

DISPLAY 12.6   Factors to Consider When Organizing Committees and
Making Appointments

- The committee should be composed of people who want to contribute in terms of commitment, energy, and time.
- The members should have a variety of work experience and educational backgrounds. Composition should, however, ensure expertise sufficient to complete the task.
- Committees should have enough members to accomplish assigned tasks but not so many that discussion cannot occur. Six to eight members is usually ideal.
- The tasks and responsibilities, including reporting mechanisms, should be clearly outlined.
- Assignments should be given ahead of time, with clear expectations that assigned work will be discussed at the next meeting.
- All committees should have written agendas and effective committee chairpersons.

committees. To compensate for some of the difficulty in organizational communication created by line and line-and-staff structures, committees are used widely to facilitate upward communication. The nature of formal organizations dictates a need for committees in assisting with management functions. Additionally, as organizations seek new ways to revamp old bureaucratic structures, committees may pave the road to increased staff participation in organization governance. Committees may be advisory or may have a coordinating or informal function. They generate ideas and creative thinking to solve operational problems or improve services and often improve the quality and quantity of work accomplished. Committees also can pool specific skills and expertise and help to reduce resistance to change.

 Because committees communicate upward and downward and encourage the participation of interested or affected employees, they assist the organization in receiving valuable feedback and important information.

However, all of these positive benefits can be achieved only if committees are appropriately organized and led. If not properly used, the committee becomes a liability to the organizing process because it wastes energy, time, and money and can defer decisions and action. One of the leadership roles inherent in organizing work is to ensure that committees are not used to avoid or delay decisions but to facilitate organizational goals. Display 12.6 lists factors to consider when organizing committees.

RESPONSIBILITIES AND OPPORTUNITIES OF COMMITTEE WORK

Committees present the leader–manager with many opportunities and responsibilities. Managers need to be well grounded in group dynamics because meetings represent a major time commitment. Managers serve as members of committees and as leaders or chairpersons of committees. Because committees make major decisions, managers should use the opportunities available at meetings to become more visible in the larger organization. The manager has a responsibility to select appropriate power strategies, such as coming to meetings well prepared, and to use skill in the group process to generate influence and gain power at meetings.

Another responsibility is to create an environment at unit committee meetings that leads to shared decision making. Encouraging an interaction free of status and power is important. Likewise, an appropriate seating arrangement, such as a circle, will increase motivation for committee members to speak up. The responsible manager is also aware that staff from different cultures may have different needs in groups, which is why multicultural committees should be the norm. In addition, because gender differences are increasingly being recognized as playing a role in problem solving, communication, and power, efforts should be made to include both men and women on committees.

When assigning members to committees, cultural and gender diversity should always be a goal.

The manager must not rely too heavily on committees or use them as a method to delay decision making. Numerous committee assignments exhaust staff, and committees then become poor tools for accomplishing work. An alternative that will decrease the time commitment for committee work is to make individual assignments and gather the entire committee only to report progress.

In the leadership role, an opportunity exists for important influence on committee and group effectiveness. A dynamic leader inspires people to put spirit into working for a shared goal. Leaders demonstrate their commitment to participatory management by how they work with committees. Leaders keep the committee on course. Committees may be chaired by an elected member of the group, appointed by the manager, or led by the department or unit manager. Informal leaders also may emerge from the group process.

It is important for the manager to be aware of the possibility for groupthink to occur in any group or committee structure. *Groupthink* occurs when group members fail to take adequate risks by disagreeing, being challenged, or assessing discussion carefully. If the manager is actively involved in the work group or on the committee, groupthink is less likely to occur. The leadership role includes teaching members to avoid groupthink by demonstrating critical thinking and being a role model who allows his or her own ideas to be challenged.

ORGANIZATIONAL EFFECTIVENESS

There is no one "best" way to structure an organization. Variables such as the size of the organization, the capability of its human resources, and the commitment level of its workers should always be considered. Regardless of what type of organizational structure is used, certain minimal requirements can be identified:

- The structure should be clearly defined so that employees know where they belong and where to go for assistance.
- The goal should be to build the fewest possible management levels and have the shortest possible chain of command. This eliminates friction, stress, and inertia.
- The unit staff need to be able to see where their tasks fit into common tasks of the organization.
- The organizational structure should enhance, not impede communication.

- The organizational structure should facilitate decision making that results in the greatest work performance.
- Staff should be organized in a manner that encourages informal groups to develop a sense of community and belonging.
- Nursing services should be organized to facilitate the development of future leaders.

Despite the known difficulties of bureaucracies, it has been difficult for some organizations to move away from the bureaucratic model. However, perhaps as a result of magnet hospital research demonstrating both improved patient outcomes and improved recruitment and retention of staff, there has been an increasing effort to redesign and restructure organizations to make them more flexible and decentralized. Still, progress toward these goals continues to be slow.

INTEGRATING LEADERSHIP ROLES AND MANAGEMENT FUNCTIONS ASSOCIATED WITH ORGANIZATIONAL STRUCTURE

Integrated leader–managers need to look at organizational structure as the road map that tells them how organizations operate. Without organizational structure, people would work in a chaotic environment. Structure becomes an important tool, then, to facilitate order and enhance productivity.

Astute leader–managers understand both the structure of the organization in which they work as well as external stakeholders. The integrated leader–manager, however, goes beyond personal understanding of the larger organizational design. The leader–manager takes responsibility for ensuring that subordinates also understand the overall organizational structure and the structure at the unit level. This can be done by being a resource and a role model to subordinates. The role modeling includes demonstrating accountability and the appropriate use of authority.

The effective manager recognizes the difficulties inherent in advisory positions and uses leadership skills to support staff in these positions. This is accomplished by granting sufficient authority to enable advisory staff to carry out the functions of their role.

Leadership requires that problems are pursued through appropriate channels, that upward communication is encouraged, and that unit structure is periodically evaluated to determine if it can be redesigned to enable increased lower-level decision making. The integrated leader–manager also facilitates constructive informal group structure. It is important for the manager to be knowledgeable about the organization's culture and subcultures. It is just as important for the leader to promote the development of a shared constructive culture with subordinates.

It is a management role to evaluate types of organizational structure and governance and to implement those that will have the most positive impact in the department. It is a leadership skill to role model the shared authority necessary to make newer models of organizational structure and governance possible.

When serving on committees, the opportunity should be used to gain influence to present the needs of patients and staff appropriately. The integrated leader–manager comes to meetings well prepared and contributes thoughtful comments and ideas. The leader's critical thinking and role-modeling behavior discourages groupthink among work groups or in committees.

Integrated leader–managers also refrain from judging and encourage all members of a committee to participate and contribute. An important management function is to see that appropriate work is accomplished in committees, that they remain productive, and that they are not used to delay decision making. A leadership role is the involvement of staff in organizational decision making, either informally or through more formal models of organizational design, such as shared governance. The integrated leader–manager understands the organization and recognizes what can be molded or shaped and what is constant. Thus, the interaction between the manager and the organization is dynamic.

Key Concepts

* Many modern health care organizations continue to be organized around a *line* or *line-and-staff* design and have many attributes of a bureaucracy; however, there is a movement toward less bureaucratic designs, such as ad hoc, matrix, or care-centered systems.
* A *bureaucracy*, as proposed by Max Weber, is characterized by a clear chain of command, rules and regulations, specialization of work, division of labor, and impersonality of relationships.
* An *organization chart* depicts formal relationships, channels of communication, and authority through line-and-staff positions, scalar chains, and span of control.
* *Unity of command* means that each person should have only one boss so that there is less confusion and greater productivity.
* *Centrality* refers to the degree of communication of a particular management position.
* In *centralized decision making,* decisions are made by a few managers at the top of the hierarchy. In *decentralized decision making,* decision making is diffused throughout the organization, and problems are solved at the lowest practical managerial level.
* Organizational structure affects how people perceive their roles and the status given to them by other people in the organization.
* Organizational structure is effective when the design is clearly communicated, there are as few managers as possible to accomplish goals, communication is facilitated, decisions are made at the lowest possible level, informal groups are encouraged, and future leaders are developed.
* The entities in an organization's environment that play a role in the organization's health and performance, or which are affected by the organization, are called *stakeholders.*
* *Authority, responsibility,* and *accountability* differ in terms of official sanctions, self-directedness, and moral integration.
* *Organizational culture* is the total of an organization's beliefs, history, taboos, formal and informal relationships, and communication patterns.
* Subunits of large organizations also have a culture. These subcultures may support or be in conflict with other cultures in the organization.
* Informal groups are present in every organization. They are often powerful, although they have no formal authority. Informal groups determine norms and assist members in the socialization process.
* *Shared governance* refers to an organizational design that empowers staff nurses by making them an integral part of patient care decision making and providing accountability and responsibility in nursing practice.
* *Magnet hospital status* is conferred by the ANCC on hospitals exemplifying well-qualified nurse executives in a decentralized environment, with organizational structures that emphasize open, participatory management. Magnet hospitals demonstrate improved patient outcomes and higher staff nurse satisfaction than nonmagnet hospitals.

* Too many committees in an organization is a sign of a poorly designed organizational structure.
* Committees should have an appropriate number of members, prepared agendas, clearly outlined tasks, and effective leadership if they are to be productive.
* *Groupthink* occurs when there is too much conformity to group norms.

ADDITIONAL LEARNING EXERCISES AND APPLICATIONS

LEARNING EXERCISE 12.5

Restructuring—In Depth

You are the supervisor at a home health agency. There are 22 RNs in your span of control. In a meeting today, John Dao, the CNO, tells you that your span of control needs adjustment to be effective. Therefore, the CNO has decided to decentralize the department. To accomplish this, he plans to designate three of your staff as shift coordinators. These shift coordinators will "schedule patient visits for all the staff on their shift and be accountable for the staff that they supervise." The CNO believes that this restructuring will give you more time for implementing a continuous quality improvement (CQI) program and promoting staff development.

Although you are glad to have the opportunity to begin these new projects, you are somewhat unclear about the role expectations of the new shift coordinators and how this will change your job description. Will these shift coordinators report to you? If so, will you have direct line authority or staff authority? Who should be responsible for evaluating the performance of the staff nurses now? Who will handle employee disciplinary problems? How involved should the shift coordinators be in strategic planning or determining next year's budget? What types of management training will be needed by the shift coordinators to prepare for their new role? Are you the most appropriate person to train them?

● ASSIGNMENT: There is great potential for conflict here. In small groups, make a list of 10 questions (not including the ones listed in the learning exercise) that you would want to ask the CNO at your next meeting to clarify role expectations. Discuss tools and skills that you have learned in the preceding units that could make this role change less traumatic for all involved.

LEARNING EXERCISE 12.6

Problem Solving: Working Toward Shared Governance

You are the supervisor of a surgical services department in a nonunion hospital. The staff on your unit have become increasingly frustrated with hospital policies regarding staffing ratios, on-call pay, and verbal medical orders but feel that they have limited opportunities for providing feedback to change the current system. You would like to explore the possibility of moving toward a shared governance model of decision making to resolve this issue and others like it but are not quite sure where to start.

(Learning Exercise continues on page 290)

● ASSIGNMENT: Assume that you are the supervisor in this case. Answer the following questions.

1. Who do I need to involve in this discussion and at what point?
2. How might I determine if the overarching organizational structure supports shared governance? How would I determine if external stakeholders would be impacted? How would I determine if organizational culture and subculture would support a shared governance model?
3. What types of nursing councils might be created to provide a framework for operation?
4. Who would be the members on these nursing councils?
5. What support mechanisms would need to be in place to ensure success of this project?
6. What would be my role as a supervisor in identifying and resolving employee concerns in a shared governance model?

LEARNING EXERCISE 12.7

Finding Direction

You are a new graduate working the 3 PM to 11 PM shift in a large, metropolitan hospital on the pediatrics unit. You feel frustrated because you had many preceptors while you were being oriented, and each told you slightly different variations of the unit routine. Additionally, the regular charge nurse has just been promoted and moved to another unit, and the charge nurse position on your unit is being filled by two part-time nurses.

You feel inadequate for the job and do not know where to turn or to whom you should direct your questions. Assuming that your organization chart resembles the one in Figure 12.1, outline a plan of action that would be appropriate to take. Share your plan with a larger group.

LEARNING EXERCISE 12.8

Thinking About Committee Work

As a writing exercise, choose one of the following to examine in depth:

1. What has contributed to the productivity of the committees on which you have served?
2. Have you ever served on a committee that made recommendations on which higher authority never acted? What was the effect on the group?

LEARNING EXERCISE 12.9

Participation and Productivity

You are a 3 PM to 11 PM charge nurse on a surgical unit. You have been selected to chair the unit's safety committee. Each month, you have a short committee meeting with the other committee members. Your committee's main responsibility is to report upward any safety issues that have been identified. Lately, you have found an increase in needle-stick incidents, and the committee has been addressing this problem.

The committee is made up of two nursing assistants, one unit clerk, two staff RNs, and two LPN/LVNs. All shifts and staff cultures are represented. Lately, you have found that the meetings are not going well because one member of the group, Mary, has begun to monopolize the meeting time. She is especially outspoken about the danger of HIV and seems more interested in pointing blame regarding the needle sticks than in finding a solution to the problem.

You have privately spoken to Mary about her frequent disruption of the committee business; although she apologized, the behavior has continued. You feel that some members of the committee are becoming bored and restless, and you believe that the committee is making little progress.

● ASSIGNMENT: Using your knowledge of committee structure and effectiveness, outline steps that you would take to facilitate more group participation and make the committee more productive. Be specific, and explain exactly what you would do at the next meeting to prevent Mary from taking over the meeting.

Web Links

American Nurses Credentialing Center
http://www.nursingworld.org/ancc/magnet.html
Frequently asked questions about magnet hospital status as well as current list of magnet hospitals.

Organizational Charts
http://ftp.fcc.gov/fccorgchart.html
Site shows a typical government (Federal Communications Commission) organization chart.

Max Weber, 1864–1920
http://cepa.newschool.edu/het/profiles/weber.htm
Photo, biography, and major works of sociologist and economist Max Weber.

References

American Nurses Credentialing Center. (2006a). *ANCC Magnet Recognition Program.* Retrieved January 7, 2007, from *http://www.nursing/world.org/MainMenuCategories/CertificationandAccreditation/Magnet-aspt*

American Nurses Credentialing Center (2006b). *Frequently asked questions.* Retrieved September 29, 2006, from *http://www.nursecredentialing.org/magnet/facilities.html.*

Black, K. (2003). Recruitment & retention report. Innovative programs grab a thumbs up. *Nursing Management, 34*(6), 19–20, 22.

Bumgarner, S. D., & Beard, E. L. (2003). The magnet application: Pitfalls to avoid. *Journal of Nursing Administration, 33*(11), 603–606.

Campbell, S. L., Fowles, E. R., & Weber, B. J. (2004). Organizational structure and job satisfaction in public health nursing. *Public Health Nursing, 21*(6), 564–571.

Caramanica, L. (2004). Shared governance: Hartford Hospital's experience. *Online Journal of Issues in Nursing, 9*(1), 1–7.

Drenkard, K. N. (2005). Sustaining magnet: Keeping forces alive. *Nursing Administration Quarterly, 29*(3), 214–222.

Fayol, H. (1949). *General and industrial management* (C. Storrs, Trans.). London: Isaac Pittman and Sons.

Hess, R. G. (2004). From bedside to boardroom—Nursing shared governance. *Online Journal of Issues in Nursing, 9*(1), 1–10.

Huston, C. (2006). The current nursing shortage: Causes, consequences and solutions. In C. Huston (Ed.), *Professional issues in nursing.* Philadelphia: Lippincott Williams & Wilkins.

Kane-Urrabazo, C. (2006). Management's role in shaping organizational culture. *Journal of Nursing Management, 14*(3), 188–194.

Kramer, M., & Schmalenberg, C. E. (2004). Essentials of a magnetic work environment: Part 2. *Nursing, 34*(7),44–47.

Kramer, M., & Schmalenberg, C. E. (2005). Best quality patient care: A historical perspective on magnet hospitals. *Nursing Administration Quarterly, 29*(3), 275–287.

Lockyer, J. (2005). An analysis of the development of a successful medical collaboration to create and sustain family physician anaesthesiology capacity in rural Canada. *Australian Journal of Rural Health, 13*(3), 178–182.

McConnell, C. R. (2005). Larger, smaller and flatter. *The Health Care Manager, 24*(2), 177–189.

Pinkerton, S. (2006). Retention and recruitment. Stories as motivators. *Nursing Economics*, 24(3), 166–167.

Upenieks, V. V. (2003). What's the attraction to magnet hospitals? *Nursing Management*, 34(2), 43–44.

Wake Forest University Baptist Medical Center. (n.d.). *Shared governance*. Retrieved November 20, 2003, from *http://www.wfubmc.edu/Nursing/Shared+Governance*.

Waters, V. L. (2004). Cultivate corporate culture and diversity: Create and maintain a thriving environment in the midst of institutional change. *Nursing Management*, 35(1), 36–37, 50.

Way, M. (2006). Organizational characteristics and their effect on health. *Nursing Economics*, 24(2), 67–77.

Waymack, P. M. (2005). Managed care. Exit strategies: planning for contract termination. *Healthcare Financial Management*, 59(11), 50–52.

Wooten, L. P., & Crane, P. (2003). Nurses as implementers of organizational culture. *Nursing Economic$*, 21(6), 275–279.

Bibliography

Anthony, M. K. (2004). Shared governance models: The theory, practice and evidence. *Online Journal of Nursing*, 9(1), 1–13.

Batson, V. (2004). Home study program. Shared governance in an integrated health care network. *AORN*, 80(3), 493–496.

Carney, M. (2004). Middle manager involvement in strategy development in not-for-profit organizations: The director of nursing perspective—How organizational structure impacts the role. *Journal of Nursing Management*, 12(1), 13–21.

Clark, M. L. (2006). The Magnet recognition program and evidence-based practice. *Journal of Perianesthesia Nursing*, 21(3), 186–189.

Gershon, R. R., Stone, P. W., Bakken, S., & Larson, E. (2004). Measurement of organizational culture and climate in healthcare. *Journal of Nursing Administration*, 34(1), 33–40.

Henderson, A., Winch, S., Henney, R., McCoy, R., & Grugan, C. (2005). Working from the inside: An infrastructure for the continuing development of nurses' professional clinical practice. *Journal of Nursing Management*, 13(2), 106–110.

Hill, V. L. (2004). Cultivate corporate culture and diversity. *Nursing Management*, 35(1), 36–37, 50.

Kerfoot, K. (2005). On leadership. Compliance leadership: the 17th century model that doesn't work. *Urological Nursing*, 25(2), 131–133.

Kroposki, M., & Alexander, J. W. (2004). Workplace variables and their relationship to quality client outcomes in home health. *Public Health Nursing*, 21(6), 555–563.

Rutherford, J., Leigh, J., Monk, J., & Murray, C. (2005). Creating an organizational infrastructure to develop and support new nursing roles—A framework for debate. *Journal of Nursing Management*, 13(2), 97–105.

Shirely, M. R. (2005). Celebrating certification in nursing: Forces of magnetism in action. *Nursing Administration Quarterly*, 29(3), 245–253.

Taylor, N. T. (2005). The magnet pull. *Nursing Management*, 36(7), 45–48.

13

Understanding Organizational, Political, and Personal Power

. . . power is a positive concept, and several types of power are prerequisite for human development and self-expression.

—Sue Thomas Hegyvary

Chapter 12 reviewed organizational structure and introduced status, authority, and responsibility at different levels of the organizational hierarchy. In this chapter, the organization is examined further, with emphasis on the management functions and leadership roles inherent in effective use of authority, establishment of a personal power base, empowerment of staff, and the impact of organizational politics on power.

The word *power* is derived from the Latin verb *potere* (to be able); thus, power may be appropriately defined as that which enables one to accomplish goals. Power can also be defined as the capacity to act or the strength and potency to accomplish something. A person or group with power can possibly influence attitudes and behaviors.

 Having power gives one the potential to change the attitudes and behaviors of individual people and groups.

Authority, or the right to command, accompanies any management position and is a source of legitimate power, although components of management, authority, and power are also necessary, to a degree, for successful leadership. The manager who is knowledgeable about the wise use of authority, power, and political strategy is more effective at meeting personal, unit, and organizational goals. Likewise, powerful leaders are able to raise morale because they delegate more and build with a team effort. Thus, their followers become part of the growth and excitement of the organization as their own status is enhanced. The leadership roles and management functions inherent in the use of authority and power are shown in Display 13.1.

DISPLAY 13.1 Leadership Roles and Management Functions Associated With Understanding Organizational, Political, and Personal Power

Leadership Roles

1. Creates a climate that promotes followership in response to authority
2. Recognizes the dual pyramid of power that exists between the organization and its employees
3. Uses a powerful persona to increase respect and decrease fear in subordinates
4. Recognizes when it is appropriate to have authority questioned or to question authority
5. Is personally comfortable with power in the political arena
6. Empowers other nurses
7. Assists staff in using appropriate political strategies

Management Functions

1. Uses authority to ensure that organizational goals are met
2. Uses political strategies that are complementary to the unit and organization's functioning
3. Builds a power base adequate for the assigned management role
4. Maintains a small authority–power gap
5. Is knowledgeable about the essence and appropriate use of power
6. Maintains personal credibility with subordinates
7. Serves as a role model of the empowered nurse

UNDERSTANDING POWER

Power may be feared, worshipped, or mistrusted. It is frequently misunderstood. Our first experience with power usually occurs in the family unit. Power, in most ordinary uses of the term, appears to be more aligned with male than with female stereotypes (Robb, 2004). Because children's roles are likened to later subordinate roles and the parental power position is similar to management, adult views of the management–subordinate relationship are influenced by how power was used in the family unit. A positive or negative familial power experience may greatly affect a person's ability to deal with power systems in adulthood.

Gender and Power

Successful leaders are aware of their views on the use and abuse of power. Some women, in particular, may hold negative connotations of power and never learn to use power constructively. Women have traditionally demonstrated, at best, ambivalence toward the concept of power, and until recently, some have openly eschewed the pursuit of power. This may have occurred because women as a whole have been socialized to view power differently than men do. For some women, power may be viewed as dominance versus submission; associated with personal qualities, not accomplishment; and dependent on personal or physical attributes, not skill. Many women may not believe that they inherently possess power but instead must rely on others to acquire it. Rather than feeling capable of achieving and managing power, some women may feel that power manages them (Huston, 2006).

However, the historical view of women as less powerful than men appears to be changing. In today's world, people are finding new ways for leaders to acquire and manage power. These changes are taking place within women, in women's view of other women holding power, in organizational hierarchies, and among male subordinates and male colleagues (Houghton, 2004; Huston, 2006).

> Today, gender differences regarding power are fading, and the corporate world is beginning to look at new ways for leaders to obtain and handle power.

Robb (2004) maintains that there is a revival among academics to show there are real differences in gender and that these differences, especially in communication styles, can help an organization be successful. It is possible that nurse–leaders in the 21st century will need to deal with organizational power and politics in a completely different way and will need to develop political strategies for team building and establishing trust. Leadership behavior that promotes group power will be especially valued as a means to gain political clout (Sieloff, 2004). Political skill in developing consensus, inclusion, and involvement are also needed—skills that have often been linked to female characteristics.

It is notable that these very attributes, which once closed corporate doors and created the barrier popularly called the *glass ceiling*, are now welcomed in the boardroom. These attributes are certainly not limited to women; many male leaders also possess these characteristics. However, despite significant gains, many women continue to remain unskilled in the art of the political process. While the view of men and women as being powerful has gradually changed over the years, it is reasonable to maintain that men are stereotypically viewed as the more powerful in health care organizations (Ceci, 2004).

LEARNING EXERCISE 13.1

Is Power Different for Men and Women?

Research studies differ on how men and women view power and how others view men and women in positions of authority. Do you think that there are gender differences in how people are viewed as being powerful? Discuss this in a group, and then go to the library or use Internet sources to see if you can find recent studies that support your views.

Politics is the art of using legitimate power wisely. It requires clear decision making, assertiveness, accountability, and the willingness to express one's own views. It also requires being proactive rather than reactive and demands decisiveness. Women in power positions in today's health care settings are more likely to recognize their innate abilities that support the effective use of power.

In determining whether power is "good" or "bad," it may be helpful to look at its opposite: *powerlessness*. Most people agree that they dislike being powerless. Everyone needs some control in life. Powerlessness tends to breed bossiness. Thus, the leader–manager who feels powerless often creates an ineffective, petty, dictatorial, and rule-minded management style. Individuals who feel powerless become bossy and rules-oriented. They may become oppressive leaders, punitive and rigid in decision making, or withhold information from others, and they become difficult to work with. Although the adage that power corrupts might be true for some, it may be more correct to say that powerlessness, not power, corrupts.

> Power is likely to bring more power in an ascending cycle, whereas powerlessness will only generate more powerlessness.

Because the powerful have credibility to support their actions, they have greater capacity to get things accomplished and can enhance their base. As managers gain power, they are less coercive and rule bound; thus, their peers and subordinates are more cooperative.

Apparently, then, power has a negative and a positive face. The negative face of power is the "I win, you lose" aspect of dominance versus submission. The positive face of power occurs when someone exerts influence on behalf of—rather than over—someone or something. Hegyvary (2003) maintains that several types of power are prerequisite for self-expression and human development. Power, therefore, is not good or evil; how it is used and for what purpose it is used determine if it is good or evil.

Types of Power

For leadership to be effective, some measure of power must often support it. This is true for the informal social group and the formal work group. French and Raven (1959), in their classic work, postulate that several bases, or sources, exist for the exercise of power: reward power, punishment or coercive power, legitimate power, expert power, and referent power.

Reward power is obtained by the ability to grant favors or reward others with whatever they value. The arsenal of rewards that a manager can dispense to get employees to work toward meeting organizational goals is very broad. Positive leadership through rewards tends to develop a great deal of loyalty and devotion toward leaders.

Punishment or *coercive power*, the opposite of reward power, is based on fear of punishment if the manager's expectations are not met. The manager may obtain compliance through threats (often implied) of transfer, layoff, demotion, or dismissal. The manager who shuns or ignores an employee is exercising power through punishment, as is the manager who berates or belittles an employee.

Legitimate power is position power. Authority also is called legitimate power. It is the power gained by a title or official position within an organization. Legitimate power has inherent in it the ability to create feelings of obligation or responsibility. As previously discussed, the socialization and culture of subordinate employees will influence to some degree how much power a manager has due to his or her position.

Expert power is gained through knowledge, expertise, or experience. Having critical knowledge allows a manager to gain power over others who need that knowledge. This type of power is limited to a specialized area. For example, someone with vast expertise in music would be powerful only in that area, not in another specialization. When Florence Nightingale used research to quantify the need for nurses in the Crimea (by showing that when nurses were present, fewer soldiers died), she was using her research to demonstrate expertise in the health needs of the wounded. Power derived from expert knowledge is fundamental for any profession (Hegyvary, 2003).

Referent power is power that a person has because others identify with that leader or with what that leader symbolizes. Referent power also occurs when one gives another person feelings of personal acceptance or approval. It may be obtained through association with the powerful. People also may develop referent power because others perceive them as powerful. This perception could be based on personal charisma, the way the leader talks or acts, the organizations to which he or she belongs, or the people with whom he or she associates. People who

TABLE 13.1 **Sources of Power**

Type	Source
Referent	Association with others
Legitimate	Position
Coercive	Fear
Reward	Ability to grant favors
Expert	Knowledge and skill
Charismatic	Personal
Informational	The need for information
Self	Maturity, ego strength

others accept as role models or leaders enjoy referent power. Physicians use referent power very effectively; society, as a whole, views physicians as powerful, and physicians carefully maintain this image.

Although correlated with referent power, *charismatic power* is distinguished by some from referent power. Referent power is gained only through association with powerful others, whereas charisma is a more personal type of power.

Heineken and McCloskey (1985) add another type of power to the French and Raven power sources by identifying *informational power*. This source of power is obtained when people have information that others must have to accomplish their goals. Morrison (1988) refers to all these types of power as patriarchal in that they imply power over others. Morrison prefers a power defined as *feminist power* or *self-power*—the power a person gains over his or her own life—and maintains that this power is a personal power that comes from maturity, ego integration, security in relationships, and confidence in one's impulse. The various sources of power are summarized in Table 13.1.

THE AUTHORITY–POWER GAP

If authority is the right to command, then a logical question is, "Why do workers sometimes not follow orders?" The right to command does not ensure that employees will follow orders. The gap that sometimes exists between a position of authority and subordinate response is called the *authority–power gap*. The term *manager power* may explain subordinates' response to the manager's authority. The more power subordinates perceive a manager to have, the smaller the gap between the right to expect certain things and the resulting fulfillment of those expectations by others.

The negative effect of a wide authority–power gap is that organizational chaos may develop. There would be little productivity if every order were questioned. The organization should rightfully expect that its goals would be accomplished. One of the core dynamics of civilization is that there will always be a few authority figures pushing the many for a certain standard of performance.

People in the United States are socialized very early to respond to authority figures. In many cases, children are conditioned to accept the directives of their parents, teachers, and community leaders. The traditional nurse–educator has been portrayed as an authoritarian who demands unconditional obedience. Educators who maintain a very narrow authority–power gap reinforce dependency and obedience by emphasizing the ultimate calamity—the death of the patient. Thus, nursing students may be socialized to be overly cautious and to hesitate when making independent nursing judgments.

Because of these types of early socialization, the gap between the manager's authority and the worker's response to that authority tends to be relatively small. In other countries, it may be larger or smaller, depending on how people are socialized to respond to authority. This authority dependence that begins with our parents and is later transferred to our employers may be an important resource to managers.

Although the authority–power gap continues to be narrow, it has grown in the last 20 years. Both the women's movement and the student unrest of the 1960s have contributed to the widening of the authority–power gap. This widening gap was evident when a 1970s college student asked her mother why she did not protest as a college student; the mother replied, "I didn't know I could."

At times, however, authority should be questioned by either the leader or the subordinates. This is demonstrated in health care by the increased questioning of the authority of physicians—many of whom feel they have the authority to command—by nurses and consumers. Figure 13.1 shows the dynamics of the relationships in the organizational authority–power response.

LEARNING EXERCISE 13.2

Power and Authority

Think back to your childhood. Who do you feel was most powerful in your family? Why do you think that person was powerful? If you are using group work, how many in your group named powerful male figures; how many named powerful female figures?

Did you grow up with a very narrow authority–power gap? Have your views regarding authority and power changed since you were a child? Do you believe that children today have an authority–power gap similar to what you had as a child? Support your answers with examples.

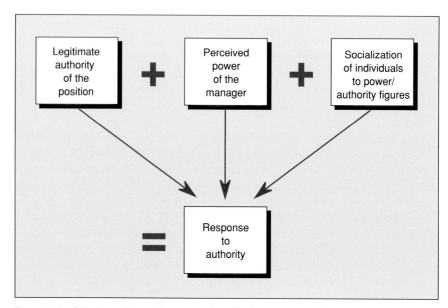

Figure 13.1   Interdependency of response to authority.

Bridging the Authority–Power Gap

Sometimes subordinates feel badgered by very visible exercises of authority (which should be used only as a last resort). Because overusing commands can stifle cooperation, outright naked commands should be used infrequently.

Visual displays of authority should be used as a last resort.

A way for the leader to bridge the gap is to make a genuine effort to know and care about each subordinate as a unique individual. This is especially important because each person has a limited tolerance of authority, and subordinates are better able to tolerate authority if they believe that the leader cares about them as individuals.

The manager needs to provide enough information about organizational and unit goals to subordinates so that they understand how their efforts and those of their manager are contributing to goal attainment. The manager will have bridged the authority–power gap if followers (a) perceive that the manager is doing a good job, (b) believe that the organization has their best interests in mind, and (c) do not feel controlled by authority.

Finally, the manager must be seen as credible for the authority–power gap not to widen. All managers begin their appointment with subordinates ready to believe them. This, again, is due to the socialization process that causes people to believe that those in power say what is true. However, the deference to authority will erode if managers handle employees carelessly, are dishonest, or seem incapable of carrying out their duties. When a manager loses credibility, the power inherent in his or her authority decreases.

Another dimension of credibility that influences the authority–power relationship is *future promising*. It is best to underpromise if promises must be made. Managers should never guarantee future rewards unless they have control of all possible variables. If managers revoke future rewards, they lose credibility in the eyes of their subordinates. However, managers should dispense present rewards to buy patronage, making the manager more believable and building greater power into his or her legitimate authority. A scenario that illustrates the difference in dispensing future and present awards follows.

An RN requests a day off to attend a wedding, and you are able to replace her. You use the power of your position to reward her and give her the day off. The RN is grateful to you, and this increases your power.

Another RN requests 3 months in advance to have every Thursday off in the summer to take a class. Although you promise this to her, on the first day of June, three nurses resign, rendering you unable to fulfill your promise. This nurse is very upset, and you have lost much credibility and, therefore, power. It would have been wiser for you to say that you could not grant her original request (underpromising) or to make it contingent on several factors. If the situation had remained the same and the nurses had not resigned, you could have granted the request. Less trust is lost between the manager and the subordinate when underpromising occurs than when a granted request is rescinded, as long as the subordinate believes that the manager will make a genuine effort to meet his or her request.

Empowering Subordinates

The empowerment of staff is a hallmark of transformational leadership. To empower means to enable, develop, or allow. *Empowerment*, as discussed in Chapter 2, can be defined as decentralization

EXAMINING THE EVIDENCE 13.1

Source: DeSisto, M. C., & DeSisto, T. P. (2004). School nurses' perceptions of empowerment and autonomy. *Journal of School Nursing, 20*(4), 228–233.

This study used Kanter's Theory of Structural Power in Organizations to determine if there was a relationship between school nurses' perception of empowerment and autonomy. The nurses perceived themselves to have a high degree of autonomy and a moderate degree of empowerment and reported that their access to informal power structures was greater than access to formal power structures in their school systems.

of power. Empowerment occurs when leaders communicate their vision, employees are given the opportunity to make the most of their talents, and learning, creativity, and exploration are encouraged. Empowerment plants seeds of leadership, collegiality, self-respect, and professionalism. Hegyvary (2003) maintains that nurses are empowered through nursing knowledge and research, which then frees staff from mechanistic thinking and encourages critical thinking, problem solving, and the application of knowledge to practice.

In their research on school nurses' perception of empowerment, DeSisto and DeSisto (2004) found that when job demands are balanced with control over decisions, job strain is decreased (Examining the Evidence 13.1). Their research suggests that empowered employees have management support, which in turn encourages them to act on their expertise and judgment.

Empowerment is not an easy one-step process but a complex process that consists of responsibility for the individual desiring empowerment as well as the organization and its leadership. Individually, all practitioners must have professional traits, including responsibility for continuing education, participation in professional organizations, political activism, and most importantly, a sense of value about their work. Additionally, the nurse must work in an environment that encourages empowerment, and the empowerment process must include an effective leadership style. The leader–manager must be someone who nurtures the development of an empowered staff. If all these elements are present, there is a greater chance that the environment will foster the empowering process, which in turn leads to a sense of autonomy (DeSisto & DeSisto, 2004).

Leaders empower subordinates when they delegate assignments to provide learning opportunities and allow employees to share in the satisfaction derived from achievement. Empowerment is not the relinquishing of rightful power inherent in a position, nor is it a delegation of authority or its commensurate responsibility and accountability. Instead, the actions of empowered staff are freely chosen, owned, and committed to on behalf of the organization without any requests or requirements to do so.

Empowerment creates and sustains a work environment that speaks to values, such as facilitating the employee's choice to invest in and own personal actions and behaviors that result in positive contributions to the organization's mission.

Valadares (2004) posits that "while the notion of employee empowerment is by itself noble, for it to succeed, health care organizations must promote a culture of psychological safety to ensure genuine commitment exists to its mission and strategies" (p. 220).

However, not having a commitment to empowerment is only one of many barriers to creating an environment for empowerment in an organization. Other barriers would include a rigid organizational belief about authority and status. As well, a manager's personal feelings regarding empowerment's potential effect on the manager's own power can also impede the empowering process.

Once organizational barriers have been minimized or eliminated, the leader–manager should develop strategies at the unit level to empower staff. The easiest strategy is to be a role model of an empowered nurse. Another strategy would be to assist staff in building their own personal power base. This can be accomplished by showing subordinates how their personal, expert, and referent power can be expanded. Empowerment also occurs when subordinates are involved in planning and implementing change; subordinates believe that they have some input in what is about to happen to them and some control over the environment in which they will work in the future.

LEARNING EXERCISE 13.3

Cultural Diversity
Do you think that cultural diversity might be a challenge when empowering nurses? Think of ways that various cultures may view power and empowerment differently. If you know people from other cultures, ask them how powerful people or those in authority positions are viewed in their culture and compare that with your own culture.

MOBILIZING THE POWER OF NURSING

Until the nursing profession has a seat at the health care policy-making table, individual nurses and leader–managers will be limited in how much personal power they will hold. Grindel (2006) feels that nursing has not been the force it could be and sites many reasons: lack of nurses' interest, interorganization power struggles, lack of leadership, and lack of insight in how to build coalitions.

Huston (2006) concurs, stating that nurses have often been reactive rather than proactive in addressing policy decisions and legislation after the fact rather than taking part in drafting and sponsoring legislation. However, she cites several driving forces that should increase nursing's power base (Display 13.2).

DISPLAY 13.2 Five Driving Forces to Increase Nursing's Power Base

1. Right timing
2. Size of the nursing profession
3. Increasing knowledge base and education for nurses
4. Nursing's unique perspective
5. Desire of consumers and providers for change

Source: Courtesy of Huston, C. (2006). The nursing profession's historic struggle to increase its power base. In C. Huston (Ed.), *Professional issues in nursing*. Philadelphia: Lippincott Williams & Wilkins. Used with permission.

- *Right timing.* The errors reported in our medical system, the numbers of uninsured, and problems with our health insurance system are all reasons that consumers and legislators are willing to listen to nurses as an attempt is made to fix the health care crisis.
- *Size of the nursing profession.* Numbers are very important in politics, and the nursing profession's size is its greatest asset. The United States has 2.7 million RNs, which represents an impressive voting block.
- *Increasing knowledge base and education for nurses.* There are more nurses being awarded master's and doctoral degrees than ever before. If knowledge is power, then those having knowledge can influence others, gain credibility, and gain power.
- *Nursing's unique perspective.* Nursing has long been recognized as having a strong caring component. Combine that with nursing's recent surge in scientific knowledge and critical thinking, and there is a blend of art and science that brings a unique perspective to the health care arena.
- *Desire of consumers and providers for change.* Health care restructuring and downsizing have sparked increasing concern among consumers. The public cares about who is taking care of them. The public wants quality care.

Huston (2006) also developed an action plan for the nursing profession to build its power base (Display 13.3 shows a summary of action). These include:

- *Place more nurses in positions that influence public policy.* Holding office is the ultimate in political activism. Nurses are uniquely qualified to hold office, and more nurses need to seek this role.
- *Stop acting like victims.* Unhappy nurses tend to look like victims. That is not to say that nurses have not been victimized in the past, but nurses need to address the cause of their unhappiness and attempt to alleviate the problem. They can confront situations, change jobs, or move into a different career path. Motivated people who care about their profession will help to bring power to nursing.
- *Become better informed about all health care policy efforts.* This means becoming involved with grassroots knowledge building—becoming better-informed consumers and providers of health care with a commitment to collective strength.
- *Build coalitions inside and outside of nursing.* There are a multitude of professional organizations related to health care and to nursing. In addition to belonging to nursing

DISPLAY 13.3 Action Plan for Increasing the Power of the Nursing Profession

1. Place more nurses in positions that influence public policy.
2. Stop nurses from acting like victims.
3. Increase level of nurses' understanding regarding all health care policy efforts.
4. Build coalitions within and outside of nursing.
5. Promote greater research to strengthen evidence-based practice.
6. Support nursing leaders.
7. Pay attention to mentoring future nurse–leaders and leadership succession.

Source: Huston, C. (2006). The nursing profession's historic struggle to increase its power base. In C. Huston (Ed.), *Professional issues in nursing. Philadelphia*: Lippincott Williams & Wilkins. Used with permission.

professional organizations, nurses need to reach out to other non-nursing groups that share the same concerns and goals. Remember, there is strength in numbers.

• *Conduct more research to strengthen evidence-based practice.* Research what nurses do that makes a difference. Use research to present the case that nursing skills are vital to competent health care. Building evidence-based practice will require a greater number of well-educated nurses prepared at the master and doctoral levels.

• *Support nursing leaders.* Rather than supporting their leaders' efforts to lead, nurses have often viewed their leaders as deviants. There is a proper arena for conflict and disagreement, but the position presented to the public must be of nursing unity and direction.

• *Mentor future nurse–leaders and plan for leadership succession.* Female-dominated professions often exemplify the *queen bee syndrome.* The queen bee is a woman who has struggled to become successful, but once successful, she refuses to help other women reach the same success. Increased and adequate empowering of others, mentoring the young, and ensuring leadership succession is clearly needed to advance nursing leadership.

STRATEGIES FOR BUILDING A PERSONAL POWER BASE

In addition to assisting with empowering the profession, nurse–leaders and nurse–managers must build a personal power base to further organizational goals, fulfill the leadership role, carry out management functions, and meet personal goals. A beginning manager or even a newly graduated nurse can begin to build a power base in many ways. Habitual behaviors resulting from early lessons, passivity, and focusing on wrong targets can be replaced with new power-gaining behaviors. The following are suggested strategies for enhancing power.

Maintain Personal Energy

Power and energy go hand in hand. Effective leaders take sufficient time to unwind, reflect, rest, and have fun when they feel tired. Managers who do not take care of themselves begin to make mistakes in judgment that may result in terrible political consequences. Taking time for significant relationships and developing outside interests are important so that other resources are available for sustenance when political forces in the organization drain energy.

Present a Powerful Picture to Others

How people look, act, and talk influence whether others view them as powerful or powerless. The nurse who stands tall and is poised, assertive, articulate, and well groomed presents a picture of personal control and power. The manager who looks like a victim will undoubtedly become one.

Pay the Entry Fee

Newcomers who stand out and appear powerful are those who do more, work harder, and contribute to the organization. They are not clock watchers or "nine-to-fivers." They attend meetings and in-service opportunities; they do committee work and take their share of night shifts and weekend and holiday assignments without complaining. A power base is not achieved by slick, easy, or quick maneuvers but through hard work.

Determine the Powerful in the Organization

Understanding and working within the formal and informal power structures are necessary. People must be cognizant of their limitations and seek counsel appropriately. One should know the names and faces of those with both formal and informal power. The powerful people in the informal structure are often more difficult to identify than those in the formal structure. When working with powerful people, look for similarities and shared values and avoid focusing on differences.

Learn the Language and Symbols of the Organization

Each organization has its own culture and value system. New members must understand this culture and be socialized into the organization if they are to build a power base. Being unaware of institutional taboos and sacred cows often results in embarrassment for the newcomer.

Learn How to Use the Organization's Priorities

Every group has its own goals and priorities for achieving those goals. Those seeking to build a power base must be cognizant of organizational goals and use those priorities and goals to meet management needs. For example, a need for a new manager in a community health service might be to develop educational programs on chemotherapy because some of the new patient caseload includes this nursing function. If fiscal management is a high priority, the manager needs to show superiors how the cost of these educational programs will be offset by additional revenues. If public relations with physicians and patients are a priority, the manager would justify the same request in terms of additional services to patients and physicians.

Increase Professional Skills and Knowledge

Because employees are expected to perform their jobs well, one's performance must be extraordinary to enhance power. One method of being extraordinary is to increase professional skills and knowledge to an expert level. Having knowledge and skill that others lack greatly augments a person's power base. Excellence that reflects knowledge and demonstrates skill enhances a nurse's credibility and determines how others view him or her.

Maintain a Broad Vision

Because people are assigned to a unit or department, they often develop a narrow view of the total organization. Power builders always look upward and outward. The successful manager recognizes not only how the individual unit fits within the larger organization but also how the institution as a whole fits into the scheme of the total community. People without vision rarely become very powerful.

Use Experts and Seek Counsel

Newcomers should seek out role models. By looking to others for advice and counsel, people demonstrate that they are willing to be team players, that they are cautious and want expert opinion before proceeding, and that they are not rash newcomers who think they have all the answers. Aligning oneself with appropriate veterans in the organization is excellent for building power.

Be Flexible

Anyone wishing to acquire power should develop a reputation as someone who can compromise. The rigid, uncompromising newcomer is viewed as being insensitive to the organization's needs.

Develop Visibility and a Voice in the Organization

Newcomers must become active in committees or groups that are recognized by the organization as having clout. When working in groups, the newcomer must not monopolize committee time. Novice leaders and managers must develop observational, listening, and verbal skills. Their spoken contributions to the committee should be valuable and articulated well.

Learn to Toot Your Own Horn

Accepting compliments is an art. One should be gracious but certainly not passive when praised for extraordinary effort. Additionally, people should let others know when some special professional recognition has been achieved. This should be done in a manner that is not bragging but reflects the self-respect of one who is talented and unique.

Maintain a Sense of Humor

Appropriate humor is very effective. The ability to laugh at oneself and not take oneself too seriously is a most important power builder.

Empower Others

Leaders need to empower others, and followers must empower their leaders. When nurses empower each other, they gain referent power. Individual nurses and the profession as a whole do not gain their share of power because they allow others to divide them and weaken them. Nurses can empower other nurses by sharing knowledge, maintaining cohesiveness, valuing the profession, and supporting each other. Power-building and political strategies are summarized in Display 13.4.

DISPLAY 13.4   Leadership Strategies: Developing Power and Political Savvy

Power-Building Strategies	Political Strategies
Maintain personal energy	Develop information acquisition skills
Present a powerful persona	Communicate astutely
Pay the entry fee	Become proactive
Determine the powerful	Assume authority
Learn the organizational culture	Network
Use organizational priorities	Expand personal resources
Increase skills and knowledge	Maintain maneuverability
Have a broad vision	Remain sensitive to people, timing, and
Use experts and seek counsel	situations
Be flexible	Promote subordinates' identities
Be visible and have a voice	Meet organizational needs
Toot your own horn	Expand personal wellness
Maintain a sense of humor	
Empower others	

LEARNING EXERCISE 13.4

Building Power as the New Nurse

You have been an RN for 3 years. Six months ago, you left your position as a day charge nurse at one of the local hospitals to accept a position at the public health agency. You really miss your friends at the hospital and find most of the public health nurses older and aloof. However, you love working with your patients and have decided that this is where you want to build a lifetime career. Although you believe you have some good ideas, you are aware that because you are new, you will probably not be able to act as change agent yet. Eventually, you would like to be promoted to agency supervisor and become a powerful force for stimulating growth within the agency. You decide that you can do a few things to build a power base. You spend a weekend plotting your political design.

● ASSIGNMENT: Make a power-building plan. Give six to ten specific examples of things you would do to build a power base in the new organization. Provide rationale for each selection. (Do not merely select from the general lists in the text. Outline specific actions that you would take.) It might be helpful to consider your own community and personal strengths when solving this learning exercise.

THE POLITICS OF POWER

Earlier in this chapter, *politics* was defined as the effective use of power or the art of using power. There continues to be a lack of empirical research to assist nurses within organizations to improve their power position; however, there are many strategies that are politically wise. Sieloff (2004) has identified two leadership behaviors (power competency and power prospective) that foster group power, and Houser (2005) addresses the power that comes with collaboration.

It is also important for managers to understand politics within the context of their employing organization. After the employee has built a power base through hard work, increased personal power, and knowledge of the organization, developing skills in the politics of power is necessary. After all, power may not be gained indefinitely; it may be fleeting. For example, people often lose hard-earned power in an organization because they make political mistakes. Even seasoned leaders occasionally blunder in this arena.

 Although power is a universally available resource, it does not have a finite quality and can be lost as well as gained.

It is useless to argue the ethics or value of politics in an organization, because politics exists in every organization. Thus, nurses waste energy and remain powerless when they refuse to learn the art and skill of political maneuvers. Politics becomes divisive only whenever gossip, rumor, or unethical strategies occur.

Much attention is given to improving competence, but little time is spent in learning the intricacies of political behavior. The most important strategy is to learn to "read the environment" (e.g., understand relationships within the organization) through observation, listening, reading, detachment, and analysis. Sieloff (2004) maintains, "When organizational and group relationships are developed and fostered in order to achieve a group's goals, these relationships increase a group's level of power. The relationships enable a group to access communication, information and resources beyond those that a group could access without those relationships" (p. 250).

Because power implies interdependence, nurses must not only understand the organizational structure in which they work but also be able to function effectively within that structure, including dealing effectively with the institution's inherent politics. Only when managers understand power and politics will they be capable of recognizing limitations and potential for change. Understanding one's own power can be frightening, especially when one considers that "attacks" (or opposition) from various fronts may reduce that power. When these attacks occur, people who hold powerful positions may undermine themselves by regressing rather than progressing and by being reactive rather than proactive. The following political strategies will help the novice manager to negate the negative effects of organizational politics:

- *Become an expert handler of information and communication.* Beware that facts can be presented seductively and out of context. Be cautious in accepting facts as presented, because information is often changed to fit others' needs. Managers must become artful at acquiring information and questioning others. Delay decisions until adequate and accurate information has been gathered and reviewed. Failing to do the necessary homework may lead to decisions with damaging political consequences. Managers must not trap themselves by discussing something about which they know very little. Political astuteness in communication is a skill to be mastered, and the politically astute manager says, "I don't know" when adequate information is unavailable. Grave consequences can result from sharing the wrong information with the wrong people at the wrong time. Determining who should know, how much they should know, and when they should know requires great finesse. One of the most politically serious errors that one can make is lying to others within the organization. Unlike withholding and refusing to divulge information, which may be good political strategies, lying destroys trust, and leaders must never underestimate the power of trust.

- *Be a proactive decision maker.* Nurses have had such a long history of being reactive that they have had little time to learn how to be proactive. Although being reactive is better than being passive, being proactive means getting the job done better, faster, and more efficiently. Proactive leaders prepare for the future instead of waiting for it. Seeing changes approaching in the health care system, they prepare to meet them, not fight them. Assuming authority is one way that nurses can become proactive. Part of power is the image of power; a powerful political strategy also involves image. Instead of asking, "May I?" leaders assume that they may. When people ask permission, they are really asking someone to take responsibility for them. If something is not expressly prohibited in an organization or a job description, the powerful leader assumes that it may be done. Politically astute nurses have been known to create new positions or new roles within a position simply by gradually assuming that they could do things that no one else was doing. In other words, they saw a need in the organization and started meeting it. The organization, through default, allowed expansion of the role. People need to be aware, however, that if they assume authority and something goes wrong, they will be held accountable; so this strategy is not without risk.

- *Expand personal resources.* Because organizations are dynamic and the future is impossible to predict, the proactive nurse prepares for the future by expanding personal resources. Personal resources include economic stability, higher education, and a broadened skill base. Some call this the political strategy of "having maneuverability," that is, the person avoids having limited options. People with "money in the bank and gas in the tank" have a political freedom of maneuverability that others do not. People lose power if others within the organization know that they cannot afford to make a job change or lack the necessary skills to do so. Those who become economically dependent on a position lose political clout. Likewise, the nurse who has not developed additional skills or sought further education loses the political strength that comes from being able to find quality employment elsewhere.

• *Develop political alliances and coalitions.* Nurses often can increase their power and influence by forming alliances with other groups, be they peers, sponsors, or subordinates. The alliances may be from within their own group or from outside the group. One of the most effective methods of forming alliances is networking. Managers can sharpen their political skills by becoming involved with peers outside the organization. In this manner, the manager keeps abreast of current happenings and consults others for advice and counsel. Although networking works among many groups, for the nurse–manager, few groups are as valuable as local and state nursing associations. *Networking*—forming coalitions and alliances—also can be effective within the organization, especially for some types of planned change. More power and political clout result from working together rather than alone. When a person faces political opposition from others in the organization, group power is very useful.

• *Be sensitive to timing.* Successful leaders are sensitive to the appropriateness and timing of their actions. The person who presents a request to attend an expensive nursing conference on the same afternoon that his or her supervisor just had extensive dental work typifies someone who is insensitive to timing. Besides being able to choose the right moment, the effective manager should develop skill in other areas of timing, such as knowing when it is appropriate to do nothing. For example, in the case of a problem employee who is 3 months from retirement, time itself will resolve the situation. The sensitive manager also learns when to stop requesting something. That time is before a superior issues a firm "no," at which point continuing to press the issue is politically unwise.

• *Promote subordinate identification.* A manager can promote the identification of subordinates in many ways. A simple "thank you" for a fine job works well when spoken in front of someone else. Calling attention to the extra efforts of subordinates says in effect, "Look what a good job we are capable of doing." Sending subordinates sincere notes of appreciation is another way of praising and promoting. Rewarding excellence is an effective political strategy.

• *View personal and unit goals in terms of the organization.* Even extraordinary and visible activities will not result in desired power unless those activities are used to meet organizational goals. Hard work purely for personal gain will become a political liability. Frequently, novice managers think only in terms of their needs and their problems rather than seeing the large picture. Moreover, people often look upward for solutions rather than attempting to find answers themselves. When problems are identified, it is more politically astute to take the problem and a proposed solution upward rather than just presenting the problem to the superior. Although the superior may not accept the solution, the effort to problem solve will be appreciated.

• *"Leave your ego at home in a jar."* Although political actions can be negative, you should make an effort not to take political muggings personally, because you may well be a bystander hit in a crossfire. Likewise, be careful about accepting credit for all political successes, because you may just have been in the right place at the right time. Be prepared as a manager to make political errors. The key to success is how quickly you rebound.

LEARNING EXERCISE 13.5

Turning Lemons into Lemonade

The following is based on a real event. The cast includes Sally Jones, the director of nursing; Jane Smith, the hospital administrator and CEO; and Bob Black, the assistant hospital administrator. Sally has been in her position at Memorial Hospital for 2 years. She has made many improvements in the nursing department and is generally respected by the hospital administrator, the nursing staff, and the physicians.

The present situation involves the newly hired Bob Black. Previously too small to have an assistant administrator, the hospital has grown, and this position was created. One of the departments assigned to Bob is the personnel and payroll department. Until now, nursing, which comprises 45 percent of all personnel, has done its own recruiting, interviewing, and selecting. Since Bob has been hired, he has shown obvious signs that he would like to increase his power and authority. Now Bob has proposed that he hire an additional clerk who will do much of the personnel work for the nursing department, although nursing administration will be able to make the final selections in hiring. Bob proposes that his department should do the initial screening of applicants, seeking references, and so on. Sally has grown increasingly frustrated in dealing with the encroachment of Bob. Having just received Bob's latest proposal, she has requested to meet with Jane Smith and Bob to discuss the plan.

● ASSIGNMENT: What danger, if any, is there for Sally Jones in Bob Black's proposal? Explain two political strategies that you believe Sally could use in the upcoming meeting. Is it possible to facilitate a win–win solution to this conflict? If so, how? If there is not a win–win solution, how much can Sally win?

Note: Attempt to solve this case before reading the solution presented in the Appendix.

INTEGRATING LEADERSHIP ROLES AND MANAGEMENT FUNCTIONS WHEN USING AUTHORITY AND POWER IN ORGANIZATIONS

A manager's ability to gain and wisely use power is critical to his or her success. Nurses will never be assured of adequate resources until they gain the power to manipulate the needed resources legitimately. To do this, managers must be able to bridge the authority–power gap, build a personal power base, and minimize the negative politics of the organization.

One of the most critical leadership roles in the use of power and authority is the empowerment of subordinates. The leader recognizes the dual pyramid of power and acknowledges the power of others, including that of subordinates, peers, and higher administrators. The key to establishing and keeping authority and power in an organization is for the leader–manager to be able to accomplish four separate tasks:

• Maintain a small authority–power gap.
• Empower subordinates whenever possible
• Use authority in such a manner that subordinates view what happens in the organization as necessary.
• When needed, implement political strategies to maintain power and authority.

Integrating the leadership role and the functions of management reduces the risk that power will be misused. Power and authority will be used to increase respect for the position and for nursing as a whole. The leader comfortable with power ensures that the goal of political maneuvers is cooperation, not personal gain. The successful manager who has integrated the role of leadership will not seek to have power over others but instead will empower others. It is imperative for leader–managers to become skillful in the art of politics and the use of political strategy if they are to survive in the corporate world of the health care industry. It is with the use of such strategies that organizational resources are obtained and goals for nursing are achieved.

Key Concepts

- *Power* and *authority* are necessary components of leadership and management.
- A person's response to authority is conditioned early through authority figures and experiences in the family unit.
- The gap that sometimes exists between a position of authority and subordinate response is called the *authority–power gap*.
- The *empowerment* of staff is a hallmark of transformational leadership. Empowerment means to enable, develop, or allow.
- Power has both a positive and a negative face.
- Traditionally, women have been socialized to view power differently than men do. However, recent studies show that gender differences regarding power are slowly changing.
- *Reward power* is obtained by the ability to grant rewards to others.
- *Coercive power* is based on fear and punishment.
- *Legitimate power* is the power inherent in one's position.
- *Expert power* is gained through knowledge or skill.
- *Referent power* is obtained through association with others.
- *Charismatic power* results from a dynamic and powerful persona.
- *Information power* is gained when someone has information that another needs.
- *Feminist power* or *self-power* is gained through maturity, ego integration, confidence, and security in relationships.
- To acquire power in an organization, the novice manager should use appropriate power-building tactics.
- Power gained may be lost because one is politically naive or fails to use appropriate political strategies.
- *Politics* exist in every organization, and leader–managers must learn the art and skills of politics.

ADDITIONAL LEARNING EXERCISES AND APPLICATIONS

LEARNING EXERCISE 13.6

Empowering Your Staff

After 5 years as a public health nurse, you have just been appointed as supervisor of the western region of the county health department. There is one supervisor for each region, a nursing director, and an assistant director. You have eight nurses who report directly to you. Your organization seems to have few barriers to prevent staff empowerment, but in talking with the staff that report to you, they frequently express feelings of powerlessness in their ability to effect lasting change in their patients or in changing policies within the organization. Your first planned change, therefore, is to develop strategies to empower them.

● ASSIGNMENT: Devise a political strategy for successfully empowering the staff that report directly to you. Consider the three elements necessary in the empowerment process: professional traits of the staff, a supportive environment, and effective leadership. Of these things, what is in your sphere of control? Where is there danger of your plan being sabotaged? What change tactics can you use to increase the likelihood of success?

LEARNING EXERCISE 13.7

Friendships and Truth

You are a middle-level manager in a public health department. One of your closest friends, Janie, is an RN under your span of control. Today, Janie calls and tells you that she injured her back yesterday during a home visit after she slipped on a wet front porch. She said that the home owners were unaware that she fell and that no one witnessed the accident. She has just returned from visiting her doctor, who advises 6 weeks of bed rest. She requests that you initiate the paperwork for workers compensation and disability, because she has no sick days left.

Shortly after your telephone conversation with Janie, you take a brief coffee break in the lounge. You overhear a conversation between Jon and Lacey, two additional staff members in your department. Jon says that he and Janie were water skiing last night, and she took a terrible fall and hurt her back. He planned to call her to see how she was feeling.

You initially feel hurt and betrayed by Janie because you believe that she has lied to you. You want to call Janie and confront her. You plan to deny her request for workers' compensation and disability. You are angry that she has placed you in this position. You also are aware that proving Janie's injury is not work related may be difficult.

● ASSIGNMENT: How should you proceed? What are the political ramifications if this incident is not handled properly? How should you use your power and authority when dealing with this problem?

LEARNING EXERCISE 13.8

Decision Making: Conflict and Dilemma

You are the director of a small Native American health clinic. Other than yourself and a part-time physician, your only professional staff members are two RNs. The remaining staff members are Native Americans and have been trained by you.

Because nurse Bennett, a 26-year-old female BSN graduate, has had several years of experience working at a large southwestern community health agency, she is familiar with many of the patients' problems. She is hard working and extremely knowledgeable. Occasionally, her assertiveness is mistaken for bossiness among the Native American workers. However, everyone respects her judgment.

The other RN, nurse Mikiou, is a 34-year-old male Native American. He started as a medic in the Persian Gulf War and attended several career-ladder external degree programs until he

(Learning Exercise continues on page 312)

was able to take the RN examination. He does not have a baccalaureate degree. His nursing knowledge is occasionally limited, and he tends to be very casual about performing his duties. However, he is competent and has never shown unsafe judgment. His humor and good nature often reduce tension in the clinic. The Native American population is very proud of him, and he has a special relationship with them. However, he is not a particularly good role model because his health habits leave much to be desired, and he is frequently absent from work.

Nurse Bennett has come to find nurse Mikiou intolerable. She believes that she has tried working with him, but this is difficult because she does not respect him. As the director of the clinic, you have tried many ways to solve this problem. You feel especially fortunate to have nurse Bennett on your staff. It is difficult to find many nurses of her quality willing to come and live on a Native American reservation. On the other hand, if the Native American health concept is really going to work, the Native Americans themselves must be educated and placed in the agencies so that one day they can run their own clinics. It is very difficult to find educated Native Americans who want to return to this reservation. Now, you are faced with a management dilemma. Nurse Bennett has said that either nurse Mikiou must go, or she will go. She has asked you to decide.

● ASSIGNMENT: List the factors bearing on this decision. What (if any) power issues are involved? Which choice will be the least damaging? Justify your decision.

LEARNING EXERCISE 13.9

Power Struggle

You are team leader on a medical unit of a small community hospital. Your shift is 3 PM to 11 PM. When leaving the report room, John, the day-shift team leader, tells you that Mrs. Jackson, a patient who is terminally ill with cancer, has decided to check herself out of the hospital "against medical advice." John states that he has already contacted Mrs. Jackson's doctor, who expressed his concern that the patient would have inadequate pain control at home and undependable family support. He believes that she will die within a few days if she leaves the hospital. He did, however, leave orders for home prescriptions and a follow-up appointment.

You immediately go into Mrs. Jackson's room to assess the situation. She tells you that the doctor has told her she will probably die within 6 weeks and that she wants to spend what time she has left at home with her little dog, who has been her constant companion for many years. In addition, she has many things "to put in order." She states that she is fully aware of her doctor's concerns and that she was already informed by the day-shift nurse that leaving "against medical advice" may result in the insurance company refusing to pay for her current hospitalization. She states that she will be leaving in 15 minutes when her ride home arrives.

When you go to the nurse's station to get a copy of the home prescriptions and follow-up doctor's appointment for the patient, the unit clerk states, "The hospital policy says that patients who leave against medical advice have to contact the physician directly for prescriptions and an appointment, because they are not legally discharged. The hospital has no obligation to provide this service. She made the choice—now let her live with it." She refuses to give a copy of the orders to you and places the patient's chart in her lap. Short of physically removing the chart from the clerk's lap, you clearly have no immediate access to the orders.

You confront the charge nurse, who is unsure what to do and who states that the hospital policy does give that responsibility to the patient. The unit director, who has been paged, appears to be out of the hospital temporarily.

You are outraged. You believe that the patient has the "right" to her prescriptions because the doctor ordered them, assuming she would receive them before she left. You also know that if the medications are not dispensed by the hospital, there is little likelihood that Mrs. Jackson will have the resources to have the prescriptions filled. Five minutes later, Mrs. Jackson appears at the nurse's station, accompanied by her friend. She states that she is leaving and would like her discharge prescriptions.

● ASSIGNMENT: The power struggle in this scenario involves you, the unit clerk, the charge nurse, and organizational politics. Does the unit clerk in this scenario have informal or formal power? What alternatives for action do you have? What are the costs or consequences of each possible alternative? What action would you take?

LEARNING EXERCISE 13.10

When a Subordinate Goes Over Your Head

You are the day-shift charge nurse for the intensive care unit. One of your nurses, Carol, has just requested a week off to attend a conference. She is willing to use her accrued vacation time for this and to pay the expenses herself. The conference is in 1 month, and you are a little irritated with her for not coming to you sooner. Carol's request conflicts with a vacation that you have given another nurse. This nurse requested her vacation 3 months ago.

You deny Carol's request, explaining that you will need her to work that week. Carol protests, stating that the educational conference will benefit the intensive care unit and repeating that she will bear the cost. You are firm but polite in your refusal. Later, Carol goes to the supervisor of the unit to request the time. Although the supervisor upholds your decision, you believe that Carol has gone over your head inappropriately in handling this matter.

● ASSIGNMENT: How are you going to deal with Carol? Decide on your approach, and support it with political rationale.

Web Links

Organizational Power
www.geocities.com/Athens/Forum/1650/htmlpower.html
Examples of coercive power in organizations.

Women Working 2006 and Beyond
http://womenworking2000.com
Website that springs from the television special, "Women Working 2000 and Beyond." Offers networking contacts, wisdom, and leadership.

Political Action Links for Nurses
http://www.academic.scranton.edu/faculty/zalonm1/political.html
Links to workplace government organizations in health care, sponsored by the University of Scranton.

References

Ceci, C. (2004). Gender, power, nursing: A case analysis. *Nursing Inquiry*, *11*(2), 72–82.

DeSisto, M. C., & DeSisto, T. P. (2004). School nurses' perceptions of empowerment and autonomy. *Journal of School Nursing*, *20*(4), 228–233.

French, J., & Raven, B. (1959). The bases of social power. In D. Cartwright (Ed.), *Studies in social power*. Ann Arbor, MI: University of Michigan.

Grindel, C. (2006). The power of nursing: Can it ever be mobilized? *Academy of Medical-Surgical Nursing*, *15*(1), 5–7.

Hegyvary, S. T. (2003). Foundations of professional power. *Journal of Nursing Scholarship*, *35*(2), 104.

Heineken, J., & McCloskey, J. (1985). Teaching power concepts. *Journal of Nursing Education*, *24*(1), 40–42.

Houghton, C .(2004). Power and gender. *Nursing Standard*, *1*(52), 27.

Houser, B. P. (2005). The power of collaboration. *Nursing Administration Quarterly*, *29*(3), 263–267.

Huston, C. (2006). The nursing profession's historic struggle to increase its power base. In C. Huston (Ed.), *Professional issues in nursing*. Philadelphia: Lippincott Williams & Wilkins.

Morrison, E. G. (1988). Power and nonverbal behavior. In J. Muff (Ed.), *Socialization, sexism, and stereotyping*. Prospect Heights, IL: Waveland Press.

Robb, M. (2004). Continuing professional development. Gender and communication. *Nursing Management*, *11*(3), 29–33.

Sieloff, C. L. (2004). Leadership behaviors that foster nursing group power. *Nursing Management*, *12*(1), 248–251.

Valadares, K. J. (2004). The practicality of employee empowerment: Supporting a psychologically safe culture. *Health Care Manager*, *23*(3), 220–224.

Bibliography

Daiski, I. (2004). Changing nurses' disempowering relationship patterns. *Journal of Advanced Nursing*, *48*(1), 43–50.

Fradd, L. (2004). Political leadership in action. *Journal of Nursing Management*, *12*(1), 242–245.

Fuimano, J. (2005). Mentors' forum. Amp up your leadership curiosity. *Nursing Management*, *36*(11), 8.

Hagbaghery, M. A., Salsali, M., & Ahmadi, F. (2004). A qualitative study of Iranian nurses' understanding and experience of professional power. *Human Resources for Health*, *2*(9). Biomed Central. Retrieved September 24, 2006, from *http://www.human-resources-health.com/search/results.asp?terms=Hagbaghery+j.&db=jou10045&searchoperator=and&usq_param1=all&Submitted=Yes&Submit.x=22&Submit.y=12*

Laschinger, H. K. (2006). The impact of staff nurse empowerment on person–job fit and work engagement/burnout. *Nursing Administration Quarterly*, *30*(4), 358–367.

Murphy, L. (2005). Transformational leadership: A cascading chain reaction. *Journal of Nursing Management*, *13*(2), 128–136.

Patrick, A. (2006). The effect of structural empowerment and perceived organizational support on middle level nurse mangers' role satisfaction. *Journal of Nursing Management*, *14*(1), 13–22.

Pierce, K. M. (2004). Insights and reflections of a congressional nurse detailee. *Policy, Politics and Nursing Practice*, *5*(2), 113–115.

Rafferty, A. M. (2004). Context, convergence and contingency: Political leadership for nursing. *Journal of Nursing Management*, *12*(1), 258–265.

Stewart, S. D., & LaCoste, J. (2004). Light at the end of the tunnel: A vision for an empowered nursing profession across the continuum of care. *Nursing Administration Quarterly*, *28*(3), 212–216.

Venamore, J. (2004). Nurse power. *LAMP*, *61*(3), 32–33.

14

Organizing Patient Care

. . . patients now more than ever need reassurance
that they are indeed the focus of the healthcare team.

—*Joan Shinkus Clark*

First- and middle-level managers generally have their greatest influence on the organizing phase of the management process at the unit or department level. It is here that managers organize how work is to be done, shape the organizational climate, and determine how patient care delivery is organized. It is the top-level manager, however, who is most likely to influence the philosophy and resources necessary for any selected care delivery system to be effective. Without a supporting philosophy and adequate resources, the most well-intentioned delivery system will fail.

The unit leader–manager determines how best to plan work activities so that organizational goals are met effectively and efficiently. This involves using resources wisely and coordinating activities with other departments. How activities are organized can impede or facilitate communication, flexibility, and job satisfaction.

For organizing functions to be productive and facilitate meeting the organization's needs, the leader must know the organization and its members well. Activities will be unsuccessful if their design does not meet group needs. The roles and functions of the leader–manager in organizing groups for patient care are shown in Display 14.1.

TRADITIONAL MODES OF ORGANIZING PATIENT CARE

The five most well-known means of organizing nursing care for patient care delivery are total patient care, functional nursing, team and modular nursing, primary nursing, and case management (Display 14.2). Each of these basic types has undergone many modifications, often resulting in new terminology. For example, primary nursing was called case method nursing in the past and is now frequently referred to as a professional practice model. Team nursing is sometimes called partners in care or patient service partners, and case managers assume different titles depending on the setting in which they provide care. When closely examined, many of the newer models of patient care delivery systems are merely recycled, modified, or retitled versions of older models. Indeed, it is sometimes difficult to find a delivery system true to its original version or one that does not have parts of others in its design. Although some of these care delivery

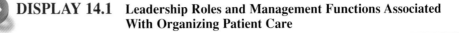

DISPLAY 14.1 Leadership Roles and Management Functions Associated With Organizing Patient Care

Leadership Roles

1. Periodically evaluates the effectiveness of the organizational structure for the delivery of patient care
2. Determines if adequate resources and support exist before making any changes in the organization of patient care
3. Examines the human element in work redesign and supports personnel during adjustment to change
4. Inspires the work group toward a team effort
5. Inspires subordinates to achieve higher levels of education, clinical expertise, competency, and experience in differentiated practice
6. Ensures that chosen nursing care delivery models advance the practice of professional nursing

Management Functions

1. Examines the unit philosophy to ensure that it supports any change in the patient care delivery system
2. Selects a patient care delivery system that is most appropriate to the needs of the patients being served
3. Uses scientific research and current literature to analyze proposed changes in nursing care delivery models
4. Uses a patient care delivery system that maximizes human and physical resources as well as time
5. Ensures that nonprofessional staff are appropriately trained and supervised in the provision of care
6. Organizes work activities to attain organizational goals
7. Groups activities in a manner that facilitates communication and coordination within and between departments
8. Organizes work so that it is as cost-effective as possible
9. Makes changes in work design to facilitate meeting organizational goals
10. Clearly delineates criteria to be used for differentiated practice roles

DISPLAY 14.2 Traditional Patient Care Delivery Methods

Total patient care
Functional nursing
Team and modular nursing
Primary nursing
Case management

systems were developed to organize care in hospitals, most can be adapted to other settings. The choice of an organization model involves staff skills, availability, resources, patient acuity, and the nature of the work to be performed.

 Choosing the most appropriate organizational model to deliver patient care for each unit or organization depends on the skill and expertise of the staff, the availability of registered professional nurses, the economic resources of the organization, the acuity of the patients, and the complexity of the tasks to be completed.

Total Patient Care Nursing or Case Method Nursing

Total patient care is the oldest mode of organizing patient care. With total patient care, nurses assume total responsibility during their time on duty for meeting all the needs of assigned patients. At the turn of the 19th century, total patient care was generally provided in the patient's home, and the nurse was responsible for cooking, house cleaning, and other activities specific to the patient and family in addition to traditional nursing care.

It is important to note that most medical and nursing care for the wealthy and middle class during this time occurred in the home; hospitals at the time were used primarily by the poor and very acutely ill. *Total patient care nursing* is sometimes referred to as the *case method of assignment* because patients were assigned as cases, much like contemporary private-duty nursing is carried out.

During the Great Depression of the 1930s, people could no longer afford home care and began using hospitals for care that had been performed by private-duty nurses in the home. During that time, nurses and students were the caregivers in hospitals and in public health agencies. As hospitals grew during the 1930s and 1940s, providing total care continued as the primary means of organizing patient care. A structural diagram of this method is shown in Figure 14.1.

This method of assignment is still widely used in hospitals and home health agencies. This organizational structure provides nurses with high autonomy and responsibility. Assigning patients is simple and direct and does not require the planning that other methods of patient care delivery require. The lines of responsibility and accountability are clear. The patient theoretically receives holistic and unfragmented care during the nurse's time on duty.

Each nurse caring for the patient can, however, modify the care regimen. Therefore, if there are three shifts, the patient could receive three different approaches to care, often resulting in confusion for the patient. To maintain quality care, this method requires highly skilled personnel and thus may cost more than some other forms of patient care. This method's opponents argue that some tasks performed by the primary caregiver could be accomplished by someone with less training and therefore at a lower cost.

The greatest disadvantage of total patient care delivery occurs when the nurse is inadequately prepared or too inexperienced to provide total care to the patient. In the early history of nursing, only RNs provided care; now, a variety of nursing care personnel, many of whom have no license and limited education, work with patients. During nursing shortages, many hospitals assign health care workers who are not RNs to provide most of the nursing care. Because the co-assigned RN may have a heavy patient load, little opportunity for supervision exists. Potentially, this could result in unsafe care.

Functional Method

The *functional method* of delivering nursing care evolved primarily as a result of World War II and the rapid construction of hospitals as a result of the Hill Burton Act. Because nurses were in

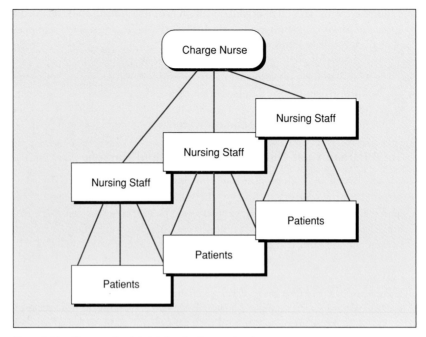

Figure 14.1   Case method or total patient care structure.

great demand overseas and at home, a nursing shortage developed and ancillary personnel were needed to assist in patient care. These relatively unskilled workers were trained to do simple tasks and gained proficiency by repetition. Personnel were assigned to complete certain tasks rather than care for specific patients. Examples of functional nursing tasks were checking blood pressures, administering medication, changing linens, and bathing patients. RNs became managers of care rather than direct care providers, and "care through others" became the phrase used to refer to this method of nursing care. Most hospitals continue to use CNAs in functional roles, such as bathing and bed making (Weitzel, Robinson, Henderson, & Anderson, 2004). Functional nursing structure is shown in Figure 14.2.

This form of organizing patient care was thought to be temporary, as it was assumed that when the war ended, hospitals would not need ancillary workers. However, the baby boom and resulting population growth immediately following World War II left the country short of nurses. Thus, employment of personnel with various levels of skill and education proliferated as new categories of health care workers were created. Currently, most health care organizations have continued this practice of employing health care workers of many educational backgrounds and skill levels.

Most administrators consider functional nursing to be an economical means of providing care. This is true if quality care and holistic care are not regarded as essential. A major advantage of functional nursing is its efficiency; tasks are completed quickly, with little confusion regarding responsibilities. Functional nursing does allow care to be provided with a minimal number of RNs. In many areas, such as the operating room, the functional structure works well and is still very much in evidence. Long-term care facilities also frequently use a functional approach to nursing care.

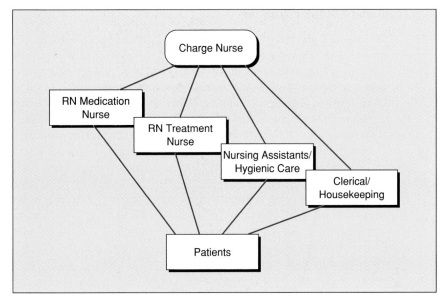

Figure 14.2 Functional nursing organization structure.

During the past decade, the use of unlicensed assistive personnel (UAP) in health care organizations has increased. Many nurse administrators believe that assigning low-skill tasks to UAPs frees the professional nurse to perform more highly skilled duties and is therefore more economical; however, others argue that the time needed to supervise the UAP negates any time savings that may have occurred. Most modern administrators would undoubtedly deny that they are using functional nursing, yet the trend of assigning tasks to workers, rather than assigning workers to the professional nurse, resembles, at least in part, functional nursing.

Functional nursing may lead to fragmented care and the possibility of overlooking patient priority needs. Because some workers feel unchallenged and understimulated in their roles, functional nursing also may result in low job satisfaction. In addition, functional nursing may not be cost-effective due to the need for many coordinators. Employees often focus only on their own efforts, with less interest in overall results.

LEARNING EXERCISE 14.1

Transitioning to Total Patient Care

Most nursing students begin their clinical training by doing some form of functional nursing care and then advancing to total patient care for a small number of patients. Reflect back to your earliest clinical experiences as a student nurse. Which tasks were easiest for you to learn? How did you gain mastery of those tasks? Was task mastery a time-consuming process for you? Was it difficult to make the transition to total patient care? If so, why? What skills were most difficult for you to learn in providing total patient care? Do you anticipate having to learn additional skills to feel comfortable in the role of total care provider as an RN? What higher level (nonfunctional) skills do you think will be the hardest to learn and be confident with?

Team and Modular Nursing

Team nursing was developed in the 1950s in an effort to decrease the problems associated with the functional organization of patient care. Many believed that despite a continued shortage of professional nursing staff, a patient care system had to be developed that reduced the fragmented care that accompanied functional nursing. Team nursing structure is illustrated in Figure 14.3.

In team nursing, ancillary personnel collaborate in providing care to a group of patients under the direction of a professional nurse. As the team leader, the nurse is responsible for knowing the condition and needs of all the patients assigned to the team and for planning individual care. The team leader's duties vary depending on the patient's needs and the workload. These duties may include assisting team members, giving direct personal care to patients, teaching, and coordinating patient activities.

Through extensive team communication, comprehensive care can be provided for patients despite a relatively high proportion of ancillary staff. This communication occurs informally between the team leader and the individual team members and formally through regular team planning conferences. A team should consist of not more than five people, or it will revert to more functional lines of organization.

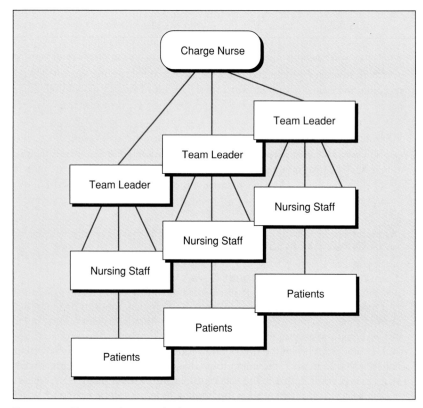

Figure 14.3   Team nursing organization structure.

Team nursing is usually associated with democratic leadership. Group members are given as much autonomy as possible when performing assigned tasks, although the team shares responsibility and accountability collectively. The need for excellent communication and coordination skills makes implementing team nursing difficult and requires great self-discipline on the part of team members.

Team nursing allows members to contribute their own special expertise or skills. Team leaders, then, should use their knowledge about each member's abilities when making patient assignments. Recognizing the individual worth of all employees and giving team members autonomy result in high job satisfaction.

Disadvantages to team nursing are associated primarily with improper implementation rather than with the philosophy itself. Frequently, insufficient time is allowed for team care planning and communication. This can lead to blurred lines of responsibility, errors, and fragmented patient care. For team nursing to be effective, the leader must be an excellent practitioner and have good communication, organizational, management, and leadership skills.

Team nursing, as originally designed, has undergone much modification in the last 30 years. Most team nursing was never practiced in its purest form but was instead a combination of team and functional structure. Recent attempts to refine and improve team nursing have resulted in the concept of *modular nursing*, which is a mini-team (two or three members) approach. Members of the modular nursing team are sometimes called *care pairs*. Keeping the team small and attempting to assign personnel to the same team as often as possible should allow the professional nurse more time for planning and coordinating team members. Additionally, a small team requires less communication, allowing members better use of their time for direct patient care activities.

Primary Nursing

Primary nursing, also known as *relationship-based nursing*, developed in the early 1970s, uses some of the concepts of total patient care, and brings the RN back to the bedside to provide clinical care. Primary nursing is one type of patient care delivery that requires a one-to-one relationship between an RN and a patient, with responsibility for planning and managing care clearly established.

As originally designed, primary nursing requires a nursing staff made up only of RNs. The RN primary nurse assumes 24-hour responsibility for planning the care of one or more patients from admission or the start of treatment to discharge or the treatment's end. During work hours, the primary nurse provides total direct care for that patient.

When the primary nurse is not on duty, *associate nurses*, who follow the care plan established by the primary nurse, provide care. Primary nursing structure is shown in Figure 14.4. Although designed for use in hospitals, this structure lends itself well to home health nursing, hospice nursing, and other health care delivery enterprises. An integral responsibility of the primary nurse is to establish clear communication among the patient, the physician, the associate nurses, and other team members. Although the primary nurse establishes the care plan, feedback is sought from others in coordinating the patient's care. The combination of clear interdisciplinary group communication and consistent, direct patient care by relatively few nursing staff allows for holistic, high-quality patient care.

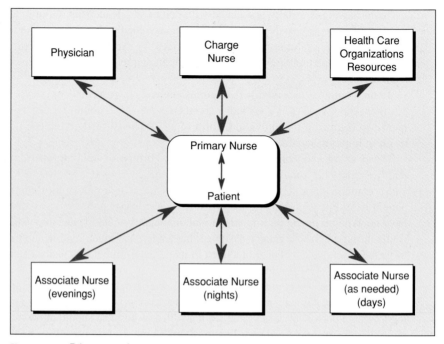

Figure 14.4   Primary nursing structure.

Although job satisfaction is high in primary nursing, this method is difficult to implement because of the degree of responsibility and autonomy required of the primary nurse. However, for these same reasons, once nurses develop skill in primary nursing care delivery, they feel challenged and rewarded.

Disadvantages to this method, as in team nursing, lie primarily in improper implementation. An inadequately prepared or incompetent primary nurse may be incapable of coordinating a multidisciplinary team or identifying complex patient needs and condition changes. Many nurses may be uncomfortable in this role or initially lack the experience and skills necessary for the role. Although an all-RN nursing staff has not been proved to be more costly than other modes of nursing, it sometimes has been difficult to recruit and retain enough RNs, especially in times of nursing shortages. Currently, LVNs and LPNs serve as associate nurses in some facilities, although the role of the primary nurse should be reserved for an experienced RN who has an appropriate scope of requisite skills for the role.

LEARNING EXERCISE 14.2

Reorganizing to Accommodate a Change in Staffing Mix
You are the head nurse of an oncology unit. At present, the patient care delivery method on the unit is total patient care. You have a staff composed of 60-percent RNs, 35-percent practical nurses (LPNs/LVNS), and 5-percent clerical staff. Your bed capacity is 28, but your average daily census is 24. An example of day-shift staffing follows:

- One charge nurse who notes orders, talks with physicians, organizes care, makes assignments, and acts as a resource person and problem solver
- Three RNs who provide total patient care, including administering all treatments and medications to their assigned patients, giving IV medications to the LVN/LPNs' assigned patients, and acting as a clinical resource person for the LVN/LPNs
- Two LPNs assigned to provide total patient care except for administering IV medications

Your supervisor has just told all head nurses that because the hospital is having difficulty recruiting nurses, it has decided to hire nursing assistants. The nurses on your unit will have to assume more supervisory responsibilities and focus less on direct care. Your supervisor has asked you to reorganize the patient care management on your unit to best use the following day-shift staffing: three RNs, which will include the present charge nurse position; two LVN/LPNs and two nursing assistants. You may delete the past charge nurse position and divide charge responsibility among all three nurses or divide up the work any way you choose.

● ASSIGNMENT: Draw a new patient care organization diagram. Who would be most affected by the reorganization? Evaluate your rationale, both for the selection of your choice and the rejection of others. Explain how you would go about implementing this planned change.

Case Management

Case management is another work design proposed to meet patient needs. Case management is defined by the Case Management Society of America (CMSA) as a collaborative process that assesses, plans, implements, coordinates, monitors, and evaluates options and services to meet an individual's health needs through communication and available resources to promote quality, cost-effective outcomes (CMSA, 2006).

> The focus in case management is on individual patients, not populations of patients.

Case managers handle each case individually, identifying the most cost-effective providers, treatments, and care settings for insured individuals. According to Harrison, Nolin, and Suero (2004), "there is increasing evidence that use of the case management process in both acute and long-term care settings has led to quantitative and qualitative improvements in health care delivery" (p. 64). While case management referrals often begin in the hospital inpatient setting, with length of stay and profit margin per confinement used as measures of efficiency, case management in the managed care era frequently extends to outpatient settings as well. Historically, however, the focus has been episodic or component-style orientation to the treatment of disease in inpatient settings and post acute-care settings for insured individuals.

Acute-care case management integrates utilization management and discharge planning functions and may be unit based, assigned by patient, disease based, or primary nurse case managed. Assignment by unit is most common, particularly in mid- to large-sized hospitals because patient units typically care for patients with like diagnoses (Smith, 2003). "The advantages of this model include additional work efficiency due to geographic proximity, but more importantly, the benefit of establishing solid working relationships with the nursing and ancillary staff working on the unit" (p. 238). In general, a case manager can handle a load of 25 patients (Smith, 2003).

EXAMINING THE EVIDENCE 14.1

Source: Harrison, J. P., Nolin, J., & Suero, E. (2004). The effect of case management on U.S. Hospitals. *Nursing Economic$, 22*(2), 64–68.

This study demonstrated that case management programs in hospitals (a) were more likely to be located in markets with higher per capita income and fewer elderly patients; (b) had a higher return on assets, higher occupancy rates, and lower operating expenses; and (c) were associated with larger institutions. The hospitals with patients having the greatest need for care management and coordination were less likely to have case management programs.

The premise of inpatient case management is that hospitals are better off "managing the demand for care" than attempting to try to increase the "supply of resources" such as beds or personnel (Smith, 2003). Case managers do this by using *critical pathways* (Chapter 10) and *multidisciplinary action plans* (MAPs) to plan patient care.

The care MAP is a combination of a *critical pathway* and a *nursing care plan*. In addition, the care MAP indicates times when nursing interventions should occur. All health care providers follow the care MAP to facilitate expected outcomes. If a patient deviates from the normal plan, a *variance* is indicated. A variance is anything that occurs to alter the patient's progress through the normal critical path.

Furlow (2003) suggests a different type of care MAP in her discussion of cycle time reduction. *Cycle time reduction* involves reviewing an existing process that provides a product or service; determining where there is wasted time or effort; and developing an improved, streamlined way to achieve the same results more efficiently.

Harrison, Nolin, and Suero (2004) compared hospitals with and without case managers and found significant advantage to having case managers. However, they also found that hospitals with the highest percentage of elderly patients were less likely to have case management programs (Examining the Evidence 14.1).

Because the role expectations and scope of knowledge required to be a case manager are extensive, some experts have argued that this role should be reserved for the advance practice nurse or RN with advanced training (Huston, 2002), although this is not usually the case in the practice setting today. Smith (2003) argues that effective case managers should have 3 to 5 years of direct care experience, preferably within the specialty area in which they case manage. They should also be extremely bright, have well-developed interpersonal skills, be able to multitask, have a strong foundation in utilization review, and understand payer–patient specifics and hospital reimbursement mechanisms.

LEARNING EXERCISE 14.3

Developing a Case Management Plan

Jimmy Jansen is a 44-year-old man with type 1 diabetes mellitus. He was recently referred to your home health agency for case management follow-up at home. He is experiencing multiple complications from his diabetes, including the recent onset of blindness and peripheral neuropathy. His left leg was amputated below the knee last year as a result of a gangrenous infection of his foot. He is unable to wear his prosthesis at present because he has a small ulcer at the stump site. His chart states that he has been only "intermittently compliant" with blood sugar testing or insulin administration in the past despite the visit of a community health nurse on a weekly basis over the past year. His renal function has become progressively worse over the past 6 months, and it is anticipated that he will need to begin hemodialysis soon.

His social history reveals that he recently separated from his wife and has no contact with an adult son who lives in another state. He has not worked for more than 10 years and has no insurance other than Medicaid. The home he lives in is small, and he says that he has not been able to keep it up with his wife gone. No formal safety assessment of his home has been conducted. He also acknowledges that he is not eating right because he now must do his own cooking. He cannot drive and states, "I don't know how I'm going to get to the clinic to have my blood cleaned by the kidney machine."

● ASSIGNMENT: Mr. Jansen has many problems that would likely benefit from case management intervention.

1. Make a list of five nursing diagnoses for Mr. Jansen that you would use to prioritize your interventions.
2. Then make a list of at least five goals that you would like to accomplish in planning Mr. Jansen's care. Make sure that these goals reflect realistic patient outcomes.
3. What referrals would you make? What interventions would you implement yourself? Would you involve other disciplines in his plan of care?
4. What is your plan for follow-up and evaluation?

DISEASE MANAGEMENT AND CASE MANAGEMENT

One role that is increasingly assumed by case managers is coordinating disease management programs. *Disease management* (DM), also known as *population-based health care* and *continuous health improvement*, is a comprehensive, integrated approach to the care and reimbursement of high-cost, chronic illnesses. The goal of DM is to address such illnesses or conditions with maximum efficiency across treatment settings regardless of typical reimbursement patterns Thus, a continuum of chronic illness care is established that includes early detection and early intervention. This prevents or reduces exacerbation of the disease, acute episodes (known as *cost drivers*), and the use of expensive resources such as hospital inpatient care, making prevention and proactive case management two important areas of emphasis (Huston, 2002). In addition, DM programs include comprehensive tracking of patient outcomes. Thus, the goals for disease management are focused on integrating components and improving long-term outcomes.

In DM programs, common high-cost, high-resource utilization diseases are identified, and population groups are targeted for implementation. This is one of the most important differences between case management and disease management. In *population-based health care*, the focus is on "covered lives" or populations of patients, rather than on the individual patient (Huston, 2002). The goal in DM is to service the optimal number of covered lives required to reach operational and economic efficiency.

Providing optimum, cost-effective care to individual patients is critical to the success of a DM program; however, the focus for planning, implementation, and evaluation is population based.

Other primary features of DM programs include the use of a multidisciplinary health care team, including specialists in the area, the selection of large population groups to reduce adverse selection, the use of standardized clinical guidelines–clinical pathways reflecting best practice research to guide provider practice, and the use of integrated data management systems to track patient progress across care settings and allow continuous and ongoing improvement of treatment algorithms (Huston, 2002). Common features of DM programs are shown in Display 14.3.

One thing is clear—DM continues to grow as a means of organizing patient care. This is particularly true in the government sector, where there was almost a complete absence of DM services in the traditional Medicare plan until early this decade (Huston, 2002). Beginning in 2000, Medicare embraced a new round of trial DM demonstration projects, many of which are now mainstream initiatives, in an effort to deliver better outcomes at better prices.

The National Committee for Quality Assurance (NCQA) accreditation process began in January 2002 for organizations that offer comprehensive DM programs with services to patients, practitioners, or both and certification for organizations that provide specific DM functions. The American Creditation Health Care Commission (URAC) announced the first six DM program accreditation recipients in August 2002, and The Joint Commission granted its first DM program certification to a diabetes DM program in April 2002 (DM Program, 2002). The use of impartial, independent, and credible third-party programs to evaluate and certify DM programs will increase the validity of such programs both to providers and consumers alike.

DM continues to hold significant promise as a strategy for promoting cost-effective, quality health care in the future, and DM programs can only be expected to expand in scope and quantity. Similarly, RNs, in their roles as case managers, will continue to experience new and expanded roles as key players in the development, coordination, and evaluation of DM programs in the future (Huston, 2002).

DISPLAY 14.3   Common Features of Disease Management Programs

1. Provide a comprehensive, integrated approach to the care and reimbursement of common, high-cost, chronic illnesses
2. Focus on prevention as well as early disease detection and intervention to avoid costly acute episodes but provide comprehensive care and reimbursement
3. Target population groups (population based) rather than individuals
4. Employ a multidisciplinary health care team, including specialists
5. Use standardized clinical guidelines–clinical pathways reflecting best practice research to guide providers
6. Use integrated data management systems to track patient progress across care settings and allow continuous and ongoing improvement of treatment algorithms
7. Frequently employ professional nurses in the role of case manager or program coordinator

LEARNING EXERCISE 14.4

Researching Disease Management Programs
Search the Internet for DM (disease management, not diabetes mellitus) programs. What chronic diseases were most commonly represented in the DM programs that you identified? What entities (private insurance companies, managed care insurers, government, pharmaceutical companies, private companies, etc.) sponsored these programs? What is the process for referral? Are the programs accredited? Are RNs used as case managers or program coordinators? What standardized clinical guidelines are used in the program, and are they evidence based?

● ASSIGNMENT: Select one of the programs that you found, and write a one-page summary regarding your findings.

DIFFERENTIATED NURSING PRACTICE

Differentiated nursing practice refers to an attempt to separate nursing practice roles based on education or experience or some combination of both. Using basic licensure as the common denominator for most nursing positions causes dissension among nurses and confusion among health care consumers (Fox, 2006). Fox states that "expecting similar performance from nurses with varying educational preparation can lead to role confusion, stress, and burnout as nurses struggle to develop role competencies for which they have not been prepared" (p. 24). The philosophy behind differentiated nursing practice is that RNs should work within the role structure and responsibilities that correspond best with their individual capabilities.

Two basic models are used to differentiate practice (Display 14.4). The older one, the education model, reflects the ADN, BSN, and MSN programs and includes three basic components of nursing: provision of care, communication, and management. The competency model is based partly on the eight American Nurses Association's Standards of Nursing and also reflects Benner's (1984) five levels of practice: novice, advanced beginner, competent, proficient, and expert. Brady and associates (2001) suggest, however, that the 21 Pew Health Professional Commission Competencies could serve as a useful tool to nurses and health system leaders as they attempt to adapt the current model of nursing practice to the demands and realities of the contemporary and continually evolving health care environment. As well, Brady and associates argue that this framework would offer an approach to rationalizing both nursing education and practice, with the potential for improving the quality of care and reducing fragmentation, cost, and public confusion about a nurse's educational preparation and scope of practice.

DISPLAY 14.4   Two Basic Differentiated Practice Models

Type	Type of Differentiation
Education Model	Role differentiation based on type of educational preparation (ADN, BSN, and MSN)
Competency Model	Role differentiation based on individual nurse skill level, expertise, experience, etc.

The rationale for differentiated practice is to match patient needs with nursing competencies; facilitate the effective and efficient use of nursing resources; provide equitable compensation based on education, productivity, and expertise; increase nurse satisfaction; build loyalty; and increase the prestige of the nursing profession. It also recognizes the broad domain of professional nursing, the multiple roles and responsibilities that nurses assume, and the contribution of all nursing personnel as valuable and unique (Blais, Hayes, Kozier, & Erb, 2002).

Since the scope and regulation of nursing practice and educational standards are controlled by each state, Fox (2006) maintains that true institutionalization of differentiated practice concepts must occur at the state level. Differentiated nursing practice is still too new to determine whether it has met the intended goals. It is hoped that the effectiveness of this concept will be thoroughly demonstrated before it is widely embraced and, if it is proven to be effective, that it be implemented correctly so that its adaptation will be successful.

LEARNING EXERCISE 14.5

Differentiating Practice at the Unit Level
You are serving on a committee of nurse–managers and staff nurses to develop guidelines and job descriptions for a new pay structure based on differentiated nursing practice. Several members of the committee are resistant to change. Your committee is now looking at four clinical levels of RNs, with different salary ranges for each level. Some believe that both education and expertise should be required for advancement from one level to the next, and others believe that it should be based only on expertise.

So far, the committee has agreed that nurses who wish to advance to the next clinical level must (a) apply for an open position at that level, (b) be recommended by their immediate supervisor and one other nurse of an advanced clinical level, and (c) possess the expertise and education necessary to fulfill the job functions. It is the third requirement that you are having difficulty. You cannot agree on the type (formal or certifications) and amount of education necessary for each level or on how you will document expertise.

● ASSIGNMENT: Write a proposal for differentiating practice at the unit level. Will you use education, years of experience, or skill level to differentiate your career ladder, or will you use some combination of the three? What would you name each of the four levels of nursing? Will your minimum requirements for each level be fixed, or will you allow for individual variations?

WHAT THE FUTURE HOLDS FOR PATIENT CARE DELIVERY MODELS

The American Organization of Nurse Executives (AONE) (2006) maintains that by 2010, there will be too few health care workers to deliver care by using the same models as are presently being used. They suggest that health care agencies begin to plan and experiment now—before, not after, all answers and solutions are established.

The future will see many attempts to deliver care in unique ways. However, a prominent characteristic among the new models being tried is the nurse as a clinical expert leading other members of a team of partners. Tornabeni, Stanhope, and Wiggins (2006) report that the membership of the American Association of Colleges of Nursing has initiated a national effort to create a new nursing role (the *clinical nurse–leader*) that is more responsive to the realities of the modern health care system.

In examining the literature for new care-delivery models, a variety of titles for a new nursing role may be found. The title of the nurse may vary from institution to institution; names such as clinical expert and advanced practice nurse may be used. Some (Sloand & Groves, 2005) call this a *primary nursing care model*. Others have had success using professional accountability through a nursing role of patient care facilitator (PCF) and using a 12-bed team approach but with the PCF maintaining a clinical, not supervisory focus (Clark, 2004).

Because health care workers may be scarce in the future, some organizations have begun using a cooperative model of care delivery. In this example, lay care partners of the client are taught to recognize systems, identify problems, and take action (Eilers, Heermann, Wilson, & Knutson, 2005). Using lay individuals as helpers in delivery of care has long been standard in other countries but is relatively new in the United States. This form of delivery of care requires that the nurse be an excellent teacher and communicator.

All of these examples call for a well-educated nurse using an evidence-based practice and having an ability to work collaboratively. This realization led AONE in 2005 to come to the conclusion that "The educational preparation of the nurse of the future should be at the baccalaureate level. This educational preparation will prepare the nurse of the future to function as an equal partner, collaborator, and manager of the complex patient care journey that is envisioned by AONE" (AONE, 2006).

It is perhaps a folly to determine a model of nursing care delivery without examining a broader picture of nursing. Reno, Cerone, Ferket, Wojcieszak, & Reshoft (2005) reported on how one community hospital developed a strategy to address its delivery of care needs. They determined that five key components were needed: (a) conversion of manual systems into automated ones, (b) differentiated levels of nursing practice, (c) increased knowledge base of nursing practitioners, (d) development of flexibility and nimbleness, and (e) attraction of nursing candidates from a more diverse pool of professionals (Reno et al., 2005).

As many forces come together to change the future of health care, it behooves all of the profession to think smarter, to think outside the box, and to discover innovative ways to organize and deliver care to clients both inside and outside the acute-care setting. AONE (2004) stresses that regardless of new models of delivery, the core of nursing must be driven by both knowledge and caring, and nursing must become partners with patient/clients in the delivery of care.

SELECTING THE OPTIMUM MODE OF ORGANIZING PATIENT CARE

Most health care organizations use one or more modes to organize patient care. While not all care must be provided by RNs, the care delivery system chosen should be based on patient acuity and not on economics alone. In addition, the knowledge and skill required for particular activities with specific populations should always be the true driver in determining appropriate care delivery models. Nursing departments need to organize delivery of patient care based on the best method for their particular situation.

 Many nursing departments have a history of selecting methods of organizing patient care based upon the most current popular mode rather than objectively determining the best method for a particular unit or department.

If evaluation of the present system reveals deficiencies, the manager needs to examine available resources and compare those with resources needed for the change. Nursing managers often elect to change to a system that requires a high percentage of RNs, only to discover resources are inadequate, resulting in a failed planned change. One of the leadership responsibilities in organizing patient care is to determine the availability of resources and support for proposed changes. There must be a commitment on the part of top-level administration and a majority of the nursing staff for a change to be successful. Because health care is multidisciplinary, the care delivery system used will have a heavy impact on many others outside the nursing unit; therefore, those affected by a system change must be involved in its planning. Change affects other departments, the medical staff, and the health care consumer.

Perhaps most importantly, the philosophy of the nursing services division must support the delivery model selected. Additionally, without support from top-level health facility administration, reorganization of patient care delivery will fail.

Another mistake frequently made when changing modes of patient care delivery is not fully understanding how the new system should function or be implemented. Managers must carry out adequate research and be well versed in the system's proper implementation if the change is to be successful. It is important also to remember that not every nurse desires a challenging job with the autonomy of personal decision making. Many forces interact simultaneously in employee job design situations. Satisfaction does not occur only because of role fulfillment but also because of social and interpersonal relations. Therefore, the nurse leader–manager needs to be aware that redesigning work that disrupts group cohesiveness may result in increased levels of job dissatisfaction.

Such change should not be taken lightly. The leader–manager should consider the following when evaluating the current system and considering a change:

- Is the method of patient care delivery providing the level of care that is stated in the organizational philosophy? Does the method facilitate or hinder other organizational goals?
- Is the delivery of nursing care organized in a cost-effective manner?
- Does the care delivery system satisfy patients and their families? (Satisfaction and quality care differ; either may be provided without the other being present.)
- Does the organization of patient care delivery provide some degree of fulfillment and role satisfaction to nursing personnel?
- Does the system allow implementation of the nursing process?
- Does the system promote and support the profession of nursing as both independent and interdependent?
- Does the method facilitate adequate communication among all members of the health care team?
- How will a change in the patient care delivery system alter individual and group decision making? Who will be affected? Will autonomy decrease or increase?
- How will social interactions and interpersonal relationships change?
- Will employees view their unit of work differently? Will there be a change from a partial unit of work to a whole unit? (For example, total patient care would be a whole unit of work, whereas team nursing would be a partial unit.)
- Will the change require a wider or more restricted range of skills and abilities on the part of the caregiver?
- Will the redesign change how employees receive feedback on their performance, either for self-evaluation or by others?
- Will communication patterns change?

INTEGRATING LEADERSHIP ROLES AND MANAGEMENT FUNCTIONS IN ORGANIZING PATIENT CARE

Organizing is an all-important management function. The work must be organized so that organizational goals are sustained. Activities must be grouped so that resources, people, materials, and time are used fully. The integrated leader–manager understands that the organization and unit's nursing philosophy and the availability of resources greatly influence the type of patient care delivery system that should be chosen and the potential success of future work redesign.

The integrated leader–manager, then, is responsible for selecting and implementing a patient care delivery system that facilitates the accomplishment of unit goals. All members of the work group should be assisted with role clarification, especially when work is redesigned or new systems of patient care delivery are implemented. This team effort in work activity increases productivity and worker satisfaction. The emphasis is on seeking solutions to poor organization of work rather than finding fault.

There is no one "best" mode for organizing patient care. Integrating leadership roles and management functions ensures that the type of patient care delivery model selected will provide quality care and staff satisfaction. It also ensures that change in the mode of delivery will not be attempted without adequate resources, appropriate justification, and attention to how it will affect group cohesiveness. Historically, nursing has frequently adopted models of patient care delivery based on societal events (e.g., a nursing shortage, a proliferation of types of health care workers) rather than upon well-researched models with proven effectiveness that promote professional practice. The leadership role demands that the primary focus of patient care delivery be on promoting a professional model of practice that also reduces costs and improves patient outcomes.

Key Concepts

* *Total patient care*, utilizing the case method of assignment, is the oldest form of patient care organization and is still widely used today.
* *Functional nursing* organization requires the completion of specific tasks by different nursing personnel.
* *Team* or *modular nursing* organization uses a leader who coordinates team members in the care of a group of patients.
* *Primary care nursing* is organized so that the patient is at the center of the structure. One nurse has 24-hour responsibility for the nursing care plan.
* *Case management* is a collaborative process that assesses, plans, implements, coordinates, monitors, and evaluates options and services to meet an individual's health needs through communication and available resources to promote quality, cost-effective outcomes.
* While the focus historically for case management has been the individual patient, the case manager employed in a *disease management program* plans the care for populations or groups of patients with the same chronic illness.
* *Differentiated nursing practice* delineates different roles for nurses based on their skill, knowledge, educational level, and motivation.
* The care *MAP (multidisciplinary action plan)* is a combination of a critical path and a nursing care plan, except that it shows times when nursing interventions should occur as well as variances.

* A new role sometimes termed *clinical nurse–leader*, an experienced nurse possessing a baccalaureate or higher degree, will facilitate care for patients in the future.
* Delivery systems may have elements of the various designs present in the system in use in any organization.
* Each unit's care delivery structure should facilitate meeting the goals of the organization, be cost-effective, satisfy the patient, provide role satisfaction to nurses, allow implementation of the nursing process, and provide for adequate communication among health care providers.
* When work is redesigned, it frequently has personal consequences for employees that must be considered. Social interactions, the degree of autonomy, the abilities and skills necessary, employee evaluation, and communication patterns are often affected by work redesign.

ADDITIONAL LEARNING EXERCISES AND APPLICATIONS

LEARNING EXERCISE 14.6

Creating a Plan to Reduce Resistance

You work in an intensive care unit where there is an RN staff. The unit works 12-hour shifts, and each nurse is assigned one or two patients, depending on the nursing needs of the patient. The unit has always used total patient care delivery assignments. Recently, your unit manager has informed the staff that all patients in the unit would be assigned a case manager in an effort to maximize the use of resources and to reduce length of stay in the unit. Many of the unit staff resent the case manager and believe that this has reduced the RN's autonomy and control of patient care. They are resistant to the need to document variances to the care MAPs and are generally uncooperative but not to the point that they are insubordinate.

Although you feel some loss of autonomy, you also think that the case manager has been effective in coordinating care to speed patient discharge. You believe that at present, the atmosphere in the unit is very stressful. The unit manager and case manager have come to you and requested that you assist them in convincing the other staff to go along with this change.

● ASSIGNMENT: Using your knowledge of planned change and case management, outline a plan for reducing resistance.

LEARNING EXERCISE 14.7

Types of Patient Care Delivery Models Used in Your Area

In a group, investigate the types of patient care delivery models used in your area. Do not limit your investigation to hospitals. One health care organization should be assigned to a group. If possible, conduct interviews with nurses from a variety of delivery systems. Share the report of your findings with your classmates. How many different models of patient care delivery did you find? What is the most widely used method in health care facilities in your area? Does this vary from models identified most frequently in current nursing literature?

LEARNING EXERCISE 14.8

Implementing a Managed Care System

You are the director of a home health agency that has recently come under a managed care system. In the past, only a physician's order was necessary for authorization from the Medicare system, but now approval must come from the managed care organization (MCO). In the past, public health certified nurses (all BSNs) have acted as case managers for their assigned caseload. Now the MCO case manager has taken over this role, creating much conflict among the staff. Additionally, there is pressure from your board to cut costs by using more nonprofessionals who are less skilled for some of the home care. You realize that unless you do so, your agency will not survive.

You have visited other home health agencies and researched your options carefully. You have decided that you must use some type of team approach.

● ASSIGNMENT: Develop a plan, objectives, and a time frame for implementation. In your plan, discuss who will be most affected by your changes. As a change agent, what will be your most important role?

Web Links

University of Colorado Health Sciences Center—Colorado Differentiated Practice Model
http://www.uchsc.edu/ahec/cando/nursing/diffpractice97.htm
Examines history, purposes, goals, and implementation of the Colorado Differentiated Practice Model for Nursing.

M. L. Birnbaum—Guidelines, Algorithms, Critical Pathways, Templates, and Evidence-Based Medicine
http://pdm.medicine.wisc.edu/birnbaum6.htm
Differentiates between standardized guidelines, algorithms, critical pathways, and templates and urges critical analysis of all these components that form the standards of practice for evidence-based medicine.

Case Management Society of America
http://www.cmsa.org/
The professional society for case management professionals. This site includes society information, links to other case management sites, and other information about case management.

American Organization of Nurse Executives
www.aone.org/aone/index.jsp
Site discusses many issue related to delivery of nursing care.

References

American Organization of Nursing Executives. (2004). *AONE guiding principles for future patient care delivery toolkit.* Retrieved September 29, 2006, from *http://www.aone.org/aone/resource/guidingprinciples.html.*

American Organization of Nursing Executives. (2006). *AONE practice and education partnership for the future.* Retrieved September 29, 2006, from *http://www.cmsa.org/ABOUTUS/DefinitionofCaseManagement/tabid/104/Default.aspx.*

Benner, P. (1984). *From novice to expert: Excellence and power in clinical nursing practice.* Menlo Park, CA: Addison-Wesley.

Blais, K. K., Hayes, J. S., Kozier, B., & Erb, G. (2002). *Professional nursing practice: Concepts and perspectives.* Fourth Edition. Upper Saddle River, NJ: Prentice Hall Health.

Brady, M., Leuner, J. D., Bellack, J. P., Loquist, R. S., Cipriano, P. F, & O'Neil, E. H. (2001). A proposed framework for differentiating the 21 Pew competencies by level of nursing education. *Nursing and Health Care Perspectives, 22*(1), 30–35.

Case Management Society of America. (2006). *Definition of case management.* Retrieved September 26, 2006, from *http://www.cmsa.org/ABOUTUS/DefinitionofCase Management/tabid/104/Default.aspx.*

Clark, J. S. (2004). An aging population with chronic disease compels new delivery systems focused on new structures and practices. *Nursing Administration Quarterly, 28*(2), 105–115.

DM program is first to be accredited by JCAHO . . . disease management. (2002). *Healthcare-Benchmarks, 9*(4), 46–47.

Eilers, J., Heermann, J. A., Wilson, M. E., & Knutson, S. (2005). Independent nursing actions in cooperative care. *Oncology Nursing Forum, 32*(4), 849–854.

Fox, S. (2006). Differentiated nursing practice: Maximizing resources or dividing an already divided profession? In C. Huston (Ed.), *Professional issues in nursing.* Philadelphia: Lippincott Williams & Wilkins.

Furlow, L. (2003). Cut the clutter with cycle time reduction. *Nursing Management, 34*(3), 42–44.

Harrison, J. P., Nolin, J., & Suero, E. (2004). The effect of case management on U.S. Hospitals. *Nursing Economic$, 22*(2), 64–68.

Huston, C. (2002). The role of the case manager in a disease management program. *Lippincott's Case Management, 7*(6), 221–227.

Reno, K., Cerone, P., Ferket, K., Wojcieszak, E., & Reshoft, M. (2005). Getting over the rainbow. *Nursing Administration Quarterly, 29*(2), 119–122.

Sloand, E., & Groves, S. (2005). A community-oriented primary care nursing model in an international setting that emphasizes partnerships. *Journal of the American Academy of Nurse Practitioners, 17* (2), 47–50.

Smith, A. P. (2003). Case management: Key to access, quality, and financial success. *Nursing Economic$, 21*(5), 237–240, 244.

Tornabeni, J., Stanhope, M., & Wiggins, M. (2006). Clinical nurse leader evolution of a revolution. The CNL vision. *Journal of Nursing Administration, 36*(3), 103–108.

Weitzel, T., Robinson, S. B., Henderson, L., & Anderson, K. (2004). Satisfaction and retention of CNAs working within a functional model of elder care. *Holistic Nursing Practice, 18*(6), 309–312.

Bibliography

Aliotta, S. (2006). The lessons of case management. *Case Manager, 17*(3), 49–52.

Allen, E. E., & Vitale-Nolen, R. A. (2005). Patient care delivery model improves nurse job satisfaction. *Journal of Continuing Education in Nursing, 36*(6), 277–282.

Boswell, A. E. (2004). The impact of staff shortages on care delivery. *Nursing Times, 100*(13), 36–39.

Grant, D., & Murphy, M. L. (2004). Building a new nursing model: Patient care services and nursing philosophy. *Stanford Nurse, 24*(1), 3–5.

Hayman, B., Cioffi, J., & Wilkes, L. (2006). Redesign of the model of nursing practice in an acute care ward: Nurses' experiences. *Collegian, 13*(1), 31–36.

Huffman, M. H., & Cowan, J. A. (2004). Redefine care delivery and documentation. *Nursing Management, 35*(2), 34–38.

Jacobson Vann, J. C. (2006). Measuring community-based case management performance: Strategies for evaluation. *Lippincott's Case Management, 11*(3), 149–159.

Kramer, M., & Schmalenberg, C. (2005). Revising the essentials of magnetism tool: There is more to adequate staffing than numbers. *Journal of Nursing Administration, 35*(4), 188–198.

Lewis-Fleming, G., Laing, D. G., & Lovelace, D. (2006). Bridging case management and primary care manager gaps in a military setting. *Case Manager, 17*(3), 66–71.

Lookinland, S., Tiedeman, M. E., & Crosson, A. E. T. (2005). Nontraditional models of care delivery: Have they solved the problems? *Journal of Nursing Administration, 35*(2), 74–80.

Mezey, M., Kobayashi, M., Grossman, S., Firpo, A., Fulmer, T., & Mitty, E. (2004). Nurses improving care to health system elders (NIVHE): Implementation of best practice models. *Journal of Nursing Administration, 34*(10), 451–457.

Ramos, E. I. (2006). Occupational health nurses and case management. *Nursing Economic$, 24*(1), 30–34.

15

Employee Recruitment, Selection, Placement, and Indoctrination

. . . recruitment and retention of staff is more than technique. It requires enthusiasm about nursing and caring for others.

—*Louis Benson*

. . . I have always surrounded myself with the best people to do their jobs, because I do not want to learn what they already know better than I do.

—*Shirley Sears Chater*

After planning and organizing, staffing is the third phase of the management process. In staffing, the leader–manager recruits, selects, places, and indoctrinates personnel to accomplish the goals of the organization. These steps, which are depicted in Display 15.1, are typically sequential, although each step has some interdependence with all staffing activities.

Staffing is an especially important phase of the management process in health care organizations because such organizations are usually labor intensive (i.e., many employees are required for an organization to accomplish its goals). In addition, many health care organizations are open 24 hours a day, 365 days a year, and client demands and needs are often variable. This large workforce must reflect an appropriate balance of highly skilled, competent professionals and ancillary support workers.

The workforce should also reflect the gender, culture, ethnicity, age, and language diversity of the communities that the organization serves. Having a staff that is both sensitive and

DISPLAY 15.1   Sequential Steps in Staffing

1. Determine the number and types of personnel needed to fulfill the philosophy, meet fiscal planning responsibilities, and carry out the chosen patient care delivery system selected by the organization.
2. Recruit, interview, select, and assign personnel based on established job description performance standards.
3. Use organizational resources for induction and orientation.
4. Ascertain that each employee is adequately socialized to organization values and unit norms.
5. Use creative and flexible scheduling based on patient care needs to increase productivity and retention.

responsive to diversity typically reflects a valuing of diversity at the highest levels of the organization. The importance of this goal cannot be overstated. Traditionally, the nursing profession comprises approximately 90 percent white women, yet more than 40 percent of the population will reflect an ethnic or racial minority by 2020 (Frusti, Niesen, & Campion, 2003).

This chapter examines national and regional trends for professional nurse staffing. It also addresses preliminary staffing functions, namely determining staffing needs and recruiting, interviewing, selecting, and placing personnel. It also reviews two employee indoctrination functions: induction and orientation. The management functions and leadership roles inherent in these staffing responsibilities are shown in Display 15.2.

PREDICTING STAFFING NEEDS

Accurately predicting staffing needs is a crucial management skill because it enables the manager to avoid staffing crises. Managers should know the source of their nursing pool, the number of students enrolled in local nursing schools, the usual length of employment of newly hired staff, peak staff resignation periods, and times when the patient census is highest. In addition, managers must consider the patient care delivery system used, the education and knowledge level of needed staff, budget constraints, historical staffing needs and availability, and the diversity of the patient population to be served.

Third-party insurer reimbursement also impacts staffing. As government and private insurer reimbursements declined in the 1990s, many health care organizations—hospitals in particular—began downsizing by replacing RN positions with unlicensed assistive personnel. Even hospitals that did not downsize during this period often did little to recruit qualified RNs. By the late 1990s, an acute shortage of RNs in many health care settings was attributed to downsizing and shortsightedness regarding recruitment and retention.

 Hospital downsizing and shortsightedness regarding recruitment and retention contributed to the beginning of an acute shortage of RNs in many health care settings by the late 1990s.

The manager also should be aware of the role that national and local economics play in staffing. Historically, nursing shortages occur when the economy is on the upswing and decline

DISPLAY 15.2 Leadership Roles and Management Functions Associated
With Preliminary Staffing Functions

Leadership Roles

1. Plans for future staffing needs proactively by being knowledgeable regarding current and historical staffing events
2. Identifies and recruits talented people to the organization
3. Seeks diversity in staffing, which reflects the diversity of the population being served
4. Is self-aware regarding personal biases during the preemployment process
5. Seeks to find the best possible fit between employees' unique talents and organizational staffing needs
6. Periodically reviews induction and orientation programs to ascertain they are meeting unit needs
7. Ensures that each new employee understands appropriate organizational policies
8. Continually aspires to create a work environment that promotes retention and worker satisfaction

Management Functions

1. Ensures that there is an adequate skilled workforce to meet the goals of the organization
2. Shares responsibility for the recruitment of staff with organization recruiters
3. Plans and structures appropriate interview activities
4. Uses techniques that increase the validity and reliability of the interview process
5. Applies knowledge of the legal requirements of interviewing and selection to ensure that the organization is not unfair in its hiring practices
6. Develops established criteria for selection
7. Uses knowledge of organizational needs and employee strengths to make placement decisions
8. Interprets information in employee handbook and provides input for handbook revisions
9. Participates actively in employee orientation

when the economy recedes, because many unemployed nurses return to the workforce and part-time nurses return to full-time employment. This is only a guideline, however, as some workforce shortages, such as the current professional nursing shortage, have occurred regardless of the economic climate.

Historically, when the economy improves, nursing shortages occur. When the economy declines, nursing vacancy rates decline as well.

THE CURRENT NURSING SHORTAGE

Health care managers have long been sensitive to the importance of physical (technology, space) and financial resources to the success of service delivery. It is the shortage of human resources, however, that likely poses the greatest challenge to most health care organizations today. This shortage is predicted to grow.

The shortage of unlicensed and licensed nursing staff is profound (indeed worldwide in the case of RNs) and is predicted to grow even larger in the coming decade.

The nursing shortage is widespread. The United States currently has about 2.9 million RNs filling about 2.4 million jobs (U.S. Department of Labor, 2006). Yet, this is not enough. The American Hospital Association (AHA) reported 118,000 RN job vacancies by late 2005, and 49 percent of hospitals reported more trouble recruiting RNs in 2005 than in 2004 (AHA, 2006). Similarly, a study released by the U.S. Health Resources and Services Administration (HRSA) in April 2006 (USDHHS, 2006) suggested that one million new nurses will be needed by 2020 and that all 50 states in the United States will experience a nursing shortage of some degree by 2015 (American Association of Colleges of Nursing [AACN], 2006a). Similarly, in 2005, the U.S. Bureau of Labor Statistics suggested that more than 1.2 million new and replacement nurses will be needed by 2014 than are currently available (Hecker, 2005).

It also seems to be clear that resolving the current shortage will require more than the short-term, quick-fix solutions that have worked in the past because there are too few nurses now, and there is a projected need for more nurses in the long term.

 The current shortage is caused by both an inadequate short-term and long-term supply of human resources as well as a projected long-term rise in demand for nursing services.

SUPPLY FACTORS

Supply factors contributing to the current nursing shortage include an aging workforce and inadequate nursing education enrollments.

The Aging Workforce

Nurses are a graying population—even more so than the population at large. This means that the nursing workforce is retiring at a rate faster than it can be replaced. The most recent national RN survey (2004 National Sample Survey of Registered Nurses), released in March 2006, indicates that the estimated average age of the RN is 46.8 years, more than a year older than the estimated average age of 45.2 years in the 2000 survey (Hart, 2006). Indeed, the average age of the working nurse has been increasing for some time. Only 26.6 percent of the RN population in the survey was under age 40; just 16.6 percent was under 30, and the age of the largest group of RNs ranged between 45 and 49 (Hart, 2006). This rising average age reflected a 2- to 3-decade trend toward older students entering nursing education programs as well as a general decline in interest in nursing as a career among younger people today.

A new 2007 study, however, suggests that this trend may be reversing. Auerbach, Buerhaus, and Staiger (2007) found that although the number of people entering nursing in their early to mid-20s remains at its lowest point in 40 years, greater numbers of individuals in their late 20s and 30s are entering the field, which should serve to decrease the age of the average nurse. In addition, the study showed that people born in the 1970s are now almost as likely to become nurses as people born during the 1950s when interest in nursing careers was at its highest. The

EXAMINING THE EVIDENCE 15.1

Source: Bernard Hodes Group. (2006). *The 2006 aging nursing workforce survey.* Retrieved December 6, 2006, from *http://www.hodes.com/publications/pdfs/ agingnurse_sep06.pdf.*

The Nursing Management Aging Workforce Survey—of nearly 1,000 nurses, predominantly nurse–managers—found that by 2010, about 20 percent of the nurse–managers will have retired, and about 35 percent of their nursing employees will have retired. By 2020, 75 percent of those nurse–leaders who completed this survey will have retired, and about 52 percent of their nursing employees will have retired.

The end result of the survey was that more than 55 percent of respondents reported intending to retire between 2011 and 2020. An additional 25.5 percent of respondents expected to leave the workplace soon after that.

The researchers concluded that in order to replace those who are retiring, "It will be necessary to bolster recruitment and hiring efforts for nurse leaders and nursing employees. In addition, efforts should be made to retain nurse leaders and nursing employees as they near retirement. It also may be beneficial to find solutions to encourage staff nurses to pursue a career in nurse management and for health care organizations to develop the educational programs to enable this goal" (p. 5).

researchers suggest that this projected increase in nursing will mitigate the severity of the nursing shortage in 2020.

Yet, retirement projections for the profession are grim. The Nursing Management Aging Workforce Survey, released in July 2006, reported that 55 percent of surveyed nurses planned to retire between 2011 and 2020 and that generally, employers were taking little action to retain aging workers (Orlovsky, 2006) (Examining the Evidence 15.1). In addition, another recent study suggested that one in three nurses under the age of 30 plans to leave the profession within a year (Health Workforce Institute, 2006).

Inadequate Nursing Education Enrollments

The current shortage is also being caused by inadequate enrollment in nursing programs. While enrollment has increased between 5 and 18 percent every year since 2001 (AACN, 2006b), the increases are insufficient to replace those nurses who will be lost to retirement. Indeed, HRSA projects that nursing school graduates would need to increase by 90 percent nationwide to adequately address the nursing shortage (USDHHS, 2006). Unfortunately, such enrollment increases are not possible without the significant boost in federal and state funding needed to prepare new faculty, enhance teaching resources, and upgrade nursing school infrastructure (AACN, 2006b).

Ironically, the problem is not a lack of nursing school applicants. The problem is that there are inadequate resources to provide nursing education to those interested in pursuing nursing as a career. Indeed, the AACN (2006b) reports that 32,323 qualified applications to entry-level baccalaureate programs were denied acceptance in 2005. Some universities have chosen to close nursing programs because of funding cuts. Others have reduced program size.

Still others turn away potential students because of a lack of faculty—a major reason for denying qualified students admission (La Rocco, 2006).

> By 2005, 75 percent of nursing schools cited faculty shortages as the major reason that they had denied qualified students admission (La Rocco, 2006). According to a 2006 survey by AACN, there were 637 faculty vacancies at 329 nursing schools with baccalaureate and/or graduate programs across the country, and an additional 55 faculty positions were needed just to accommodate student demand (AACN, 2006c). This translates into approximately 1.9 faculty vacancies per school.

The "graying" of the nursing faculty also contributes to the current nursing shortage. With the average age of PhD-prepared nurse educators being almost 54 years and the average retirement age for nursing faculty being 62.5 (La Rocco, 2006), one must question where the faculty will come from to teach the new nurses needed to solve the current shortage (Huston, 2006a). In addition, with only 13 percent of nurses holding earned master's or doctoral degrees (HRSA, 2006) and the lag time required to educate master's- or doctorally prepared faculty, the faculty shortage may end up being the greatest obstacle to solving the nursing shortage.

DEMAND FACTORS

The U.S. Department of Labor (2006) predicts an increased demand for professional nurses in both the short- and long-term future. In fact, employment of RNs is expected to grow much faster than average for all occupations through 2014 and will create the second largest number of new jobs among all occupations (U.S. Department of Labor, 2006).

At least part of this increased demand will be driven by technological advances in patient care and by the increasing emphasis on preventive health care. In addition, the growing elderly population will require more nursing care (U.S. Department of Labor, 2006).

Acting to Resolve the Current Nursing Shortage

Federal moneys for nursing education have increased. The passage of legislation, such as the 2002 Nurse Reinvestment Act, has encouraged more students to choose nursing as a career and helps students financially to complete their education. It also encourages graduate students to complete their studies and assume teaching positions in nursing schools. In addition, many states have introduced or passed legislation designed to improve working conditions or attract more nurses.

Some experts suggest, however, that too much emphasis is placed on recruiting new nurses to solve the current shortage and that supply could more easily be increased by bringing unemployed or part-time nurses back to nursing full-time (Huston, 2006a)—or by enticing nurses back into nursing who are now working in non-nursing positions (Duffield et al., 2006). Indeed, about one of four nurses works part-time (U.S. Department of Labor, 2006). The reality is, however, that 81.7 percent, or 2,201,813 of active licensed RNs, are already employed in nursing (USDHHS, 2001).

Other experts suggest that more attention be given to retaining older workers or bringing retired nurses back into the workforce. Cyr (2005) agrees, suggesting that while many nurses

DISPLAY 15.3 Strategies for Retaining Older Workers

- Offer flexible shifts: options of 4, 6, and 8 hours as well as job-sharing.
- Cluster patient assignments, and keep supplies and equipment in central locations to avoid extensive walking.
- Use lift teams, special beds, and equipment to curtail work-related injuries and physical strain.
- Review and adapt benefits packages to accommodate different needs.
- Use older nurses for nonphysical work, such as patient admissions and discharges.
- Move older nurses and other allied health professionals into areas and positions maximizing their expertise while minimizing physical stress.
- Use older staff as mentors and preceptors.

Source: Hart, K. A. (2006). *The aging workforce: Implications for recruiters.* Retrieved December 6, 2006, from *http://www.hodes.com/publications/talentmatters/archives/hcmatters_jul06.asp.*

retire because they are financially independent, some would consider delaying retirement if the work environment were altered to support older nurses. The Bernard Hodes Group (2006) agrees, suggesting that employers must be able to accommodate aging workers with technology aimed at reducing physical strain, such as electric beds, bariatric equipment, and mechanical lift devices. Other strategies suggested for retaining aging nurses include flexible scheduling and benefits, continuing education aid, and wellness programs (Bernard Hodes Group, 2006). These strategies and others are summarized in Display 15.3.

Another short-term solution to the current shortage has been the importation of foreign nurses, particularly by developed countries from developing countries. While such importation can result in positive global economic, social, and professional development, many of the donor countries, who can least afford it, are experiencing a substantial "brain and skills drain." Huston (2006b) goes so far as to suggest that recruiting foreign nurses to solve acute staffing shortages "may be a poorly thought out, quick fix to a much greater problem and that in doing so, not only are donor nations harmed, the issues that led to the shortage in the first place are never addressed" (p. 113).

Clearly, long-term planning and aggressive intervention will be needed for some time to ensure that an adequate, highly qualified nursing workforce will be available to meet the health care needs of U.S. citizens.

RECRUITMENT

Recruitment is the process of actively seeking out or attracting applicants for existing positions, and it should be an ongoing process.

 Although at any given time an organization may have an adequate supply of RNs to meet demand, recruitment should be an ongoing process.

In complex organizations, work must be accomplished by groups of people; wise managers, therefore, try to surround themselves with people of ability, motivation, and promise. Unfortunately, some managers feel threatened by bright and talented people and surround themselves with mediocrity. The organization's ability to meet its goals and objectives relates directly to the quality of its employees.

The Nurse Recruiter

The manager may be greatly or minimally involved with recruiting, interviewing, and selecting personnel depending on (a) the size of the institution, (b) the existence of a separate personnel department, (c) the presence of a nurse recruiter within the organization, and (d) the use of centralized or decentralized nursing management.

Generally speaking, the more decentralized nursing management and the less complex the personnel department, the greater the involvement of lower-level managers in selecting personnel for individual units or departments. When deciding whether to hire a nurse–recruiter or decentralize the responsibility for recruitment, the organization needs to weigh benefits against costs. Costs include more than financial considerations. For example, an additional cost to an organization employing a nurse–recruiter might be the eventual loss of interest by managers in the recruiting process. The organization loses if managers relegate their collective and individual responsibilities to the nurse–recruiter.

When organizations use nurse–recruiters, a collaborative relationship must exist between managers and recruiters. Managers must be aware of recruitment constraints, and the recruiter must be aware of individual department needs and culture. Both parties must understand the organization's philosophy, benefit programs, salary scale, and other factors that influence employee retention.

Recruitment and Retention

Recruiting adequate numbers of nurses is less difficult if the organization is located in a progressive community with several schools of nursing and if the organization has a good reputation for quality patient care and fair employment practices. It will likely be much more difficult to recruit nurses to rural areas that historically have experienced less appropriation of health care professionals per capita than urban areas.

Because most recruiting methods are expensive, health care organizations often seek less costly means of recruitment. One of the best ways to maintain an adequate employee pool is by word of mouth; the recommendation of the organization's own satisfied and happy staff. Recruitment, however, is not the key to adequate staffing in the long term. Retention is and only occurs when the organization is able to create a work environment that makes staff want to stay.

Some turnover, however, is normal and, in fact, desirable. Turnover infuses the organization with fresh ideas. It also reduces the probability of groupthink, in which everyone shares similar thought processes, values, and goals. However, excessive or unnecessary turnover reduces the ability of the organization to produce its end product and is expensive.

Atencio, Cohen, and Gorenberg (2003) suggest that the cost of turnover is up to twice a nurse's annual salary, or $92,422 for a medical–surgical nurse. The costs of replacing a specialty nurse could be as high as $145,000 (Atencio et al., 2003). Such costs generally include human resource expenses for advertising and interviewing; recruitment fees such as sign-on bonuses; increased use of traveling nurses, overtime, and temporary replacements for the lost worker; lost productivity; and the costs of training time to bring the new employee up to desired efficiency.

Clearly, the manager must recognize the link between retention and recruitment. Some health care organizations find it necessary to do external recruitment, partly because of their lack of attention to retention. Atencio and colleagues (2003) suggest that the social climate of the workplace is the primary initiator of a nurse's intent to stay or leave and that this social climate may reflect either work frustration or work excitement. Research by Strachota, Normandin, O'Brien, Clary, and Krukow (2003) concur, citing work hours (having to work the majority of holidays, every other weekend, nights with no possibility of changing to day shift, and lack of scheduling flexibility) as the number one reason that nurses leave their position. Similarly, Lynn and Redman (2005) suggest that retention programs must focus on both organizational commitment and work and professional satisfaction. The middle level manager has the greatest impact in addressing these concerns and creating a positive social climate.

 It is critical that the manager recognize the link between retention and recruitment.

In addition, the closer the fit between what the nurse is seeking in employment and what the organization can offer, the greater the chance that the nurse will be retained. Often, those recruiting during a nursing shortage inadvertently misrepresent the organization. At times, this behavior borders on unethical conduct but most often occurs because of the recruiter's overzealousness.

LEARNING EXERCISE 15.1

Examining Recruitment Advertisements
Select one of the following:
1. In small groups, examine several nursing journals that carry job advertisements. Select three ads that particularly appeal to you. What do these advertisements say, or what makes them stand out? Are similar key words used in all three ads? What bonuses or incentives are being offered to attract qualified professional nurses?
2. Select a health care agency in your area. Write an advertisement or recruitment poster that accurately depicts the agency and the community. Compare your completed advertisement or recruitment flyer with those created by others in your group.

THE INITIAL CONTACT

Many prospective employees will make their first contact with an organization through the human resources department or the recruiter. Generally, these individuals are directed to complete an application and set up an appointment for an interview. Research by Kalisch (2003) suggests, however, that this process is often fraught with problems and that up to 25 percent of potential employees never receive a response to letters, or they end up in an extensive and frustrating "telephone tag" (83 percent). In 21 of the 122 hospitals in Kalisch's study, the applications or résumés provided by the applicant were lost either temporarily or permanently. Interview wait times ranged from 1 to 90 minutes, and interview length ranged from 5 to 95 minutes. Only two applicants were offered coffee or refreshments of any kind, and 32 percent reported reluctance or refusal to set up an appointment for an interview by the human resources secretary. Clearly, this conveys a lack of valuing of the potential employee, and most health care institutions cannot afford this neglect of common courtesy in an era of nursing shortages.

INTERVIEWING AS A SELECTION TOOL

An *interview* may be defined as a verbal interaction between individuals for a particular purpose. Although other tools such as testing and reference checks may be used, the interview is frequently accepted as the foundation for hiring. The purposes or goals of the selection interview are threefold: (a) the interviewer seeks to obtain enough information to determine the applicant's suitability for the available position; (b) the applicant obtains adequate information to make an intelligent decision about accepting the job, should it be offered; and (c) the interviewer seeks to conduct the interview in such a manner that regardless of the interview's result, the applicant will continue to have respect for and goodwill toward the organization.

Interviews may be unstructured or structured. The unstructured interview requires little planning because the goals for hiring may be unclear, questions are not prepared in advance, and often the interviewer does more talking than the applicant. The structured interview requires greater planning time because questions must be developed in advance that address the specific job requirements, information must be offered about the skills and qualities being sought, examples of the applicant's experience must be received, and the willingness or motivation of the applicant to do the job must be determined. The interviewer who uses a structured format would ask the same essential questions of all applicants.

Limitations of Interviews

The major defect of the interview is subjectivity. Most interviewers feel confident that they can overcome this subjectivity and view the interview as a reliable selection tool, whereas most interviews still have an element of subjectivity. The applicant, trying to create a favorable impression, also may be unduly influenced by the interviewer's personality.

Research findings regarding the validity and reliability of interviews have been inconsistent. However, the following findings are generally accepted:

- The same interviewer will consistently rate the interviewee the same. Therefore, the *intra-rater reliability* is said to be high.
- If two different interviewers conduct unstructured interviews of the same applicant, their ratings will not be consistent. Therefore, the *inter-rater reliability* is extremely low in unstructured interviews.
- Inter-rater reliability is satisfactory if the interview is *structured* and the same format is used by both interviewers.
- Even if the interview has *reliability* (i.e., it measures the same thing consistently), it still may not be valid. *Validity* occurs when the interview measures what it is supposed to measure, which in this case is the potential for productivity as an employee. Structured interviews have greater validity than unstructured interviews. Thus, the structured interview was found to be a much better predictor of job performance and overall effectiveness than the unstructured interview.
- High interview assessments are not related to subsequent high-level job performance.
- Validity increases when there is a team approach to the interview.

- The attitudes and biases of interviewers greatly influence how candidates are rated. Although steps can be taken to reduce subjectivity, it cannot be eliminated entirely.
- The interviewer is more influenced by unfavorable information than by favorable information. Negative information is weighed more heavily than positive information about the applicant.
- Interviewers tend to make up their minds about hiring applicants very early in the job interview. Decisions are often formed in the first few minutes of the interview.
- In unstructured interviews, the interviewer tends to do most of the talking, whereas in structured interviews, the interviewer talks less. The goal should always be to have the interviewee do most of the talking.

As a predictor of job performance and overall effectiveness, the structured interview is much more reliable than the unstructured interview.

Regardless of inherent defects, interviewing continues to be widely used as a selection tool. By knowing the limitations of interviews and using findings from current research evidence, interviewers should be able to conduct interviews so that they will have an increased predictive value.

Overcoming Interview Limitations

Interview research has helped managers to develop strategies for overcoming its limitations. The following strategies will assist the manager in developing an interview process with greater reliability and validity.

Prepare for the Interview

Asselin (2006) suggests that managers should "have a complete and clear understanding of the open position" before interviewing a candidate (p. 42). This includes obtaining a copy of the job description and knowing the educational and experiential requirements for the position. The manager should also create a list of competencies that are essential for success on the job as well as the professional values, characteristics, and behaviors that are most likely to ensure success in the position (Asselin, 2006).

Use a Team Approach

Having more than one person interview the job applicant reduces individual bias. Staff involvement in hiring can be viewed on a continuum from no involvement to a team approach, using unit staff for the hiring decisions. When hiring a manager, using a staff nurse as part of the interview team is effective, especially if the staff nurse is mature enough to represent the interests and needs of the unit rather than his or her own self-interests.

Develop a Structured Interview Format for Each Job Classification

Because each job has different position requirements, interviews must be structured to fit the position. The same structured interview should be used for all employees applying for the same job classification. A well-developed structured interview uses open-ended questions and provides ample opportunity for the interviewee to talk. The structured interview is advantageous because it allows the interviewer to be consistent and prevents the interview from becoming sidetracked. Display 15.4 is an example of a structured interview.

DISPLAY 15.4   **Sample Structured Interview**

Motivation

Why did you apply for employment with this company?

Physical

Do you have any physical limitations that would prohibit you from accomplishing the job?
How many days have you been absent from work during the last year of employment?

Education

What was your grade point average in nursing school?
What were your extracurricular activities, offices held, awards conferred?
For verification purposes, are your school records listed under the name on your application form?

Professional

In what states are you licensed to practice?
Do you have your license with you?
What certifications do you hold?
What professional organizations do you currently participate in that would be of value in the job for which you are applying?

Military Experience

What are your current military obligations?
Which military assignments do you think have prepared you for this position?

Present Employer

How did you secure your present position?
What is your current job title? What was your title when you began your present position?
What supervisory responsibilities do you currently have?
How would you describe your immediate supervisor?
What are some examples of success at your present job?
How do you get along with your present employer?
How do you get along with your present colleagues?
What do you like most about your present job?
What do you like least about your present job?
May we contact your present employer?
Why do you want to change jobs?
For verification purposes only, is your name the same as it was while employed with your current employer?

Previous Position(s)

Ask similar questions about recent past employment. Depending on the time span and type of other positions held, the interviewer does not usually review employment history that took place beyond the position just previous to the current one.

Specific Questions for RNs

What do you like most about nursing?
What do you like least about nursing?
What is your philosophy of nursing?

Personal Characteristics

Which personal characteristics are your greatest assets?
Which personal characteristics cause you the most difficulty?

Professional Goals

What are your career goals?
Where do you see yourself 10 years from now?

Contributions to Organization

What can you offer this company?

General Questions

What questions do you have about the organization?
What questions do you have about the position?
What other questions do you have?

LEARNING EXERCISE 15.2

Creating Additional Interview Criteria

You are a home health nurse with a large caseload of low-income, inner-city families. Because of your spouse's job transfer, you have just resigned from your position of 3 years to take a similar position in another public health district. Your agency supervisor has asked that you assist her with interviewing and selecting your replacement. Five applicants meet the minimum criteria. They each have at least 2 years of acute-care experience, a baccalaureate nursing degree, and a state public health credential. Because you know the job requirements better than anyone, your supervisor has asked that you develop additional criteria and a set of questions to ask each applicant.

● ASSIGNMENT:
  1. Use a decision grid (see Fig. 1.3 on page 120) to develop additional criteria. Weight the criteria so that the applicants will have a final score.
  2. Develop an interview guide of six appropriate questions to ask the applicants.

Use Scenarios to Determine Decision-Making Ability

Use scenarios to determine decision-making ability. In addition to obtaining answers to a particular set of questions, the interview also should be used to determine the applicant's decision-making ability. This can be accomplished by designing scenarios that require problem-solving and decision-making skills. The same set of scenarios should be used with each category of employee.

For example, a set could be developed for new graduates, critical care nurses, unit secretaries, and practical nurses. Patient care situations, as shown in Display 15.5, require clinical judgment and are very useful for this purpose.

Conduct Multiple Interviews

Candidates should be interviewed more than once on separate days. This prevents applicants from being accepted or rejected merely because they were having a good or bad day. Regardless of the number of interviews held, the person should be interviewed until all the interviewers' questions have been answered, and they feel confident that they have enough information to make the right decision.

Provide Training in Effective Interviewing Techniques

Training should focus on communication skills and advice on planning, conducting, and controlling the interview. It is unfair to expect a manager to make appropriate hiring decisions if he or she has never had adequate training in interview techniques. Unskilled interviewers often allow subjective data rather than objective data affect their hiring evaluation. In addition, unskilled interviewers may ask questions that could be viewed as discriminatory or that are illegal.

Planning, Conducting, and Controlling the Interview

Planning the interview in advance is vital to its subsequent success as a selection tool. If other interviewers are to be present, they should be available at the appointed time. The plan also should include adequate time for the interview. Before the interview, all interviewers should review the application, noting questions concerning information supplied by the applicant. Although it takes

DISPLAY 15.5   **Sample Interview Questions Using Case Situations**

Each recent graduate applying for a position at Country Hospital will be asked to respond to the following:

Case 1

You are working on the evening shift of a surgical unit. Mr. Jones returned from the postanesthesia care unit following a hip replacement 2 hours ago. While in the recovery room, he received 10 mg of morphine sulfate intravenously for incisional pain. Thirty minutes ago, he complained of mild incisional pain but then drifted off to sleep. He is now awake and complaining of moderate to severe incisional pain. His orders include the following pain relief order: morphine sulfate 8–10 mg, IV push every 3 hours for pain. It has been 2½ hours since Mr. Jones' last pain medication. What would you do?

Case 2

One of the LPNs/LVNs on your team seems especially tired today. She later tells you that her new baby kept her up all night. When you ask her about the noon finger-stick blood glucose level on Mrs. White (82 years old), she looks at you blankly and then says quickly that it was 150. Later, when you are in Mrs. White's room, she tells you that she doesn't remember anyone checking her blood glucose level at noon. What do you do?

considerable practice, consistently using a planned sequence in the interview format will eventually yield a relaxed and spontaneous process. The following is a suggested interview format:

1. Introduce yourself, and greet the applicant.
2. Make a brief statement about the organization and the available positions.
3. Ascertain the position for which the person is applying.
4. Discuss the information on the application, and seek clarification or amplification as necessary.
5. Discuss employee qualifications, and proceed with the structured interview format.
6. If the applicant appears qualified, discuss the organization and the position further.
7. Explain the subsequent procedures for hiring, such as employment physicals, and hiring date. If the applicant is not hired at this time, discuss how and when he or she will be notified of the interview results.
8. Terminate the interview.

Try to create and maintain a comfortable environment throughout the interview, but do not forget that the interviewer is in charge of the interview. If the interview has begun well and the applicant is at ease, the interview will usually proceed smoothly. During the meeting, the manager should pause frequently to allow the applicant to ask questions. The format should always encourage and include ample time for questions from the applicant. Often, interviewers are able to infer much about applicants by the types of questions that they ask.

Remember that the interviewer should have control of the interview and set the tone.

Moving the conversation along, covering questions on a structured interview guide, and keeping the interview pertinent but friendly becomes easier with experience. Methods that help to reach the goals of the interview follow:

- Ask only job-related questions.
- Use open-ended questions that require more than a "yes" or "no" answer.
- Pause a few seconds after the applicant has seemingly finished before asking the next question. This gives the applicant a chance to talk further.
- Return to topics later in the interview on which the applicant offered little information initially.
- Ask only one question at a time.
- Restate part of the applicant's answer if you need elaboration.
- Ask questions clearly, but do not verbally or nonverbally indicate the correct answer. Otherwise, by watching the interviewer's eyes and observing other body language, the astute applicant may learn which answers are desired.
- Always appear interested in what the applicant has to say. The applicant should never be interrupted, nor should the interviewer's words ever imply criticism of or impatience with the applicant.
- Language should be used that is appropriate for the applicant. Terminology or language that makes applicants feel the interviewer is either talking down to them or talking over their heads is inappropriate.
- A written record should be kept of all interviews. Note taking ensures accuracy and serves as a written record to recall the applicant. Keep note taking or use of a checklist, however, to a minimum so that you do not create an uncomfortable climate.

As the interview draws to a close, the interviewer should make sure that all questions have been answered and that all pertinent information has been obtained. Usually, applicants are not offered a job at the end of a first interview unless they are clearly qualified and the labor market is such that another applicant would be difficult to find. In most cases, interviewers need to analyze their impressions of the applicant, compare these perceptions with members of the selection team, and incorporate those impressions with other available data about the applicant. It is important, however, to let applicants know if they are being seriously considered for the position and how soon they can expect to hear a final outcome.

When the applicant is obviously not qualified, the interviewer needs to be extremely tactful. The interviewer should not give false hope but should advise the person as soon as possible that he or she does not have the proper qualifications for the position. Such applicants should believe that they have been treated fairly. The interviewer should, however, maintain records of the exact reasons for rejection in case of later discrimination charges.

Evaluation of the Interview

Interviewers should plan postinterview time to evaluate the applicant's interview performance. Interview notes should be reviewed as soon as possible and necessary points clarified or amplified. Using a form to record the interview evaluation is a good idea. The final question on the interview report form is a recommendation for or against hiring. In answering this question, two aspects must carry the most weight:

- *The requirements for the job.* Regardless of how interesting or friendly people are, unless they have the basic skills for the job, they will not be successful at meeting the expectations of the position. Likewise, those overqualified for a position will usually be unhappy in the job.
- *Personal bias.* Because completely eliminating the personal biases inherent in the interview is impossible, it is important for the interviewer to examine any negative feelings that occurred during the interview. Often, the interviewer discovers that the negative feelings have no relation to the criteria necessary for success in the position.

Legal Aspects of Interviewing

The organization must ascertain that the application form does not contain questions that violate various employment acts. Likewise, managers must avoid unlawful inquiries during the interview. Inquiries cannot be made regarding age, marital status, children, race, sexual preference, financial or credit status, national origin, or religion.

 Interview inquiries regarding age, marital status, children, race, sexual preference, financial or credit status, national origin, or religion are illegal because they are deemed discriminatory.

In addition to federal legislation, many states have specific laws pertaining to information that can and cannot be obtained during the process. For example, some states prohibit asking about a woman's ability to reproduce or her attitudes toward family planning. Table 15.1 lists subjects that are most frequently part of the interview process or applicant form, with examples of acceptable and unacceptable inquiries.

Managers who maintain interview records and receive applicants with an open and unbiased attitude have little to fear regarding charges of discrimination. Remember that each applicant

TABLE 15.1   Acceptable and Unacceptable Interview Inquiries

Subject	Acceptable Inquiries	Unacceptable Inquiries
Name	If applicant has worked for the organization under a different name. If school records are under another name. If applicant has another name.	Inquiries about name that would indicate lineage, national origin, or marital or criminal status.
Marital and family status	Whether applicant can meet specified work schedules or has commitments that may hinder attendance requirements. Inquiries as to anticipated stay in the position.	Any question about applicant's marital status or number or age of children. Information about child care arrangements. Any questions concerning pregnancy.
Address or residence	Place of residence and length resided in city or state.	Former addresses, names or relationships of people with whom applicant resides, or if owns or rents home.
Age	If over 18 or statement that hire is subject to age requirement. Can ask if applicant is between 18 and 70.	Inquiry of specific age or date of birth.
Birthplace	Can ask for proof of U.S. citizenship.	Birthplace of applicant or spouse or any relative.
Religion	No inquiries allowed.	
Race or color	Can be requested for affirmative action but not as employment criteria.	All questions about race are prohibited.
Character	Inquiry into actual convictions that relate to fitness to perform job.	Questions relating to arrests or conviction of a crime.
Relatives	Relatives employed in organization. Names and addresses of parents if applicant is a minor.	Questions about who applicant lives with or number of dependents.
Notify in case of emergency	Name and address of a *person* to be notified.	Name and address of a *relative* to be notified.
Organizations	Professional organizations.	Requesting a list of all memberships.
References	Professional or character reference.	Religious references.
Physical condition	All applicants can be asked if they are able to carry out the physical demands of the job.	Employers must be prepared to justify any mental or physical requirements. Specific questions regarding handicaps are forbidden.

(continued)

TABLE 15.1   **Acceptable and Unacceptable Interview Inquiries** (continued)

Subject	Acceptable Inquiries	Unacceptable Inquiries
Photographs	Statement that a photograph may be required *after* employment.	Requirement that a photograph be taken *before* interview or hiring.
National origin	If necessary to perform job, languages applicant speaks, reads, or writes.	Inquiries about birthplace, native language, ancestry, date of arrival in United States, or native language.
Education	Academic, vocational, or professional education. Schools attended. Ability to reads, speak, and write foreign languages.	Inquiries into racial or religious affiliation of a school. Inquiry into dates of schooling.
Sex	Inquiry or restriction of employment is only for bona fide occupational qualification, which is interpreted very narrowly by the courts.	Cannot ask sex on application. Sex cannot be used as a factor for hiring decisions.
Credit rating	No inquiries.	Questions about car or home ownership also are prohibited.
Other	Notice may be given that misstatements or omissions of facts may be cause for dismissal.	

should feel good about the organization when the interview concludes and be able to recall the experience as a positive one. It is a leadership responsibility to see that this goal is accomplished.

TIPS FOR THE INTERVIEWEE

Just as there are things that the interviewer should do to prepare and conduct the interview, there are things that interviewees should do to increase the likelihood that the interview will be a mutually satisfying and enlightening experience (Display 15.6). The interviewee must also prepare in advance for the interview. Obtaining copies of the philosophy and organization chart of the organization to which you are applying should give you some insight as to the organization's priorities and help you to identify questions to ask the interviewer. Speaking to individuals who already work at the organization should be helpful in determining whether the organization philosophy is implemented in practice.

Schedule an appointment for the interview. Do not allow yourself to be drawn into an impromptu interview when you are dropping off an application or seeking information from the human resource department. You will want to be professionally dressed and will likely need time to reflect and prepare for the interview.

Practice responses to potential interview questions, such as your philosophy of nursing or your goals and strengths.

DISPLAY 15.6 Interviewing Tips for Applicants

1. Prepare in advance for the interview.
2. Obtain copies of the philosophy and organization chart of the organization to which you are applying.
3. Schedule an appointment for the interview.
4. Dress professionally and conservatively.
5. Practice responses to potential interview questions in advance.
6. Arrive early on the day of the interview.
7. Greet the interviewer formally, and do not sit down before he or she does unless given permission to do so.
8. Shake the interviewer's hand upon entering the room and smile.
9. During the interview, sit quietly, be attentive, and take notes only if absolutely necessary.
10. Do not chew gum, fidget, slouch, or play with your hair, keys, or writing pen.
11. Ask appropriate questions about the organization or the specific job for which you are applying.
12. Avoid a "what can you do for me?" approach, and focus instead on whether your unique talents and interests are a fit with the organization.
13. Answer interview questions as honestly and confidently as possible.
14. Shake the interviewer's hand at the close of the interview, and thank him or her for his or her time.
15. Send a brief, typed thank-you note to the interviewer within 24 hours of the interview.

It is difficult to spontaneously answer interview questions about your personal philosophy of nursing, your individual strengths and weaknesses, and your career goals if you have not given them advance thought.

On the day of the interview, arrive about 10 minutes early to allow time for you to collect your thoughts and be mentally ready. Anticipate some nervousness (this is perfectly normal). Greet the interviewer formally (not by first name), and do not sit down before the interviewer does unless given permission to do so. Be sure to shake the interviewer's hand upon entering the room and to smile. Smiling will reduce both your anxiety and that of the interviewer. Remember that many interviewers make up their mind early in the interview process, so first impressions count a lot.

During the interview, sit quietly, be attentive, and take notes only if absolutely necessary. Do not chew gum, fidget, slouch, or play with your hair, keys, or writing pen. Dress conservatively and make sure that you are neatly groomed. Ask appropriate questions about the organization or the specific job for which you are applying. Questions about wages, benefits, and advancement opportunities should likely come later in the interview. Avoid a "what can you do for me?" approach, and focus instead on whether your unique talents and interests are a fit with the organization. Answer interview questions as honestly and confidently as possible. Avoid rambling and never lie. If you do not know the answer to a question, say so. Also, if you need a few moments to reflect on a complex question before answering, state that as well.

At the close of the interview, shake the interviewer's hand and thank him or her for taking time to talk with you. It is always appropriate to clarify at that point when hiring decisions will be made and how you will be notified about the interview's outcome. You may want to send a brief thank-you note to the interviewer as well.

SELECTION

After applicants have been recruited, have completed their applications, and have been interviewed, the next step in the preemployment staffing process is selection. *Selection* is the process of choosing from among applicants the best-qualified individual or individuals for a particular job or position. This process involves verifying the applicant's qualifications, checking his or her work history, and deciding if a good match exists between the applicant's qualifications and the organization's expectations. Determining whether a "fit" exists between an employee and an organization is seldom easy.

Educational and Credential Requirements

Consideration should be given to educational requirements and credentials for each job category as long as a relationship exists between these requirements and success on the job. If requirements for a position are too rigid, the job may remain unfilled for some time. Additionally, people who might be able to complete educational or credential requirements for a position are sometimes denied the opportunity to compete for the job. Therefore, many organizations have a list of *preferred criteria* for a position and a second list of *minimal criteria*. Frequently, organizations will accept *substitution criteria* in lieu of preferred criteria. For example, a position might require a bachelor's degree, but a master's degree is preferred. However, 5 years of nursing experience could be substituted for the master's degree.

It is very important to check the academic and professional credentials of all job applicants. In a competitive job market, candidates may succumb to the pressure of "embroidering" their qualifications.

Reference Checks

All applications should be examined to see if they are complete and to ascertain that the applicant is qualified for the position. At this point, references are requested, and employment history is verified. According to Asselin (2006), the manager should always be cognizant of red flags in applications such as "unexplained gaps in employment history or frequent changes of employer without acceptable explanation" (p. 45). Similarly, "listing 'personal' as a reason for leaving prior positions, having blanks on the application form, questions, and noting dates that don't match, are additional warning signs" (p. 45).

Clearly, a strong application and excellent references do not necessarily guarantee excellent job performance; however, carefully reviewing applications and checking references may help to prevent a bad hiring decision. Ideally, whenever possible, these actions as well as verifying work experience and credentials should be done before the interview. Some managers prefer to interview first so that time is not wasted in processing the application if the interview results in a decision not to hire, and this is a personal choice. Not until applications have been verified and references obtained is a position offered.

 Positions should never be offered until information on the application has been verified and references have been checked.

Occasionally, reference calls will reveal unsolicited information about the applicant. Information obtained by any method may not be used to reject an applicant unless a justifiable reason for disqualification exists. For example, if the applicant volunteers information about his or her driving record or if this information is discovered by other means, it cannot be used to reject a potential employee unless the position requires driving.

Preemployment Testing

Preemployment testing is used only when such testing is directly related to the ability to perform a specific job. Although testing is not a stand-alone selection tool, it can, when coupled with excellent interviewing and reference checking, provide additional information about a candidate to make the best selection.

Lawsuits resulting from allegedly improper implementation and interpretation of preemployment testing have made employers shy away from preemployment testing. Some major corporations, but few health care organizations, still use testing as a selection tool. Some health care organizations, however, do use postemployment testing to determine learning needs or skill deficiencies.

Physical Examination as a Selection Tool

A medical examination is often a requirement for hiring. This examination determines if the applicant can meet the requirements for a specific job and provides a record of the physical condition of the applicant at the time of hiring. The physical examination also may be used to identify applicants who will potentially have unfavorable attendance records or may file excessive future claims against the organization's health insurance.

Only those selected for hire can be required to have a physical examination, which is nearly always conducted at the employer's expense. If the physical examination reveals information that disqualifies the applicant, he or she is not hired. Most employers make job offers contingent on meeting certain health or physical requirements.

Making the Selection

When determining the most appropriate person to hire, the manager must be sure that the same standards are used to evaluate all candidates. Final selection should be based on established criteria, not on value judgments and personal preferences.

Frequently, managers fill positions with internal applicants. These positions might be entry level or management. Applicants are interviewed in the same manner as newcomers to the organization; however, some organizations give special consideration and preference to their own employees. Every organization should have guidelines and policies regarding how transfers and promotions are to be handled. Transfers and promotions were discussed more fully in Chapter 11.

Finalizing the Selection

Once a final selection has been made, the manager is responsible for closure of the preemployment process as follows:

1. Follow up with applicants as soon as possible, thanking them for applying and informing them when they will be notified about a decision.
2. Candidates not offered a position should be notified of this as soon as possible. Reasons should be provided when appropriate (e.g., insufficient education or work experience), and candidates should be told whether their application will be considered for future employment or if they should reapply.
3. Applicants offered a position should be informed in writing of the benefits, salary, and placement. This avoids misunderstandings later regarding what employees think they were promised by the nurse–recruiter or the interviewer.

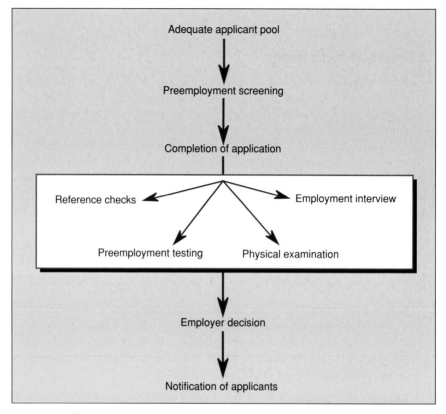

Figure 15.1 The selection process.

4. Applicants who accept job offers should be informed as to preemployment procedures such as physical examinations and supplied with the date to report to work.
5. Applicants who are offered positions should be requested to confirm in writing their intention to accept the position.

Because selection involves a process of reduction (i.e., diminishing the number of candidates for a particular position), the person making the final selection has a great deal of responsibility. These decisions have far-reaching consequences, both for the organization and for the people involved. For these reasons, the selection process should be as objective as possible. The selection process is shown in Figure 15.1.

LEARNING EXERCISE 15.3

Making a Hiring Selection and Assessing Its Impact
You are the head nurse of a surgical unit, a position that you have held for 6 years. You are comfortable with your role and know your staff well. Recently, the day charge nurse resigned. Two of your staff, Nancy and Sally, have applied for the position.

Nancy, an older nurse, has been with the organization for 8 years but has been assigned to your department for only 5 years. She has 12 years of experience in acute-care nursing. She performs her job competently and has good interpersonal relationships with the other staff and with patients and physicians. Although her motivation level is adequate for her current job, she has demonstrated little creativity or initiative in helping the surgical unit to establish a reputation for excellence. Nor has she demonstrated specific skills in predicting or planning for the future.

Sally, a nurse in her mid-30s, has been with the organization and the unit for 3 years. She has been a positive driving force behind many of the changes that have occurred. She is an excellent clinician and is highly respected by physicians and staff. The older staff, however, appear to resent her because they feel she attempted too much change before "paying her dues."

Both nurses have baccalaureate degrees and meet all the position qualifications for the job. Both nurses can be expected to work at least another 5 years in the new position. There is no precedent for your decision.

You must make a selection. If you do not use seniority as a primary selection criterion, many of the long-term employees may resent both Sally and you, and they may become demotivated. You are aware that Nancy is limited in her futuristic thinking and that the unit may not grow and develop under her leadership as it could under that of Sally.

● ASSIGNMENT: Identify how your own values will affect your decision. Rank your selection criteria, and make a decision about what you will do. Determine the personal, interpersonal, and organizational impact of your decision.

PLACEMENT

The astute leader is able to assign a new employee to a position within his or her sphere of authority where the employee will have a reasonable chance for success. Nursing units and departments develop subcultures that have their own norms, values, and methods of accomplishing work. It is possible for one person to fit in well with an established group, whereas another equally qualified person would never become part of that group.

Additionally, many positions within a unit or department require different skills. For example, in a hospital, decision-making skills might be more important on a shift where leadership is less strong; communication skills might be the most highly desired skill on a shift where there is a great deal of interaction among a variety of nursing personnel.

Frequently, newcomers suffer feelings of failure because of inappropriate placement within the organization. This can be as true for the newly hired experienced employee as for the novice nurse. Appropriate placement is as important to the organization's functioning as it is to the new employee's success. Faulty placement can result in reduced organizational efficiency, increased attrition, threats to organizational integrity, and frustration of personal and professional ambitions.

Conversely, proper placement fosters personal growth, provides a motivating climate for the employee, maximizes productivity, and increases the probability that organizational goals will be met. Managers who are able to match employee strengths to job requirements facilitate unit functioning, accomplish organizational goals, and meet employee needs.

LEARNING EXERCISE 15.4

Which Two Grads Would You Choose—and Why?

You are the supervisor of a critical care surgical unit. For the past several years, you have been experimenting with placing four newly graduated nurses directly into the unit, two from each spring and fall graduating class. These nurses are from the local BSN program. You consult closely with the nursing faculty and their former employers before making a selection.

Overall, this experiment has worked well. Only two new graduates were unable to develop into critical care nurses. Both of these nurses later transferred back into the unit after 2 years in a less intensive medical–surgical area.

Because of the new graduates' motivation and enthusiasm, they have complemented your experienced critical care staff nicely. You believe that your success with this program has been due to your well-planned and structured 4-month orientation and education program, careful selection, and appropriate shift placement.

This spring, you have narrowed the selection down to four acceptable and well-qualified candidates. You plan to place one on the 3 PM to 11 PM shift and one on the 11 PM to 7 PM shift. You sit in your office and review the culture of each shift and your notes on the four candidates. You have the following information:

3 PM to 11 PM shift: A very assertive, all-female staff; 85 percent RNs and 15 percent LPNs/LVNs. This is your most clinically competent group. They are highly respected by everyone, and although the physicians often have confrontations with them, the physicians also tell you frequently how good they are. The nurses are known as a group that lacks humor and does not welcome newcomers. However, once the new employee earns their trust, they are very supportive. They are intolerant of anyone not living up to their exceptionally high standards. Your two unsuccessful new graduate placements were assigned to this shift.

11 PM to 7 AM shift: A very cohesive and supportive group. Although overall these nurses are competent, this shift has some of your more clinically weak staff. However, it also is the shift that rates the highest with families and patients. They are caring and compassionate. Every new graduate that you have placed on this shift has been successful. Of the nurses on this shift, 30 percent are men. The group tends to be very close and has a number of outside social activities.

Your four applicants consist of the following:

- *John:* A 30-year-old married man without children. He has had a great deal of emergency room experience as a medical emergency technician. He appears somewhat aloof. His definite career goals are 2 years in critical care, 3 years in emergency room, and then flight crew. Instructors praise his independent judgment but believe that he was somewhat of a loner in school. Former employers have rated him as an independent thinker and very capable.
- *Sally:* A 22-year-old unmarried woman. She is at the top of her class clinically and academically. She has not had much work experience other than the last 2 years as a summer nursing intern at a medical center, where her performance appraisal was very good. Instructors believe that she lacks some maturity and interpersonal skills but praise her clinical judgment. She does not want to work in a regular medical–surgical unit. She believes that she can adapt to critical care.
- *Joan:* A mature, divorced 38-year-old woman. She has no children. She has had a great deal of health-related work experience in counseling and has had limited clinical work experience (only nursing school). Former employers praise her attention to detail and her general competence. Instructors praise her interpersonal skills, maturity, and intelligence.

She is quite willing to work elsewhere if not selected. She has a long-term commitment to nursing.
- *Mary:* A dynamic, 28-year-old married mother of two. She was previously an LPN/LVN and returned to school to get her degree. She did not do as well academically due to working and family commitments. Former employers and instructors speak of her energy, organization, and interpersonal skills. She appears to have fewer independent decision-making skills than the others do. She previously worked in a critical care unit.

● ASSIGNMENT: Select the two new graduates, and place them on the appropriate shift. Support your decisions with rationale.

INDOCTRINATION

As a management function, *indoctrination* refers to the planned, guided adjustment of an employee to the organization and the work environment. Although the words "induction" and "orientation" are frequently used to describe this function, the indoctrination process includes three separate phases: induction, orientation, and socialization. Because socialization is part of the staff development and team-building process, it will be covered in the next chapter.

Indoctrination denotes a much broader approach to the process of employment adjustment than either induction or orientation. It seeks to (a) establish favorable employee attitudes toward the organization, unit, and department; (b) provide the necessary information and education for success in the position; and (c) instill a feeling of belonging and acceptance. Effective indoctrination programs result in higher productivity, fewer rule violations, reduced attrition, and greater employee satisfaction. The employee indoctrination process begins as soon as a person has been selected for a position and continues until the employee has been socialized to the norms and values of the work group. An example of employee indoctrination content is shown in Display 15.7. Effective indoctrination programs assist employees in having a successful employment tenure.

Induction

Induction, the first phase of indoctrination, takes place after the employee has been selected but before performing the job role. The induction process includes all activities that educate the new employee about the organization and employment and personnel policies and procedures.

Induction activities are often performed during the placement and preemployment functions of staffing or may be included with orientation activities. However, induction and orientation are often separate entities, and new employees suffer if content from either program is omitted. The most important factor is to provide the employee with adequate information.

Employee handbooks, an important part of induction, are usually developed by the personnel department. Managers, however, should know what information the employee handbooks contain and should have input into their development. Most employee handbooks contain a form that must be signed by the employee, verifying that he or she has received and read it. The signed form is then placed in the employee's personnel file.

DISPLAY 15.7   **Employee Indoctrination Content**

1. Organization history, mission, and philosophy
2. Organization service and service area
3. Organizational structure, including department heads, with an explanation of the functions of the various departments
4. Employee responsibilities to the organization
5. Organizational responsibilities to the employee
6. Payroll information, including how increases in pay are earned and when they are given (progressive or unionized companies publish pay scales for all employees)
7. Rules of conduct
8. Tour of the facility and of the assigned department
9. Work schedules, staffing and scheduling policies
10. When applicable, a discussion of the collective bargaining agreement
11. Benefit plans, including life insurance, health insurance, pension, and unemployment
12. Safety and fire programs
13. Staff development programs, including in-service, and continuing education for relicensure
14. Promotion and transfer policies
15. Employee appraisal system
16. Workload assignments
17. Introduction to paperwork/forms used in the organization
18. Review of selection in policies and procedures
19. Specific legal requirements, such as maintaining a current license, reporting of accidents, and so forth
20. Introduction to fellow employees
21. Establishment of a feeling of belonging and acceptance, showing genuine interest in the new employee

Note: Much of this content could be provided in an employee handbook, and the fire and safety regulations could be handled by a media presentation. *Appropriate* use of videotapes or film strips can be very helpful in the design of a good orientation program. All indoctrination programs should be monitored to see if they are achieving their goals. Most programs need to be revised at least annually.

The handbook is important because employees cannot assimilate all the induction information at one time, so they need a reference for later. However, providing an employee with a personnel handbook is not sufficient for real understanding. The information must be followed with discussion by various people during the employment process, such as the personnel manager and staff development personnel during orientation. The most important link in promoting real understanding of personnel polices is the first-level manager.

Orientation

Induction provides the employee with general information about the organization, whereas *orientation* activities are more specific for the position. A sample 2-week orientation schedule is shown in Display 15.8. Organizations may use a wide variety of orientation programs. For example, a first-day orientation could be conducted by the hospital's personnel department, which could include a tour of the hospital and all of the induction items listed in Display 15.7.

DISPLAY 15.8 **Sample Two-Week Orientation Schedule for Experienced Nurses**

Week One

Day 1, Monday:

8:00 AM–10:00 AM	Welcome by personnel department; employee handbooks distributed and discussed
10:00 AM–10:30 AM	Coffee and fruit served; welcome by staff development department
10:30 AM–12:00 PM	General orientation by staff development
12:00 PM–12:30 PM	Tour of the organization
12:30 PM–1:30 PM	Lunch
1:30 PM–3:00 PM	Fire and safety films; body mechanics demonstration
3:00 PM–4:00 PM	Afternoon tea and introduction to each unit supervisor

Day 2, Tuesday:

8:00 AM–10:00 AM	Report to individual units
	Time with unit supervisor; introduction to assigned preceptor
10:00 AM–10:30 AM	Coffee with preceptor
10:30 AM–12:00 PM	General orientation of policies and procedures
12:00 PM–12:30 PM	Lunch
12:30 PM–4:30 PM	CPR recertification
Day 3, Wednesday:	Assigned all day to unit with preceptor
Day 4, Thursday:	Assigned all day to unit with preceptor
Day 5, Friday:	Morning with preceptor, afternoon with supervisor and staff development for wrap-up

Week Two

Monday to Wednesday:	Work with preceptor on shift and unit assigned, gradually assuming greater responsibilities
Thursday:	Assign 80 percent of normal assignment with assistance and supervision from preceptor
Friday:	Carry normal workload. Have at least a 30-minute meeting with immediate supervisor to discuss progress

The next phase of the orientation program could take place in the staff development department, where aspects of concern to all employees such as fire safety, accident prevention, and health promotion, would be presented The third phase would be the individual orientation for each department. At this point, specific departments such as dietary, pharmacy, and nursing would each be responsible for developing their own programs. A sample distribution of responsibilities for orientation activities is shown in Display 15.9.

Because induction and orientation involve many different people from a variety of departments, they must be carefully coordinated and planned to achieve preset goals. The overall goals of induction and orientation include helping employees by providing them with information that will smooth their transition into the new work setting and health care team.

DISPLAY 15.9 **Responsibilities for Orientation**

1. **Personnel or Human Resources Department:** Performs salary and payroll functions, insurance forms, physical exams, income withholding forms, tour of the organization, employee responsibilities to the organization and vice versa, additional labor–management relationships, and benefit plan.
2. **Staff Development Department:** Hands out and reviews employee handbook; discusses organizational philosophy and mission; reviews history of the organization; shows media presentation of various departments and how they function (if a media presentation is not available, introduces various department heads and shares how departments function); discusses organizational structure, fire and safety programs, CPR certification, and verifications; discusses available educational and training programs and reviews selected policies and procedures, including medication, treatment, and charting policies.
3. **The Individual Unit:** Tour of the department, introductions, review of specific unit policies that differ in any way from general policies, review of unit scheduling and staffing policies and procedures, work assignments, promotion and transfer policies, and establishment of a feeling of belonging, acceptance, and socialization.

 The purpose of the orientation process is to make the employee feel like a part of the team. This will reduce burnout and help new employees become independent more quickly in their new roles.

It is important to look at productivity and retention as the orientation program is planned, structured, and evaluated. Organizations should periodically assess their induction and orientation program in light of organizational goals; programs that are not meeting organizational goals should be restructured. For example, if employees consistently have questions about the benefit program, this part of the induction process should be evaluated.

Too often, various people having partial responsibility for induction and orientation "pass the buck" regarding failure of or weaknesses in the program. It is the joint responsibility of the personnel/human resources department, the staff development department, and each nursing service unit to work together to provide an indoctrination program that meets the needs of employees and the organization.

For some time, managers in health care organizations, especially hospitals, did not fulfill their proper role in the orientation of new employees. Managers assumed that between the personnel/human resources and staff development, or in-service, departments, the new employee would become completely oriented. This often frustrated new employees because although they received an overview of the organization, they received little orientation to the specific unit. Because each unit has many idiosyncrasies, the new employee was left feeling inadequate and incompetent. The latest trend in orientation is for the nursing unit to take a greater responsibility for individualizing orientation.

The unit manager must play a key role in the orientation of the new employee. An adequate orientation program minimizes the likelihood of rule violations, grievances, and misunderstandings; fosters feelings of belonging and acceptance; and promotes enthusiasm and morale.

INTEGRATING LEADERSHIP ROLES AND MANAGEMENT FUNCTIONS IN EMPLOYEE RECRUITMENT, SELECTION, PLACEMENT, AND INDOCTRINATION

Productivity is directly related to the quality of an organization's personnel. Active recruitment allows institutions to bring in the most-qualified personnel for a position. After those applicants have been recruited, managers—using specified criteria—have a critical responsibility to see that the best applicant is hired. To ensure that all applicants are evaluated by using the same standards and that personal bias is minimized, the manager must be skilled in interviewing and other selection processes.

Leadership roles in preliminary staffing functions include planning for future staffing needs and keeping abreast of changes in the health care field. Leadership also is necessary in the interview process to ensure that all applicants are treated fairly and that the interview terminates with applicants having positive attitudes about the organization. Because leaders are fully aware of nuances, strengths, and weaknesses within their sphere of authority, they are able to assign newcomers to areas that offer the greatest potential for success.

The integration of leadership roles and management functions in the organization ensures positive public relations because applicants know that they will be treated fairly. In addition, there is greater likelihood that the pool of applicants will be sufficient because future needs are planned for proactively. The leader–manager uses the selection and placement process as a means to increase productivity and retention, accomplish the goals of the organization, and meet the needs of new employees.

The integrated leader–manager also knows that a well-planned and implemented induction and orientation program is a wise investment of organizational resources. It provides the opportunity to mold a team effort and infuse employees with enthusiasm for the organization. New employees' impressions of an organization during this period will stay with them for a long time. If the impressions are positive, they will be remembered in the difficult times that will ultimately occur during any long tenure of employment.

Key Concepts

* The first step in the staffing process is to determine the type and number of personnel needed.
* A number of factors have contributed to a severe nursing shortage, particularly in acute-care hospitals, in the early 21st century. These factors include a nationwide downsizing of hospitals in the 1990s, the aging of the nursing workforce, accelerating demand for professional nursing services, and inadequate enrollment in nursing programs of study.
* Successfully *recruiting* an adequate workforce depends on many variables, including financial resources, an adequate nursing pool, competitive salaries, the organization's reputation, the location's desirability, and the status of the national and local economy.
* Effective recruiting methods include advertisements, career days, literature, and the informal use of members of the organization as examples of satisfied employees.
* Despite their limitations, interviews are widely used as a method of selecting employees for hire.
* The interview should meet the goals of both the applicant and the manager.
* Managers must be skilled in planning, conducting, and controlling interviews.
* Due to numerous federal acts that protect the rights of job seekers, managers must be cognizant of the legal constraints on interviews.

* *Selection* should be based on the requirements necessary for the job; these criteria should be developed before beginning the selection process.
* Managers should seek to proactively recruit and hire staff that represent age, gender, cultural, ethnic, and language diversity in response to the rapidly increasing diversity of the communities that they serve.
* Managers should place new employees on units, departments, and shifts where they have the best chance of succeeding.
* *Indoctrination* consists of induction, orientation, and socialization of employees.
* A well-prepared and executed orientation program educates the new employee about the desired behaviors and expected goals of the organization and actively involves the new employee's immediate supervisor.

ADDITIONAL LEARNING EXERCISES AND APPLICATIONS

LEARNING EXERCISE 15.5

Assessing Personal Bias in Interviewing

You are a new evening charge nurse on a medical floor in an acute-care hospital. This is your first management position. You graduated 18 months ago from the local university with a bachelor's degree in nursing. Your immediate supervisor has asked you to interview two applicants who will be graduating from nursing school in 3 months. Your supervisor believes that they both are qualified. Because the available position is on your shift, she wants you to make the final hiring decision.

Both applicants seem equally qualified in academic standing and work experience. Last evening, you interviewed Lisa and were very impressed. Tonight, you interviewed John. During the meeting, you kept thinking that you knew John from somewhere but could not recall where. The interview went well, however, and you were equally impressed with John.

After John left, you suddenly remembered that one of your classmates used to date him and that he had attended some of your class parties. You recall that on several occasions, he appeared to abuse alcohol. This recollection bothers you, and you are not sure what to do. You know that tomorrow your supervisor wants to inform the applicants of your decision.

● ASSIGNMENT: Decide what you are going to do. Support your decision with appropriate rationale. Explain how you would determine which applicant to hire. How great a role did your personal values play in your decision?

LEARNING EXERCISE 15.6

How Would You Strengthen This Orientation Process?

As a new head nurse, one of your goals is to reduce attrition. You plan to do this by increasing retention, thus reducing costs for orienting new employees. In addition, you believe that the increased retention will provide you with a more stable staff.

In studying your notes from exit interviews, it appears that new employees seldom develop a loyalty to the unit but instead use the unit to gain experience for other positions. You believe that one difficulty with socializing new employees might be your unit's orientation program. The agency allows 2 weeks of orientation time (80 hours) when the new employee is not counted in the nursing care hours. These are referred to as *nonproductive hours* and are charged to the education department. Your unit has the following 2-week schedule for new employees:

Week One

Monday, Tuesday	9 AM to 5 PM	Classroom
Wednesday, Thursday, Friday	7 AM to 11 AM	Assigned to work with someone on the unit

Week Two

Monday, Tuesday	7 AM to 3:30 PM	Assigned to unit with an employee
Wednesday, Thursday, Friday		Assigned to shift they will be working for orientation to shift

Following this 2-week orientation, the new employee is expected to function at 75-percent productivity for 2 or 3 weeks and then perform at full productivity. The exception to this is the new graduate (RN) orientation. These employees spend one extra week on 7 AM to 3 PM and one extra week assigned to their particular shift before being counted as staff.

Your nursing administrator has stated that you may alter the orientation program in any way you wish as long as you do not increase the nonproductive time and you ensure that the employee receives information necessary to meet legal requirements and to function safely.

● ASSIGNMENT: Is there any way for you to strengthen the new employee orientation to your unit? Outline your plans (if any), and state the rationale for your decision.

LEARNING EXERCISE 15.7

Choosing Your Place in the Workforce

You are a baccalaureate nursing student who will graduate in 3 months. You are aware that there are multiple vacancies at almost every acute-care hospital in the area as well as more limited openings in home health, public health, community health, telehealth, and case management. The local community hospital is offering a significant sign-on bonus for new graduates who are willing to sign a 2-year contract. This would be helpful in paying off school loans that you have accrued.

You really enjoyed, however, the autonomy and patient interaction that you experienced in your public health practicum as part of school, and the Monday to Friday work schedule of the public health nurses appeals to you since you have small children. The salary, however, would be significantly lower than if you worked in an acute-care setting. Moreover, the orientation period at the public health facility is fairly brief.

Finally, you have always had an interest in pediatric oncology, a specialty not available to you unless you relocate to a regional medical center. No sign-on bonus is available at the medical center; however, there are more opportunities for advancement and professional development there. Your spouse is willing to make this move if this is what you really want.

● ASSIGNMENT:
1. Determine how you will move forward in making a decision about where you will seek employment.
2. Make a list of 10 factors that you need to consider in weighting conflicting wants, needs, and obligations.
3. What evaluation criteria can you generate to look at both the process you used to make your decision as well as the decision itself?

LEARNING EXERCISE 15.8

Ethical Issues in Hiring

You are the head nurse of an intensive care unit and are interviewing Sam, a prospective charge nurse for your evening shift. Sam is currently the unit supervisor at Memorial Hospital, which is the other local hospital and your organization's primary competitor. He is leaving Memorial Hospital for personal reasons.

Sam, well qualified for the position, has strong management and clinical skills. Your evening shift needs a strong manager with the excellent clinical skills, which Sam also has. You feel fortunate that Sam is applying for the position.

Just before the close of the interview, however, Sam shuts the door, lowers his voice secretively, and tells you that he has vital information regarding Memorial's plans to expand and reorganize its critical care unit. He states that he will share this information with you if you hire him.

● ASSIGNMENT: How would you respond to Sam? Should you hire him? Identify the major issues in this situation. Support your hiring decision with rationale from this chapter and other readings.

(Web Links)

Interviewing Tips
http://www.careercc.com/interv3.shtml
This site includes general interviewing tips, questions that the interviewer might ask applicants, and questions that the applicant should consider asking the interviewer.

Monster Career Center—Interview Tips
http://content.monster.com/jobinfo/interview/
Includes a practice virtual interview, questions to ask the interviewer, and an interview planner.

Monster Resume Center
http://resume.monster.com/
Includes résumé writing tips as well as a link to more articles on résumé writing.

HRSA—Bureau of Health Professions, National Sample Survey of Registered Nurses
http://bhpr.hrsa.gov/healthworkforce/reports/rnpopulation/preliminaryfindings.htm
The nation's most extensive and comprehensive source of statistics on nurses with current licenses to practice in the United States.

(References)

American Association of Colleges of Nursing. (2006a). *Nursing shortage.* Retrieved January 11, 2007, from *http://www.aacn.nche.edu/Media/FactSheets/NursingShortage.htm.*

American Association of Colleges of Nursing. (2006b). *Student enrollment rises in U.S. nursing colleges and universities for the 6th consecutive year.* Retrieved January 11, 2007, from *http://www.aacn.nche.edu/Media/NewsReleases/06Survey.htm.*

American Association of Colleges of Nursing. (2006c). *Nursing faculty shortage.* Retrieved January 11, 2007, from *http://www.aacn.nche.edu/Media/FactSheets/FacultyShortage. htm.*

American Hospital Association. (2006). *The state of America's hospitals: Taking the pulse.* Retrieved January 11, 2007, from *http://www.aha.org/aha/content/2006/PowerPoint/ StateHospitalsChartPack2006.PPT.*

Asselin, M. E. (2006). Strategies for effective interviews. *Nursing Management, 37*(8), 42–47.

Atencio, B. L., Cohen, J., & Gorenberg, B. (2003). Nurse retention: Is it worth it? *Nursing Economic$, 21*(6), 262–268.

Auerbach, D. I., Buerhaus, P. I., & Staiger, D. O. (2007). Better late than never: Workforce supply implications of later entry into nursing. *Health Affairs, 26*(1), 178–185.

Bernard Hodes Group. (2006). *The 2006 aging nursing workforce survey.* Retrieved December 6, 2006, from *http://www.hodes.com/publications/pdfs/agingnurse_sep06. pdf.*

Cyr, J. P. (2005). Retaining older hospital nurses and delaying their retirement. *Journal of Nursing Administration, 35*(12), 563–567.

Duffield, C., O'Brien-Pallas, L., Aitken, L., Roche, M., & Merrick, E. T. (2006). Recruitment of nurses working outside nursing. *Journal of Nursing Administration, 36*(2), 58–62.

Frusti, D. K., Niesen, K. M., & Campion, J. K. (2003). Creating a culturally competent organization. *Journal of Nursing Administration, 33*(1), 31–38.

Hart, K. A. (2006). *The aging workforce: Implications for recruiters.* Retrieved December 6, 2006, from *http:// www.hodes.com/publications/talentmatters/archives/ hcmatters_jul06.asp.*

Health Workforce Institute. (2006). *Supply & demand: Registered nurses.* Retrieved January 20, 2007, from *http://www.healthcarepersonnel.org/supply/regnurses.htm.*

Hecker, D. E. (2005, November). Employment outlook: 2004–2014. Occupational employment projections to 2014.

Monthly Labor Review, 70–101. Retrieved January 11, 2007, from *http://www.bls.gov/opub/mlr/2005/11/art5full.pdf.*

Huston, C. (2006a). Chapter 5. The current nursing shortage. In *Professional issues in nursing.* Philadelphia: Lippincott Williams & Wilkins.

Huston, C. (2006b). Chapter 6. Importing foreign nurses to meet America's demand for nurses. In *Professional issues in nursing.* Philadelphia: Lippincott Williams & Wilkins.

Kalisch, B. J. (2003). Recruiting nurses. The problem is the process. *Journal of Nursing Administration, 33*(9), 408–477.

La Rocco, S. A. (2006, May-June). Who will teach the nurses? *Academe.* Retrieved January 16, 2007, from *http://www.aaup. org/publications/Academe/2006/06mj/06mjlaro.htm.*

Lynn, M. R., & Redman, R. W. (2005). Faces of the nursing shortage. *Journal of Nursing Administration, 35*(5), 264–270.

Orlovsky, C. (2006). *Mass nurse retirement expected in 2011: Survey.* Retrieved December 6, 2006, from *http://www. amnhealthcare.com/News.aspx?id=15444.*

Strachota, E., Normandin, P., O'Brien, N., Clary, M., & Krukow, B. (2003). Reasons registered nurses leave or change employment status. *Journal of Nursing Administration, 33*(2), 111–117.

U.S. Department of Health and Human Services Administration. (2006). *What is behind HRSA's projected supply, demand, and shortage of registered nurses?* Retrieved January 11, 2007, from *http://bhpr.hrsa.gov/healthworkforce/reports/ behindrnprojections/index.htm.*

U.S. Department of Health and Human Services, Bureau of Health Professions, Division of Nursing. (2001). The registered nurse population: National sample survey of registered nurses, March 2000. Preliminary Findings, February 2001. *Nurse Week.* Retrieved April 18, 2004, from *http://www.nurseweek.com/ nursingshortage/rnsurvey.asp.*

U.S. Department of Labor (2006, August 6). *Registered nurses.* Retrieved January 11, 2007, from *http://www.bls.gov/ oco/ocos083.htm.*

⟨Bibliography⟩

Baggot, D. M., Dawson, C., Valdes, M. S., & Zaim, S. (2005). Management issues. Rethinking nurse recruitment: A return-on-investment approach. *Journal of Nursing Administration, 35*(10), 424–427.

Butler, M. R., & Felts, J. (2006). Tool kit for the staff mentor: Strategies for improving retention. *Journal of Continuing Education in Nursing, 37*(5), 210–213.

Dixon, A. (2006, October). Preceptor program and new grad retention. *Nursing News, 30*(4), 18.

Ellerbe, S., Ostermeier, L., & Shelley, S. (2006). Redesigning the recruitment function: Winning at recruitment and retention of critical health care professionals. *Nurse Leader, 4*(4), 38–41.

Flexible schedules, safe workplace help retain veteran nurses. (2006). *OR Manager, 22*(8), 32.

Flynn, L. (2005). The importance of work environment: Evidence-based strategies for enhancing nurse retention. *Home Healthcare Nurse, 23*(6), 366–371, 385–387.

Innovation aids nurse recruitment, retention: Re-entry RNs are untapped source. (2005, October). *Hospital Home Health, 22*(10), 116–117.

Kennedy, M. S. (2006). In the news. The case for retaining experienced RNs: Recruitment alone won't solve the nursing shortage. *American Journal of Nursing, 106*(8), 20.

Kubar, P. A., Miller, D., & Spear, B. T. (2004). The meaningful retention strategy inventory. *Journal of Nursing Administration, 34*(1), 10–18.

Lehna, C., Sheaffer, J., Andrade-Pulido, M., Martinez, A., & Bishop, B. (2006). Clinical practice column. Using nurse shadowing as the focus for a recruitment program. *Journal of Pediatric Nursing, 21*(1), 73–79.

Manderson, L., Bennett, E., & Andajani-Sutjahjo S. (2006) The social dynamics of the interview: Age, class, and gender. *Qualitative Health Research, 16*(10), 1317–1334.

Retaining older nurses in bedside practice. (2006). *Nurse Educator, 31*(6), 206.

Shermont, H., & Krepcio, D. (2006). The impact of culture change on nurse retention. *Journal of Nursing Administration, 36*(9), 407–415.

Silkman, S. M., Palazzo, L., Keepnews, D., & Hart, L. G. (2006). Characteristics of registered nurses in rural versus urban areas: Implications for strategies to alleviate nursing shortages in the United States. *Journal of Rural Health, 22*(2), 151–157.

Xu, Y., & Zhang, J. (2005). One size doesn't fit all: Ethics of international nurse recruitment from the conceptual framework of stakeholder interests. *Nursing Ethics, 12*(6), 571–581.

16

Socializing and Educating Staff for Team Building

. . . environments rich in continuing education ripen staff development, morale and retention.

—*Diane Postlen-Slattery and Kathryn Foley*

. . . as part of the lifelong learning process, nurse leaders will increasingly use mentors and personal coaches to help them refine their tools and skills and to identify new lenses through which to view current concerns or issues.

—*Karen S. Haase-Herrick*

Health care organizations face major challenges in upgrading skills of the workforce and in maintaining a competent staff. Staff development has always been important, but in times of exploding knowledge and technology, educating staff has become critical. Kramer and Schmalenberg (2004) state that educational support is essential for creating a magnetic work environment. Educational needs of staff are partially dependent on the staffing mix and position responsibilities that were developed during the organizing and planning phases of management. For example, the more experienced and educated the staff, the less educational and training needs they will have.

This chapter begins by introducing the concept of the learning organization and then examines the various components of staff development. Staff development is a broad area of responsibility and is borne by many people in the organization. Topics covered in this chapter are the delineation between education and training as well as the differences between role models, preceptors, and mentors in the socialization process. The needs of the adult learner are explored, and the concept of coaching as a staff development tool is introduced. There is an emphasis on how organizations, leader–managers, and staff development departments can best support evidence-based practice. Last, the need to build a cohesive team, including the needs of a culturally diverse workforce, is explored. The leadership roles and management functions in staff development are shown in Display 16.1.

DISPLAY 16.1   Leadership Roles and Management Functions Associated With Socializing and Educating Staff for Team Building

Leadership Roles

1. Clarifies department norms and values to all new employees
2. Infuses a team spirit among employees
3. Serves as a role model to all employees and a mentor to select employees
4. Encourages mentorship between senior staff and junior employees
5. Observes carefully for signs of knowledge or skill deficit in new employees and intervenes appropriately
6. Assists employees in developing personal strategies to cope with role transition
7. Applies adult learning principles when helping employees learn new skills or information
8. Coaches employees spontaneously regarding knowledge and skill deficits
9. Is sensitive to the unique socialization and education needs of a culturally and ethnically diverse staff
10. Continually promotes aspects of the learning organization to employees
11. Assists nursing staff in overcoming organization barriers to effective evidence-based practice

Management Functions

1. Is aware of and clarifies organizational and unit goals for all employees
2. Clarifies role expectations for all employees
3. Uses positive and negative sanctions appropriately to socialize new employees
4. Carefully selects preceptors and encourages role modeling of the senior staff
5. Provides methods of meeting the special orientation needs of new graduates, international nurses, and experienced nurses changing roles
6. Works with the education department to delineate shared and individual responsibility for staff development
7. Ensures that there are adequate resources for staff development and makes appropriate decisions regarding resource allocation during periods of fiscal restraint
8. Assumes responsibility for quality and fiscal control of staff development activities
9. Ensures that all staff are competent for roles assigned
10. Provides input in formulating staff development policies
11. Ensures that the organization provides resources to promote evidence-based nursing practice

THE LEARNING ORGANIZATION

A growing body of literature supports the concept that learning should go beyond the boundaries of individual learning and that organizations that desire to have learning as a major part of their philosophy will be more successful. This concept was first introduced by Senge (1994), who called such organizations *learning organizations* (LOs).

The key characteristics of Senge's model include the following:

• *Open systems thinking.* The organization encourages staff to see themselves as connected to the whole organization. Work activities are seen as having an impact beyond the individual.

- *Improving the capabilities of individuals.* Each member of the staff has a commitment to improve his or her personal abilities. This personal and professional learning is then integrated into the team and organization.
- *Team learning.* It is teams that allow LOs to achieve their goals. Learning together benefits both the team and its individuals.
- *Updating mental models.* Assumptions held by individuals must be challenged and changed. Encouraging new assumptions releases individuals from traditional thinking and promotes the full potential of individuals to learn.
- *A cohesive vision.* This acts as a guide to individuals working within the organization and assists everyone to work to achieve the same goals.

Wilkinson, Rushmer, and Davies (2004) suggest that since Senge's first exploration of LOs, many theorists have contributed to our understanding of the most relevant features of such organizations. Among their observations are that LOs can adapt to change, exploit opportunities for development, learn from errors, improve quality, and maximize the contributions of human resources. They also report that common features of LOs include (a) celebration of success, (b) absence of complacency, (c) tolerance of mistakes, (d) belief in human potential, (e) recognition of tacit knowledge, (f) openness, (g) trust, and (h) outward looking.

In LOs, there is recognition that learning is a part of quality. Learning is seen as the key to a better future, not only for individuals but also for organizations. Organizational learning emphasizes individual internalized changes in ways of thinking. The challenge for leader–managers in such organizations is to manage tensions arising from the "bottom up" of the LO with the "top down" hierarchy of most bureaucracies (Wilkinson, Rushmer, & Davies, 2004).

STAFF DEVELOPMENT

The leader–manager has a responsibility for maintaining a competent staff, but this responsibility is shared with other members of the organization. An organization's commitment to learning is often demonstrated by its commitment to staff development. An LO does not just meet licensure requirements for education and training but encourages individual growth and supports staff development activities both financially and philosophically.

Education and training are two components of staff development that occur after an employee's indoctrination. Early staff development emphasized orientation and in-service training. In the last 20 years, however, other forms of education have become common in health care organizations. The staff's knowledge level and capabilities are a major factor in determining the number of staff required to carry out unit goals. The better trained and more competent the staff, the fewer staff required, which in turn saves the organization money and raises productivity.

Staff development is a cost-effective method of increasing productivity.

Training Versus Education

Managers have a greater responsibility for seeing that staff is properly trained than they do for meeting educational needs. *Training* may be defined as an organized method of ensuring that people have knowledge and skills for a specific purpose and that they have acquired the necessary knowledge to perform the duties of the job. The knowledge may require increased affective, motor, or cognitive skills. It is expected that acquiring new skills will increase productivity or create a better product.

Education is more formal and broader in scope than training. Whereas training has an immediate use, education is designed to develop individuals in a broader sense. Recognizing educational needs and encouraging educational pursuits are roles and responsibilities of the leader. Managers may appropriately be requested to teach classes or courses; however, unless they have specific expertise, managers would not normally be responsible for an employee's formal education.

Responsibilities of the Education Department

Most education departments on the organization chart are depicted as having staff or advisory authority rather than line authority. Difficulties inherent in staff positions were discussed in Chapter 12. Because staff positions do not have line authority, education personnel generally have little or no authority over those for whom they are providing educational programs. Likewise, the unit manager has no authority over personnel in the education department. Because of the ambiguity of overlapping roles and difficulties inherent in line and staff positions, educating and training employees may be neglected. So when it *is* undertaken, it is important that those responsible for educating and training be identified and given the authority to carry out the programs.

 If staff development activities are to be successful, it is necessary to delineate and communicate the authority and responsibility for all components of education and training.

Other difficulties arising from the shared responsibility among managers, personnel department staff, and educators for the indoctrination, education, and training of personnel are a frequent lack of cost-effectiveness evaluation and little accountability for the quality and outcomes of the educational activities. The following suggestions can help overcome the difficulties inherent in a staff development system in which there is shared authority:

- The nursing department must ensure that all parties involved in the indoctrination, education, and training of nursing staff understand and carry out their responsibilities in that process.
- If the nursing department is not directly responsible for the staff development department (in large institutions, a non-nursing administrator may have authority for this department), there must be input from the nursing department in formulating staff development policies and delineating duties.
- An advisory committee should be formed with representatives from top-, middle-, and first-level management; staff development; and the human resource department. Representatives from all classifications of employees receiving training or education should be part of this committee.
- Accountability for various parts of the staff development program must be clearly communicated.
- Some method of determining the cost and benefits of various programs should be used.

THEORIES OF LEARNING

All levels of management have a responsibility to improve employee performance through teaching. Therefore, they must be familiar with basic learning theories. Understanding teaching–learning theories allows managers to structure training and use teaching techniques to change employee behavior and improve competence, which is the goal for all staff development.

Adult Learning Theory

Many managers attempt to teach adults by using pedagogical or child-learning strategies, the same method used in school. This type of teaching is usually ineffective for mature learners because adults have special needs. Knowles (1970) developed the concept of *androgogy*, or adult learning, to separate adult learner strategies from *pedagogy*, or child learning. Adult learners are mature, self-directed people who have learned a great deal from life experiences and are focused toward solving problems that exist in their immediate environments.

Adult learning theory has contributed a great deal to the manner in which adults are taught. Display 16.2 depicts the obstacles and assets to adult learning, and Table 16.1 shows how the child and adult (pedagogical and androgogical) learning environments should differ. Knowles' studies have the following implications for trainers and educators:

- A climate of openness and respect will assist in the identification of what the adult learner wants and needs to learn.
- Adults enjoy taking part in and planning their learning experiences.
- Adults should be involved in the evaluation of their progress.
- Experiential techniques work best with adults.
- Mistakes are opportunities for adult learning.
- If the value of the adult's experience is rejected, the adult will feel rejected.
- Adults' readiness to learn is greatest when they recognize that there is a need to know (such as in response to a problem).
- Adults need the opportunity to apply what they have learned very quickly after the learning.
- Assessment of need is imperative in adult learning.

DISPLAY 16.2 Obstacles and Assets to Adult Learning

Obstacles to Learning

Institutional barriers
Time
Self-confidence
Situational obstacles
Family reaction
Special individual obstacles

Assets for Learning

High self-motivation
Self-directed
A proven learner
Knowledge experience reservoir
Special individual assets

TABLE 16.1   **Characteristics and Learning Environment of Pedagogy and Androgogy**

Pedagogy	Androgogy
Characteristics	
Learner is dependent.	Learner is self-directed.
Learner needs external rewards and punishment.	Learner is internally motivated.
Learner's experience is inconsequential or limited.	Learner's experiences are valued and varied.
Subject centered.	Task or problem centered.
Teacher directed.	Self-directed.
Learning Environment	
The climate is authoritative.	The climate is relaxed and informal.
Competition is encouraged.	Collaboration is encouraged.
Teacher sets goals.	Teacher and class set goals.
Decisions are made by teacher.	Decisions are made by teacher and students.
Teacher lectures.	Students process activities and inquire about projects.
Teacher evaluates.	Teacher, self, and peers evaluate.

Social Learning Theory

Social learning theory builds on reinforcement theory as part of the motivation to learn and has many of the same components as the theories of socialization discussed in previous chapters. Bandura (1977) suggests that people learn most behavior by direct experience and observation, and behaviors are retained or not retained based on positive and negative rewards. Social learning theory involves four separate processes. First, people learn as a result of the direct experience of the effects of their actions. Second, knowledge is frequently obtained through vicarious experiences, such as by observing someone else's actions. Third, people learn by judgments voiced by others, especially when vicarious experience is limited. Fourth, people evaluate the soundness of the new information by reasoning through inductive and deductive logic. Social learning theory also acknowledges that anticipation of reinforcement influences what is observed and what goes unnoticed (Bandura, 1977). Figure 16.1 depicts the social learning theory process.

 Because the cognitive process is very much a part of social learning, observational learning will be more effective if the learner is informed in advance of the benefits of adopting a role model's behavior.

Other Learning Theories

The following learning concepts may also be helpful to the leader–manager in meeting the learning needs of staff:

- *Readiness to learn.* This refers to the maturational and experiential factors in the learner's background that influence learning and is not the same as motivation to learn. *Maturation* means that the learner has received the prerequisites for the next stage of learning. The prerequisites could be behaviors or prior learning. *Experiential factors* are skills previously acquired that are necessary for the next stage of learning.

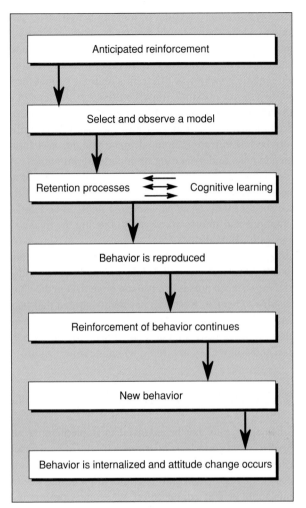

Figure 16.1   The social learning theory process.

- *Motivation to learn.* If learners are informed in advance about the benefits of learning specific content and adopting new behaviors, they are more likely to be motivated to attend the training sessions and learn. Telling employees why and how specific educational or training programs will benefit them personally is a vital management function in staff development.
- *Reinforcement.* Because a learner's first attempts are often unsuccessful, a preceptor is essential. Good preceptors can reinforce desired behavior. Once the behavior or skill is learned, it needs continual reinforcement until it becomes internalized.
- *Task learning.* The learning of complex tasks is facilitated when tasks are broken into parts, beginning with the simplest and continuing to the most difficult. It is necessary, however, to combine *part learning* with *whole learning*. When learning motor skills, *spaced practice* is more effective than *massed practice*.

- *Transfer of learning.* The goal of training is to transfer new learning to the work setting. For this to occur, there should first be as much similarity between the training context and the job as possible. Second, adequate practice is mandatory, and *overlearning* (learning repeated to the degree that it is difficult to forget) is recommended. Third, the training should include a variety of different situations so that the knowledge is generalized. Fourth, whenever possible, important features or steps in a process should be identified. Finally, the learner must understand the basic principles underlying the tasks and how a variety of situations will modify how the task is accomplished. Learning in the classroom will not be transferred without adequate practice in a simulated or real situation and without an adequate understanding of underlying principles.
- *Span of memory.* The effectiveness of staff development activities depends to some extent on the ability of the participants to retain information. Effective strategies include the chance for repeated rehearsal, grouping items to be learned (three or four items for oral presentations and four to six visually), having the material presented in a well-organized manner, and *chunking.*
- *Chunking.* This occurs when two independent items of information are presented and then grouped together into one unit. While the mind can remember only a limited number of chunks of data, experienced nurses can include more data in the chunks than can novice nurses.
- *Knowledge of results.* Research has demonstrated that people learn faster when they are informed of their progress. The knowledge of results must be automatic, immediate, and meaningful to the task at hand. People need to experience a feeling of progress, and they need to know how they are doing when measured against expected outcomes.

ASSESSING STAFF DEVELOPMENT NEEDS

Although managers may not be involved in implementing all educational programs, they are responsible for identifying learning needs. If educational resources are scarce, staff desires for specific educational programs may need to be sacrificed to fulfill competency and new learning needs. Because managers and staff may identify learning needs differently, an educational needs assessment should be carried out before developing programs.

 Staff development activities are normally carried out for one of three reasons: to establish competence, to meet new learning needs, and to satisfy interests the staff may have in learning in specific areas.

Many staff development activities are generated to ensure that workers at each level are competent to perform the duties assigned to the position. *Competence* is defined as having the abilities to meet the requirements for a particular role. Health care organizations use many resources to determine competency. State board licensure, national certification, and performance review are some of the methods used to satisfy competency requirements (Huston, 2006a). Other methods are self-administered checklists, record audits, and peer evaluation. Many of these methods are explained in Unit VII. For staff development purposes, it is important to remember that in the case of deficient competencies, some staff development activity must be implemented to correct the deficiencies. Another learning need that frequently affects health care organizations is the need to meet new technological and scientific challenges. Much of a manager's educational resources will be used to meet these new learning needs.

Medical technology and science are developing rapidly, resulting in the need to learn new skills and procedures and acquire the knowledge necessary to operate complex equipment.

Some organizations implement training programs because they are faddish and have been advertised and marketed well. Educational programs are expensive, however, and should not be undertaken unless a demonstrated need exists. Educational resources should be able to be justified. In addition to developing rationale for education programs, the use of an assessment plan will be helpful in meeting learner needs. The following plan outlines the sequence that should be used in developing an educational program:

1. Identify the desired knowledge or skills that the staff should have.
2. Identify the present level of knowledge or skill.
3. Determine the deficit of desired knowledge and skills.
4. Identify the resources available to meet needs.
5. Make maximum use of available resources.
6. Evaluate and test outcomes after use of resources.

EVALUATION OF STAFF DEVELOPMENT ACTIVITIES

Because staff development includes participation and involvement from many departments, it is very difficult to control this important function effectively. Controlling, the evaluation phase of the management process, becomes extremely difficult when accountability is shared. It is very easy for the personnel department, middle-level managers, and the education department to "pass the buck" among one another for accountability regarding staff development activities.

Currently, in most organizations, responsibility for staff development is decentralized and includes the nurse–manager. This has occurred as a result of fiscal concerns, the awareness of the need to socialize new employees at the unit level, and recognition of the relationship between employee competence and productivity. It is generally accepted that the ultimate responsibility for staff training and education rests with the manager, although the manager does not personally provide all aspects of staff development. Some difficulties associated with decentralized staff development include the conflict created by *role ambiguity* whenever two people share responsibility. Role ambiguity is sometimes reduced when staff development personnel and managers delineate the difference between training and education.

Evaluation of staff development consists of more than merely having class participants fill out an evaluation form at the end of the class session, signing an employee handbook form, or assigning a preceptor for each new employee. Evaluation of staff development should include the following four criteria:

- *Learner's reaction.* How did the learner perceive the orientation, the class, the training, or the preceptor?
- *Behavior change.* What behavior change occurred as a result of the learning? Was the learning transferred? Testing someone at the end of a training or educational program does not confirm that the learning changed behavior. There needs to be some method of follow-up to observe if behavior change occurred.
- *Organizational impact.* Although it is often difficult to measure how staff development activities affect the organization, efforts should be made to measure this criterion. Examples of

EXAMINING THE EVIDENCE 16.1

Source: East, D., & Jacoby, K. (2005). The effect of a nursing staff education program on compliance with central line care policy in the cardiac intensive care unit. *Pediatric Nursing*, 31(3), 182–184.

The purpose of this research was to demonstrate the effectiveness of an education module on staff compliance. A quasi-experimental pre- and post-test design was conducted. Pre- and post-test results were used to analyze the effectiveness of the education module. Compliance with central line care policy was based upon 10 observable policy requirements. Data were collected on 47 patients over a 1- to 2-month period before and after intervention. Results showed a marked improvement with compliance to policy.

measurements are assessing quality of care, medication errors, accidents, quality of clinical judgment, turnover, and productivity.

• *Cost-effectiveness*. All staff development activities should be quantified in some manner. This is perhaps the most neglected aspect of accountability in staff development. All staff development activities should be evaluated for quality control, impact on the institution, and cost-effectiveness. This is true regardless of whether the education and training activities are carried out by the manager, the preceptor, the personnel department, or the education department. An example of a quantified evaluation of an education program can be found in Examining the Evidence 16.1, which reports on the effectiveness of an educational program to reduce central venous line complications.

LEARNING EXERCISE 16.1

Designing a Teaching Plan

You have been working in a home health agency for 3 years. During that time, the acuity of your caseload has increased dramatically, and you find that teaching home health aides has become more difficult, as the equipment they need to use has become more complex. The home health aides seem motivated to learn, but you believe that part of the difficulty lies with how you are presenting the material. Many of them have a limited knowledge of nursing procedures.

One of your clients is Mr. Jones, who has no family. His insurance company has approved a visit from a home health aide every other day to bathe him and help him ambulate with a walker. Because of his chronic severe respiratory disease, he must be ambulated with oxygen but does not need it when resting. Today, you have scheduled a session with Mr. Jones' home health aide for a demonstration and return demonstration on how to connect and disconnect the oxygen and how to use the walker. The aide is very competent in basic hygiene skills but has not always used good body mechanics when providing patient care, and she seems intimidated by new equipment.

● ASSIGNMENT: Using your knowledge of the learning theories presented in this chapter, construct a teaching plan for this aide. Support your plan with appropriate rationale.

SHARED RESPONSIBILITY FOR IMPLEMENTING EVIDENCE-BASED PRACTICE

Chapter 11 discussed the individual's responsibility for a professional practice that was evidenced based. However, the organization, as well as the individual, has a responsibility to promote best practices. One way that health care organizations can demonstrate their commitment to becoming a learning organization is to promote and facilitate professional practice that is evidenced based, since nurses often find that barriers to evidence-based practices exist within organizations.

In discussing such organizational constraints, Prevost (2006) delineates various difficulties that nurses face in their attempt to use best practices. Although nurses face difficulties, they need to realize that evidence-based practice is not only a responsibility of RNs but also of the organization and various staff members, including the staff development and education departments. Included among the barriers were accessibility of research findings and administrative support.

 Facilitating evidence-based practice is, therefore, a shared responsibility of the professional nurse, the organization, leader–managers and the education or staff development department.

Prevost suggests numerous strategies that the organization can use to encourage best practices:
- Develop and refine research-based policies and procedures.
- Build consensus from the interdisciplinary team through the development of protocols, decision trees, standards of care and institutional clinical practice guidelines and other such mechanisms.
- Make research findings accessible through libraries and computer resources.
- Provide organization support such as time to do research and educational assistance in showing staff how to interpret research statistics and use findings.
- Encourage cooperation among professionals.
- When possible, hire nurse researchers or consultants to assist staff.

Although, much progress has been made in developing research experts to collect and critique findings to adopt evidence-based practice, much still needs to be done by organizations and staff development departments. "Organizational cultures may not support the nurse who seeks out and uses research to change long-standing practices rooted in tradition" (Prevost, 2006, p. 61).

Echoing the need for organizational support, McAllister and Osborne (2005) maintain that nurse educators are the key change agents in the organization to bring about a research-based culture that improves professional nursing practice.

SOCIALIZATION AND RESOCIALIZATION

Responsibilities of the leader–manager include socializing employees to their roles and the organization as well as educating and training them. It should be noted, however, that the leader–manager is not alone in socializing new employees. The education department, especially during orientation, other employees, and many members of an organization also assist with employee socialization.

There is no single theory of socialization. Among sociologists, the phenomenon of socialization has generally focused on *role theory*—that is, the behaviors that accompany each role are learned socially and by instruction, observation, and trial and error. The first *socialization* to the nursing role occurs during nursing school and continues after graduation. Because nurse administrators and nursing faculty have been found to hold different values and both of these groups assist in socializing the new nurse, there is potential for the new nurse to develop conflict and frustration. However, less research exists on the unique resocialization needs of nurses as they change roles throughout their professional careers.

Resocialization occurs when individuals are forced to learn new values, skills, attitudes, and social rules as a result of changes in the type of work they do, the scope of responsibility they hold, or in the work setting itself. Individuals who frequently need resocialization include new graduates leaving nursing school and entering the work world; experienced nurses who change work settings, either within the same organization or in a new organization; and nurses who undertake new roles. Some employees adapt easily to resocialization, but most experience some stress with *role change*. Organizations can plan in advance to ease the stress of resocialization by the conscious use of appropriate interventions.

 Perhaps one of the best uses of a leader–manager's time in staff development is facilitating the socialization of new employees and the resocialization of employees in new roles.

Clarifying Role Expectations Through Role Models, Preceptors, and Mentors

The soundness of social learning theory, discussed earlier in this chapter, is demonstrated by the effectiveness of role models, preceptors, and mentors to clarify role expectations. Although all three clarify roles through social interaction and educational processes, each has a different focus and uses different mechanisms. All have an appropriate place in employee socialization and resocialization.

A *role model* is defined as someone worthy of imitation (Hyperdictionary, 2003). Role models in nursing are experienced, competent employees. The relationship between the new employee and the role model is a passive one (i.e., employees see that role models are skilled and attempt to emulate them, but the role model does not actively seek this emulation). One of the exciting aspects of role models is their cumulative effect. The greater the number of excellent role models available for new employees to emulate, the greater the possibilities for new employees to perform well.

The educational process in role modeling is passive, but the preceptor role is active and purposeful. The assumption that a one-on-one relationship increases learning is the basis for the use of preceptors. A *preceptor* is an experienced nurse who provides knowledge and emotional support, as well as a clarification of role expectations, on a one-to-one basis. An effective preceptor can role model and adjust teaching to each learner as needed.

Occasionally, the fit between a preceptor and preceptee is not good. This risk is lower if preceptors willingly seek out this responsibility and if they have attended educational courses outlining preceptor duties and responsibilities. In addition, preceptors need to have an adequate knowledge of adult learning theory. Organizations that use preceptors to help new employees clarify their roles and improve their skill level should be careful not to overuse preceptors to the point that that they become tired or demotivated. In addition, workload assignments for the preceptor should be decreased whenever possible so that adequate time can be devoted to helping the preceptee problem solve and learn. Incentive pay for preceptors reinforces that the organization values this role.

LEARNING EXERCISE 16.2

Criteria for Preceptorship

You have been selected to represent your unit on a committee to design a preceptor program for the nursing department. One of the committee's first goals is to develop criteria for the selection of preceptors.

● ASSIGNMENT: In groups, select a minimum of five and a maximum of eight criteria that would be appropriate for selecting preceptors on your unit. Would you have minimum education or experience requirements? What personality or behavioral traits would you seek? Which of the criteria that you identified are measurable?

Mentors take on an even greater role in using education as a means for role clarification. Madison (2006) describes mentoring as a distinctive interactive relationship between two individuals, occurring most commonly in a professional setting. Some individuals use the terms *preceptor* and *mentor* interchangeably. While a preceptor takes on some of the roles of a mentor, they are not the same. For example, preceptors are usually assigned, but true mentors freely choose who they will mentor. The mentor makes a conscious decision to assist the protégé in attaining expert status and in furthering his or her career development. Preceptors have a relatively short relationship with the person to whom they have been assigned, but the relationship between the mentor and mentee is longer and more intense.

Hurst and associates (2002) maintain that there are four phases in mentoring relationships. The first phase, *initiation*, occurs when the relationship is established. The second phase, *cultivation*, is characterized by coaching, protection, and sponsorship as well as counseling, acceptance, and the creation of a sense of competence. During this phase, the relationship develops through established meeting times to share and evaluate progress (Pinkerton, 2003). The third phase is *separation*, and the fourth is *redefinition*, in which the relationship takes on a new form or ends. Separation and redefinition are often difficult, as the mentor and mentee may share different perceptions about whether it is time to separate and what their new relationship should be. Separation and redefinition are critical, however, as mentees should outgrow the need for such intense coaching if the mentor has done a good job of cultivation. Madison (2006) maintains that the mentoring process is part of the interactional work that is essential for socialization and career development. Display 16.3 depicts the stages of the mentoring relationship.

Mentors serve a particularly useful role in acclimating nurses to management roles. Although many nurses will not have a mentor, those lucky enough to find a mentor as they move into roles with increased responsibilities and status will find that resocialization will be smoother.

> Not every nurse will be fortunate to have a mentor to facilitate each new career role. Most nurses will be lucky if they have one or two mentors throughout their lifetimes.

A mentor, as no other, is able to instill the values and attitudes that accompany each role. This is because mentors lead by example. A mentor's strong moral and ethical fiber

DISPLAY 16.3   **Stages of the Mentoring Relationship**

1. Initiation
2. Cultivation
3. Separation
4. Redefinition

encourages mentees to think critically and take a stand on ethical dilemmas in the workplace. Becoming a mentor requires committing to a personal relationship. It also requires teaching skills and a genuine interest and belief in the capabilities of others. A mentor may have various roles in the mentor–mentee relationship. The mentor is often a role model and a visionary for the mentee. Mentors may also open doors in the organization, be someone who the mentee can use to bounce ideas off, or be a supporter or problem solver. The mentor is often a teacher or counselor, especially in career advice. Last, Madison (2006) states that the relationship may even at times be similar to a parent–child relationship. It is both intense and caring.

Assistance in Meeting Role Demands

When meeting role demands, people generally need assistance in two areas: the specific skills and knowledge requirements for the role and the values and attitudes that accompany any given role. To assist the employee in meeting the demands of the job, the manager needs to determine what those needs are. This requires more than just asking employees about their knowledge deficits or giving employees a skills checklist or test; it requires careful observation by the manager and preceptor so that deficiencies are identified and corrected before they handicap the employee's socialization. Careful observation is a leadership role. When such deficiencies are not corrected early, other employees often create a climate of nonacceptance that prevents assimilation of the new employee. The second area in which employees often need assistance is in meeting value and attitude requirements for their roles which may produce conflict in the process.

⊕ Values and attitudes may be a source of conflict as nurses learn new roles.

Organizations can assist new employees in meeting this requirement of socialization. Useful strategies are providing role models; providing a safe climate for new employees to ventilate their frustration with value conflicts; clarifying differing role expectations that are held by physicians, patients, and other staff; and assisting new employees in developing strategies to cope with and resolve value and attitude conflicts.

Overcoming Motivational Deficiencies

Sometimes, difficulties in socialization or resocialization occur because of motivational deficiencies. A planned program should be implemented to correct the deficiencies by using positive and negative sanctions.

Positive Sanctions

Positive sanctions can be used as an interactional or educational process of socialization. If deliberately planned, they become educational. However, sanctions given informally through the group process, or reference group, use the social interaction process. The reference group sets norms of behavior and then applies sanctions to ensure that new members adopt the group norms before acceptance into the group. These informal sanctions offer an extremely powerful tool for socialization and resocialization in the workplace. Managers should become aware of what role behavior they reward and what new employee behavior the senior staff is rewarding.

Negative Sanctions

Negative sanctions, like rewards, provide cues that enable people to evaluate their performance consciously and to modify behavior when needed. For positive or negative sanctions to be effective, they must result in the role learner internalizing the values of the organization.

　　Negative sanctions are often applied in very subtle and covert ways. Making fun of a new graduate's awkwardness with certain skills or belittling a new employee's desire to use nursing care plans is a very effective negative sanction that may be used by group members to mold individual behavior to group norms. This is not to say that negative sanctions should never be used. New employees should be told when their behavior is not an acceptable part of their role. However, the sanctions used should be constructive and not destructive.

 The manager should know what the group norms are, be observant of sanctions used by the group to make newcomers conform, and intervene if group norms are not appropriate.

LEARNING EXERCISE 16.3

Great Influences
Who or what has been the greatest influence on your socialization to the nursing role? Were positive or negative sanctions used? Write a short essay (three or four paragraphs) describing this socialization. If appropriate, share this in a group.

EMPLOYEES WITH UNIQUE SOCIALIZATION NEEDS

The previous discussion focused on the problems that frequently occur in role adaptation for all new employees. However, some employees have unique problems in socializing to new roles. These include the new nurse, the international nurse, new managers, and the experienced nurse in role transition. Managers who provide appropriate socialization assistance for these groups increase the chance of a positive employment outcome.

The New Nurse

One group with unique socialization needs is the new nursing graduate. Kramer (1974) described special fears and difficulties in adapting to the work setting that are common to new graduate nurses and named this fear *reality shock* because it occurs as a result of conflict between a new graduate's expectations of the nursing role and the reality of the actual role in the work setting.

Schmalenberg and Kramer (1979) built on this original work in their assertion that there are four phases of role transition from student nurse to staff nurse: the *honeymoon phase*, followed by the *shock*, *recovery*, and *resolution* phases. As long as the novice nurse is sincerely welcomed into the workplace, the new nurse has little difficulty in the honeymoon phase. During the second phase of reality shock, however, there is often great personal conflict as the nurse discovers that many nursing school values are not prized in the workplace. The organization and the manager then must take sufficient action during the recovery and resolution phases if the new graduate is to be successfully socialized.

Managers can use several mechanisms to ease the role transition of new graduates. *Anticipatory socialization* carried out in educational settings will help prepare new nurses for their professional role. However, managers should not assume that such anticipatory socialization has occurred. Instead, they should build opportunities for sharing and clarifying values and attitudes about the nursing role into orientation programs. Use of the group process is an excellent mechanism to promote the sharing that provides support for new graduates and assists them in recovering from reality shock.

Additionally, managers should be alert for signs and symptoms of the shock phase of role transition; they should intervene by listening to new graduates and helping them cope in the real world. Managers must recognize the intensity of new nurses' practice experience, encourage them to have a balanced life, foster a work environment that has zero tolerance for disrespect, and strive to create work relationship models that promote interdependency of physicians and nursing staff.

> It is important to remember that no one is immune to a loss of idealism and commitment in response to stress in the workplace.

Managers should also ensure that some of the new nurse's values are supported and encouraged so that work and academic values can blend. New professionals need to understand the universal nature of role transition and know that it is not limited to nurses. Providing a class on role transition also may assist new graduates in socialization.

To combat reality shock, some hospitals have developed prolonged orientation periods for new graduates that last from 6 weeks to 6 months. This extended orientation, or *internship*, contrasts sharply with the routine 2-week orientation that is normal for most other employees. During this time, graduate nurses are usually assigned to work with a preceptor and gradually take on a patient assignment equal to that of the preceptor.

Many of the potential hazards of internship (and preceptorship) programs can be overcome by (a) carefully selecting the preceptors, (b) selecting only preceptors who have a strong desire to be role models, (c) preparing preceptors for their role by giving formal classes in adult learning and other social learning concepts, and (d) having either experienced staff development or supervisory personnel monitor the preceptor and new graduate closely to ensure that the relationship continues to be beneficial and growth producing for both.

LEARNING EXERCISE 16.4

Investigating Reality Shock

Talk with at least four nursing graduates who have been working as nurses for anywhere from 3 months to 3 years. Make sure at least two of them are recent graduates and two of them have been working at least 18 months. Ask them about their socialization to nursing after graduation. Did any of them experience reality shock? How long did it last? Did they recover from the shock? If so, how? Share your findings with other members of your group.

International Nurses

One solution to the current nursing shortage has been the active recruitment of nurses from overseas. Ryan (2003) suggests that socialization to the professional nursing role is one of four basic needs that must be addressed if foreign nurses are to adapt successfully to American workplaces. Ryan suggests that initially, foreign nurses must be introduced to American jargon and variations in nursing practice delivery. Then, many must be supported through a period of cultural, professional, and psychological dissonance that is associated with anxiety, homesickness, and isolation. Finally, these nurses must be integrated within the institution so that they develop a sense of community life on the nursing unit.

Bola, Driggers, Dunlap, and Ebersole (2003) state that international nurses also frequently experience culture shock regarding nonverbal communication that may interfere with their assimilation. "Patients or staff with limited cultural competence may interpret nonverbal communication, such as eye contact or smiling, as disrespectful" (Bola et al., p. 41). Ryan (2003) suggests that using a *cultural diversity enhancement group* (CDEG) and a *buddy program* may assist in socializing these international nurses. The CDEG includes staff nurses and management personnel from varied ethnic backgrounds who agree to buddy with the international nurses to make them feel welcomed in the organizational culture and to assist them regarding basic services, places, or necessary items that they need to know about or have. Bola and colleagues (2003) concur, suggesting that without a support system, international nurses may question their ability to solve problems and function successfully since the values and behaviors helpful in solving problems in their home country may not be helpful in the United States.

Dumpel (2005) says that international nurses need the same socialization as other transition groups such as mentors and preceptors, support groups, and good orientation programs. However, he maintains that they also need language classes, cultural classes, and assistance with life activities, such as finding living quarters.

New Managers

Probably no other aspect of an employee's work life has as great an influence on productivity and retention as the quality of supervision exhibited by the immediate manager. Unfortunately, the orientation of new managers is often neglected by organizations. A qualitative study undertaken by Sullivan, Bretschneider, and McCausland (2003) found that many new managers perceived themselves as lacking basic and introductory managerial skills related to communication, conflict resolution, role transitioning, scheduling, budgeting and payroll management, performance evaluation, and staff counseling. This lack of skills may result in management errors.

Additionally, many restructured hospital organizational designs have created different and expanded roles for existing managers without ensuring that managers are adequately prepared for these new roles. Indeed, Kleinman (2003) argues that nurse–managers are often less well prepared to manage the business activities than the clinical activities and that organizations must develop strategies to help nurse–managers develop the business knowledge and skills essential for the role.

 There is a growing recognition that good managers do not emerge from the workforce without a great deal of conscious planning on the part of the organization.

A management development program should be ongoing, and individuals should receive some management development instruction before their appointment to a management position. In speaking to the issue of opportunities for stewardship of the nursing profession, Haase-Herrick (2005) states that "the most obvious opportunity lies in succession planning to develop a future generation of diverse nurse leaders" (p. 118). When an individual is filling a position where the previous manager is still available for orientation, the orientation period should be relatively short. The previous manager usually spends no longer than 1 week working directly with the new manager, especially when the new manager is familiar with the organization. A short orientation by the outgoing manager allows the newly appointed manager to gain control of the unit quickly and establish his or her own management style. If the new manager has been recruited from outside the organization, the orientation period may need to be extended.

Frequently, a new manager will be appointed to a vacant or newly established position. In either case, no one will be readily available to orient the new manager. In such cases, the new manager's immediate superior appoints someone to assist the new manager in learning the role. This could be a manager from another unit, the manager's supervisor, or someone from the unit who is familiar with the manager's duties and roles.

A new manager's orientation does not cease after the short introduction to the various tasks. Every new manager needs guidance, direction, and continued orientation and development during the first year in this new role. This direction comes from several sources in the organization:

- *The new manager's immediate superior.* This could be the unit supervisor if the new manager is a charge nurse, or it could be the chief nursing executive if the new manager is a unit supervisor. The immediate superior should have regularly scheduled sessions with the new manager to continue the ongoing orientation process.
- *A group of the new manager's peers.* There should be a management group in the organization with which the new manager can consult. The new manager should be encouraged to use the group as a resource.
- *A mentor.* If someone in the organization decides to mentor the new manager, it will undoubtedly benefit the organization. Although mentors cannot be assigned, the organization can encourage experienced managers to seek out individuals to mentor.

Clinical nurses who have recently assumed management roles often experience guilt when they decrease their involvement with direct patient care. When employees and physicians see a nurse–manager assuming the role of caregiver, they often make disparaging remarks such as, "Oh, you're working as a real nurse today." This tends to reinforce the nurse's value conflict in the new role.

Nurses moving into positions of increased responsibility also experience *role stress* created by *role ambiguity* and role overload. Role ambiguity describes the stress that occurs when job expectations are unclear. *Role overload* occurs when the demands of the role are excessive. Role overload is a major source of stress for nurse–managers. In addition, as nurses move into positions with increased status, their job descriptions tend to become increasingly vague. Therefore, clarifying job roles becomes an important tool in the resocialization process.

The Experienced Nurse in a New Position

For many reasons, nurses make frequent career moves. Experienced nurses often make lateral transfers within the same organization. Others take new positions that are quite different from their previous role; these new positions may be in their present organization or with a new one. Specific orientation needs arise for these nurses:

- *Transition from expert to novice.* This is a very difficult role transition. Many nurses transfer or change jobs because they no longer find their present job challenging. However, this results in the necessity of assuming a learning role in their new environment. The employee assigned to orient the nurse in role transition should be aware of the difficulties that this nurse will experience. Transferred employees' lack of knowledge in the new area should never be belittled; whenever possible, the special expertise that they bring from their former work area should be acknowledged and utilized.
- *Transition from the familiar to the unfamiliar.* In the old surroundings, the employee knew everyone and where everything was located. In the new position, the employee will not only be learning new job skills but will also be in an unfamiliar environment. Special orientation materials should be developed and made available in departments to which nurses transfer more often than others. In addition to providing necessary staff development content, these orientation programs should focus on efforts to promote the self-esteem of these nurses as they learn the skills necessary for their new role. The unique socialization needs of these new employees are often overlooked; these people need special attention that many organizations neglect.

> The managers of departments that receive frequent transfers should prepare a special orientation for experienced nurses transferring to the department.

Transitioning into a new job would result in less role strain if programs were designed to facilitate role modification and role expansion. For example, when a nurse moves from a medical floor to labor and delivery, the nurse does not know the group norms, is unsure of expected values and behaviors, and goes from being an expert to being a novice. All of this creates a great deal of role strain. This same type of role stress occurs when experienced nurses move from one organization to another or from an inpatient setting to a community setting. Often, nurses feel powerless during role transitions, which may culminate in anger and frustration as they seek socialization to a different role.

Assisting the Experienced Nurse in Role Transition

Programs designed to assist the nurse with the transition to a new position should do more than just provide an orientation to the new position; they also should address specific values and behaviors necessary for the new roles. The values and attitudes expected in a hospice nursing role may be quite different from those expected of a trauma nurse. Managers should not assume that the experienced nurse is aware of the new role's expected attitudes. Excellent companies have leaders who take responsibility for shaping the values of new employees. By instilling and clarifying organizational values, managers promote a homogeneous staff that functions as a team.

Employees adopting new values often experience role strain because they may need to give up a former value. Managers need to support employees during this value resocialization. Members of the reference group often use negative sanctions. For example, saying things like, "Well, we don't believe in doing that here" can make new, experienced employees feel as though the values held in other nursing roles were bad or wrong. Therefore, the manager should make efforts to see that formerly held values are not belittled.

Coaching as a Teaching Strategy

Coaching as a means to develop and train employees is a teaching strategy rather than a learning theory. Coaching is one of the most important tools for empowering subordinates, changing behavior, and developing a cohesive team. It is perhaps the most difficult role for a manager to master. *Coaching* is one person helping the other to reach an optimum level of performance. The emphasis is always on assisting the employee to recognize greater options, to clarify statements, and to grow. Haase-Herrick (2005) suggests that coaching is part of a renewing and productive process.

Coaching may be long term or short term. *Short-term coaching* is effective as a teaching tool, for assisting with socialization, and for dealing with short-term problems. *Long-term coaching* as a tool for career management and in dealing with disciplinary problems is different and is discussed in other chapters. Short-term coaching frequently involves spontaneous teaching opportunities. Learning Exercise 16.5 is an example of how a manager can use short-term coaching to guide an employee in a new role.

LEARNING EXERCISE 16.5

Paul's Complaint
Paul is the charge nurse on a surgical floor from 3 PM to 11 PM. One day, he comes to work a few minutes early, as he occasionally does, so that he can chat with his supervisor, Mary, before taking patient reports. Usually, Mary is in her office around this time. Paul enjoys talking over some of his work-related management problems with her because he is fairly new in the charge nurse role, having been appointed 3 months ago. Today, he asks Mary if she can spare a minute to discuss a personnel problem.

Paul: Sally is becoming a real problem to me. She is taking long break times and has not followed through on several medication order changes lately.

Mary: What do you mean by "long breaks" and not following through?

Paul: In the last 2 months, she has taken an extra 15 minutes for dinner three nights a week and has missed changes in medication orders eight times.

Mary: Have you spoken to Sally?

Paul: Yes, and she said that she had been an RN on this floor for 4 years, and no one had ever criticized her before. I checked her personnel record, and there is no mention of those particular problems, but her performance appraisals have only been mediocre.

Mary: What do you recommend doing about Sally?

Paul: I could tell her that I won't tolerate her extended dinner breaks and her poor work performance.

Mary: What are you prepared to do if her performance does not improve?

Paul: I could give her a written warning notice and eventually fire her if her work remains below standard.

Mary: Well, that is one option. What are some other options available to you? Do you think that Sally really understands your expectations? Do you feel that she might resent you?

Paul: I suppose I should sit down with Sally and explain exactly what my expectations are. Since my appointment to charge nurse, I've talked with all the new nurses as they have come on shift, but I just assumed that the old-timers knew what was expected on this unit. I've been a little anxious about my new role; I never thought about her resenting my position.

Mary: I think that is a good first option. Maybe Sally interpreted your not talking with her, as you did all the new nurses, as a rejection. After you have another talk with her, let me know how things are going.

Analysis: The supervisor has coached Paul toward a more appropriate option as a first choice in solving this problem. Although Mary's choice of questions and guidance assisted Paul, she never "took over" or directed Paul but instead let him find his own better solution. As a result of this conversation, Paul had a series of individual meetings with all his staff and shared with them his expectations. He also enlisted their assistance in his efforts to have the shift run smoothly. Although he began to see an improvement in Sally's performance, he realized that she was a marginal employee who would need a great deal of coaching. He reported back to Mary and outlined his plans for improving Sally's performance further. Mary reinforced Paul's handling of the problem by complimenting his actions.

MEETING THE EDUCATIONAL NEEDS OF A CULTURALLY DIVERSE STAFF

In the 21st century, nurse–leaders should expect to work with a more diverse workforce. According to Huston (2006b), there are three main types of diversity in the workforce: ethnicity, gender, and generational. Creating an organization that celebrates a diverse workforce rather than merely tolerating it requires well-planned learning activities. There should also be sufficient opportunity for small groups so that personnel can begin recognizing their own biases and prejudices. This type of learning activity is especially important as more unlicensed assistive personnel (UAP) are added to the staff. Education to support cultural diversity should be part of the staff development of RNs and UAP to facilitate their learning to work together in teams.

Heterogeneity of staff in a teaching–learning setting may add strength or create difficulty. Factors such as gender, age, English language proficiency, and culture may affect success and cooperative learning of groups. Although meeting the educational needs of a heterogeneous staff may be more time consuming and beset with communication problems, the educational needs must be met. The ability of all nurses to work well with a culturally diverse staff is essential. Managers should respect cultural diversity and recognize the desirability of having nurses from numerous cultures on their staff.

Education staff should be aware that learners with diverse learning styles and cultural backgrounds may perceive both the classroom and instruction different from learners who have never experienced a culture different from that of the mainstream United States. Managers should also consider older nurses' learning styles and preceptor needs. Older nurses learn in a different manner than do new graduates and respond well to sharing anecdotal case histories.

Whether teaching in a classroom or at the bedside, there are several things that staff development personnel can do to facilitate the learning process, such as giving the learner plenty of time to respond to questions and restating information that is not understood.

LEARNING EXERCISE 16.6

Cultural Considerations in Teaching
You are the evening charge nurse for a large surgical unit. Recently, your long-time and extremely capable unit clerk retired, and the manager of the unit replaced the clerk with 23-year-old Nan, who does not have a health care background and is a recent immigrant. She speaks English with an accent but can be easily understood. She appears highly intelligent but shy and unassertive.

Nan received a 2-week unit clerk orientation that consisted of actual classroom time and working directly with the retiring clerk. She has been functioning on her own for 2 weeks, and you realize that her orientation was insufficient. Last evening, after her tenth mistake, you became rather sharp with her, and she broke down in tears.

You are frustrated by this situation. Your unit is very busy in the evening with returning surgeries and surgeons making rounds and leaving a multitude of orders. On the other hand, you believe that Nan has great potential. You realize that there is much to learn in this job and, for a person without a health care background, that learning the terminology, physicians' names, and unit routine is difficult. You spend the morning devising a training plan for Nan.

● ASSIGNMENT: Using your knowledge of learning theories, explain your teaching plan, and support your plan with appropriate rationale. How might Nan's lack of an American education and socialization influence her learning?

BUILDING TEAM UNITY THROUGH STAFF DEVELOPMENT AND SOCIALIZATION

The new momentum in organizations is toward encouraging a team effort through team building and providing a continual supportive learning environment. Health care science and technology change so rapidly that without adequate teaching–learning skills and educational services, organizations will get left behind. Likewise, it has become obvious in the new millennium that teams, rather than individuals, function more efficiently. Slowikowski (2005) states, "A true leader knows the keys for inspiring and influencing team members. If a leader can instill the desire to excel in team members, then the team as a whole will succeed" (p. 835).

A premise of the learning organization is that learning itself enhances the team. Learning together and for the organization makes the sum of the team more important than the individual. Greggs-McQuilkin (2004) says that successful teams require individuals to be adaptable, to embrace change and cultural diversity, and allow everyone to have a voice. The workplace becomes more productive when there is team compatibility.

INTEGRATING LEADERSHIP AND MANAGEMENT IN TEAM BUILDING THROUGH SOCIALIZING AND EDUCATING STAFF FOR TEAM BUILDING

The recent emphasis on learning in organizations is seen as a way for organizations to improve quality. The many components of staff development are of critical importance for the fast-changing health care environment. There is constant development of new technology and continual need to absorb new information and knowledge. The integrated leader–manager knows that a well-planned and well-implemented staff development program is a wise investment of organizational resources. It provides the opportunity to mold a team effort and infuse employees with enthusiasm for the organization.

The manager recognizes the ultimate responsibility for staff development and uses appropriate teaching theories to assist with teaching and training staff. There is a shared responsibility for assessing educational needs, educational quality, and fiscal accountability of all staff development activities.

The leader uses knowledge of androgogy in dealing with all employees; coaches spontaneously and effectively; and seeks opportunities to be personally involved with teaching, training, and staff development. By integrating the leadership role with the management functions of staff development, the manager is able to collaborate with education personnel and others so that the learning needs of unit employees are met.

The manager ensures that resources for staff development are used wisely. A focus of staff development should be keeping staff updated with new knowledge and ascertaining that all personnel remain competent to perform their roles. The integrated leader–manager is the role model of a good teacher, using teaching–learning theory to empower staff.

The integrated leader–manager is also one who encourages continuous learning from all individuals in the organization and is a role model of the lifelong learner. This is especially important in promoting evidence-based nursing practice. The nurse–leader should use evidence-based practice and make research resources available to the staff. He or she understands that by building and supporting a knowledgeable team, the collective knowledge generated will be greater than any single individual's contribution.

There is perhaps no other part of management that has as great an influence on reducing burnout as successful socializing new employees to the values of the organization. Socialization, a critical component of introducing the employee into the organization, is a complex process directed at the acquisition of appropriate attitudes, cognition, emotions, values, motivations, skills, knowledge, and social patterns necessary to cope with the social and professional environment. Socialization differs from and has a greater impact than either induction or orientation on subsequent productivity and retention. It can also help to build loyalty and team spirit. This is the time to instill the employee with pride in the organization and the unit. This type of affective learning becomes the foundation for subsequent increased satisfaction and motivation.

The integrated leader–manager supports employees during difficult role transitions. Mentoring and role modeling are encouraged, and role expectations are clarified. The manager recognizes that employees who are not supported and socialized to the organization will not develop the loyalty necessary in the competitive marketplace. Leaders understand that creating a positive work environment where there is interdisciplinary respect will assist employees in their role transitions.

Key Concepts

* The socialization of people into roles occurs with all professions and is a normal socio-logical process.
* *Socialization* and *resocialization* are often neglected areas of the indoctrination process.
* The terms *role model*, *preceptor*, and *mentor* are not synonymous, and all play an important role in assisting with the socialization of employees.
* New graduates, international nurses, new managers, and experienced nurses in new roles have unique socialization needs.
* Difficulties with resocialization usually centers on unclear role expectations (*role ambiguity*), an inability to meet job demands, or deficiencies in motivation. *Role strain* and *role overload* contribute to the problem.
* *Training* and *education* are important parts of staff development.
* Managers and education department staff have a shared responsibility for the education and training of staff.
* Theories of learning and principles of teaching must be considered if staff development activities are to be successful.
* *Social learning theory* suggests that people learn most behavior by direct experience and observation.
* People from different cultures and age groups may have different socialization and learning needs.
* All staff development activities should be evaluated for quality control and fiscal accountability.
* The leader is a role model of the lifelong learner.
* The philosophy of *learning organizations* is the concept that collective learning goes beyond the boundaries of individual learning and releases gains for both the individual and the organization.
* There is a shared responsibility for the promotion of evidence-based nursing practice.

ADDITIONAL LEARNING EXERCISES AND APPLICATIONS

LEARNING EXERCISE 16.7

Accepting Additional Responsibility

You are an experienced staff nurse on an inpatient specialty unit. Today, a local nursing school instructor approaches you and asks if you would be willing to become a preceptor for a nursing student as part of his 10-week leadership–management clinical rotation. The instructor relays that there will be no instructor on site and that the student has had only minimal exposure to acute-care clinical skills. The student will have to work very closely with you on a one-to-one basis. The school of nursing can offer no pay for this role, but the instructor states that she would be happy to write a thank-you letter for your personnel file and that she would be available at any time to address questions that might arise.

The unit does not reduce workload for preceptors, although credit for service is given on the annual performance review. The unit supervisor states that the choice is yours but warns that you may also be called upon to assist with the orientation of a nurse who will transfer to the unit in 6-weeks time. You have mixed feelings about whether to accept this role. Although you enjoy having students on the unit and being in the teaching role, you are unsure if you can do both your normal, heavy workload as well as give the students the time that they will undoubtedly need to learn. You do feel a "need to give back to your profession" and personally believe that nurses need to be more supportive of each other, but you are significantly concerned about role overload.

● ASSIGNMENT: Decide if you will accept this role. Would you place any constraints upon the instructor, the student, or your supervisor as a condition of accepting the role? What were the strongest driving forces for your decision? What were the greatest restraining forces? What evaluation criteria would you develop to assess whether your final decision was a good one?

LEARNING EXERCISE 16.8

Addressing Resocialization Issues

You are one of the care coordinators for a home health agency. One of your duties is to orient new employees to the agency. Recently, the chief nursing executive hired Brian, an experienced acute-care nurse, to be one of your team members. Brian seemed eager and enthusiastic. He confided in you that he was tired of acute care and wanted to be more involved with long-term patient and family caseloads.

During Brian's orientation, you became aware that his clinical skills were excellent, but his therapeutic communication skills were inferior to those of the rest of your staff. You discussed this with Brian and explained how important communication is in gaining the trust of agency patients and that trust is necessary if the needs of the patients and the goals of the agency are to be met. You referred Brian to some literature that you believed might be helpful to him.

After a 3-week orientation program, Brian began working unsupervised. It is now 4 weeks later. Recently, you received a complaint from one of the other nurses and one from a patient regarding Brian's poor communication skills. Brian seems frustrated and has not gained acceptance from the other nurses in your work group. You suspect that some of the nurses resent Brian's superior clinical skills, whereas others believe that he does not understand his new role, and they are becoming impatient with him. You are genuinely concerned that Brian does not seem to be fitting in.

● ASSIGNMENT: Could this problem have been prevented? Decide what you should do now. Outline a plan to resocialize Brian into his new role and make him feel like a valued part of the staff.

LEARNING EXERCISE 16.9

Effective Interpersonal Problem Solving

You have been working at Memorial Hospital for 3 months and have begun to feel fairly confident in your new role. However, one of the older nurses working on your shift constantly belittles your nursing education. Whenever you request assistance in problem solving or in learning a new skill, she says, "Didn't they teach you anything in nursing school?" Your charge nurse has given you a satisfactory 3-month evaluation, but you are becoming increasingly defensive regarding the comments of the other nurse.

● ASSIGNMENT: Explain how you plan to evaluate the accuracy of the older nurse's comments. Might you be contributing to the problem? How will you cope with this situation? Would you involve others? What efforts can you make to improve your relationship with this co-worker?

LEARNING EXERCISE 16.10

Changing Learning Needs

Learning needs and the maturity of those in a class often influence course content and teaching methods. Look back at how your learning needs and maturity level have changed since you were a beginning nursing student. When viewed as a whole, were you and the other beginning nursing students child or adult learners? Compare Knowles's (1970) pedagogy and androgogy characteristics to determine this.

Are pedagogical teaching strategies appropriate for beginning nursing students? If so, when does the nursing student make a transition from child to adult learner? What teaching modes do you believe would be most conducive to learning for a beginning nursing student? Would this change as students progressed through the nursing program? Support your beliefs with rationale.

(Web Links)

Multicultural Pavilion
http://curry.edschool.virginia.edu/go/multicultural
Provides instructional resources for those creating a multicultural curriculum, along with a discussion board dealing with diversity.

Free Learning Games and Tips for Staff Development Educators
http://www.nurselearn.com/free_game_&_tips.htm
Includes word games, word searches, and crossword puzzles for use as staff development pretests or posttests with a classroom presentation, self-study program, poster presentation, and the like.

Nursing Center for Staff Development
http://www.nursingcenter.com/library/journalarticleprint.asp?
A monthly column on best practices in staff development administration.

References

Bandura, A. (1977). *Social learning theory.* Englewood Cliffs, NJ: Prentice-Hall.

Bola, T. V., Driggers, K., Dunlap, C., & Ebersole, M. (2003). Foreign-educated nurses. Strangers in a strange land. *Nursing Management, 34*(7), 39–42.

Dumpel, H. (2005). Contemporary issues facing international nurses: Adopting a CAN/NNOC code of practice for international nurse recruitment. *California Nurse, 101*(9), 18–23.

Haase-Herrick, K. S. (2005). The opportunities of stewardship. *Nursing Administration Quarterly, 29*(2), 115–118.

Hurst, S., Koplin-Baucum, S., Wilkins, B., Merkel, D., Lujan, L., Helmich, C., Henry, C., & Mosesman, A. (2002). *Mentoring program.* Phoenix, AZ: Good Samaritan Regional Medical Center.

Huston, C. (2006a). Assuring provider competence through licensure, continuing education and certification. In C. Huston (Ed.), *Professional issues in nursing.* Philadelphia: Lippincott Williams & Wilkins.

Huston, C. (2006b). Diversity in the nursing workforce. In C. Huston (Ed.), *Professional issues in nursing.* Philadelphia: Lippincott, Williams & Wilkins.

Hyperdictionary. (2003). Retrieved January 2, 2004, from *http://www.hyperdictionary.com/.*

Kleinman, C. S. (2003). Leadership roles, competencies, and education. How prepared are our nurse managers? *Journal of Nursing Administration, 33*(9), 451–455.

Knowles, M. (1970). *The modern practice of adult education: Androgogy versus pedagogy.* New York: Association Press.

Kramer, M. (1974). *Reality shock: Why nurses leave nursing.* St. Louis, MO: C.V. Mosby.

Kramer, M., & Schmalenberg, C. (2004). Essentials of a magnetic work environment. *Nursing2004, 34*(6), 50–54.

Madison, J. (2006). Socialization and mentoring. In C. Huston (Ed.), *Professional issues in nursing.* Philadelphia: Lippincott, Williams & Wilkins.

McAllister, M., & Osborne, S. R. (2005). Teaching and learning practice development for change. *Journal of Continuing Education in Nursing, 37*(4), 154–159.

Pinkerton, S. E. (2003). Mentoring new graduates. *Nursing Economic$, 21*(4), 202–203.

Postlen-Slattery, D., & Foley, K. (2003). The fruits of lifelong learning. *Nursing Management, 34*(2), 35–37.

Prevost, S. S. (2006). Defining evidence-based best practices. In C. Huston (Ed.), *Professional issues in nursing.* Philadelphia: Lippincott Williams & Wilkins.

Ryan, M. (2003). A buddy program for international nurses. *Journal of Nursing Administration, 33*(6), 350–352.

Schmalenberg, C., & Kramer, M. (1979). *Coping with reality shock.* Wakefield, MA: Nursing Resources.

Senge, P. (1994). *The fifth discipline: The art and practice of the learning organization.* New York: Currency Doubleday.

Slowikowski, M. K. (2005). Using the DISC behavioral instrument to guide leadership and communication. *AORN Journal, 82*(5), 835, 841–843.

Sullivan, J., Bretschneider, J., & McCausland, M. P. (2003). Designing a leadership development program for nurse managers. *Journal of Nursing Administration, 33*(10), 544–549.

Wilkinson, J. E., Rushmer, R. K., & Davies, T. O. (2004). Clinical governance and the learning organization. *Journal of Nursing Management, 12*(1), 105–113.

Bibliography

Bunkers, S. S. (2005). Teaching-learning processes. The quality of a teaching-learning organization and the novice nurse. *Nursing Science Quarterly, 18*(3), 215.

Chang, E. M., Hancock, K. M., Johnson, A., Daly, J., & Jackson, D. (2005). Role stress in nurses: Review of related factors and strategies for moving forward. *Nursing and Health Sciences, 7*(1), 57–65.

Davis, E. (2005). Home study program. Educating perioperative managers about materials and financial management. *AORN Journal, 81*(4), 798–801.

Elcock, K. (2006). Good mentors are the key to effective learning. *Nursing Standard, 20*(36), 38.

Fleck, C. (2005). Can we talk? Pass it on: The power of mentors. *Ostomy Wound Management, 51*(11), 64.

Gallagher, R. M. (2005). National quality efforts: What continuing and staff development educators need to know. *Journal of Continuing Education, 36*(1), 39, 42–45.

Guttman, M. S. (2004). Increasing the linguistic competence of the nurse with limited English proficiency. *Journal of Continuing Education in Nursing, 35*(6), 264–269.

Hofler, L. D. (2006). Learning from the best: The benefits of a structured health policy fellowship in developing nursing health policy leaders. *Politics and Nursing Practice, 7*(2), 110–113.

Lloyd, S., & Bristol, S. (2006). Modeling mentorship and collaboration for BSN and MSN students in a community clinical practicum. *Journal of Nursing Education, 45*(4), 129–132.

Lynn, M. R. (2006). Research reflections. Mentoring the next generation of systems researchers. *Journal of Nursing Administration, 36*(6), 288–291.

McKenna, H. P., Ashton, S., & Keeney, S. (2004). Barriers to evidence-based practice in primary care. *Journal of Advanced Nursing, 45*(2), 178–189.

McCloskey, A. (2005). Peer presence: Tips for top challenges. Staff or team: What does it mean? *Nursing Management, 36*(7), 72.

McNamara, S. A. (2005). President's message. Teaching others the "why" of what we do. *AORN Journal, 82*(1), 9–11.

Metcalfe, J., & Garrett, S. (2005). Team esteem. *Nursing Standard, 19*(21), 88.

Olade, R. (2004). Evidence-based practice and research utilization activities among rural nurses. *Journal of Nursing Scholarship, 36*(3), 220–225.

Strasser, P. B. (2005). Management file. Competency based occupational health nurse orientation. *AAOHN Journal, 53*(8), 338–339.

Van Sell, S., Johnson-Russell, J., & Kindred, C. (2006). The teaching power of high-tech dummies. *RN, 69*(4), 30–35.

Vander Woude, D. L., & Letcher, D. C. (2005). Teaching-learning processes. Becoming a living-learning organization. *Nursing Science Quarterly, 19*(1), 24–30.

Wachs, J. E. (2005). Building the occupational health team: Keys to successful interdisciplinary collaboration. *AAOHN Journal, 53*(4), 166–171.

Winkelmann-Gleed, A., & Seeley, J. (2005). International nursing. Strangers in a British world? Integration of international nurses. *British Journal of Nursing, 14*(18), 954–961.

West, E., Barron, D. N., & Reeves, R. (2005). Overcoming the barriers to patient-centered care: Time, tools and training. *Journal of Clinical Nursing, 14*(4), 435–443.

17

Staffing Needs and Scheduling Policies

. . . accurate definition and quantification of the work of nursing is critical to the identification of appropriate nursing resource requirements.

—Graf, Millar, Feilteau, Coakley, and Erickson (2003)

In addition to selecting, developing, and socializing staff, the manager must ascertain that adequate numbers and an appropriate mix of personnel are available to meet daily unit needs and organizational goals. Because staffing patterns and scheduling policies directly affect the daily lives of all personnel, it is important that they be administered fairly as well as economically. This chapter examines different methods for determining staffing needs, communicating staffing plans, and developing and communicating scheduling policies. Unit fiscal responsibility is discussed, with sample formulas and instructions for calculating daily staffing needs.

The manager's responsibility for adequate and well-communicated staffing and scheduling policies is stressed, as is the need for periodic re-evaluation of staffing philosophy to meet stated care delivery. There is a focus on the leadership responsibility for developing trust through fair staffing and scheduling procedures. Recent legislation regarding mandatory staffing requirements is also discussed, including the manager's role for ensuring that the organization can facilitate the changes required by law. The leadership roles and management functions inherent in staffing and scheduling are shown in Display 17.1.

UNIT MANAGER'S RESPONSIBILITIES IN MEETING STAFFING NEEDS

The requirement for night, evening, weekend, and holiday work that is frequently necessary in health care organizations is stressful and frustrating for some nurses. Inflexible scheduling and extended work schedules are major contributors to job dissatisfaction and turnover on the part of nurses (Trinkoff et al., 2006). Managers should do whatever they can to see that employees feel they have some control over scheduling, shift options, and staffing policies.

DISPLAY 17.1 **Leadership Roles and Management Functions Associated With Staffing and Scheduling**

Leadership Roles

1. Identifies creative and flexible staffing methods to meet the needs of patients, staff, and the organization
2. Is knowledgeable regarding contemporary methods of scheduling and staffing
3. Assumes a responsibility toward staffing that builds trust and encourages a team approach
4. Periodically examines the unit standard of productivity to determine if changes are needed
5. Is alert to extraneous factors that have an impact on staffing
6. Is ethically accountable to patients and employees for adequate and safe staffing
7. Plans for staffing shortages so that patient care goals will be met
8. Assesses if and how workforce intergenerational values impact staffing needs and responds accordingly

Management Functions

1. Provides adequate staffing to meet patient care needs according to the philosophy of the organization
2. Uses organizational goals and patient classification tools to minimize understaffing and overstaffing as patient census and acuity fluctuate
3. Schedules staff in a fiscally responsible manner
4. Develops and implements fair and uniform scheduling policies and communicates these clearly to all staff
5. Ascertains that scheduling policies are not in violation of state and national labor laws, organizational policies, or union contracts
6. Assumes accountability for quality and fiscal control of staffing
7. Evaluates scheduling and staffing procedures and policies on a regular basis

Although many organizations now use staffing clerks and computers to assist with staffing, the overall responsibility for scheduling continues to be an important function of first- and middle-level managers. Each organization has different expectations regarding the unit manager's responsibility in long-range human resource planning and in short-range planning for daily staffing.

CENTRALIZED AND DECENTRALIZED STAFFING

Some organizations decentralize staffing by having unit managers make scheduling decisions. Other organizations use *centralized staffing*, where staffing decisions are made by personnel in a central office or staffing center. Such centers may or may not be staffed by RNs, although someone in authority would be a nurse even when a staffing clerk carries out the day-to-day activity.

In organizations with *decentralized staffing*, the unit manager is often responsible for covering all scheduled staff absences, reducing staff during periods of decreased patient census or acuity, adding staff during periods of high patient census or acuity, preparing monthly unit schedules, and preparing holiday and vacation schedules. Nursing management is highly decentralized in most hospitals, with considerable variation found in staffing among patient care units. This means that many nurse–managers have some control over factors that affect cost on their specific units.

Advantages of decentralized staffing are that the unit manager understands the needs of the unit and staff intimately, which leads to the increased likelihood that sound staffing decisions will be made. Additionally, the staff feels more in control of their work environment because they are able to take personal scheduling requests directly to their immediate supervisor. Also, decentralized scheduling and staffing leads to increased autonomy and flexibility, thus decreasing nurse attrition. In a survey of nurses, Buerhaus, Donelan, Ulrich, Norman, and Dittus (2006) found that 60% of nurses felt that frontline managers recognized the importance of RNs' personal and family life and incorporated that into the scheduling. This research supports the advantages of decentralized staffing.

Decentralized staffing, however, carries the risk that employees will be treated unequally or inconsistently. Additionally, the unit manager may be viewed as granting rewards or punishments through the staffing schedule. Decentralized staffing also is time-consuming for the manager and often promotes more "special pleading" than centralized staffing. However, undoubtedly, the major difficulty with decentralized staffing is ensuring high-quality staffing decisions throughout the organization.

In centralized staffing, the manager's role is limited to making minor adjustments and providing input. For example, the manager would communicate special staffing needs and assist with obtaining staff coverage for illness and sudden changes in patient census. Therefore, the manager in centralized staffing continues to have ultimate responsibility for seeing that adequate personnel are available to meet the needs of the organization.

Centralized staffing is fairer to all employees because policies tend to be employed more consistently and impartially. In addition, centralized staffing frees the middle-level manager to complete other management functions. Centralized staffing also allows for the most efficient (cost-effective) use of resources because the more units that can be considered together, the easier it is to deal with variations in patient census and staffing needs. Centralized staffing, however, does not provide as much flexibility for the worker, nor can it account as well for a worker's desires or special needs. Additionally, managers may be less responsive to personnel budget control if they have limited responsibility in scheduling and staffing matters. It is important to remember that centralized and decentralized staffing is not synonymous with centralized and decentralized decision making. For example, a manager can work in an organization that has centralized staffing but decentralized organizational decision making.

 Regardless of whether the organization has centralized or decentralized staffing, all unit managers should understand scheduling options and procedures and accept fiscal responsibility for staffing.

MANAGING A DIVERSE STAFF

Managers must also be cognizant of the need to have an ethnically and culturally diverse staff to meet the needs of an increasingly diverse patient population. Indeed, national standards for providing culturally and linguistically appropriate services in health care were released by the Department of Health and Human Services Office of Minority Health in 2000 (DHHS Minority

Health, 2007). Of the 14 standards put forth, several directly address the need for cultural and linguistic diversity in staffing. For example, Standard 4 requires that health care organizations offer language assistance services, including bilingual staff and interpreter services, at no cost to clients with limited English proficiency. Standard 6 ensures the competency of this language assistance by interpreters and bilingual staff, and Standard 5 requires that all verbal offers and written notices regarding patients' access to these services be available to patients in their preferred languages. Indeed, Malloch, Davenport, and Hatler (2003) suggest that the importance of providing culturally competent caregivers cannot be overstated, as health care congruent with cultural beliefs and values is essential for optimal outcomes.

 Managers must clearly understand the unique cultural and linguistic needs represented in their patient population and try to address these needs through an appropriately diverse staff.

COMPLYING WITH STAFFING MANDATES

As the current health care system is evaluated, nurse–managers must be cognizant of new recommendations and legislation affecting staffing. There has been movement in at least 28 states to impose *mandatory staffing requirements* (Huston, 2006a), and one state (California) has already enacted legislation requiring mandatory staffing rates that affect hospitals and long-term care facilities. Under Assembly Bill 394, passed in 1999 and crafted by the California Nurses Association, all hospitals in California had to comply with the minimum staffing ratios shown in Display 17.2 by January 1, 2004 (California Nurses Association, 2003). These ratios, developed by the California Department of Health Services, represent the maximum number of patients an RN can be assigned to care for under any circumstance. Other states—Massachusetts, New York, Florida, and Michigan—are also in the process of enacting legislation (Leighty, 2004).

Proponents of legislated minimum staffing ratios say that ratios are needed because many hospitals' current staffing levels are so low that both RNs and their patients are negatively affected (Huston, 2006a). In addition, numerous articles have appeared in the media attesting to grossly inadequate staffing in hospitals and nursing homes, and professional nursing organizations such as the American Nurses Association (ANA) have expressed concern about the effect poor staffing has on nurses' health and safety and on patient outcomes. This concern has been echoed by the Institute of Medicine in its recommendations regarding the working environment for nurses (Trinkoff et al., 2006). Adequate staffing, then, is needed to ensure that care provided is at least safe and hopefully more. Proponents of state regulation of RN-to-patient ratios suggest that such ratios protect the most basic elements of the public health we take for granted and argue that the government must take on this responsibility to ensure that safe health care is provided to all Americans (Huston, 2006a).

However, there are arguments against staffing ratios. Huston (2006a) lists numerous such arguments. The current nursing shortage makes it difficult to fill the slots when ratios exist, and the ratios may merely serve as a Band-Aid to the greater problems of quality of care. Additionally, numbers alone do not ensure improved patient care, as not all RNs have equivalent clinical experience and skill levels. There is also the argument that staffing may actually decline with ratios since they might be used as the ceiling or as ironclad criteria if institutions are not willing to make adjustments for patient acuity or RN skill level. Some critics suggest that mandatory staffing ratios create significant opportunity costs that may restrict employers

DISPLAY 17.2   **Minimum Staffing Ratios for Hospitals in California Effective January 2004**

Unit	Nurse–Patient Ratio
Critical Care/ICU	1:2
Neonatal ICU	1:2
Operating Room	1:1
Labor & Delivery	1:2
Antepartum	1:4
Postpartum couplets	1:4
Postpartum women only	1:6
Pediatrics	1:4
Step-down (initial)	1:4
Step-down (in 2008)	1:3
Medical–Surgical (initial)	1:6
Medical–Surgical (deferred from 2005 to 2008)	1:5
Oncology (initial)	1:5
Oncology (in 2008)	1:4
Psychiatry	1:6
Emergency Room	1:4
Telemetry and specialty units (to be enacted in 2008)	1:4

Source: California Nurses Association. (2007). Ratio Basics by Unit. Retrieved January 5, 2007, from *http://www.calnurses.org/nursing-practice*.

and payers from responding to market forces; subsequently, they may be unable to take advantage of improved technological support or respond to changes in patient acuity.

The bottom line, however, is that minimum staffing ratios would not have been proposed in the first place had staffing abuses and the resultant declines in the quality of patient care not occurred in the past. The implementation and subsequent evaluation of mandatory staffing ratios in states having such ratios should provide greater insight to the ongoing debate about the need for mandatory staffing ratios.

LEARNING EXERCISE 17.1

Comparing Staffing Ratios

Now that some states are moving toward or have already enacted mandatory staffing, the rest of the nation will be monitoring the implementation of minimum staffing ratios and assessing outcomes of such legislation.

● ASSIGNMENT: Compare the current staffing ratios used at the facility in which you work or do clinical practicums with those shown in Display 17.2. How do they compare? Is there an effort to legislate minimum staffing ratios in the state in which you live? Who or what would you anticipate to be the greatest barrier to implementation of staffing ratios in your state?

STAFFING AND SCHEDULING OPTIONS

Because it is beyond the scope of this book to discuss all of the creative staffing and scheduling options available, only a few are discussed here. Some of the more frequently used creative staffing and scheduling options include:

- 10- or 12-hour shifts
- Premium pay for weekend work
- Part-time staffing pool for weekend shifts and holidays
- Cyclical staffing, which allows long-term knowledge of future work schedules because a set staffing pattern is repeated every few weeks. Figure 17.1 shows a master staffing pattern that repeats every 4 weeks.
- Job sharing
- Allowing nurses to exchange hours of work among themselves
- Flextime
- Use of supplemental staffing from outside registries and float pools
- Staff self-scheduling
- Shift bidding, which allows nurses to bid for shifts rather than requiring mandatory overtime

There are advantages and disadvantages to each type of scheduling. Because extending the workday with 10- or 12-hour shifts may require overtime pay, the resultant nurse satisfaction must be weighed against the increased costs.

		Week I							Week II							Week III							Week IV						
Position	Name	S	M	T	W	T	F	S	S	M	T	W	T	F	S	S	M	T	W	T	F	S	S	M	T	W	T	F	S
Full-time	RN 1				X		X		X					X					X		X	X	X					X	
Full-time	RN 2	X				X					X			X	X	X				X					X			X
Full-time	RN 3		X				X	X	X			X					X				X	X	X			X		
Full-time	RN 4	X			X					X				X	X	X		X				X						X
Full-time	RN 5			X		X	X	X				X					X		X	X	X					X	
Full-time	RN 6	X			X				X					X	X		X				X			X				X
Full-time	RN 7		X				X	X	X			X				X				X	X	X			X		
Full-time	RN 8	X				X					X			X	X	X			X					X				X
Part-time	8 hrs/wk RN 9	On													On	On												On
Part-time	8 hrs/wk RN 10							On	On													On	On					
Part-time	8 hrs/wk RN 11	On													On	On												On
Part-time	8 hrs/wk RN 12							On	On													On	On					
Total RNs on duty each day		6	7	7	6	6	6	6	6	7	7	6	6	6	6	6	7	7	6	6	6	6	6	7	6	7	6	6	6

Elements: Every other weekend off   Number of split days off each period: 2   X: Scheduled day off
Maximum days worked: 4   Operates in multiples of 4, 8, 12 . . .
Minimum days worked: 2   Schedule repeats itself every 4 weeks

Figure 17.1   Four-week cycle master time sheet.

Extending the length of shifts may result in increased judgment errors as nurses tire. For this reason, many organizations limit the number of consecutive 10- or 12-hour days a nurse can work or the number of hours that can be worked in a given day.

LEARNING EXERCISE 17.2

Choosing Eight- or Twelve-Hour Shifts
You are the manager of an intensive care unit. Many of the nurses have approached you requesting 12-hour shifts. Other nurses have approached you stating that they will transfer out of the unit if 12-hour shifts are implemented. You are exploring the feasibility and cost-effectiveness of using both 8-hour and 12-hour shifts so that staff could select which type of scheduling they wanted.

● ASSIGNMENT: Would this create a scheduling nightmare? Will you limit the number of 12-hour shifts that staff could work in a week? Would you pay overtime for the last 4 hours of the 12-hour shift? Would you allow staff to choose freely between 8- and 12-hour shifts? What other problems may result from mixing 8- and 12-hour shifts?

Another increasingly common staffing and scheduling alternative is the use of supplemental nursing staff such as *agency nurses* or *travel nurses*. These nurses are usually directly employed by an external nursing broker and work for premium pay (often two to three times that of a regularly employed staff nurse), without benefits. While such staff provide scheduling relief, especially in response to unanticipated increases in census or patient acuity, their continuous use is expensive and can result in poor continuity of nursing care.

Some hospitals have created their own internal supplemental staff by hiring per-diem employees and creating *float pools*. Per-diem staff generally have the flexibility to choose if and when they want to work. In exchange for this flexibility, they receive a higher rate of pay but usually no benefits. Float pools are generally composed of employees who agree to cross train on multiple units so that they can work additional hours during periods of high census or worker shortages. Float pools are adequate for filling intermittent staffing holes but, like agency or registry staff, are not an answer to the ongoing need to alter staffing according to census. In addition, they result in a lack of staff continuity.

Some organizations have made an effort to meet the needs of a diverse workforce by using flextime and self-scheduling. *Flextime* is a system that allows employees to select the time schedules that best meet their personal needs while still meeting work responsibilities. In the past, most flextime has been possible only for nurses in roles that did not require continuous coverage. However, staff nurses recently have been able to take part in a flextime system through prescheduled shift start times. Variable start times may be longer or shorter than the normal 8-hour workday. When a hospital uses flextime, units have employees coming and leaving the unit at many different times. Although flextime staffing creates greater employee choices, it may be difficult for the manager to coordinate and could easily result in overstaffing or understaffing.

Self-scheduling allows nurses in a unit to work together to construct their own schedules rather than have schedules created by management. With self-scheduling, employees typically are given 4- to 6-week schedule worksheets to fill out several weeks in advance of when the schedule is to begin. The nurse–manager then reviews the worksheet to make sure that all guidelines or requirements have been met. Although self-scheduling offers nurses greater control over their work environment, it is not easy to implement. Success depends on the leadership skills of the manager to support the staff and demonstrate patience and perseverance throughout the implementation.

One of the newer methods of reducing staff shortages and also allowing nurses some control over scheduling extra shifts and to reduce mandatory overtime is *shift bidding*. In shift bidding, the organization sets the opening price for a shift. For example, this may be at a higher rate of pay than the hourly wage of some nurses, and nurses may bid down the price in order to be assigned the overtime shift. Generally, the organization will choose the nurse to work the shift who bid lowest, but some organizations may deny bids to nurses who work too much overtime (Huston, 2006b).

Obviously, all scheduling and staffing patterns, from traditional to creative, have shortcomings. Therefore, any changes in current policies should be evaluated carefully as they are implemented. Because all scheduling and staffing patterns have a heavy impact on employees' personal lives, productivity, and budgets, it is wise to have a 6-month trial of new staffing and scheduling changes, with an evaluation at the end of that time to determine the impact on financial costs, retention, productivity, risk management, and employee and patient satisfaction.

LEARNING EXERCISE 17.3

Self-Scheduling Holiday Dilemma

You graduated last year from your nursing program and were excited to obtain the job that you wanted most. The unit where you work has a very progressive supervisor who believes in empowering the nursing staff. Approximately 6 months ago, after considerable instruction, the unit began self-scheduling. You have enjoyed the freedom and control that this has given you over your work hours. There have been some minor difficulties among staff, and occasionally the unit was slightly overstaffed or understaffed. However, overall, the self-scheduling has seemed to work well.

Today (September 15), you come to work on the 3 PM to 11 PM shift after 2 days off and see that the schedule for the upcoming Thanksgiving and Christmas holiday period has been posted, and many of the staff have already scheduled their days on and their days off. When you take a close look, it appears that no one has signed up to work Christmas Eve, Thanksgiving Day, or Christmas Day. You are very concerned, because self-scheduling includes responsibility for adequate coverage. There are still a few nurses, including yourself, who have not added their days to the schedule, but even if all of the remaining nurses work all three holidays, it will provide only scant coverage.

● ASSIGNMENT: What leadership role (if any) should you take in solving this dilemma? Should you ignore the problem and schedule yourself for only one holiday and let your supervisor deal with the issue? Remember, you are a new nurse, both in experience and on this unit. List the options for decision making available to you and, using rationale to support your decision, plan a course of action.

WORKLOAD MEASUREMENT TOOLS

Requirements for staffing are based on whatever standard unit of measurement for productivity is used in a given unit. A formula for calculating nursing care hours per patient-day (NCH/PPD) is reviewed in Figure 17.2. This is the simplest formula in use and continues to be used widely. In this formula, all nursing and ancillary staff are treated equally for determining hours of nursing care, and no differentiation is made for differing acuity levels of patients. These two factors alone may result in an incomplete or even inaccurate picture of nursing care needs, and the use of NCH/PPD as a workload measurement tool may be too restrictive, since it may not represent the reality of today's inpatient care setting, where staffing fluctuates not only among shifts but within shifts as well.

As a result, *patient classification systems* (PCS), also known as workload management, or *patient acuity tools*, were developed in the 1960s. A PCS groups patients according to specific characteristics that measure acuity of illness in an effort to determine both the number and mix of the staff needed to adequately care for those patients. Because other variables within the system have an impact on nursing care hours, it is usually not possible to transfer a PCS from one facility to another. Instead, each basic classification system must be modified to fit a specific institution.

Adomat and Hewison (2004) suggest that most PCSs can be classified as robust measures for severity of illness. However, they maintain that although they are helpful, they are not accurate tools for determining nurse–patient ratios, and that all PCS measurements tools need nursing input if they are to measure nurse–patient needs accurately.

There are several types of PCS measurement tools. The *critical indicator* PCS uses broad indicators such as bathing, diet, intravenous fluids and medications, and positioning to categorize patient care activities. The *summative task* type requires the nurse to note the frequency of occurrence of specific activities, treatments, and procedures for each patient. For example, a summative task–type PCS might ask the nurse whether a patient required nursing time for teaching, elimination, or hygiene. Both types of PCSs are generally filled out prior to each shift, although the summative task type typically has more items to fill out than the critical incident or criterion type.

Once an appropriate PCS is adopted, hours of nursing care must be assigned for each patient classification. Although an appropriate number of hours of care for each classification is generally suggested by companies marketing PCSs, each institution is unique and must determine to what degree that classification system must be adapted for that institution. White (2003) suggests that each patient population is different and that each unit must examine clinical profiles of patients, average length of stay, and practitioner specialty in defining its patient population. In addition, staff competency, core staff versus visiting staff, and skill mix must be considered (White, 2003).

It is a mistake for managers to think that PCSs will solve all staffing problems, as all systems have special features and faults as well. Although such systems provide a better definition of problems, it is up to people in the organization to make judgments and use the information obtained by the system appropriately to solve staffing problems. A sample classification system is illustrated in Table 17.1.

Figure 17.2 Standard formula for calculating nursing care hours (NCH) per patient-day (PPD).

$$\text{NCH/PPD} = \frac{\text{Nursing Hours Worked in 24 Hours}}{\text{Patient Census}}$$

TABLE 17.1 Patient Care Classification Using Four Levels of Nursing Care Intensity

Area of Care	Category 1	Category 2	Category 3	Category 4
Eating	Feeds self or needs little food	Needs some help in preparing food tray; may need encouragement	Cannot feed self but is able to chew and swallow	Cannot feed self and may have difficulty swallowing
Grooming	Almost entirely self-sufficient	Needs some help in bathing, oral hygiene, hair combing, and so forth	Unable to do much for self	Completely dependent
Excretion	Up and to bathroom alone or almost alone	Needs some help in getting up to bathroom or using urinal	In bed, needs bedpan or urinal placed; may be able to partially turn or lift self	Completely dependent
Comfort	Self-sufficient	Needs some help with adjusting position or bed (e.g., tubes, IVs)	Cannot turn without help, get drink, adjust position of extremities, and so forth	Completely dependent
General health	Good—in for diagnostic procedure, simple treatment, or surgical procedure (D & C, biopsy, minor fracture)	Mild symptoms—more than one mild illness, mild debility, mild emotional reaction, mild incontinence (not more than once per shift)	Acute symptoms—severe emotional reaction to illness or surgery, more than one acute illness, medical or surgical problem, severe or frequent incontinence	Critically ill—may have severe emotional reaction
Treatments	Simple—supervised ambulation, dangle, simple dressing, test procedure preparation not requiring medication, reinforcement of surgical dressing, x-pad, vital signs once per shift	Any category 1 treatment more than once per shift, Foley catheter care, I & O; bladder irrigations, sitz bath, compresses, test procedures requiring medications or follow-ups, simple enema for evacuation, vital signs every 4 hours	Any treatment more than twice per shift, medicated IVs, complicated dressings, sterile procedures, care of tracheostomy, Harris flush, suctioning, tube feeding, vital signs more than every 4 hours	Any elaborate or delicate procedure requiring two nurses, vital signs more often than every 2 hours

Area of Care	Category 1	Category 2	Category 3	Category 4
Medications	Simple, routine, not needing pre-evaluation or post evaluation; medications no more than once per shift	Diabetic, cardiac, hypotensive, hypertensive, diuretic, anticoagulant medications, prn medications, more than once per shift, medications needing pre-evaluation or postevaluation	High amount of category 2 medications; control of refractory diabetes (need to be monitored more than every 4 hours)	Extensive category 3 medications; IVs with frequent, close observation and regulation
Teaching and emotional support	Routine follow-up teaching; patients with no unusual or adverse emotional reactions	Initial teaching of care of ostomies; new diabetics; tubes that will be in place for periods of time; conditions requiring major change in eating, living, or excretory practices; patients with mild adverse reactions to their illness (e.g., depression, overly demanding)	More intensive category 2 items; teaching of apprehensive or mildly resistive patients; care of moderately upset or apprehensive patients; confused or disoriented patients	Teaching of resistive patients, care and support of patients with severe emotional reaction

 Any PCS has many variables, and all systems have their faults.

The middle-level manager must be alert to internal or external forces affecting unit needs that may not be reflected in the organization's patient care classification system. Examples of such forces could be a sudden increase in nursing or medical students using the unit, a lower skill level of new graduates, or cultural and language difficulties of recently hired foreign nurses. The organization's classification system may prove to be inaccurate, or the hours allotted for each category or classification of patient may be inadequate. This does not imply that unit managers should not be held accountable for the standard unit of measurement; rather, they must be cognizant of justifiable reasons for variations.

Some futurists have suggested that eventually *workload measurement systems* may replace acuity-based staffing systems. Workload measurement is a relatively new technique that evaluates work performance as well as necessary resource levels (Walsh, 2003). Therefore, it goes beyond patient diagnosis or acuity level and examines the specific number of care hours needed to meet a given population's care needs. Thus, workload measurement systems capture census data, care hours, patient acuity, and patient activities. This tool, while more complicated, holds great promise for better predicting the nursing resources needed to staff hospitals effectively.

Regardless of the workload measurement tool used (NCH/PPD, PCS, workload measurement system, etc.), the units of workload measurement that are used need to be reviewed periodically and adjusted as necessary. This is both a leadership role and a management responsibility.

LEARNING EXERCISE 17.4

Calculating Staffing Needs

You use a PCS to assist you with your daily staffing needs. The following are the hours of nursing care needed for each acuity level patient per shift:

	Category I Acuity Level	Category II Acuity Level	Category III Acuity Level	Category IV Acuity Level
NCH/PPD needed for day shift	2.3	2.9	3.4	4.6
NCH/PPD needed for PM shift	2.0	2.3	2.8	3.4
NCH/PPD needed for night shift	0.5	1.0	2.0	2.8

When you came on duty this morning, you had the following patients:
    1 patient in category I acuity level
    2 patients in category II acuity level
    3 patients in category III acuity level
    1 patient in category IV acuity level
    Note that you must be overstaffed or understaffed by more than half of the hours a person is working to reduce or add staff. For example, for nurses working 8-hour shifts, the staffing must be over or under more than 4 hours to delete or add staff.

● ASSIGNMENT: Calculate your staffing needs for the day shift. You have on duty one RN and one LVN/LPN working 8-hour shifts and a ward clerk for 4 hours. Are you understaffed or overstaffed?

If you had the same number of patients but the acuity levels were the following, would your staffing needs be the same?
    2 patients in category I acuity level
    3 patients in category II acuity level
    2 patients in category III acuity level
    0 patients in category IV acuity level

THE RELATIONSHIP BETWEEN NURSING CARE HOURS, STAFFING MIX, AND QUALITY OF CARE

It is difficult to pick up a nursing journal today that does not have at least one article that speaks to the relationship between nursing care hours, staffing mix, quality of care, and patient outcomes. This has occurred in response to the "restructuring" and "re-engineering" boom that occurred in many acute-care hospitals in the 1990s. Restructuring and re-engineering was done to reduce costs, increase efficiency, decrease waste and duplication, and reshape the way that care was delivered (Huston, 2006c).

Given that health care is labor intensive, cost cutting under restructuring and re-engineering often included staffing models that reduced RN representation in the staffing mix and increased the use of unlicensed assistive personnel (UAP). This fairly rapid and dramatic shift in both RN care hours and staffing mix provided fertile ground for comparative studies that examined the relationship between nursing care hours, staffing mix, and patient outcomes.

Although early research on nursing care hours, staffing mix, and patient outcomes lacked standardization in terms of tools used and measures examined, nationwide attention shifted to this issue and a plethora of better-funded and more-rigorous scientific study followed.

 A current review of the literature consistently and overwhelmingly demonstrates that as RN hours decrease in NCH/PPD, adverse patient outcomes increase, including increased medication errors and patient falls and decreased patient satisfaction with pain management (Seago, Williamson, & Atwood, 2006).

Unit managers must understand the effect that major restructuring and redesign have on their staffing and scheduling policies as well. As new practice models are introduced, there must be a simultaneous examination of the existing staff mix and patient care assessments to ensure that appropriate changes are made in staffing and scheduling policies.

For example, decreasing licensed staff, increasing numbers of UAP, and developing new practice models have a tremendous impact on patient care assignment methods. Past practices of relying on part-time staff, responding to staff preferences for work, and providing a variety of shift lengths and shift rotations may no longer be enough. Administrative practices also have saved money in the past by sending people home when there was low census; they have also floated them to other areas to cover other unit needs, not scheduled staff for consecutive shifts because of staff preferences, and had scheduling polices that were unreasonably accommodating. Finally, often patient assignments in the past were made without attention to patient continuity and were assigned by numbers rather than workload. Some of these past practices benefited staff, and some benefited the organization, but few of them benefited the patient. Indeed, assigning a different nurse to care for a patient each day of an already reduced length of stay may contribute to negative patient outcomes.

Therefore, an honest appraisal of current staffing, scheduling, and assignment policies is needed at the same time that organizations are restructured and new practice models are engineered. Changing these policies often has far-reaching consequences, but this must be done for new models of care to be successfully implemented. For example, if primary nursing is to be effective, then nurses must work a number of successive days with a client to ensure that there is time to formulate and evaluate a plan of care. In this example, floating policies and requests for days off may need to be changed or modified to fit the philosophy of primary nursing care delivery.

Ascertaining an appropriate skill mix depends on the patient care setting, acuity of patients, and other factors. There is no national standard to determine whether staffing decisions are suitable for a given setting. Additionally, many of the tools and methods used to determine staffing have been unreliable and invalid, either in their development or their application. However, some formulas allow for adjustment for variations in the skill mix of staff. These formulas are still relatively new but may be a better tool to use when making staffing decisions. Having an adequate number of knowledgeable, trained nurses is imperative to attaining desired patient outcomes.

Buerhaus and colleagues (2006) maintain that although the present nursing shortage seems to have eased, several factors remain that will affect staffing and the nursing work environment in the coming decade. These factors include an aging workforce and the need for more diversity in nursing in all areas, including age, gender, race, and ethnicity.

GENERATIONAL CONSIDERATIONS FOR STAFFING

Some researchers suggest that the different generations represented in nursing today have different value systems, which may impact staffing (Display 17.3). Hill (2004) describes the *veteran generation* as those nurses born between 1925 and 1942. Having lived through several international military conflicts (World War II, the Korean War, and Vietnam), they are often adverse to risks regarding personal finances; they are respectful of authority, supportive of hierarchy, and disciplined (Hill, 2004). Therefore, these nurses may be less likely to question staffing assignments and may work best in a more structured patient care delivery system. However, most of this generation of workers are either retired or nearing retirement age.

McNeese-Smith and Crook (2003) posit that the *boom generation* (born between 1943 and the early 1960s) and the *silent generation* (born between 1925 and 1942) have more traditional work values and ethics; however, the boomers are more materialistic and are willing to work long hours at their jobs. Hill (2004) points out, however, that many nurses in the boomer group have been taught from a young age to think as individuals and to express themselves creatively. These nurses, then, may be best suited for staffing assignments that require flexibility, independent thinking, and creativity.

DISPLAY 17.3   Generational Work Groups

Generation	Year of Birth
Silent Generation or Veteran Generation	1925 to 1942
Baby Boomer or Boom	1943 to early 1960s
Generation X	Early 1960s to 1980
Generation Y	Late 1970s to 1986

Source: Adapted from Hill, K. S. (2004). Defy the decades with multigenerational teams. *Nursing Management, 35*(1), 32–35; McNeese-Smith, D. K., & Crook, M. (2003). Nursing values and a changing nurse workforce: Values, age, and job stages. *Journal of Nursing Administration, 33*(5), 260–270; Martin, C. A. (2003, April). Transcend generational timelines. *Nursing Management, 34*(4), 25–26, 28.

Generation Xers (born between the early 1960s and 1980), in contrast, may lack the interest in lifetime employment at one place that prior generations have valued. Instead, this generation values the more flexible part-time and 12-hour shift options (McNeese-Smith & Crook, 2003). Hill (2004) argues that this is because family structure changed during this generation's values-formative years. Many were raised as latchkey children because both parents worked outside the home and were disillusioned with the values of corporate America. Thus, members of this generation, while no less interested in success than the workers of generations preceding them, typically choose to define success in their own terms.

Generation Y (born between the late 1970s and 1986) represents the first cohort of truly global citizens. Generation Yer's frequently seek roles that will push their limits (Martin, 2003). They are also optimistic, upbeat, self-confident, volunteer-minded, and socially conscious, all of which have staffing implications. Clearly, the astute leader–manager must be able to assess if and how intergenerational values impact the staffing needs of their units and respond accordingly.

THE IMPACT OF A SHORTAGE OF NURSING STAFF UPON STAFFING

As discussed in Chapter 15, shortages of nurses have always occurred periodically, whether nationally, regionally, or locally. It has been difficult for the profession as a whole to accurately predict exactly when and where there will be a short supply of professional nurses, but all nurse–managers will at some time face a short supply of staff—both RNs and others.

Health care organizations have used many solutions to combat this problem. Such things as advanced planning and recruitment have already been discussed. Another long-term solution to a shortage of staff is *cross-training*. Cross-training involves giving personnel with varying educational backgrounds and expertise the skills necessary to take on tasks normally outside their scope of work and to move between units and function knowledgeably. These are all good solutions for long-term problem solving and show vision on the part of the leader–manager.

However, staffing shortages frequently occur on a day-to-day basis. These occur because of an increase in patient census, an unexpected increase in client needs, or an increase in staff absenteeism or illness. Health care organizations have used many methods to deal with an unexpected short supply of staff. Chief among the solutions are closed-unit staffing, drawing from a central pool of nurses for additional staff, requesting volunteers to work extra duty, and mandatory overtime.

Closed-unit staffing occurs when the staff members on a unit make a commitment to cover all absences and needed extra help themselves in return for not being pulled from the unit in times of low census. In *mandatory overtime*, employees are forced to work additional shifts, often under threat of patient abandonment, should they refuse to do so. Some hospitals routinely use mandatory overtime in an effort to keep fewer people on the payroll.

A health care worker who is in an exhausted state represents a risk to public health and patient safety. In a study by Rogers, Wei-Ting, Scott, Aiken, and Dinges (2004), working overtime increased the odds of nurses making errors (Examining the Evidence 17.1). These findings were reinforced by the Institute of Medicine (IOM) report on patient safety (IOM, 2004). While mandatory overtime is neither efficient nor effective in the long term, it has an even more devastating short-term impact with regard to staff perceptions of a lack of control and its subsequent impact on mood, motivation, and productivity. Nurses who are forced to work overtime do so

EXAMINING THE EVIDENCE 17.1

Source: Rogers, A., Wie-Ting, H., Scott, L. D., Aiken, L. H., & Dinges, D. F. (2004). The working hours of hospital staff nurses and patient safety. *Health Affairs, 23*(4), 202–212.

Logbooks completed by 393 staff showed that working hours of 40% of the participants exceeded 12 hours in a given day. Fourteen percent of the respondents worked at least 16 consecutive hours at least once during the 4-week period studied.

The study found that the risk of making an error greatly increased when nurses had to work shifts that were longer than 12 hours, when they worked significant overtime, or when they worked more than 40 hours per week. Nurses who worked 12.5 hours or longer were three times more likely to make errors than those who worked an 8.5-hour day. Working overtime increased the odds of making at least one error, regardless of how long the shift was originally scheduled.

under the stress of competing duties—to their job, their family, their own health, and their patient's safety (Huston, 2006b). Clearly, mandatory overtime should be a last resort, not standard operating procedure because an institution does not have enough staff.

However, Manthey (2006) suggests that nurses themselves, as well as employing organizations, need to become smarter about workload issues. She maintains that intermittent peak workload issues should not be solved by adding personnel but should be solved by prioritizing what can get done in a shift that will meet patient critical needs and learning what is not critical to be done. Manthey maintains that we should stop the all-or-none thinking that has led nursing staff to feel angry regarding staffing issues.

Regardless of how the manager chooses to deal with an inadequate number of staff, certain criteria must be met:

- Decisions made must meet state and federal labor laws and organizational policies.
- Staff must not be demoralized or excessively fatigued by frequent or extended overtime requests.
- Long-term as well as short-term solutions must be sought.
- Patient care must not be jeopardized.

FISCAL AND ETHICAL ACCOUNTABILITY FOR STAFFING

Regardless of inherent difficulties, PCSs and the assignment of nursing care hours remain a method for controlling the staffing function of management. As long as managers realize that all systems have weaknesses and as long as they periodically evaluate the system, managers will be able to initiate needed change. It is crucial, however, for managers to make every effort to base unit staffing on their organization's PCS. Nursing care remains labor intensive, and the manager is fiscally accountable to the organization for appropriate staffing. Accountability for a prenegotiated budget is a management function.

Growing federal and state budget deficits have resulted in increased pressure for all health care organizations to reduce costs. Because personnel budgets are large in health care organizations, a small percentage cut in personnel may result in large savings. Thus, managers must increase staffing when patient acuity rises as well as decrease staffing when acuity is low; to do otherwise is demoralizing to the unit staff. It is important for managers to use staff to provide safe and effective care economically.

Fiscal accountability to the organization for staffing is not incompatible with ethical accountability to patients and staff. The manager's goal is to stay within a staffing budget *and* meet the needs of patients and staff.

Some organizations require only that managers end the fiscal year within their budgeted nursing care hours and pay less attention to daily or weekly nursing care hours. Shift staffing based on a patient acuity system does, however, allow for more consistent staffing and is better able to identify overstaffing and understaffing on a more timely basis. In addition, this is a fairer method of allocating staff.

The disadvantage of shift-based staffing is that it is time-consuming and somewhat subjective, because acuity or classification systems leave much to be determined by the person assigning the acuity levels. The greater the degree of objectivity and accuracy in any system, the longer the time required to make staffing computations. Perhaps the greatest danger in staffing by acuity is that many organizations are unable to supply the extra staff when the system shows unit understaffing. However, the same organization may use the acuity-based staffing system to justify reducing staff on an overstaffed unit. Therefore, a staffing classification system can be demotivating if used inconsistently or incorrectly.

Employees have the right to expect a reasonable workload. Managers must ensure that adequate staffing exists to meet the needs of staff and patients. Managers who constantly expect employees to work extra shifts, stay overtime, and carry unreasonable patient assignments are not being ethically accountable.

Effective managers, however, do not focus totally on numbers of personnel but look at all components of productivity. They examine nursing duties, job descriptions, patient care organization, staffing mix, and staff competencies. Such managers also use every opportunity to build a productive and cohesive team.

Uncomplaining nursing staff have often put forth superhuman efforts during periods of short staffing simply because they believed in their supervisor and in the organization. However, just as often, the opposite has occurred: Nurses on units that were only moderately understaffed spent an inordinate amount of time and wasted energy complaining about their plight. The difference between the two examples has much to do with trust that such conditions are the exception, not the norm; that real solutions and not Band-Aid approaches to problem solving will be used to plan for the future; that management will work just as hard as the staff in meeting patient needs; and that the organization's overriding philosophy is based on patient interest and not financial gain.

DEVELOPING STAFFING AND SCHEDULING POLICIES

Nurses will be more satisfied in the workplace if staffing and scheduling policies and procedures are clearly communicated to all employees. Written policies provide a means for greater consistency and fairness. Personnel policies represent the standard of action that is communicated in advance so that employees are not caught unaware regarding personnel matters. In addition to being standardized, personnel policies should be written in a manner that allows some flexibility. A leadership challenge for the manager is to develop policies that focus on outcomes rather than constraints or rules that limit responsiveness to individual employee needs.

Scheduling and staffing policies should be reviewed and updated periodically. When formulating policies, management must examine its own philosophy and consider prevailing community practices. Unit-level managers will seldom have complete responsibility for formulating organizational personnel policies but should have some input as policies are reviewed. There are, however, nursing department and unit personnel policies that supervisors develop and implement.

The policies in Display 17.4 should be formalized by the manager and communicated to all personnel. To ensure that unit-level staffing policies do not conflict with higher-level policies, there should be adequate input from the staff, and they should be developed in collaboration with personnel and nursing departments. For example, some states have labor laws that prohibit 12-hour shifts. Other states allow workers to sign away their rights to overtime pay for shifts greater than 8 or 12 hours. Additionally, in organizations with union contracts, many staffing and scheduling policies are incorporated into the union contract. In such cases, staffing changes might need to be negotiated at the time of contract renewal.

DISPLAY 17.4   Unit Checklist of Employee Staffing Policies

1. Name of the person responsible for the staffing schedule and the authority of that individual if it is other than the employee's immediate supervisor
2. Type and length of staffing cycle used
3. Rotation policies, if shift rotation is used
4. Fixed shift transfer policies, if fixed shifts are used
5. Time and location of schedule posting
6. When shift begins and ends
7. Day of week schedule begins
8. Weekend off policy
9. Tardiness policy
10. Low census procedures
11. Policy for trading days off
12. Procedures for days-off requests
13. Absenteeism policies
14. Policy regarding rotating to other units
15. Procedures for vacation time requests
16. Procedures for holiday time requests
17. Procedures for resolving conflicts regarding requests for days off, holidays, or requested time off
18. Emergency request policies
19. Policies and procedures regarding requesting transfer to other units
20. Mandatory overtime policy

INTEGRATING LEADERSHIP ROLES AND MANAGEMENT FUNCTIONS IN STAFFING AND SCHEDULING

The manager is responsible for providing adequate staffing to meet patient care needs. Attention must be paid to fluctuations in patient census and workload units to ensure that understaffing or overstaffing is minimized and to ensure fiscal accountability to the organization. The prudent manager involves employees when developing unit staffing and scheduling policies and ascertains that adopted policies are not in violation of organizational policies, union contracts, or labor laws.

When leadership roles are integrated with management functions, creative staffing and scheduling options can occur. Knowing that staff needs are in part related to work design, the prudent leader–manager looks for ways to redesign work to reduce staffing needs.

The leader keeps abreast of changes in community and national trends and uses contemporary methods of staffing and scheduling. The leader also assumes an ethical accountability to patients and employees for adequate and appropriate staffing. Unit policies are reviewed and revised on a timely basis. Additionally, the leader is alert for factors that affect the standard of productivity and negotiates changes in the standard when appropriate.

The effective leader–manager knows that establishing trust helps to build the team spirit needed to deal with temporary staff shortages. The leader also looks for innovative methods to overcome staffing difficulties.

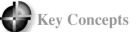 Key Concepts

- The manager has both a fiscal and ethical duty to plan for adequate staffing to meet patient care needs.
- Innovative and creative methods of staffing and scheduling should be explored to avoid understaffing and overstaffing as patient census and acuity fluctuate.
- Staffing and scheduling policies must not violate labor laws, state or national laws, or union contracts.
- Workload measurement tools include *NCH/PPD, PCS,* and *workload measurement systems.* All workload measurement tools should be periodically reviewed to determine if they are a valid and reliable tool for measuring staffing needs in a given organization.
- *Mandatory overtime* should be a last resort, not standard operating procedure because an institution does not have enough staff.
- Research clearly shows that as RN representation in the *skill mix* increases, patient outcomes improve and adverse incidents decline.
- Those with staffing responsibility must remain cognizant of *mandatory staffing ratios* and comply with such mandates.
- Managers should attempt to have a diverse staff that will meet the cultural and language needs of the patient population.
- Fair and uniform staffing and scheduling policies and procedures must be written and communicated to all staff.
- Existing staffing policies must be examined periodically to determine if they still meet the needs of the staff and the organization.

ADDITIONAL LEARNING EXERCISES AND APPLICATIONS

LEARNING EXERCISE 17.5

Implementing a New Nursing Care Delivery Model

You are serving on an ad hoc committee to examine ways to improve the continuity of patient assignments because your unit is thinking about switching from total patient care to a primary nursing care delivery model. The committee is having a difficult time formulating policies because you currently have a great number of nurses who work part-time, 2 days on and 2 days off. Additionally, your unit has a census that goes up and down unexpectedly, resulting in nurses being floated out of the unit often. The committee is committed to providing continuity of care in the new patient care delivery system.

● ASSIGNMENT: Develop some scheduling and staffing policies that have the probability of increasing continuity of assignment and will not result in a financial liability to the unit. How will these polices be fairly executed, and do they have the potential to cause staff to leave the unit?

LEARNING EXERCISE 17.6

Making Sound Staffing Decisions

You are the staffing coordinator for a small community hospital. It is now 12:30 PM, and your staffing plan for the 3 to 11 PM shift must be completed no later than 1 PM. (The union contract stipulates that any "call offs" that must be done for low census must be done at least 2 hours before the shift begins; otherwise, employees will receive a minimum of 4 hours of pay.) You do, however, have the prerogative to call off staff for only half a shift (4 hours). If they are needed for the last half of the shift (7 to 11 PM), you must notify them by 5 PM tonight. A local outside registry is available for supplemental staff; however, their cost is two and a half times that of your regular staff, so you must use this resource sparingly. Mandatory overtime is also used but only as a last resort.

The current hospital census is 52 patients, although the emergency department (ED) is very busy and has four possible patient admissions. There are also two patients with confirmed discharge orders and three additional potential discharges on the 3 to 11 PM shift. All units have just submitted their PCS calculations for that shift.

You have five units to staff: the ICU, pediatrics, obstetrics (includes labor, delivery, and postpartum), medical, and surgical departments. The ICU must be staffed with a minimum of a 1:2 nurse–patient ratio. The pediatric unit is generally staffed at a 1:4 nurse–patient ratio and the medical and surgical departments at a 1:6 ratio. In obstetrics, a 1:2 ratio is used for labor and delivery, and a 1:6 ratio is used in postpartum. On reviewing the staffing, you note the following:

ICU

Census = 6. Unit capacity = 8. The PCS shows a current patient acuity level requiring 3.2 staff. One of the potential admissions in the ED is a patient who will need cardiac monitoring. One patient, however, will likely be transferred to the medical unit on 3 to 11 PM shift. Four RNs are assigned for that shift.

Pediatrics

Census = 8. Unit capacity = 10. The PCS shows a current acuity level requiring 2.4 staff. There are two RNs and one CNA assigned for the 3 to 11 PM shift. There are no anticipated discharges or transfers.

Obstetrics

Census = 6. Unit capacity = 8. Three women are in active labor, and three women are in the postpartum unit with their babies. Two RNs are assigned to the obstetrics department for the 3 to 11 PM shift. There are no in-house staff on that shift who have been cross trained for this unit.

Medical Floor

Census = 19. Unit capacity = 24. The PCS shows a current acuity level requiring 4.4 staff. There are two RNs, one LVN, and two CNA assigned for the 3 to 11 PM shift. Three of the potential ED admissions will come to this floor. Two of the potential patient discharges are on this unit.

Surgical Floor

Census = 13. Unit capacity = 18. The PCS shows a current acuity level requiring 3.6 staff. Because of sick calls, you have only one RN and two CNAs assigned for the 3 to 11 PM shift. Both confirmed patient discharges as well as one of the potential discharges are from this unit.

● ASSIGNMENT: Answer the following questions:
  1. Which units are overstaffed, and which are understaffed?
  2. Of those units that are overstaffed, what will you do with the unneeded staff?
  3. How will you staff units that are understaffed? Will outside registry or mandatory overtime methods be used?
  4. How did staffing mix and PCS acuity levels factor into your decisions, if at all?
  5. What safeguards can you build into the staffing plan for unanticipated admissions or changes in patient acuity during the shift?

LEARNING EXERCISE 17.7

Reviewing Pros and Cons of Staffing Solutions

You are serving on a committee to help resolve a chronic problem with short staffing on your unit, which is a pediatric ICU. Volunteer overtime, cross training with the regular non-intensive care pediatric unit, and closed-unit staffing have been suggested as possible solutions.

● ASSIGNMENT: Make a list of the pros and cons of each of these suggestions to bring back to the committee for review. Share your list with group members.

LEARNING EXERCISE 17.8

Choosing a Delivery Care Model and Staffing Pattern

You have been hired as the unit supervisor of the new rehabilitation unit at Memorial Hospital. The hospital decentralizes the responsibility for staffing, but you must adhere to the following constraints:
  1. All staff must be licensed.
  2. The ratio of LVNs/LPNs to RNs is 1:1.

(Learning Exercise continues on page 418)

3. An RN must always be on duty.
4. Your budgeted NCH/PPD is 8.2.
5. You are not counted into the NCH/PPD, but ward clerks are counted.
6. Your unit capacity is seven patients, and you anticipate a daily average census of six patients.
7. You may use any mode of patient care organization.

Your patients will be chronic, not acute, but will be admitted for an active 2- to 12-week rehabilitation program. The emphasis will be in returning the patient home with adequate ability to perform activities of daily living. Many other disciplines, including occupational and physical therapy, will be part of the rehabilitation team. A waiting list for the beds is anticipated because this service is needed in your community. You anticipate that most of your patients will have had cerebrovascular accidents, spinal cord injuries, other problems with neurologic deficits, and amputations.

You have hired four full-time RNs and two part-time RNs. The part-time RNs would like to have at least 2 days of work in a 2-week pay period; in return for this work guarantee, they have agreed to cover for most sick days and vacations and some holidays for your regular RN full-time staff.

You also have hired three full-time LVNs/LPNs and two part-time LVNs/LPNs. However, the part-time LVNs/LPNs would like to work at least 3 days per week. You have decided not to hire a ward clerk but to use the pediatric ward clerk for 4 hours each day to assist with various duties. Therefore, you need to calculate the ward clerk's 4 hours into the total hours worked.

You have researched various types of patient care delivery models (Chapter 14) and staffing patterns. Your newly hired staff is willing to experiment with any type of patient care delivery model and staffing pattern that you select.

● ASSIGNMENT: Determine which patient care delivery model and staffing pattern you will use. Explain why and how you made the choice your choice. Next, show a 24-hour and 7-day staffing pattern. Were you able to create a schedule that adhered to the given constraints? Was this a time-consuming process?

Web Links

California Nurses Association Position Statement on RN Staffing Ratio
http://www.calnurses.org/nursing-practice
Argues in support of CA AB 394 and differentiates between scope of practice of RNs and LVNs in staffing ratios.

American Nurses Association—Background Information and Legislative Maps, Nurse Staffing Plans and Ratios
http://www.nursingworld.org/SpecialPages/Search.aspx?SearchPhrase=Staffing+ratios
Addresses need for nurse staffing ratios.

National Academies Press
http://www.nap.edu/books/0309053986/html/241.html
Information regarding the congressionally mandated study of the adequacy of nurse staffing in hospitals and nursing facilities by the Institute of Medicine, entitled. Nursing Staff in Hospitals and Nursing Homes: Is It Adequate? (1996).

References

Adomat, R., & Hewison, A. (2004). Assessing patient category/dependence systems for determining the nurse/patient ration in ICU and HDU: A review of approaches. *Journal of Nursing Management, 12*(5), 299–308.

Buerhaus, P. I., Donelan, K., Ulrich, B. T., Norman, L., & Dittus, R. (2006). State of the registered nurse workforce in the United States. *Nursing Economics, 24*(1), 6–12.

California Nurses Association. (2003). RN staffing ratios: It's the law. Retrieved November 26, 2003, from *http://www.calnurse.org/nursing-practice.*

Department of Health and Human Services (DHHS) Office of Minority Health. (2007). National standards for providing culturally and linguistically appropriate services (CLAS) in health care. Retrieved September 14, 2007, from *http://www.omhrc.gov/templates/browse.aspx?lvl=28lvlid=15.*

Graf, C. M., Millar, S., Feilteau, C., Coakley, P. J., & Erickson, J. I. (2003). Patients' needs for nursing care. *Journal of Nursing Administration, 33*(2), 76–81.

Hill, K. S. (2004). Defy the decades with multigenerational teams. *Nursing Management, 35*(1), 32–35.

Huston, C. (2006a). Mandatory staffing ratios: Are they working? In C. Huston (Ed.), *Professional issues in nursing.* Philadelphia: Lippincott Williams & Wilkins.

Huston, C. (2006b). Mandatory overtime in nursing: How much? How often? In C. Huston (Ed.), *Professional issues in nursing.* Philadelphia: Lippincott Williams & Wilkins.

Huston, C. (2006c). Unlicensed assistive personnel and the registered nurse. In C. Huston (Ed.), *Professional issues in nursing.* Philadelphia: Lippincott Williams & Wilkins.

Institute of Medicine. (2004). *Keeping patients safe: Transforming the work environment for nurses.* Washington, DC: National Academic Press.

Leighty, J. (2004). Unchartered waters. *Nurseweek, 17*(5), 14–16.

Malloch, K., Davenport, S., & Hatler, C. (2003). Nursing workforce management. Using benchmarking for planning and outcomes monitoring. *Journal of Nursing Administration, 33*(10), 538–543.

Manthey, M. (2006). *Getting smart about workload issues.* Marie Manthey's nursing salon. Retrieved January 3, 2007, from *http://radio.weblogs.com/0149034/.*

Martin, C. A. (2003). Transcend generational timelines. *Nursing Management, 34*(4), 25–26, 28.

McNeese-Smith, D. K., & Crook, M. (2003). Nursing values and a changing nurse workforce: Values, age, and job stages. *Journal of Nursing Administration, 33*(5), 260–270.

Rogers, A., Wie-Ting, H., Scott, L. D., Aiken, L. H., & Dinges, D. F. (2004). The working hours of hospital staff nurses and patient safety. *Health Affairs, 23*(4), 202–212.

Seago, J. A., Williamson, A., & Atwood, C. (2006). Longitudinal analyses of nurse staffing and patient outcomes: More about failure to rescue. *Journal of Nursing Administration, 36*(1), 13–21.

Trinkoff, A., Geiger-Brown, J., Brady, B., Lipscomb, J., & Muntaner, C. (2006). How long and how much are nurses now working? Too long, too much and without enough rest between shifts, a study finds. *American Journal of Nursing, 106*(4), 60–72.

Walsh, E. (2003). Get real with workload measurement. *Nursing Management, 34*(2), 38–42.

White, K. (2003). Effective staffing as a guardian of care. *Nursing Management, 34*(7), 20–24.

Bibliography

Choi, J., Bakken, S., Larson, E., Du, Y., & Stone, P. W. (2004). Perceived nursing work environment of critical care nurses. *Nursing Research, 53*(6), 370–378.

Ericksen, A. B. (2005). Foreign nurses: A viable alternative? Evaluating immigration issues when importing care. *Health care Staffing and Management Solutions, 3*(1), 5.

Gran-Moravec, M. B., & Hughes, C. M. (2005). Nursing time allocation and other considerations for staffing. *Nursing and Health Sciences, 7*(2), 126–133.

Harrington, C. (2005). Nursing counts. Addressing the dramatic decline in RN staffing in nursing homes. *American Journal of Nursing, 105*(9), 25.

Hogle, W. P. (2004). Disturbing statistics reported for patients admitted to hospitals on weekends. *Clinical Journal of Oncology Nursing, 8*(6), 587.

Lake, E. T., & Friese, C. R. (2005). Variations in nursing practice environments: Relation to staffing and hospital characteristics. *Nursing Research, 55*(1), 1–9.

Malloch, K. Staffing ratios and patient classification systems: Mutually exclusive in a rational world. *Arizona Nurse, 57*(5), 7.

Maxwell, M. (2004). HR help for religious holiday scheduling, behavior issues, and turnover. *Nursing Economic$, 22*(1), 39–40.

McGillis, L., Doran, D., & Pink, G. H. (2004). Nurse staffing models, nursing hours, and patient safety outcomes. *Journal of Nursing Administration, 34*(1), 41–45.

Moore, M., & Hastings, C. (2006). The evolution of an ambulatory nursing intensity system: Measuring workload in a day hospital setting. *Journal of Nursing Administration, 36*(5), 241–248.

Scott, L. D., Rogers, A. E., Hwang, W., & Zhang, Y. (2006). Effects of critical care nurses' work hours on vigilance and patients' safety. *American Journal of Critical Care, 15*(1), 30–37.

Spetz, J. (2005). Public policy and nurse staffing: What approach is best? *Journal of Nursing Administration, 35*(1), 14–16.

Ward, C. W. (2005). Ethics, law and policy. Registered Nurse Safe Staffing Act of 2005: Part 1. *MEDSURG Nursing, 14*(5), 338–340.

Welton, J. M., Unruh, L., & Halloran, E. J. (2006). Nurse staffing, nursing intensity, staff mix, and direct nursing care costs across Massachusetts hospitals. *Journal of Nursing Administration, 36*(9), 416–425.

18

Creating a Motivating Climate

. . . how we feel about and enjoy our work is crucial to how we perceive the quality of our lives.

—*Jo Manion*

. . . whether you think you can or whether you think you can't, you're right.

—*Henry Ford*

This unit reviews the fourth phase of the management process: *directing*. This phase also may be referred to as *coordinating* or *activating*. Regardless of the nomenclature, this is the "doing" phase of management, requiring the leadership and management skills necessary to accomplish the goals of the organization. Managers direct the work of their subordinates during this phase. Components of the directing phase discussed in this unit include creating a motivating climate, establishing organizational communication, managing conflict, facilitating collaboration, negotiating, and understanding the impact of collective bargaining and employment laws on management.

In planning and organizing, managers attempt to establish an environment that is conducive to getting work done. In directing, the manager sets those plans into action. This chapter focuses on creating a motivating climate as a critical element in meeting employee and organizational goals.

The amount and quality of work accomplished by managers directly reflect their motivation and that of their subordinates. Why are some managers or employees more motivated than others? How do demotivated managers affect their subordinates? What can the manager do to help the employee who is demotivated? The motivational problems frequently encountered by the manager are complex. To respond to demotivated staff, managers need an understanding of the relationship between motivation and behavior.

Motivation is the force within the individual that influences or directs behavior. Because motivation comes from within the person, managers cannot directly motivate subordinates. The humanistic manager can, however, create an environment that maximizes the development of human potential. Management support, collegial influence, and the interaction of personalities in the work group can have a synergistic effect on motivation. The leader–manager must identify those components and strengthen them in hopes of maximizing motivation at the unit level.

All human beings have needs that motivate them. The leader focuses on the needs and wants of individual workers and uses motivational strategies appropriate for each person and situation. McConnell (2005) states that "there is no better or more useful knowledge for the manager to possess than to know the employees as individuals and know what is important to each of them" (p. 291). Leaders should apply techniques, skills, and knowledge of motivational theory to help nurses achieve what they want out of work. At the same time, these individual goals should complement the goals of the organization. The manager bears primary responsibility for meeting organizational goals, such as reaching acceptable levels of productivity and quality.

The leader–manager, then, must create a work environment in which both organizational and individual needs can be met. Adequate tension must be created to maintain productivity while encouraging subordinates' job satisfaction. Thus, while the worker is achieving personal goals, organizational goals are being met. The leadership roles and management functions inherent in creating such an environment are included in Display 18.1.

This chapter examines motivational theories that have guided organizational efforts and resource distribution for the last 80 years. Special attention is given to the concepts of intrinsic versus extrinsic motivation and organizational motivation versus self-motivation.

INTRINSIC VERSUS EXTRINSIC MOTIVATION

Motivation involves the action people take to satisfy unmet needs. It is the willingness to put effort into achieving a goal or reward to decrease the tension caused by the need. *Intrinsic motivation* comes from within the person, driving him or her to be productive. To be intrinsically motivated at work, the worker must value job performance and productivity.

Parents and peers play major roles in shaping a person's values about what he or she wants to do and be. Parents who set high but attainable expectations for their children, and who constantly encourage them in a nonauthoritative environment, tend to impart strong achievement drives in their children. Cultural background also has an impact on intrinsic motivation; some cultures value career mobility, job success, and recognition more than others.

Rewards resulting from *extrinsic motivation* (which is motivation that is enhanced by the work evironment) occur after the work has been completed. Although all people are intrinsically motivated to some degree, it is unrealistic for the organization to assume that all workers have adequate levels of intrinsic motivation to meet organizational goals. Thus, the organization must provide a climate that stimulates both extrinsic and intrinsic drives.

 The intrinsic motivation to achieve is directly related to a person's level of aspiration. Extrinsic motivation is motivation enhanced by the job environment or external rewards.

DISPLAY 18.1 Leadership Roles and Management Functions Associated With Creating a Motivating Work Climate

Leadership Roles

1. Recognizes each worker as a unique individual who is motivated by different things
2. Identifies the individual and collective value system of the unit and implements a reward system that is consistent with those values
3. Listens attentively to individual and collective work values and attitudes to identify unmet needs that can cause dissatisfaction
4. Encourages workers to "stretch" themselves in an effort to promote self-growth and self-actualization
5. Maintains a positive and enthusiastic image as a role model to subordinates in the clinical setting
6. Encourages mentoring, sponsorship, and coaching with subordinates
7. Devotes time and energy to create an environment that is supportive and encouraging to the discouraged individual
8. Develops a unit philosophy that recognizes the unique worth of each employee and promotes reward systems that make each employee feel like a winner
9. Demonstrates through actions and words a belief in subordinates that they desire to meet organizational goals
10. Is self-aware regarding own enthusiasm for work and takes steps to remotivate self as necessary

Management Functions

1. Uses legitimate authority to provide formal reward systems
2. Uses positive feedback to reward the individual employee
3. Develops unit goals that integrate organizational and subordinate needs
4. Maintains a unit environment that eliminates or reduces job dissatisfiers
5. Promotes a unit environment that focuses on employee motivators
6. Creates the tension necessary to maintain productivity while encouraging subordinate job satisfaction
7. Clearly communicates expectations to subordinates
8. Demonstrates and communicates sincere respect, concern, trust, and a sense of belonging to subordinates
9. Assigns work duties commensurate with employee abilities and past performance to foster a sense of accomplishment in subordinates
10. Identifies achievement, affiliation, or power needs of subordinates and develops appropriate motivational strategies to meet those needs

LEARNING EXERCISE 18.1

Thinking About Motivation

Think back to when you were a child. What rewards did your parents use to promote good behavior? Was your behavior more intrinsically or extrinsically motivated? Were strong achievement drives encouraged and supported by your family? If you have children, what rewards do you use to influence their behavior? Are they the same rewards that your parents used? Why or why not?

Because people have constant needs and wants, they are always motivated to some extent. In addition, because all human beings are unique and have different needs, they are motivated differently. The difference in motivation can be explained in part by our large- and small-group cultures. For example, because American culture values material goods and possessions more highly than many other cultures, rewards in this country are frequently tied to those values.

 Because motivation is so complex, the leader faces tremendous challenges in accurately identifying individual and collective motivators.

Organizations also have cultures and values. Motivators vary among organizations as well as among units in organizations. Even in similar or nearly identical work environments, large variations in individual and group motivation often exist. Much research has been undertaken by behavioral, psychological, and social scientists to develop theories and concepts of motivation. Economists and engineers have focused on extrinsic fiscal rewards to improve performance and productivity, whereas human relations scientists have stressed intrinsic needs for recognition, self-esteem, and self-actualization. To better understand the current view that both extrinsic and intrinsic rewards are necessary for high productivity and worker satisfaction, one needs to look at how motivational theory has evolved over time.

MOTIVATIONAL THEORY

Chapter 2 introduced traditional management philosophy, which emphasizes paternalism, worker subordination, and bureaucracy as a means to predictable but moderate productivity. In this philosophy, high productivity means greater monetary incentives for the worker, and workers are viewed as being motivated primarily by economic factors. This traditional management philosophy is still in use today. Many factory and assembly-line production jobs as well as jobs that use production incentive pay are based on these principles. The shift from traditional management philosophy to a greater focus on the human element and worker satisfaction as factors in productivity began during the human relations era (1930–1970). The best-known human motivation studies in this era were the Hawthorne studies conducted by Elton Mayo (1953).

Maslow

Continued focus on human motivation did not occur until Abraham Maslow's work in the 1950s. Most nurses are familiar with Maslow's *hierarchy of needs* and theory of human motivation. Maslow (1970) believed that people are motivated to satisfy certain needs, ranging from basic survival to complex psychological needs, and that people seek a higher need only when the lower needs have been predominantly met. Maslow's hierarchy of needs is depicted in Figure 18.1.

Although Maslow's work helps to explain personal motivation, his early work, unfortunately, was not applied to motivation in the workplace. His later work, however, offers much insight into motivation and worker dissatisfaction. In the workplace, Maslow's work contributed to the recognition that people are motivated by many needs other than economic security.

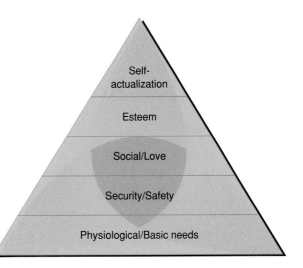

Figure 18.1   Maslow's hierarchy of needs.

 Because of Maslow's work, managers began to realize that people are complex beings, not solely economic animals, and that they have many needs motivating them at any one time.

It also became clear that motivation is internalized and that if productivity is to increase, management must help employees meet lower-level needs. The shifting focus on what motivates employees has tremendously affected how organizations value workers today.

Skinner

B. F. Skinner was another theorist in this era who contributed to the understanding of motivation, dissatisfaction, and productivity. Skinner's (1953) research on *operant conditioning* and *behavior modification* demonstrated that people could be conditioned to behave in a certain way based on a consistent reward or punishment system. Behavior that is rewarded will be repeated, and behavior that is punished or goes unrewarded is extinguished. Skinner's work continues to be reflected today in the way many managers view and use discipline and rewards in the work setting.

Herzberg

Frederick Herzberg (1977) believed that employees can be motivated by the work itself and that there is an internal or personal need to meet organizational goals. He believed that separating personal motivators from job dissatisfiers was possible. This distinction between *hygiene* or *maintenance factors* and *motivator factors* was called the Motivation–Hygiene theory or Two Factor theory. Display 18.2 lists motivator and hygiene factors identified by Herzberg.

Herzberg maintained that motivators or job satisfiers are present in work itself; they give people the desire to work and to do that work well. Hygiene or maintenance factors keep employees from being dissatisfied or demotivated but do not act as real motivators. It is important to remember that the opposite of dissatisfaction may not be satisfaction. When hygiene factors are met, there is a lack of dissatisfaction, not an existence of satisfaction. Likewise, the absence of motivators does not necessarily cause dissatisfaction.

DISPLAY 18.2   Herzberg's Motivators and Hygiene Factors

Motivators	Hygiene Factors
Achievement	Salary
Recognition	Supervision
Work	Job security
Responsibility	Positive working conditions
Advancement	Personal life
Possibility for growth	Interpersonal relationships and peers
	Company policy
	Status

For example, salary is a hygiene factor. Although it does not motivate in itself, when used with other motivators such as recognition or advancement, it can be a powerful motivator. If, however, salary is deficient, employee dissatisfaction can result. Some argue that money can truly be a motivator, as evidenced by people who work insufferable hours at jobs they truly do not enjoy. Some theorists would argue that money in this case might be taking the place of some other unconscious need.

Some people in Herzberg's studies, however, did report job satisfaction solely from hygiene or maintenance factors. Herzberg asserts that these people are only temporarily satisfied when hygiene factors are improved, show little interest in the kind and quality of their work, experience little satisfaction from accomplishments, and tend to show chronic dissatisfaction with other hygiene factors such as salary, status, and job security.

Herzberg's work suggests that although the organization must build on hygiene or maintenance factors, the motivating climate must actively include the employee. The worker must be given greater responsibilities, challenges, and recognition for work well done. The reward system must meet both motivation and hygiene needs, and the emphasis given by the manager should vary with the situation and employee involved. Although hygiene factors in themselves do not motivate, they are needed to create an environment that encourages the worker to move on to higher-level needs. Hygiene factors also combat employee dissatisfaction and are useful in recruiting an adequate personnel pool. Vaughn's (2003) study showed that among the numerous retention factors suggested by Herzberg's Two Factor theory, nurses most desired a sense of recognition and achievement.

Vroom

Victor Vroom (1964), another motivational theorist in the human relations era, developed an *expectancy model*, which looks at motivation in terms of the person's valence, or preferences based on social values. In contrast to *operant conditioning*, which focuses on observable behaviors, the expectancy model says that a person's expectations about his or her environment or a certain event will influence behavior. In other words, people look at all actions as having a cause and effect; the effect may be immediate or delayed, but a reward inherent in the behavior exists to motivate risk taking. In Vroom's expectancy model (Figure 18.2), people make conscious decisions in anticipation of reward; in operant conditioning, people react in a stimulus–response mode. Managers using the expectancy model must become personally involved with their employees to understand better the employees' values, reward systems, strengths, and willingness to take risks.

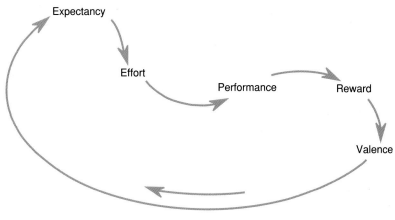

Figure 18.2 Vroom's expectancy model.

McClelland

David McClelland (1971) examined what motives guide a person to action, stating that people are motivated by three basic needs: achievement, affiliation, and power. *Achievement-oriented* people actively focus on improving what is; they transform ideas into action, judiciously and wisely, taking risks when necessary. In contrast, *affiliation-oriented* people focus their energies on families and friends; their overt productivity is less because they view their contribution to society in a different light from those who are achievement oriented. Research shows that women generally have greater affiliation needs than men and that nurses generally have high affiliation needs. *Power-oriented* people are motivated by the power that can be gained as a result of a specific action. They want to command attention, get recognition, and control others. McClelland theorizes that managers can identify achievement, affiliation, or power needs of their employees and develop appropriate motivational strategies to meet those needs.

LEARNING EXERCISE 18.2

Identifying Goals and Motivation
List six goals that you hope to accomplish in the next 5 years. Identify which goals are most related to achievement needs, affiliation needs, and power needs. Remember that most people are motivated in part by all three needs, and no one motivational need is better than the others. However, each person must recognize and understand which basic needs motivate him or her most.

Gellerman

Saul Gellerman (1968), another humanistic motivational theorist, has identified several methods to motivate people positively. One such method, *stretching*, involves assigning tasks that are more difficult than what the person is used to doing. Stretching should not, however, be a routine or daily activity but an activity used to help the employee grow. Martin (2005) maintains that the manager's role should be "I'm not out to get you. I'm out to make you better" (p. 42).

EXAMINING THE EVIDENCE 18.1

Source: Mrayyan, M. T. (2004). Nurses autonomy: Influence of nurse manager's actions. *Journal of Advanced Nursing, 45*(3), 326–336.

The aim of this study was to examine the role that nurse–managers have in enhancing staff autonomy. The study used a comparative descriptive survey design. Of the 317 hospital nurses participating, 264 were from the United States. Three important variables that were reported by nurses to increase autonomy were (a) supportive management, (b) education, and (c) experience. The three most important factors decreasing autonomy were (a) autocratic management, (b) doctors, and (c) workload. The conclusions of the study were that nurses have moderate autonomy that could be increased by effective support form nurse–managers.

> The challenge of "stretching" is to energize people to enjoy the beauty of pushing themselves beyond what they think they can do.

Another method, *participation*, entails actively drawing employees into decisions affecting their work. Gellerman strongly believed that motivation problems usually stem from the way the organization manages and not from the staff's unwillingness to work hard. According to Gellerman, most managers "overmanage"—they make the employee's job too narrow and fail to give the employee any decision-making power. Indeed, nursing autonomy in decision making was shown to be only moderate in a study of 317 nurses by Mrayyan (2004), who concluded that autonomy could be increased by effective management support (Examining the Evidence 18.1).

McGregor

Douglas McGregor (1960) examined the importance of a manager's assumptions about workers on the intrinsic motivation of the workers. These assumptions, which McGregor labeled *Theory X* and *Theory Y* (depicted in Display 18.3), led to the realization in management science that how the manager views, and thus treats, the worker will have an impact on how well the organization functions.

DISPLAY 18.3 McGregor's Theory X and Theory Y

Theory X Employees	Theory Y Employees
Avoid work if possible	Like and enjoy work
Dislike work	Are self-directed
Must be directed	Seek responsibility
Have little ambition	Are imaginative and creative
Avoid responsibility	Have underutilized intellectual capacity
Need threats to be motivated	Need only general supervision
Need close supervision	Are encouraged to participate in problem
Are motivated by rewards and punishment	solving

McGregor did not consider Theory X and Theory Y as opposite points on the spectrum but rather as two points on a continuum extending through all perspectives of people. McGregor believed that people should not be artificially classified as always having Theory X or Theory Y assumptions about others; instead, most people belong on some point on the continuum. Likewise, McGregor did not promote either Theory X or Theory Y as being the one superior management style, although many managers have interpreted Theory Y as being the ultimate management model. No one style is effective in all situations, at all times, and with all people. McGregor, without making value judgments, simply stated that in any situation, the manager's assumptions about people, whether grounded in fact or not, affect motivation and productivity.

The work of all these theorists has added greatly to the understanding of what motivates people in and out of the work setting. Research reveals that motivation is extremely complex and that there is tremendous variation in what motivates different people. Therefore, managers must understand what can be done at the unit level to create a climate that allows the worker to grow, increases motivation and productivity, and eliminates dissatisfiers that drain energy and promote frustration.

CREATING A MOTIVATING CLIMATE

Because the organization has such an impact on extrinsic motivation, it is important to examine organizational climates or attitudes that directly influence worker morale and motivation. For example, organizations frequently overtly or covertly reinforce the image that each employee is expendable and that individual recognition is in some way detrimental to the employee and his or her productivity within the organization. Just the opposite is true, because employees are an organization's most valuable asset.

McConnell (2005) maintains that employees want achievement, recognition and feedback, interesting work, the opportunity to assume responsibility, a chance for advancement, fairness, good leadership, job security and acceptance, and adequate monetary compensation. All of these things create a motivating climate and lead to satisfaction in the workplace. Nurses who experience satisfaction stay where they are, contributing to an organization's retention.

Some organizations however, erroneously believe that if a small reward results in desired behavior, then a larger reward will result in even more of the desired behavior. Thus, an employee's motivation should increase proportionately with the amount of the incentive or reward. This simply is not true. There appears to be a perceived threshold beyond which increasing the incentive results in no additional meaning or weight. Therefore, organizations need to develop incentive systems that consistently align with the values of the employees.

Organizations must be cognizant of the need to offer incentives at a level where employees value them. This requires that the organization and its managers understand employees' collective values and devise a reward system that is consistent with that value system.

Managers also must be cognizant of an employee's individual values and attempt to reward each worker accordingly. McConnell (2005) states that people vary considerably in how they respond to needs. So, the manager must assess individual employee values and needs as well as organization values and then use his or her authority to bring these values together. The ability to recognize each worker as a unique person who is motivated differently and then to act upon those differences is a leadership skill. Besides the climate created by the organization's beliefs and attitudes, the unit supervisor or unit manager also has a tremendous impact on motivation at the unit level. McConnell (2005) states that "at the level of the first-line manager, it should be evident that employees want recognition and feedback, two need-fulfilling activities over which the manager has a great deal of control" (p. 292).

The interpersonal relationship between an employee and his or her supervisor is critical to the employee's motivation level. We often forget that the only way to achieve our goals is through the people who work with us. Therefore, although managers cannot directly motivate employees, they can create a climate that demonstrates positive regard for their employees, encourages open communication as well as growth and productivity, and recognizes achievement.

LEARNING EXERCISE 18.3

The Strongest Motivator
Identify the greatest motivator in your life at this time. Has it always been the strongest motivator? Could you list the strongest motivator for the significant others in your life? If so, have you ever used this awareness to motivate those people to do something specific?

One of the most powerful, yet frequently overlooked or underused, motivators the manager can use to create a motivating climate is *positive reinforcement*. Connellan (2003) refers to such reinforcement as positive feedback and calls it energizing because it validates workers' effort. On the other hand, negative feedback makes workers feel as if they are being punished for trying, and if negative feedback is consistently provided, the person will give up trying. Connellan identified the following simple approaches for an effective reward–feedback system that uses positive reinforcement:

- Positive reinforcement must be specific or relevant to a particular performance. The manager should praise an employee for a specific task accomplished or goal met. This praise should not be general. For example, saying "Your nursing care is good" has less meaning and reward than "The communication skills you showed today as an advocate for Mr. Jones were excellent. I think you made a significant difference in his care."
- Positive reinforcement must occur as close to the event as possible.
- Reinforce any improvement, not just excellence. Both large and small achievements should be recognized or rewarded in some way.
- Rewards should be intermittent.
- Reinforcement of new behaviors should be continuous.

When rewards lack consistency, there is greater risk that the reward itself will become a source of competition and thereby lower morale. An attitude prevails that "a limited number of awards are available, and an award received by anyone else limits the chances of my getting one; thus, I cannot support recognition for my peers." Likewise, rewarding one person's behavior and not the behavior of another who has accomplished a similar task at a similar level promotes jealousy and can demotivate. Rewards and praise should be spontaneous and not relegated to predictable events, such as routine annual performance reviews or recognition dinners. Rewards and praise should be given whenever possible and whenever they are deserved.

If positive reinforcement and rewards are to be used as motivational strategies, then rewards must represent a genuine accomplishment on the part of the person and should be somewhat individual in nature. For example, many managers erroneously consider annual merit pay increases as rewards that motivate employees. Most employees, however, recognize annual merit pay increases as a universal "given"; thus, this reward has little meaning and little power to motivate.

Although, managers should promote excellence within achievable goals, people who are making a genuine effort to do things better, even if they have not reached excellence, also need encouragement. All of us need or appreciate a pat on the back, and once people get to a certain level of performance, they begin to reinforce themselves (Connellan, 2003). These are the cardinal elements for a successful motivation–reward system for the organization. Through shared governance, empowerment, and participative management, managers can have a direct impact on motivation at the unit level.

 All nurse–managers can enhance the work of their subordinates by providing them with more opportunities to experience the challenges that make their jobs exciting.

FINDING JOY AT WORK: A SHARED RESPONSIBILITY

For many in today's health care organizations, some of the joy has gone from work. Yet, joy can be rekindled and staff nurses and leaders can rediscover true joy in their work. Manion (2003) says that positive mood is directly linked to many different performance-related behaviors, including enhanced creativity, greater helping behavior, integrative thinking, inductive reasoning, more efficient decision making, greater cooperation, and the use of more successful negotiation strategies.

Effect of Joy at Work

Manion elaborates by saying that joyful people positively affect relationships and make the workplace more appealing. How is joy found in work? In Manion's (2003) study, most of the participants felt that joy was an individual element. However, her findings strongly suggested that the organization played a role in setting a climate for joy to occur in work. Creating a positive work environment, hiring and retaining good people, ensuring adequate benefits and compensation, providing adequate resources, and living up to the organization's mission were identified as factors contributing to a joy in work.

Pathways to Joy

Manion (2003) found that there were several personal pathways that individuals used to find joy in their work (Display 18.4). These pathways, summarized below, closely coincide with Herzberg and Maslow's theories of motivation.

- *Connections pathway*. This pathway is based on relationships, which was the primary source of joy for all participants in the study. This relationship connection occurred with colleagues, patients, and families. Caring for, talking with, relating to, and helping others exemplified this pathway to joy.
- *Love of work pathway*. This is the pathway that is based on the joy found in one's work itself. There was a strong connection and identification with the work that resulted in excitement and enthusiasm that brought joy to the participants.

DISPLAY 18.4   **Pathways to Joy**

Personal pathway via connections
Love of work pathway via the work itself
Achievement pathway via goal accomplishment and attainment
Recognition pathway via acknowledgement of good work by others

- *Achievement pathway*. Achievement, accomplishments, and positive work outcomes brought joy to some participants in the study. There was a sense of pride for a job well done or for being a successful change agent. Personal assessment of achievement was also more important than external rewards for achievement.
- *Recognition pathway*. Recognition and appreciation also brought people joy in their work. The recognition could be attained through a patient's gratitude, patient's families' appreciation, or though praise or thanks from colleagues or the organization.

STRATEGIES FOR CREATING A MOTIVATING CLIMATE

In addition to providing a climate that promotes joy in people's work, the leader–manager can do many other things that create an environment that is motivating. Sometimes, fostering a subordinate's motivation is as simple as establishing a supportive and encouraging environment. The cost of this strategy is only the manager's time and energy. The strategies outlined in Display 18.5 should be used consistently to create a motivating climate.

DISPLAY 18.5   **Strategies to Create a Motivating Climate**

1. Have clear expectations for workers, and communicate these expectations effectively.
2. Be fair and consistent when dealing with all employees.
3. Be a firm decision maker using an appropriate decision-making style.
4. Develop the concept of teamwork. Develop group goals and projects that will build a team spirit.
5. Integrate the staff's needs and wants with the organization's interests and purpose.
6. Know the uniqueness of each employee. Let each know that you understand his or her uniqueness.
7. Remove traditional blocks between the employee and the work to be done.
8. Provide experiences that challenge or "stretch" the employee and allow opportunities for growth.
9. When appropriate, request participation and input from all subordinates in decision making.
10. Whenever possible, give subordinates recognition and credit.
11. Be certain that employees understand the reason behind decisions and actions.
12. Reward desirable behavior; be consistent in how you handle undesirable behavior.
13. Let employees exercise individual judgment as much as possible.
14. Create a trustful and helping relationship with employees.
15. Let employees exercise as much control as possible over their work environment.
16. Be a role model for employees.

LEARNING EXERCISE 18.4

Write a Detailed Plan to Motivate—Quickly!

You are the manager of a medical unit in a community hospital. The hospital has faced extreme budget cuts during the last 5 years as a result of decreased reimbursement. Your unit used to be a place where nurses wanted to work, and you rarely had openings for long, even though it was necessary for the hospital to contain costs and shorten nursing care hours per patient-day. However, recently, there has been a severe nursing shortage in your community, and it seems to have accelerated worker dissatisfaction in your staff.

In the last week, five of the unit nurses, all excellent long-time employees, have stopped by your office either in tears, anger, or frustration. Their various comments have included, "Working here is no longer fun," "I used to love my job," "I am tired of working with incompetent people," and "I am sick to death of calling for supplies that should be stocked on the floor." You know that funding will not increase in the near future, but you think that perhaps there are things you could do to make the situation better for your staff.

● ASSIGNMENT: In examining the strategies for creating a motivating climate and the atmosphere that supports finding joy in work, decide what you as an individual unit manager can do to provide a more positive work environment. Avoid taking items from the list in Display 18.5, but write a detailed plan that is feasible, that could be implemented fairly quickly, and that would have the potential to turn this situation around.

PROFESSIONAL SUPPORT SYSTEMS FOR THE MANAGER

Managers also can create a motivating climate by being a positive and enthusiastic role model in the clinical setting. Managers who frequently project unhappiness to subordinates contribute greatly to low unit morale. A burned-out, tired manager will develop a lethargic and demotivated staff. Therefore, managers must constantly monitor their own motivational level and do whatever is necessary to restore their motivation to be role models to staff.

> The attitude and energy level of managers directly affect the attitude and productivity of their employees.

Managers must be internally motivated before they can motivate others. It is imperative that discouraged managers acknowledge their own feelings and seek assistance accordingly. Managers are responsible to themselves and to subordinates to remain motivated to do the best job possible. McConnell (2005) maintains that there is little difference between workers and their managers when it comes to consideration of what motivates them to work.

Nursing is a stressful profession, and managers must practice health-seeking behaviors and find social supports when confronted with stress or else risk burnout as a result. Weber (2004) states that "good leaders recognize what motivates and drives them not only in their professional but also in their personal lives and have discovered that mastering personal leadership is an essential ingredient in leading others" (p. 91).

Burnout and other forms of work-related stress are related to negative organizational outcomes such as illness, absenteeism, turnover, performance deterioration, decreased productivity, and job dissatisfaction. These outcomes cost the organization and impede quality of care. Davidhizar and

Hart (2006) maintain that there are many ways managers can take responsibility for their own happiness, such as keeping appropriate humor in the workplace, practicing joy building, and keeping the work environment fun and comfortable. These activities can be self-motivating and great antidotes to the burnout and negativism that befall many managers.

Perhaps the most important strategy for avoiding burnout and maintaining a high motivation level is self-care. For self-care, the manager should seek time off on a regular basis to meet personal needs, seek recreation, form relationships outside the work setting, and have fun. Friends and colleagues are essential for emotional support, guidance, and renewal. A proper diet and exercise are important to maintain physical health as well as emotional health. Finally, the manager must be able to separate his or her work life and personal life; the manager should remember that there is life outside of work and that time should be relished and protected. Ultimately, the decision to practice self-care rests with each nurse.

INTEGRATING LEADERSHIP ROLES AND MANAGEMENT FUNCTIONS IN CREATING A MOTIVATING CLIMATE AT WORK

Most human behavior is motivated by a goal that the person wants to achieve. Identifying employee goals and fostering their attainment allow the leader to motivate employees to reach personal and organizational goals. The motivational strategy that the leader uses should vary with the situation and the employee involved; it may be formal or informal. It may be extrinsic, although because of a limited formal power base, the leader generally focuses on other aspects of motivation. The leader must listen, support, and encourage the discouraged employee. However, perhaps the most important role that the leader has in working with the demotivated employee is that of role model. Davidhizar and Hart (2006) state that managers should not avoid employees when times are tough but instead should demonstrate a positive attitude. Leaders who maintain a positive attitude and high energy levels directly and profoundly affect the attitude and productivity of their followers.

When creating a motivating climate, the manager uses formal authority to reduce dissatisfiers at the unit level and to implement a reward system that reflects individual and collective value systems. This reward system may be formalized, or it may be as informal as praise. Managers, by virtue of their position, have the ability to motivate subordinates by "stretching" them intermittently with increasing responsibility and assignments that they are capable of achieving. The manager's role, then, is to create the tension necessary to maintain productivity while encouraging subordinates' job satisfaction. Therefore, the success of the motivational strategy is measured by increased productivity and benefit to the organization and by growth in the person, which motivates him or her to accomplish again.

Key Concepts

* Because human beings have constant needs and wants, they are always motivated to some extent. However, human beings are motivated differently.
* Managers cannot intrinsically motivate people, because motivation comes from within the person. The humanistic manager can, however, create an environment in which the development of human potential can be maximized.

* Maslow stated that people are motivated to satisfy certain needs, ranging from basic survival to complex psychological needs, and that people seek a higher need only when the lower needs have been predominantly met.
* Skinner's research on *operant conditioning* and *behavior modification* demonstrates that people can be conditioned to behave in a certain way based on a consistent reward or punishment system.
* Herzberg maintained that *motivators*, or *job satisfiers*, are present in the work itself and encourage people to want to work and to do that work well. *Hygiene* or *maintenance factors* keep the worker from being dissatisfied or demotivated but do not act as true motivators for the worker.
* Vroom's *expectancy model* says that people's expectations about their environment or a certain event will influence their behavior.
* McClelland's studies state that all people are motivated by three basic needs: *achievement*, *affiliation*, and *power*.
* Gellerman states that most managers in organizations overmanage, making the responsibilities too narrow and failing to give employees any decision-making power or to stretch them often enough.
* McGregor shows the importance of a manager's assumptions about workers on the intrinsic motivation of the worker.
* There appears to be a perceived threshold beyond which increasing reward incentives results in no additional meaning or weight in terms of productivity.
* *Positive reinforcement* is one of the most powerful motivators the manager can use and is frequently overlooked or underused.
* The supervisor or manager's personal motivation is an important factor affecting staff's commitment to duties and morale.
* The success of a motivational strategy is measured by the increased productivity and benefit to the organization and by the growth in the person, which motivates him or her to accomplish again.
* Managers must show their own positive attitude to demonstrate to employees that there is joy in work.

ADDITIONAL LEARNING EXERCISES AND APPLICATIONS

LEARNING EXERCISE 18.5

Create a Plan to Remotivate a New Employee

You are a county public health coordinator. You have grown concerned about the behavior of one of the new RNs assigned to work in the agency. This new nurse, Sally Brown, is a recent graduate of a local BSN program. She came to work for the agency immediately after her graduation 6 months ago and for the first few months appeared to be extremely hard working,

(Learning Exercise continues on page 436)

knowledgeable, well liked, and highly motivated. Recently, though, several small incidents involved Sally. The agency's medical director became very angry with her over a medication error that she had made. Sally was already feeling badly about the careless error. Soon after, a patient's husband began disliking Sally for no discernible reason and refused Sally entrance to his home to care for his wife. Then, 2 weeks ago, a diabetic patient died fairly suddenly from renal failure, and although no one was to blame, Sally thought that if she had been more observant and skilled in assessment, she would have detected subtle changes in the patient's condition sooner.

Although you have been supportive of Sally, you recognize that she is in danger of becoming demotivated. Her once-flawless personal appearance now borders on being unkempt, she is frequently absent from work, and her once-pleasant personality has been exchanged for withdrawal from her coworkers.

● ASSIGNMENT: Using your knowledge of new role identification, assimilation, and motivational theory, develop a plan to assist this young nurse. What can you do to provide a climate that will remotivate her and decrease her job dissatisfaction? Explain what you think is happening to this nurse and the rationale behind your plan, which should be realistic in terms of the time and energy that you have to spend on one employee. Be sure to identify the responsibilities of the employee as well.

LEARNING EXERCISE 18.6

A Nursing Officer's Dilemma

You are the chief nursing officer of County Hospital. Dr. Martin Jones, a cardiologist, has approached you about having an ICU/CCU nurse make rounds with him each morning on all of the patients in the hospital with a cardiac-related diagnosis. He believes that this will probably represent a 90-minute commitment of nursing time daily. He is vague about the nurse's exact role or purpose, but you believe that there is great potential for better and more consistent patient education and care planning.

Beth, one of your finest ICU/CCU nurses, agrees to assist Dr. Jones. Beth has always wanted to have an expanded teaching role. However, for various reasons, she has been unable to relocate to a larger city where there are more opportunities for teaching. You warn Beth that it might be some time before this role develops into an autonomous position, but she is eager to assist Dr. Jones. The other ICU/CCU staff agree to cover Beth's patients while she is gone, although it is obviously an extension of an already full patient load.

After 3 weeks of making rounds with Dr. Jones, Beth comes to your office. She tearfully reports that rounds frequently take 2 to 3 hours and that making rounds with Dr. Jones amounts to little more than "carrying his charts, picking up his pages, and being a personal handmaiden." She has assertively stated her feelings to him and has attempted to demonstrate to Dr. Jones how their allegiance could result in improved patient care. She states that she has not been allowed any input into patient decisions and is frequently reminded of "her position" and his ability to have her removed from her job if she does not like being told what to do. She is demoralized and demotivated. In addition, she believes that her peers resent having to cover her workload because it is obvious that her role is superficial at best.

You ask Beth if she wants you to assign another nurse to work with Dr. Jones, and she says that she would really like to make it work but does not know what action to take that would improve the situation.

You call Dr. Jones, and he agrees to meet with you at your office when he completes rounds the following morning. At this visit, Dr. Jones confirms Beth's description of her role but justifies his desire for the role to continue by saying, "I bring $10 million of business to this hospital every year in cardiology procedures. The least you can do is provide the nursing assistance I am asking for. If you are unable to meet this small request, I will be forced to consider taking my practice to a competitive hospital." However, after further discussion, he does agree that eventually he would consider a slightly more expanded role for the nurse after he learns to trust her.

● ASSIGNMENT: Do you meet Dr. Jones's request? Does it make any difference whether Beth is the nurse, or can it be someone else? Does the revenue that Dr. Jones generates supersede the value of professional nursing practice? Should you try to talk Beth into continuing the position for a while longer? While trying to reach a goal, people must sometimes endure a difficult path, but at what point does the means not justify the end? Be realistic about what you would do in this situation. What do you perceive to be the greatest obstacles in implementing your decision?

LEARNING EXERCISE 18.7

To Work or Not to Work?

You are a nurse in a long-term care facility. The facility barely meets minimum licensing standards for professional nursing staffing. Although agency recruiters have been actively seeking to hire more licensed staff, pay at the facility for professional staff is less than at local acute-care hospitals and the patient–nurse ratio is significantly higher. There appears to be little chance of improving the RN staffing mix in your agency in the near future. The nursing administrator is extremely supportive of the staff's efforts but can do little to ease the current workload for licensed staff other than to turn away patients or close the agency. As a result, all of the nurses on the unit have been working at least 48 hours per week during the last 6 months; many have been working several double shifts and putting in many overtime hours each pay period.

Morale is deteriorating, and the staff has begun to complain. Most of the licensed staff are feeling burned out and demotivated. Many have started refusing to work overtime or to take on extra shifts. You feel a responsibility to the patients, community, and organization and have continued to work the extra hours but you are exhausted as well.

Today is your first evening off in 6 days. At 2 PM, the phone rings, and you suspect that it is the agency calling you to come in to work. You delay answering while you decide what to do. The answering machine turns on, and you hear your administrator's voice. She says that they are desperate. Two new patients were admitted during the day, and the facility is full. She says that she appreciates all the hours you have been working but needs you once again, although she is unable to give you tomorrow off in compensation. You feel conflicting loyalties to the unit, patients, supervisor, and yourself.

● ASSIGNMENT: Decide what you will do. Will you agree to work? Will you return the administrator's telephone call or pretend that you are not at home? When do your loyalties to your patients and the organization end and your loyalties to yourself begin? Is the administrator taking advantage of you? Are the other staff being irresponsible? What values have played a part in your decision making?

LEARNING EXERCISE 18.8

Remotivating Oneself

You are a school nurse and have worked in the same school for 2 years. Before that time, you were a staff nurse at a local hospital working in pediatrics and later for a physician. You have been an RN for 6 years.

When you began your job, it was exciting. You believed that you were really making a difference in children's lives. You started several good health promotion programs and worked hard upgrading your health aides' education and training.

Several months ago, funding for the school was drastically cut, and several of your favorite programs were eliminated. You have been depressed about this and lately have been short-tempered at work. Today, one of your best health aides gave you her 2-week notice and said, "This isn't a good place to work anymore." You realize that many of the aides and several of the schoolteachers have picked up your negative attitude.

There is much that you still love about your job, and you are not sure if the budget problems are temporary or long term. You go home early today and contemplate what to do.

● ASSIGNMENT: Should you stay in this job or leave? If you stay, how can you get remotivated? Can you remotivate yourself if the budget cuts are long term? Make a plan about what to do.

LEARNING EXERCISE 18.9

Downsizing Panic and Anxiety

As the result of rising costs and shrinking reimbursement, many hospitals downsized their staffs in an effort to shrink costs. Because the hospital where you are the chief nursing administrator is faced with mandatory staffing ratios, it is impossible to cut further staff nurse positions and meet requirements for state licensing.

Therefore, the CEO of the hospital has mandated that management positions be reduced by 30% throughout the hospital. The CEO has decided that department heads can reduce management positions by any method they choose as long as it is done in 6 months. Job duties are to be reassigned among the remaining managers.

This affects you significantly, as nursing has more managers than any other department. It does not appear that attrition, or turnover, rates in the next months will be adequate to eliminate the need for some reassignments, demotions, or termination of your group of 17 managers. This includes both house supervisors and unit managers.

The news travels rapidly through the hospital grapevine. Semihysteria prevails, with many managers consulting you regarding whether their position is in jeopardy and what they can to do to increase the likelihood of their retention. Morale is rapidly plummeting, and relationships are becoming increasingly competitive rather than cooperative.

● ASSIGNMENT: Determine how you will handle this situation. What strategies might you implement to reduce the immediate anxiety level? What advice can you give to staff who may face either a layoff or a demotion? Is it possible to preserve the morale of your managers in an uncertain situation such as this?

Web Links

Landmark Education—Motivation
http://www.landmarkeducation.com
The Landmark Forum is a collaborative seminar focused on motivation.

Motivation Theory—The Theorists and Their Theories
http://www.accel-team.com/motivation/theory_01.html
Reviews the work of theorists Simon, McGregor, Maslow, Herzberg, Argyris, Likert, Luthans, Vroom, Mayo, and McClelland.

Theories About the Need for Achievement
http://mentalhelp.net/psyhelp/chap4/chap4j.htm
A psychological self-help site dedicated to the achievement needs to succeed and excel.

Strategies for Life
http://www.yourbestyear.com
Offers proven methods for setting and achieving your goals for the coming year.

References

Connellan, T. K. (2003). *Bringing out the best in others! Three keys for business leaders, educators, coaches and parents.* Austin, TX: Brad Press.

Davidhizar, R., & Hart, A. (2006). Are you born a happy person or do you have to make it happen? *Health Care Manager, 25*(1), 64–69.

Gellerman, S. W. (1968). *Management by motivation.* American Management Association.

Herzberg, F. (1977). One more time: How do you motivate employees? In L. Carroll, R. Paine, & A. Miner (Eds.), *The management process* (2nd ed.). New York: Macmillan.

Manion, J. (2003). Joy at work! Creating a positive workplace. *Journal of Nursing Administration, 33*(12), 652–659.

Martin, C. A. (2005). Leadership: Make it H.O.T. *Nursing Management, 36*(9), 38–45.

Maslow, A. (1970). *Motivation and personality* (2nd ed.). New York: Harper & Row.

Mayo, E. (1953). *The human problems of an industrialized civilization.* New York: Macmillan.

McClelland, D. C. (1971). *Assessing human motivation.* Morristown, NJ: General Learning Press.

McConnell, C. R. (2005). Motivating your employees and yourself. *Health Care Manager, 24*(3), 284–292.

McGregor, D. (1960). *The human side of enterprise.* New York: McGraw-Hill.

Mrayyan, M. T. (2004). Nurses autonomy: Influence of nurse manager's actions. *Journal of Advanced Nursing, 45*(3), 326–336.

Skinner, B. F. (1953). *Science and human behavior.* New York: Free Press.

Vaughn, G. R. M. (2003). Motivators get creative. *Nursing Management, 34*(4), 12–14.

Vroom, V. (1964). *Work and motivation.* New York: John Wiley and Sons.

Weber, B. (2004). Leadership: Do you have the motivation? *Plastic Surgical Nursing, 24*(3), 91.

Bibliography

Curtin, L. (2004). Editorial opinion. Leadership of the spirit. . . . *Journal of Clinical Systems Management, 6*(12), 5–19.

DiMichele, C., & Gaffney, L. (2005). Notes from the field. Proactive teams yield exceptional care. *Nursing Management, 36*(5), 61–62, 64.

Drach-Zahavy, A. (2004). Primary nurses' performance: Role of supportive management. *Journal of Advanced Nursing, 45*(1), 7–16.

Heckerson, E. W. (2006). Nurse leader as coach. *Nurse Leader, 4*(1), 29–31.

Herbert, R., & Edgar, L. (2004). Innovation in leadership. Emotional intelligence: A primal dimension of nursing leadership? *Canadian Journal of Nursing Leadership*, *17*(4), 56–63.

Hill, K. S. (2004). Defy the decades with multigenerational teams: Learn what motivates veteran, baby boomer, generation X and generation Y employees. *Nursing Management*, *35*(1), 32–35.

Jooste, K. (2004). Leadership: A new perspective. *Journal of Nursing Management*, *12*(3), 217–223.

Laschinger, H. (2004). Making a case for shared accountability. *Journal of Nursing Administration*, 34, 354–364.

Leichtling, B. (2004). Leadership & management. Motivation, inspiration and relation: The three-legged stool for retaining quality staff. *Caring*, *23*(4), 46–47.

Odom-Forren, J. (2004). The back page: The melodious bell: The joy of work. *Journal of Perianesthesia Nursing*, *19*(6), 443.

Pinkerton, S. (2006). Retention and recruitment. Stories as motivators. *Nursing Economics*, *24*(3), 166–167.

Sherman, R. O. (2005). Growing our future nursing leaders. *Nursing Administration Quarterly*, *29*(2), 125–132.

19

Organizational, Interpersonal, and Group Communication

. . . effective communication is the lifeblood of a successful organization. It reinforces the organization's vision, connects employees to the business, fosters process improvement, facilitates change and drives business results by changing employee behavior.

—*Watson Wyatt Worldwide (2007)*

. . . the difference between the right word and the almost right word is the difference between lightning and a lightning bug.

—*Mark Twain*

Although some functions of management such as planning, organizing, and controlling can be reasonably isolated, communication impacts all management activities and cuts across all phases of the management process. It is also the core of the nurse–patient, nurse–nurse, and nurse–physician relationship (Manning, 2006).

Because most managerial communication time is spent speaking and listening, it is clear that in a leadership role, one must have excellent interpersonal communication skills. These are perhaps the most critical leadership skills. The nurse–leader communicates with clients, colleagues, superiors, and subordinates. In addition, because nursing practice tends to be group oriented, interpersonal communication among group members is necessary for continuity and productivity. The leader is responsible for developing a cohesive team to meet organizational goals. To do this, the leader must articulate issues and concerns so that workers will not become confused about priorities. The ability to communicate effectively often determines success as a leader–manager.

Organizational communication is even more complex than interpersonal or group communication, as there are more communication channels, more individuals to communicate with, and more information to transmit. Thus, organizational communication is a high-level management

EXAMINING THE EVIDENCE 19.1

Source: Watson Wyatt Worldwide. (2007). *Effective communication: A leading indicator of financial performance—2005/2006. Communication ROI Study.* Retrieved January 19, 2007, from *http://www.watsonwyatt.com/research/resrender.asp?id=w-868&page=1.*

Watson Wyatt Worldwide serves as a business partner to many of the world's leading organizations on people and financial issues. In 2005–2006, a survey was undertaken to determine how communication impacted organizational turnover and financial performance. Key findings included:

- Companies that communicate effectively have a 19.4% higher market premium than companies that do not.
- Shareholder returns for organizations with the most effective communication were over 57% higher over the last 5 years (2000–2004) than were returns for firms with less effective communication.
- Communication effectiveness is a leading indicator of financial performance.
- Firms that communicate effectively are 4.5 times more likely to report high levels of employee engagement than those that communicate less effectively.
- Companies that are highly effective communicators are 20% more likely to report lower turnover rates than their peers.

function; it must be systematic, have continuity, and be appropriately integrated into the organizational structure, encouraging an exchange of views and ideas. Organizational communication is complex, however, and communication failure occurs frequently as a result of the interruptions associated with hectic, noisy, and distracting clinical care environments (Manning, 2006). Such communication failure often results in a failure to meet organizational goals.

Hamm (2006) agrees, arguing that the most effective CEOs "understand that the risks of miscommunication are very high, and ask themselves the following questions on their way to work: What needs to happen today so that we can get where we want to go? Where is there confusion in my company? What vague belief or notion can I clarify or debunk today? What have I not communicated completely or clearly? What kinds of things are people taking for granted?"

Developing expertise in all aspects of communication, then, is critical to managerial success. Indeed, a 2005–2006 study by Watson Wyatt Worldwide (2007), as discussed in Examining the Evidence 19.1, confirmed a correlation between communication effectiveness, organizational turnover, and financial performance. Indeed, effective communication was the leading indicator of an organization's financial performance. Hamm (2006) agrees, arguing that "a CEO who communicates precisely to 10 direct reports, each of whom communicates with equal precision to 40 other talented employees, effectively aligns the organization's commitment and energy around a clear, well-understood, shared vision of the company's real goals, priorities, and opportunities. He or she saves the company time, money, and resources and allows extraordinary things to happen."

Leadership skills and management functions inherent in organizational, interpersonal, and group communication are listed in Display 19.1. This chapter examines these forms of communication. Barriers to communication in large organizations and managerial strategies to overcome those difficulties are presented. Channels and modes of communication are compared, and guidelines are given for managerial selection of the optimum channel or mode. In addition, assertiveness, nonverbal behavior, and active listening as interpersonal communication factors

DISPLAY 19.1 **Leadership Roles and Management Functions Associated With Organizational, Interpersonal, and Group Communication**

Leadership Roles

1. Understands and appropriately uses the informal communication network in the organization
2. Communicates clearly and precisely in language that others will understand
3. Is sensitive to the internal and external climate of the sender or receiver and uses that awareness in interpreting messages
4. Appropriately observes and interprets the verbal and nonverbal communication of followers
5. Role-models assertive communication and active listening
6. Demonstrates congruency in verbal and nonverbal communication
7. Recognizes status, power, and authority as barriers to manager–subordinate communication; uses communication strategies to overcome those barriers
8. Maximizes group functioning by keeping group members on course, encouraging the shy, controlling the garrulous, and protecting the weak
9. Seeks a balance between technological communication options and the need for human touch, caring, and one-on-one, face-to-face interaction

Management Functions

1. Understands and appropriately uses the organization's formal communication network
2. Determines the appropriate communication mode or combination of modes for optimal distribution of information in the organizational hierarchy
3. Prepares written communications that are clear and uses language that is appropriate for the message and the receiver
4. Consults with other departments or disciplines in coordinating overlapping roles and group efforts
5. Differentiates between "information" and "communication" and appropriately assesses the need for subordinates to have both
6. Prioritizes and protects client and subordinate confidentiality
7. Ensures that staff and self are trained to appropriately and fully utilize technological communication tools
8. Uses knowledge of group dynamics for attaining goals and maximizing organizational communication

are discussed. The chapter also includes a discussion of how technology continues to alter communication in health care settings and the ever-increasing challenge of maintaining confidentiality in a system where so many people have access to so much information.

THE COMMUNICATION PROCESS

Answers.com provides a definition of *communication* as "the exchange of thoughts, messages, or information, by speech, signals, writing, or behavior" (Answers.com, n.d., para 1). Communication can also occur on at least two levels: *verbal* and *nonverbal*. Thus, whenever two or more people are aware of each other, communication begins.

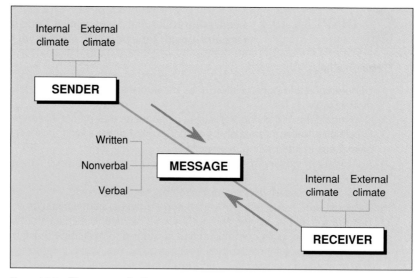

Figure 19.1 The communication process.

Communication begins the moment that two or more people become aware of each other's presence.

What happens, however, when the thoughts, ideas, and information exchanged do not have the same meaning for both the sender and the receiver of the message? What if the verbal and nonverbal messages are incongruent? Does communication occur if an idea is transmitted but not translated into action? Because communication is so complex, many models exist to explain how organizations and individuals communicate. Basic elements common to most models are shown in Figure 19.1. In all communication, there is at least one sender, one receiver, and one message. There also is a mode or medium through which the message is sent—for example, spoken, written, or nonverbal.

An internal and an external climate also exist in communication. The *internal climate* includes the values, feelings, temperament, and stress levels of the sender and the receiver. Weather conditions, temperature, timing, and the organizational climate itself are parts of the external climate. The *external climate* also includes status, power, and authority as barriers to manager–subordinate communication.

Both the sender and the receiver must be sensitive to the internal and external climate, because the perception of the message is altered greatly depending upon the climate that existed at the time the message was sent or received. For example, an insecure manager who is called to meet with superiors during a period of stringent layoffs will probably view the message with more trepidation than a manager who is secure in his or her role.

Because each person is different and thus makes decisions and perceives differently, assessing external climate is usually easier than internal climate. In assessing internal climate, remember that the human mind perceives only what it expects to perceive. The unexpected is generally ignored or misunderstood. In other words, receivers cannot communicate if the message is incompatible with their expectations. If senders want communication to be effective, they need to decide what the receiver will see or hear.

 Effective communication requires the sender to validate what receivers see and hear.

VARIABLES AFFECTING ORGANIZATIONAL COMMUNICATION

Formal organizational structure has an impact on communication. People at lower levels of the organizational hierarchy are at risk for inadequate communication from higher levels. This occurs because of the number of levels that communication must filter through in large organizations. As the number of employees increases (particularly more than 1,000 employees), the quantity of communication generally increases; however, employees may perceive it as increasingly closed. In large organizations, it is impossible for individual managers to communicate personally with each person or group involved in organizational decision making. Not only is spatial distance a factor, but the presence of subgroups or subcultures also affects what messages are transmitted and how they are perceived.

LEARNING EXERCISE 19.1

Large Organization Communication
Have you ever been employed in a large organization? Was the communication within that organization clear and timely? What or who was your primary source of information? Were you a part of a subgroup or subculture? If so, how did that affect communication?

Gender is also a significant factor in organizational communication, as men and women communicate and use language differently. Indeed, Rudan's (2003) study of gender differences in team building showed that leadership style was an extension of communication style. He found that when conducting business meetings, males were "all business" while females discussed other personal and social issues with team members. Men also frequently held "meetings before the meeting" where things were agreed upon, and women were not present at these small meetings.

Similarly, Grossman and Valiga (2005), in summarizing benchmark research on gender and leadership, suggest that men tend to see the world as more black and white, whereas women tend to see the world as gray. In addition, men tend to be more competitive and to exercise more overt power in their communications whereas women are more often supportive, future oriented, and nurturing. This has implications for communication patterns; men tend to be more hierarchical in their communication and women tend to be more connective with an almost weblike communication network (Grossman & Valiga, 2005).

Complicating the picture further is the historical need in the health care industry for a predominantly male medical profession to closely communicate with a predominantly female nursing profession. In addition, the majority of health care administrators continue to be male. Therefore, male physicians and male administrators may feel little incentive to seek a collaborative approach in communication that female nurses often desire. The quality of organizational and unit-level communication continues to be affected by differences in gender, power, and status.

 Differences in gender, power, and status significantly affect the types and quality of organizational and unit-level communication.

ORGANIZATIONAL COMMUNICATION STRATEGIES

Although organizational communication is complex, the following strategies can increase the likelihood of clear and complete communication:

- *Managers must assess organizational communication.* Who communicates with whom in the organization? Is the communication timely? Does communication within the formal organization concur with formal lines of authority? Are there conflicts or disagreements about communication? What modes of communication are used?
- *Managers must understand the organization's structure and recognize who will be affected by decisions.* Both formal and informal communication networks need to be considered. *Formal communication networks* follow the formal line of authority in the organization's hierarchy. *Informal communication networks* occur among people at the same or different levels of the organizational hierarchy but do not represent formal lines of authority or responsibility. For example, an informal communication network might occur between a hospital's CEO and her daughter, who is a clerk on a medical wing. Although there may be a significant exchange of information about unit or organizational functioning, this communication network would not be apparent on the organization chart. It is imperative, then, that managers be very careful about what they say and to whom until they have a good understanding of the formal and informal communication networks.
- *Communication is not a one-way channel.* If other departments or disciplines will be affected by a message, the manager must consult with those areas for feedback before the communication occurs.
- *Communication must be clear, simple, and precise.* Manning (2006) suggests that standardized approaches and tools may provide potential solutions to improve the quality of communication. For example, he suggests that a standardized tool such as *SBAR* (Situation-Background, Assessment-Recommendation/Request) is an easy to remember tool that provides a structured, orderly approach in providing accurate, relevant information, especially in emergent patient situations (Display 19.2).
- *Senders should seek feedback regarding whether their communication was accurately received.* One way to do this is to ask the receiver to repeat the communication or instructions. In addition, the sender should continue follow-up communication in an effort to determine if the communication is being acted upon.

 The sender is responsible for ensuring that the message is understood.

- *Multiple communication methods should be used, when possible, if a message is important.* Using a variety of communication methods in combination increases the likelihood that everyone in the organization who needs to hear the message actually will hear it.

DISPLAY 19.2   **SBAR as a Communication Tool**

S	Situation	Introduce yourself, and briefly state the issue that you want to discuss.
B	Background	Describe the background or context.
A	Assessment	State what you think the problem is.
R	Recommendation	State what you would like to do to address the problem.

Source: Adapted from Haig, K. M., Sutton, S., & Whittington, J. (2006). SBAR: A shared mental model for improving communication between clinicians. *Joint Commission Journal on Quality and Patient Safety, 32*(6), 167–175.

> • *Managers should not overwhelm subordinates with unnecessary information. Information is formal, impersonal, and unaffected by emotions, values, expectations, and perceptions. Communication,* on the other hand, involves perception and feeling. It does not depend on information and may represent shared experiences. In contrast to information sharing, superiors must continually communicate with subordinates.

Although information and communication are different, they are interdependent.

Most staff need little information about ordering procedures or organizational supply vendors as long as supplies are adequate and appropriate to meet unit needs. If, however, a vendor is temporarily unable to meet unit supply needs, the use of supplies by staff becomes an issue requiring close communication between managers and subordinates. The manager must communicate with the staff about which supplies will be inadequately stocked and for how long. The manager also may choose to discuss this inadequacy of resources with the staff to identify alternative solutions.

THE IMPACT OF TECHNOLOGY ON CONTEMPORARY ORGANIZATIONAL COMMUNICATION

Technology has dramatically changed how nurses communicate and perform their work. Younger generations of nurses, who grew up using computers, cell phones, and instant messaging, recognize that technology has given us the potential for instant information access and exchange. These nurses approach and accept technology as an adjunct to their nursing cognizance and do not question its presence or use.

Telecommunication and Email

It is clear that the telecommunication technology growth experienced in the late 20th century is continuing to proliferate even more rapidly in the 21st century. This advancing technology may help to balance the constraints being placed on other patient care resources. Technologies such as email, faxes, teleconferences, and CD-ROMs are increasing the potential for effective and efficient communication throughout the organization. The use of *hospital information system* (HIS) configurations such as stand-alone systems, on-line interactive systems, networked systems, and integrative systems has also increased.

Nurse–managers are increasingly using the *Internet* as both a communication tool and an information source. As a communication tool, the Internet provides access to electronic mail, file transfer protocol, and the World Wide Web. As an information source, the Internet allows nurses to access the latest research and best practice information so that their care can be evidence based. Huston (2006) suggests that computers and computerized charting are increasingly a part of interdisciplinary team communication and care documentation in acute-care hospitals. Moreover, *personal digital assistants* (PDAs), which give users access to text-based information, are becoming commonplace as are institutionwide documentation systems whereby everyone uses the same documentation software, and the information is transferred to and retrieved from a central server via "*hot synching*" (putting the PDA into a cradle or connecting it via cable to the central server). In addition, the PDA can serve as a reference library, especially for drug information and as a calculator for computing drug dosages.

The use of *wireless, local area networking* (WLAN) is also growing. WLAN uses spread-spectrum radio frequency modulation technology instead of hardwired systems or paper-based records and allows caregivers to access, update, and transmit critical patient and treatment information when hardwiring is impractical or impossible (Huston, 2006). However, even the most advanced communication technology cannot replace the human judgment needed by leaders and managers to use that technology appropriately. Examples of the type of communication challenges that managers face in such a rapidly evolving technological society include:

- Determining which technological advances can and should be used at each level of the organizational hierarchy to promote efficiency and effectiveness of communication
- Assessing the need for and providing workers with adequate training to appropriately and fully utilize the technological communication tools that may become available to them
- Aligning communication technology with the organizational mission
- Finding a balance between technological communication options and the need for human touch, caring, and one-on-one, face-to-face interaction.

Electronic Health Records

Even health records have changed as a result of technology. The Electronic Health Record Vendors Association (EHRVA, 2006) defines the *electronic health record* (EHR) as a "longitudinal electronic record of patient health information produced by encounters in one or more care settings. Included in this information are patient demographics, progress notes, problems, medications, vital signs, past medical history, immunizations, laboratory data and radiology reports" (para 2). As such, the EHR can streamline a clinician's workflow, provide a complete patient record, and support activities related to decision support and quality control (EHRVA, 2006).

CHANNELS OF COMMUNICATION

Because large organizations are so complex, communication channels used by the manager may be upward, downward, horizontal, diagonal, or through the "grapevine." In *upward communication*, the manager is a subordinate to higher management. Needs and wants are communicated upward to the next level in the hierarchy. Those at this higher level make decisions for a greater segment of the organization than the lower-level manager.

In *downward communication*, the manager relays information to subordinates. This is a traditional form of communication in organizations and helps to coordinate activities in various levels of the hierarchy.

In *horizontal communication*, managers interact with others on the same hierarchical level as themselves who are managing different segments of the organization. The need for horizontal communication increases as departmental interdependence increases.

In *diagonal communication*, the manager interacts with personnel and managers of other departments and groups such as physicians, who are not on the same level of the organizational hierarchy. Although these people have no formal authority over the manager, this communication is vital to the organization's functioning. Diagonal communication tends to be less formal than other types of communication.

The most informal communication network is often called the *grapevine*. *Grapevine communication* flows quickly and haphazardly among people at all hierarchical levels and usually involves three or four people at a time. Senders have little accountability for the message, and often the message is distorted as it speeds along. Given the frequency of grapevine communication in all organizations, all managers must attempt to better understand how the grapevine works in their own organization as well as who is contributing to it.

 Grapevine communication is subject to error and distortion because of the speed at which it passes and because the sender has little formal accountability for the message.

LEARNING EXERCISE 19.2

When and How Will You Tell?
Assume that you are the project director of a small family planning clinic. You have just received word that your federal and state funds have been slashed and that the clinic will probably close in 3 months. Although an additional funding source may be found, it is improbable that it will occur within that time period. The board of directors informed you that this knowledge is not to be made public at this time.

You have five full-time employees at the clinic. Because two of these employees are your close friends, you feel some conflict about withholding this information from them. You are aware that another clinic in town currently has job openings and that the positions are generally filled quickly.

● ASSIGNMENT: It is important that you staff the clinic for the next 3 months. When will you notify the staff of the clinic's intent to close? Will you communicate the closing to all staff at the same time? Will you use downward communication? Should the grapevine be used to leak news to employees? When might the grapevine be appropriate to pass on information?

COMMUNICATION MODES

A message's clarity is greatly affected by the mode of communication used. In general, the more direct the communication, the greater the probability that it will be clear. The more people involved in filtering the communication, the greater the chance of distortion. The manager must evaluate each circumstance individually to determine which mode or combination of modes is optimal for each situation. The manager uses the following modes of communication most frequently:

- *Written communication.* Written messages (including email, which will be discussed later in this chapter) allow for documentation. They may, however, be open to various interpretations and generally consume more managerial time. Most managers are required to do a considerable amount of this type of communication and therefore need to be able to write clearly.
- *Face-to-face communication.* Oral communication is rapid but may result in fewer people receiving the information than necessary. Managers communicate verbally upward and downward and formally and informally. They also communicate verbally in formal meetings, with people in peer work groups, and when making formal presentations.
- *Nonverbal communication.* Nonverbal communication includes facial expression, body movements, and gestures and is commonly referred to as *body language*. Nonverbal communication is considered more reliable because it conveys the emotional part of the message. There is significant danger, however, in misinterpreting nonverbal messages if they are not assessed in context with the verbal message. Nonverbal communication occurs any time managers are seen (e.g., messages are transmitted to subordinates every time the manager communicates verbally or just walks down a hallway).

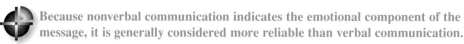 Because nonverbal communication indicates the emotional component of the message, it is generally considered more reliable than verbal communication.

- *Telephone communication.* A telephone call is rapid and allows the receiver to clarify the message at the time it is given. It does not, however, allow the receipt of nonverbal messages for either the sender or receiver of the message. Accents may be difficult to understand as well in a multicultural workforce. Because managers today use the telephone so much, it has become an important communication tool, but it does have limits as an effective communication device.

LEARNING EXERCISE 19.3

Your Communication Style
Which communication modes do you use most frequently? Which is your preferred mode and why? Which modes are the most difficult for you to use and why?

WRITTEN COMMUNICATION WITHIN THE ORGANIZATION

Although communication may take many forms, written communication is used most often in large organizations. The written communication issued by the manager reflects greatly on both the manager and the organization. Thus, the manager must be able to write clearly and professionally and to use understandable language. Many types of written communication are used in organizations. Organizational policy, procedures, events, and change may be announced in writing. Job descriptions, performance appraisals, and letters of reference also are forms of written communication.

Often, though, the written communication used most by managers in their daily worklife is the *memo*. Perkins (2007) suggests that business memos have a twofold purpose: They bring attention to problems, and they solve problems. Thus, it is important to choose the audience of a memo wisely and to ensure that everyone on the distribution list of the memo actually needs to read it. Typically, memos should be sent to only a small to moderate number of people. In addition, memos should not be used for highly sensitive messages, which are better communicated face-to-face or by telephone (Perkins, 2007).

Because writing is a learned skill that improves with practice, Writing Help Central (2006) suggests the following in writing professional correspondence:

- Keep your message short and concise. Less than one page is always preferred.
- Focus on the recipient's needs. Make sure that your communication addresses the recipient's expectations and what he or she needs to know.
- Use simple language so that the message is clear. Keep paragraphs to less than three or four sentences.
- Review the message and revise as needed. Almost all important communication requires several drafts. Always re-read the written communication before sending it. Look for areas that might be misunderstood. Pay attention to tone. Have all of the key points been made?
- Use spelling and grammar checks to be sure that the communication looks professional. Remember that your document is a direct reflection of you, and even the most important message will likely be ignored if the communication is perceived as unprofessional.

Thompson (2007) adds the following additional suggestions for writing effective memos in business communication:

- Make sure that you have addressed the reader(s) by his or her correct name. Add a job title along with the name if the memo is more formal.
- Include a subject line, when appropriate, to summarize the purpose of the memo.
- Keep the memo concise, clear, and to the point and include bullets or headings to emphasize key points.
- Do not include salutations or complimentary closings in memos.
- Use the first paragraph to express the context or purpose of the memo and to introduce the problem. In next paragraphs, address what has been done or needs to be done to address the problem at hand. In the closing, clarify what the reader is expected to do.
- Add a conclusion to summarize the memo and to address any attachments that are a part of the memo.

Perkins (2007) suggests that these segments should be allocated in the following manner:

- *Header* (includes the to, from, date, and subject lines): 1/8 of the memo
- *Opening, context, and task* (includes the purpose of the memo, the context and problem, and the specific assignment or task): 1/4 of the memo
- *Summary, discussion segment* (the details that support your ideas or plan): 1/2 of the memo
- *Closing segment, necessary attachments* (the action that you want your reader to take and a notation about what attachments are included): 1/8 of the memo

LEARNING EXERCISE 19.4

Revising a Formal Business Letter
Read the following formal business letter, and assess the quality of the writing. Rewrite the letter so that it is clearly written and professional in nature. Be prepared to read your letter to the class.

Mrs. Joan Watkins
October 19, 2008
Brownie Troop 407
Anywhere, USA 00000

Dear Mrs. Watkins:

I am the official Public Relations Coordinator for County Hospital and serve as correspondence officer for requests from public service groups. We have more than 100 requests such as yours every year, so I have a very busy job! You are welcome to come and visit our hospital anytime. My assistant told me you called yesterday and wondered whether we provide tours. There is no charge for our tours. My assistant also told me the average age of your Brownies is 8 years, so it might be most appropriate to have them visit our NICU, PICU, and ER. Please tell the girls about the units in advance so they'll be better prepared for what they will see. The philosophy at our hospital promotes community involvement, so this is one way we attempt to meet this goal. I'll be sure to arrange to have a nursing manager escort the group on your tour. Please call when you have a date and time in mind. I was a Brownie myself when I was 7 years old, so I think this is a terrific idea on your part.

Sincerely,

Ima Verbose, MSN
Public Relations Coordinator
County Hospital

ELEMENTS OF NONVERBAL COMMUNICATION

Much of our communication occurs through nonverbal channels that must be examined in the context of the verbal content. Generally, if verbal and nonverbal messages are incongruent, the receiver will believe the nonverbal message. Because nonverbal behavior can be and frequently is misinterpreted, receivers must validate perceptions with senders. The incongruence between verbal and nonverbal leads to many communication problems. The following section identifies nonverbal clues that can occur with or without verbal communication.

Space

The study of how space and territory affect communication is called *proxemics* (Loo, n.d.). All of us have an invisible zone of psychological comfort that acts as a buffer against unwanted touching and attacks. The degree of space we require depends on who we are talking to as well as the situation we are in (Loo, n.d.). It also varies according to cultural norms. Some cultures require greater space between sender and receiver than others. In the United States, between 0 and 18 inches of space is typically considered appropriate only for intimate relationships;

between 18 inches and 4 feet is appropriate for personal interactions; between 4 and 12 feet is common for social exchanges, and more than 12 feet is a public distance (Loo, n.d.). Most Americans claim a territorial personal space of about 4 feet.

Proxemics, then, may contribute to the message being sent. Distance may imply a lack of trust or warmth; whereas inadequate space, as defined by cultural norms, may make people feel threatened or intimidated. Likewise, the manager who sits beside employees during performance appraisals sends a different message than the manager who speaks to the employee from the opposite side of a large and formal desk. In this case, distance increases power and status on the part of the manager; however, the receptivity to distance and the message that it implies varies with the culture of the receiver.

Environment

The area where communication takes place is an important part of the communication process. Communication that takes place in a superior's office is generally taken more seriously than that which occurs in the cafeteria.

Appearance

Much is communicated by our clothing, hairstyle, use of cosmetics, and attractiveness. Care should be exercised, however, to be sure that organizational policies regarding desired appearance are both culturally and gender sensitive.

Eye Contact

This nonverbal clue is often associated with sincerity. Eye contact invites interaction. Likewise, breaking eye contact suggests that the interaction is about to cease. Blinking, staring, or looking away when speaking makes it difficult to connect with others emotionally. However, the manager must be aware that like space, the presence or absence of eye contact is strongly influenced by cultural standards.

Posture

Posture and the way that you control the other parts of your body are extremely important. Slouching may be inferred as indifference, and crossing arms across one's chest may suggest defensiveness or aggressiveness. Moreover, the weight of a message is increased if the sender faces the receiver; stands or sits appropriately close; and, with head erect, leans toward the receiver.

Gestures

A message accented with appropriate gestures takes on added emphasis. Too much gesturing can, however, be distracting. For example, hand movement can emphasize or detract from the message. Gestures also have a cultural meaning. Some cultures are more tactile than others. Indeed, the use of touch is one gesture that often sends messages that are misinterpreted by receivers from different cultures.

Facial Expression and Timing

Effective communication requires a facial expression that agrees with your message. Staff perceive managers who present a pleasant and open expression as approachable. Likewise, a nurse's facial expression can greatly affect how and what clients are willing to relate. On the other hand, hesitation often diminishes the effect of your statement or implies untruthfulness.

Vocal Expression

Vocal clues such as tone, volume, and inflection add to the message being transmitted. Tentative statements sound more like questions than statements, leading listeners to think that you are unsure of yourself, and speaking quickly may be interpreted as being nervous. The goal, then, should always be to convey confidence and clarity.

All nurses must be sensitive to nonverbal clues and their importance in communication. This is especially true for nursing leaders. Effective leaders make sure that both verbal and nonverbal communications agree.

 Effective leaders are congruent in their verbal and nonverbal communication so that followers are clear about the messages they receive.

Likewise, leaders are sensitive to nonverbal and verbal messages from followers and look for inconsistencies that may indicate unresolved problems or needs. Often, organizational difficulties can be prevented because leaders recognize the nonverbal communication of subordinates and take appropriate and timely action.

VERBAL COMMUNICATION SKILLS

Highly developed verbal communication skills are critical for the leader–manager. One of the most important verbal communication skills is the art of *assertive communication*. *Assertive behavior* is a way of communicating that allows people to express themselves in direct, honest, and appropriate ways that do not infringe on another person's rights. A person's position is expressed clearly and firmly by using "I" statements. In addition, assertive communication always requires that verbal and nonverbal messages be congruent. To be successful in the directing phase of management, the leader must have well-developed skills in assertive communication.

There are many misconceptions about assertive communication. The first is that all communication is either assertive or passive. Actually, at least four possibilities for communication exist: passive, aggressive, indirectly aggressive or passive–aggressive, or assertive. *Passive communication* occurs when a person suffers in silence although he or she may feel strongly about the issue. *Aggressive* people express themselves in a direct and often hostile manner that infringes on another person's rights; this behavior is generally oriented toward "winning at all costs" or demonstrating self-excellence. *Passive–aggressive communication* is an aggressive message presented in a passive way. It generally involves limited verbal exchange (with incongruent nonverbal behavior) by a person who feels strongly about a situation. This person feigns withdrawal in an effort to manipulate the situation.

The second misconception is that those who communicate or behave assertively get everything they want. This is untrue. Being assertive involves both rights and responsibilities.

The third misconception about assertiveness is that it is unfeminine. Although the role of women in society in general has undergone tremendous change in the last 100 years, some individuals continue to find great difficulty in accepting that the nurse plays an assertive, active, decision-making role. Assertive communication involves conveying a message that insists on being heard.

An assertive communication model helps people to unlearn common self-deprecating speech patterns that signal insecurity and a lack of confidence. The nursing profession must be more assertive in its need to be heard. Eventually, a form of peer pressure can emerge that reshapes others and results in an assertive nursing voice.

> Assertive communication is not rude or insensitive behavior; rather, it is having an informed voice that insists on being heard.

A fourth misconception is that the terms *assertive* and *aggressive* are synonymous. To be assertive is to not be aggressive, although some cultures find the distinction blurred. Even when faced with someone else's aggression, the assertive communicator does not become aggressive. When under attack by an aggressive person, an assertive person can do several things:

- *Reflect.* Reflect the speaker's message back to him or her. Focus on the affective components of the aggressor's message. This helps the aggressor to evaluate whether the intensity of his or her feelings is appropriate to the specific situation or event. For example, assume that an employee enters a manager's office and begins complaining about a newly posted staff schedule. The employee is obviously angry and defensive. The manager might use reflection by stating, "I understand that you are very upset about your schedule. This is an important issue, and we need to talk about it."
- *Repeat the assertive message.* Repeated assertions focus on the message's objective content. They are especially effective when the aggressor overgeneralizes or seems fixated on a repetitive line of thinking. For example, if a manager requests that an angry employee step into his or her office to discuss a problem, and the employee continues his or her tirade in the hallway, the manager might say, "I am willing to discuss this issue with you in my office. The hallway is not the appropriate place for this discussion."
- *Point out the implicit assumptions.* This involves listening closely and letting the aggressor know that you have heard him or her. In these situations, managers might repeat major points or identify key assumptions to show that they are following the employee's line of reasoning.
- *Restate the message by using assertive language.* Rephrasing the aggressor's language will defuse the emotion. Paraphrasing helps the aggressor to focus more on the cognitive part of the message. The manager might use restating by changing a "you" message to an "I" message.
- *Question.* When the aggressor uses nonverbal clues to be aggressive, the assertive person can put this behavior in the form of a question as an effective means of helping the other person become aware of an unwarranted reaction. For example, the desperate, angry employee may imply threats about quitting or transferring to another unit. The manager could appropriately confront the employee about his or her implied threat to see if it is real or simply a reflection of the employee's frustration.

> As in nonverbal communication, the verbal communication skills of the leader–manager in a multicultural workplace require cultural sensitivity.

Even when dealing with staff from the same cultural background, assertive communication requires administrative skill to decide whether to speak face-to-face, send an electronic or paper memo, telephone, or not to communicate about a particular matter at all.

LISTENING SKILLS

Research shows that most people hear or actually retain only a small amount of the information given to them. Generally, although the average person spends more than half of his or her time listening, only one third of the messages sent are retained. It is important that the leader–manager approach listening as an opportunity to learn.

To become better listeners, leaders must first become aware of how their own experiences, values, attitudes, and biases affect how they receive and perceive messages. Second, leaders must overcome the information and communication overload inherent in the middle-management role. It is easy for overwhelmed managers to stop listening actively to the many subordinates who need and demand their time simultaneously.

Finally, the leader must continually work to improve listening skills by giving time and attention to the message sender. The leader's primary purpose is to receive the message being sent rather than forming a response before the transmission of the message is complete.

 The leader who actively listens gives genuine time and attention to the sender, focusing on verbal and nonverbal communication.

GROUP COMMUNICATION

Managers must communicate with large and small groups as well as with individual employees. Because a group communicates differently than individuals do, it is essential that the manager has an understanding of group dynamics, including the sequence that each group must go through before work can be accomplished. Tuckman and Jensen (1977) labeled these stages *forming*, *storming*, *norming*, and *performing*.

When people are introduced into work groups, they must go through a process of meeting each other: the *forming* stage. They then progress through a stage where there is much competition and attempts at the establishment of individual identities: the *storming* stage. Next, the group begins to establish rules and design its work: the *norming* stage. Finally, during the *performing* stage, the work actually gets done. Table 19.1 summarizes each stage.

Some experts suggest that there is another phase: *termination* or *closure*. In this phase, the leader guides members to summarize, express feelings, and come to closure. A celebration at the end of committee work is a good way to conclude group effort.

Because a group's work develops over time, the addition of new members to a committee can slow productivity. It takes some time for the group to accept new members. Some developmental stages will be performed again or delayed if several new members join a group. Therefore, it is important when assigning members to a committee to select those who can remain until the work is finished or until their appointment time is over.

GROUP DYNAMICS

In addition to forming, storming, and norming, two other functions of groups are necessary for work to be performed. One has to do with the task or the purpose of the group, and the other has to do with the maintenance of the group or support functions. Managers should understand how groups carry out their specific tasks and roles.

TABLE 19.1   **Stages of Group Process**

Group Development Stage	Group Process	Task Process
Forming	Testing occurs to identify boundaries of interpersonal behaviors, establish dependency relationships with leaders and other members, and determine what is acceptable behavior.	Testing occurs to identify the tasks, appropriate rules, and methods suited to the task's performance.
Storming	Resistance to group influence is evident as members polarize into subgroups; conflict ensues and members rebel against demands imposed by the leader.	Resistance to task requirements and the differences surface regarding demands imposed by the task.
Norming	Consensus evolves as group cohesion develops; conflict and resistance are overcome.	Cooperation develops as differences are expressed and resolved.
Performing	Interpersonal structure focuses on task and its completion; roles become flexible and functional; energies are directed to task performance.	Problems are solved as the task performance improves; constructive efforts are undertaken to complete task; more of group energies are available for the task.

Group Task Roles

There are 11 tasks that each group performs. A member may perform several tasks, but for the work of the group to be accomplished, all of the necessary tasks will be carried out either by members or by the leader. These roles or tasks follow:

1. *Initiator.* Contributor who proposes or suggests group goals or redefines the problem. There may be more than one initiator during the group's lifetime.
2. *Information seeker.* Searches for a factual basis for the group's work.
3. *Information giver.* Offers an opinion of what the group's view of pertinent values should be.
4. *Opinion seeker.* Seeks opinions that clarify or reflect the value of other members' suggestions.
5. *Elaborator.* Gives examples or extends meanings of suggestions given and how they could work.
6. *Coordinator.* Clarifies and coordinates ideas, suggestions, and activities of the group.
7. *Orienter.* Summarizes decisions and actions; identifies and questions departures from predetermined goals.
8. *Evaluator.* Questions group accomplishments and compares them with a standard.
9. *Energizer.* Stimulates and prods the group to act and raises the level of its actions.
10. *Procedural technician.* Facilitates group action by arranging the environment.
11. *Recorder.* Records the group's activities and accomplishments.

B. T. Chapman suggests a different taxonomy for labeling the roles that are often held by individuals in groups, particularly in terms of having productive meetings (Urseny, 2007). Chapman suggests that there must always be someone in charge who can act as the *group facilitator*. In

DISPLAY 19.3   **B. T. Chapman's Group Roles Taxonomy for Productive Meetings**

- **Facilitator:** Creates the final meeting agenda and estimates the time for each agenda item. Runs the meeting and gives notice when a decision is to be made or when future action is needed.
- **Minutes keeper:** Records the meeting's minutes but does not take down every word. Records directions given, decisions, or actions made and approved by the group.
- **Time keeper:** Keeps the group on schedule by tracking the time allotted for each issue on the agenda. Seeks agreement from the group before allowing discussion on an issue to go over the predesignated time limit.
- **Next agenda person:** Records issues for the next meeting and helps to create the following agenda. Includes on the next agenda who is responsible for what issue and the time that should be allowed for discussion.
- **Action plan keeper:** Records decisions for action in two ways; 30 days or long term. If something must be done before the next meeting, it goes on the 30-day list. More complex projects go on the long-term list, which is reviewed at each meeting.

Source: Urseny, L. (2007, January 26). Sticking to the agenda. *Chico Enterprise Record,* Section E, 4E.

addition, there must be a *minutes keeper, time keeper, next agenda person,* and *action plan keeper.* These roles are further defined in Display 19.3.

Group Building and Maintenance Roles

Group task roles contribute to the work to be done; group-building roles provide for the care and maintenance of the group. Examples of group-building roles include:

- *Encourager.* Accepts and praises all contributions, viewpoints, and ideas with warmth and solidarity.
- *Harmonizer.* Mediates, harmonizes, and resolves conflict.
- *Compromiser.* Yields his or her position in a conflict situation.
- *Gatekeeper.* Promotes open communication and facilitates participation by all members.
- *Standard setter.* Expresses or evaluates standards to evaluate group process.
- *Group commentator.* Records group process and provides feedback to the group.
- *Follower.* Accepts the group's ideas and listens to discussion and decisions.

Organizations need to have a mix of members—enough people to carry out the work but also people who are good at team building. One group may perform more than one function and group-building role.

Individual Roles of Group Members

Group members also carry out roles that serve their own needs. Group leaders must be able to manage member roles so that individuals do not disrupt group productivity. The goal, however, should be management and not suppression. Not every group member has a need that results in the use of one of these roles. The eight individual roles follow:

- *Aggressor.* Expresses disapproval of others' values or feelings through jokes, verbal attacks, or envy.

- *Blocker*. Persists in expressing negative points of view and resurrects dead issues.
- *Recognition seeker*. Works to focus positive attention on himself or herself.
- *Self-confessor*. Uses the group setting as a forum for personal expression.
- *Playboy*. Remains uninvolved and demonstrates cynicism, nonchalance, or horseplay.
- *Dominator*. Attempts to control and manipulate the group.
- *Help seeker*. Uses expressions of personal insecurity, confusion, or self-deprecation to manipulate sympathy from members.
- *Special interest pleader*. Cloaks personal prejudices or biases by ostensibly speaking for others.

 Managers must be well grounded in group dynamics and group roles because of the need to facilitate group communication and productivity within the organization.

While managers must understand group dynamics and roles to facilitate communication and productivity, leaders tend to make an even greater impact on group effectiveness. Dynamic leaders inspire followers toward participative management by how they work and communicate in groups. Leaders keep group members on course, draw out the shy, politely cut off the garrulous, and protect the weak.

LEARNING EXERCISE 19.5

Identifying Group Stages and Roles
Compile a list of the various groups with which you are currently involved. Describe the stage of each one. Did it take longer for some of your groups to get to the performing stage than others? If membership in the group changed, describe what happened to the productivity level. Can you identify which individuals in the group are fulfilling group task roles? Group maintenance and building roles? Individual roles?

COMMUNICATION AND CONFIDENTIALITY

Nurses have a duty to maintain confidential information revealed to them by their patients. This *confidentiality* can be breached legally only when one provider must share information about a patient so that another provider can assume care. In other words, there must be a legitimate professional need to know. The same level of confidentiality that is required to protect patient rights is expected regarding sensitive personal communications between managers and subordinates.

 Confidentiality can be breached legally only when one provider must share information about a patient so that another provider can assume care.

The *1996 Health Insurance Portability and Accountability Act* (HIPAA) calls for strict protections and privacy of medical information. Enactment of HIPAA requires putting in place mechanisms and accountabilities to protect patients' privacy. Violations of HIPAA can result in significant fines for a facility. There is an ethical duty to maintain confidentiality as well. Curtin

(2007), however, suggests that at times, this is more difficult than it sounds. She then recounts a case study whereby a nurse, in assessing whether or not to admit a patient with a history of extreme violence to a mental health unit, contacted other health care facilities in the area to solicit that patient's history of violence toward staff. In soliciting these comments as part of the admission decision, the nurse violated not only HIPAA but also the American Nurses Association Code of Ethics. She also may have violated her nurse practice act. Clearly, the nurse was concerned that the patient's right to privacy could endanger staff and that neither physicians nor nurses should have to make decisions in a vacuum. Yet, legal and professional expectations are clear: The patient's right to privacy must be protected, especially since the nurse already had adequate information about the patient's prior history of violence to know that precautions needed to be taken to protect both the patient and personnel (Curtin, 2007).

Protecting confidentiality and privacy of personal or patient information becomes even more difficult as a result of increased electronic communication because the information available by electronic communication is typically easier to access than traditional information-retrieval methods and because computerized databases are unable to distinguish whether the user has a legitimate right to such information. For example, the federal government has mandated computerized patient records, and many health care organizations are beginning to implement this mandate. Unfortunately, the discussion and determination of who in the organization should have access to what information are often inadequate before such hardware is put in place, and great potential exists for violations of confidentiality. Clearly, any nurse–manager working with clinical information systems has a responsibility to see that confidentiality is maintained and that any breaches in confidentially are dealt with swiftly and appropriately.

LEARNING EXERCISE 19.6

When Personal and Professional Obligations Conflict

You are an RN employed by an insurance company that provides workers' compensation coverage for large companies. Your job requires that you do routine health screening on new employees to identify personal and job-related behaviors that may place these clients at risk for injury or illness and then to counsel them appropriately regarding risk reduction.

One of the areas that you assess during your patient history is high-risk sexual behavior. One of the clients you saw today expressed concern that he might be positive for HIV because a former girlfriend, with whom he had unprotected sex, recently tested positive for HIV. He tells you that he is afraid to be tested "because I don't want to know if I have it." He seems firm on his refusal to be tested. You go ahead and provide him information about HIV testing and what he can do in the future to prevent transmission of the virus to himself and others.

Later that evening, you are having dinner with your 26-year-old sister, and she reveals that she has a "new love" in her life. When she tells you his name and where he works, you immediately recognize him as the client you counseled in the office today.

● ASSIGNMENT: What will you do with the information you have about this client's possible HIV exposure? Will you share it with your sister? What are the legal and ethical ramifications inherent in violating this patient's confidentiality? What are the conflicting personal and professional obligations? Would your action be the same if a casual acquaintance revealed to you that this client was her new boyfriend? Be as honest as possible in your analysis.

INTEGRATING LEADERSHIP AND MANAGEMENT IN ORGANIZATIONAL, INTERPERSONAL, AND GROUP COMMUNICATION

Communication is critical to successful leadership and management. A manager has the formal authority and responsibility to communicate with many people in the organization. Cultural diversity and rapidly flourishing communication technologies also add to the complexity of this organizational communication. Because of this complexity, the manager must understand each unique situation well enough to be able to select the most appropriate internal communication network or channel.

After selecting a communication channel, the manager faces an even greater challenge in communicating the message clearly, either verbally or in writing, in a language appropriate for the message and the receiver. To select the most appropriate communication mode for a specific message, the manager must determine what should be told, to whom, and when. Because communication is a learned skill, managers can improve their written and verbal communication with repetition.

The interpersonal communication skills are more reflective of the leadership role. Sensitivity to verbal and nonverbal communication; recognition of status, power, and authority as barriers to manager–subordinate communication; and consistent use of assertiveness techniques are all leadership skills. Nurse–leaders who are perceptive and sensitive to the environment and people around them have a keen understanding of how the unit is functioning at any time and are able to intervene appropriately when problems arise. Through consistent verbal and nonverbal communication, the nurse–leader is able to be a role model for subordinates.

The integrated leader–manager also uses groups to facilitate communication. Group work is a tool for increasing productivity. All members of work groups should be assisted with role clarification and productive group dynamics.

Organizational communication requires both management functions and leadership skills. Management functions in communication ensure productivity and continuity through appropriate sharing of information. Leadership skills ensure appraisal and intervention in meeting expressed and tacit human resource needs. Leadership skills in communication also allow the leader–manager to clarify organizational goals and direct subordinates in reaching those goals. Communication within the organization would fail if both leadership skills and management functions were not present.

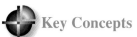 Key Concepts

* *Communication* forms the core of management activities and cuts across all phases of the management process. It is also the core of the nurse–patient, nurse–nurse, and nurse–physician relationship.
* Depending on the manager's position in the hierarchy, the overwhelming majority of managerial time is often directed at some type of organizational communication; thus, organizational communication is a high-level management function.

* Because most managerial communication time is spent speaking and listening, managers must have excellent interpersonal communication skills.
* Communication in large organizations is particularly difficult due to their complexity and size.
* Managers must understand the structure of the organization and recognize whom their decisions will affect. Both formal and informal communication networks need to be considered.
* The clarity of the message is significantly affected by the mode of communication used. In general, the more direct the communication, the greater the probability of clear communication. The more people involved in filtering the communication, the greater the chance of distortion.
* *Written communication* is used most often in large organizations.
* A manager's written communication reflects greatly on both the manager and the organization. Thus, managers must be able to write clearly and professionally and use understandable language.
* The incongruence between verbal and nonverbal messages is the most significant barrier to effective interpersonal communication.
* Effective leaders are congruent in their *verbal* and *nonverbal* communication so that followers are clear about the messages they receive. Likewise, leaders are sensitive to nonverbal and verbal messages from followers and look for inconsistencies that may indicate unresolved problems or needs.
* To be successful in the directing phase of management, the leader must have well-developed skills in *assertive communication.*
* Most people hear or retain only a small amount of the information given to them.
* *Active listening* is an interpersonal communication skill that improves with practice.
* Adding new members to an established group disrupts productivity and group development.
* Group members perform certain important tasks that facilitate work.
* Group members also perform roles that assist with group-building activities.
* Some group members will perform roles to meet their individual needs.
* Rapidly flourishing communication technologies have great potential to increase the efficiency and effectiveness of organizational communication. They also, however, pose increasing challenges to patient confidentiality.

ADDITIONAL LEARNING EXERCISES AND APPLICATIONS

LEARNING EXERCISE 19.7

Writing a Memo

You are a school nurse. In the last 2 weeks, nine cases of head lice have been reported in four different classrooms. The potential for spread is high, and both the teachers and parents are growing anxious.

● ASSIGNMENT: Compose a memo for distribution to the teachers. Your goals are to inform, reassure, and direct future inquiries.

LEARNING EXERCISE 19.8

Identifying and Rephrasing Nonassertive Responses

Decide if the following responses are an example of assertive, aggressive, passive–aggressive, or passive behavior. Change those that you identify as aggressive, passive–aggressive, or passive into assertive responses.

Situation	Response
1. A co-worker withdraws instead of saying what is on his mind. You say:	"I guess you are uncomfortable talking about what's bothering you. It would be better if you talked to me."
2. This is the third time in 2 weeks that your co-worker has asked for a ride home because her car is not working. You say:	"You're taking advantage of me, and I won't stand for it. It's your responsibility to get your car fixed."
3. An attendant at a gas station neglected to replace your gas cap. You return to inquire about it. You say:	"One of the guys here forgot to put my gas cap back on! I want it found now, or you'll buy me a new one."
4. You would like to have a turn at being in charge on your shift. You say to your head nurse:	"Do you think that, ah, you could see your way clear to letting me be in charge once in a while?"
5. A committee meeting is being established. The proposed time is convenient for other people but not for you. The time makes it impossible for you to attend meetings regularly. When you are asked about the time, you say:	"Well, I guess it's OK. I'm not going to be able to attend very much, but it fits into everyone else's schedule."
6. In a conversation, a doctor suddenly asks, "What do you women libbers want anyway?" You respond:	"Fairness and equality."
7. An employee makes a lot of mistakes in his work. You say:	"You're a lazy and sloppy worker!"
8. You are the only woman in a meeting with seven men. At the beginning of the meeting, the Chair asks you to be the secretary. You respond:	"No. I'm sick and tired of being the secretary just because I'm the only woman in the group."
9. A physician asks to borrow your stethoscope. You say:	"Well, I guess so. One of you doctors walked off with mine last week, and this new one cost me $65. Be sure you return it, OK?"
10. You are interpreting the I & O sheet for a physician, and he interrupts you. You say:	"You could understand this if you'd stop interrupting me and listen."

LEARNING EXERCISE 19.9

Memo to Chief Executive Officer Leads to Miscommunication

Carol White, the coordinator for the multidisciplinary mental health outpatient services of a 150-bed psychiatric hospital, feels frustrated because the hospital is very centralized. She

(Learning Exercise continues on page 464)

believes that this keeps the hospital's therapists and nurse–managers from being as effective as they could if they had more authority. Therefore, she has worked out a plan to decentralize her department, giving the therapists and nurse–managers more control and new titles. She sent her new plan to CEO Joe Short and has just received this memo in return.

Dear Ms. White:

The Board of Directors and I met to review your plan and think it is a good one. In fact, we have been thinking along the same lines for quite some time now. I'm sure you must have heard of our plans. Because we recently contracted with a physician's group to cover our crisis center, we believe this would be a good time to decentralize in other ways. We suggest that your new substance abuse coordinator report directly to the new chief of mental health. In addition, we believe your new director of the suicide prevention center should report directly to the chief of mental health. He then will report to me.

I am pleased that we are both moving in the same direction and have the same goals. We will be setting up meetings in the future to iron out the small details.

Sincerely,

Joe Short, CEO

● ASSIGNMENT: How and why did Carol's plan go astray? How did her mode of communication affect the outcome? Could the outcome have been prevented? What communication mode would have been most appropriate for Carol to use in sharing her plan with Joe? What should be her plan now? Explain your rationale.

LEARNING EXERCISE 19.10

Writing a Letter of Reference

Unit managers are frequently asked to write letters of reference for employees who have been terminated. The information used in writing these letters comes from performance evaluations, personal interviews with staff and patients, evidence of continuing education, and personal observations. Assume that you are a unit manager and that you have collected the following information on Mary Doe, an RN who worked at your facility for 3 months before abruptly resigning with 48 hours' notice.

Performance Evaluation

Three-month evaluation scant.
- The following criteria were marked "competent": amount of work accomplished, relationships with patients and co-workers, work habits, and basic skills.
- The following criteria were identified as "needing improvement": quality of work, communication skills, and leadership skills.
- No criteria were marked unsatisfactory or outstanding.
- Narrative comments were limited to the following: "has a bit of a chip on her shoulder," "works independently a lot," and "assessment skills improving."

Interviews with Staff
- Co-worker RN Judy: "She was OK. She was a little strange—she belonged to some kind of traveling religious cult. In fact, I think that's why she left her job."

- Co-worker LVN/LPN Lisa: "Mary was great. She got all her work done. I never had to help her with her meds or AM care. She took her turn at floating, which is more than I can say for some of the other RNs."
- Co-worker RN John: "When I was the charge nurse, I found I needed to seek Mary out to find out what was going on with her patients. It made me real uncomfortable."
- Co-worker LVN/LPN Joe: "Mary hated it here—she never felt like she belonged. The charge nurse was always hassling her about little things, and it really seemed unfair."

Patient Comments
- "She helped me with my bath and got all my pills on time. She was a good nurse."
- "I don't remember her."
- "She was so busy—I appreciated how efficient she was at how she did her job."
- "I remember Mary. She told me she really liked older people. I wish she had had more time to sit down and talk to me."

Notes from Personnel File
Twenty-four years old. Graduated from three-year diploma school two years ago. Has worked in three jobs since that time.

Continuing Education
Current CPR card. No other continuing education completed at this facility.

● ASSIGNMENT: Mary Doe's prospective employer has requested a letter of reference to accompany Mary's application to become a hospice nurse/counselor. No form has been provided, so you must determine an appropriate format. Decide which information you should include in your letter and which should be omitted. Will you weigh some information more heavily than other information? Would you make any recommendations about Mary Doe's suitability for the hospice job? Be prepared to read your letter aloud to the class, and justify your rationale for the content that you included.

LEARNING EXERCISE 19.11

Bringing a Group Together
You are the evening charge nurse of a medical unit. The staff on your unit has voiced displeasure in how requests for days off are handled. Your manager has given you the task of forming a committee and reviewing the present policy regarding requests for days off on the unit. On your committee are four LVNs, three CNAs, and five RNs. All shifts are represented. There are three men among the group members, and there is a fairly broad range of ethnic and cultural groups.

Tomorrow will be your fourth meeting, and you are becoming a bit frustrated because the meetings do not seem to be accomplishing much to reach the objectives that the group was charged to meet. The objective was to develop a fair method to handle special requested days off that were not part of the normal rotation.

On your first meeting, you spent time getting to know the members and identified the objective. Various committee members contacted other hospitals, and others did a literature search to determine how other institutions handled this matter. During the second meeting,

(Learning Exercise continues on page 466)

this material was reviewed by all members. At the last meeting, the group was very contentious. In fact, several raised their voices. Others sat quietly, and some seemed to pout. Only the three men could agree upon anything. One LVN thought that the RNs were too overly represented. One RN thought that the policy for day-off requests should be separated into three different policies—one for each classification. You are not sure how to bring this committee together or what, if any, action you should take.

● ASSIGNMENT: Review the section in this chapter about how groups work. Write a one-page essay on what is happening in the group, and answer the following questions. Should you add members to the committee? Does your group have too many task members and not enough team-building members? What should be your role in getting the group to perform its task? What could be some strategies you could use that would perhaps bring the group together?

Web Links

Communication Test
http://www.queendom.com/tests/relationships/communication_skills_r_access.html
This 34-question communication test takes 15 to 20 minutes to complete and is designed to evaluate your general level of communication skills.

University of Wisconsin Eau-Claire, Counseling Office
http://www.uwec.edu/Counsel/pubs/assertivecommunication.htm
This site provides a self-help introduction to assertive communication skills.

Dictionary of Gestures, Signs, and Body Language Cues
http://members.aol.com/nonverbal2/diction1.htm
This is a nonverbal dictionary of gestures, signs, and body language cues.

References

Answers.com. (n.d.). *Definition of communication.* Retrieved January 26, 2007, from *http://www.answers.com/topic/communication.*

Curtin, L. (2007). When patient privacy endangers staff. *American Nurse Today, 2*(1), 16–18.

Electronic Health Record Vendors Association (EHRVA). (2006, October). *HIMSS EHRVA definitional model and application process.* Retrieved January 30, 2007, from *http://www.himssehrva.org/docs/EHRVA_application.pdf.*

Grossman, S. C., & Valiga, T. M. (2005). *The new leadership challenge. Creating the future of nursing* (2nd ed.). Philadelphia: FA Davis Co.

Hamm, J. (2006, May). The five messages leaders must manage. *Harvard Business Review–Online Version.* Retrieved February 9, 2007, from *http://harvardbusinessonline.hbsp.harvard.edu/hbsp/hbr/articles/article.jsp?ml_action=getarticle&articleID-*

R0605G &ml_issueid=BR0605&ml_page=1&ml_subscriber= true& productId=R0605G&_requestid=48306.

Huston, C. J. (2006). Technology in the health care workplace: Benefits, limitations, and challenges. In *Professional issues in nursing: Challenges and opportunities.* Philadelphia: Lippincott Williams & Wilkins.

Loo, T. (n.d.) *How to communicate using space.* Retrieved January 29, 2007, from *http://hodu.com/space.shtml.*

Manning, M. L. (2006). Improving clinical communication through structured conversation. *Nursing Economics, 24*(5), 268–271.

Perkins, C. (2007, January 11). *Memo writing.* The OWL at Purdue. Retrieved February 21, 2007, from *http://owl.english.purdue.edu/owl/resource/590/01/.*

Rudan, V. T. (2003). The best of both worlds: A consideration of gender in team building. *Journal of Nursing Administration, 33*(3), 179–186.

Thompson, S. (2007, January 21). *Tips for writing a good memo in business communication*. EZine Articles. Retrieved February 29, 2007, from *http://ezinearticles.com/?Tips-for-Writing-a-Good-Memo-in-Business-Communication&id=424965*.

Tuckman, B. W., & Jensen, M. A. C. (1977). Stages of small group development revisited. *Group and Organization Studies, 2*(4), 419.

Urseny, L. (2007, January 26). Sticking to the agenda. *Chico Enterprise Record*, Section E, 4E.

Watson Wyatt Worldwide. (2007). *Effective communication: A leading indicator of financial performance—2006/2006. Communication ROI Study*. Retrieved January 19, 2007, from *http://www.watsonwyatt.com/research/resrender.asp?id=w-868&page=1*.

Writing Help Central. (2006). *Letter writing tips and resources*. Retrieved February 20, 2007, from *http://www.writinghelp-central.com/letter-writing.html*.

Bibliography

Andrade, P. D. (2006, August-October). Effective communication in palliative care: A nurse's responsibility and privilege. *DNA Reporter, 31*(3), 16.

Ang, R. (2006, Spring). SBAR: A communications framework and technique . . . situation, background, assessment, and recommendation. *SCI Nursing, 23*(1).

Clarke A., & Ross H. (2006, March). Influences on nurses' communications with older people at the end of life: Perceptions and experiences of nurses working in palliative care and general medicine. *International Journal of Older People Nursing, 1*(1), 34–43.

Drapkin, J. (2005, November-December). The fine art of gossip. *Psychology Today, 38*(6), 58, 60.

Duda, J. M. (2006, May 8). Learn to listen: Why communication skills are essential. *NurseWeek California, 19*(10), 56–58.

Friedman, N. (2006, August). The telephone doctor. How to handle the foreign accent. *Podiatry Management, 25*(6), 253–254.

Gaddis, S. (2006, April-June). Direct versus indirect communication: How to choose the style that's right for you. *New Mexico Nurse, 51*(2), 11.

Henwood, S. (2006, October). The key to communication. *Synergy*, 20–25.

Ishikawa, H., Hashimoto, H., Kinoshita, M., Fujimori, S., Shimizu, T., & Yano, E. (2006, December). Evaluating medical students' non-verbal communication during the objective structured clinical examination. *Medical Education, 40*(12), 1180–1187.

Krupat, E., Frankel, R., Stein T., & Irish J. (2006, July). The four habits coding scheme: Validation of an instrument to assess clinicians' communication behavior. *Patient Education and Counseling, 62*(1), 38–45.

Lobchuk, M. M. (2006, May). Concept analysis of perspective-taking: Meeting informal caregiver needs for communication competence and accurate perception. *Journal of Advanced Nursing, 54*(3), 330–341.

Lorin, S., Rho, L., Wisnivesky, J. P., & Nierman, D. M. (2006, September). Improving medical student intensive care unit communication skills: A novel educational initiative using standardized family members. *Critical Care Medicine, 34*(9), 2386–2391.

McCarthy, A., Lee, K., Itakura, S., & Muir D. W. (2006, November). Cultural display rules drive eye gaze during thinking. *Journal of Cross-Cultural Psychology, 37*(6), 717–722.

Miller, S. (2006). *Conversation: A history of a declining art.* New Haven, CT: Yale University Press.

Nishizawa, Y., Saito, M., Ogura, N., Kudo, S., Saito K., & Hanaya M. (2006, June). The non-verbal communication skills of nursing students: Analysis of interpersonal behavior using videotaped recordings in a 5-minute interaction with a simulated patient. *Japan Journal of Nursing Science, 3*(1), 15–22.

Patten, C. W. Jr., & Kammer, R. M. (2006, May). Better communication with minority patients: Seven strategies for achieving cultural competency. *Community Oncology, 3*(5), 295–298, 302.

Pew Internet project report on bloggers. (2006, September-October). *CIN: Computers, Informatics, Nursing, 24*(5), 246–247.

Röndahl, G., Innala, S., & Carlsson, M (2006, November). Heterosexual assumptions in verbal and non-verbal communication in nursing. *Journal of Advanced Nursing, 56*(4), 373–381.

Sitzman, K. (2006, May). Reducing negative workplace gossip. *AAOHN Journal, 54*(5), 240.

Thornby, D. (2006, July-September). Beginning the journey to skilled communication. *AACN Advanced Critical Care, 17*(3), 266–271.

20

Delegation

. . . delegation is both an art and a science. It includes cognitive, affective, and intuitive dimensions.

—*Marjorie Barter (2002)*

. . . at its most basic, delegation is empowering one person to act for another.

—*Susanne A. Quallich (2005)*

Delegation can be defined simply as getting work done through others or as directing the performance of one or more people to accomplish organizational goals. More complex definitions of delegation, supervision, and assignment, however, have been created by the American Nurses Association (ANA) and the National Council of State Boards of Nursing (NCBSN) in response to the emerging complexity of delegation in today's health care arena, where increasing numbers of unlicensed and relatively untrained workers provide direct patient care. Both the ANA and the NCBSN have defined delegation differently (Huston, 2006).

The ANA defines delegation as the transfer of responsibility for the performance of a task from one person to another. The NCBSN defines delegation as transferring to a competent individual the authority to perform a selected nursing task in a selected situation. This second definition suggests that delegation is complex, requiring insight and judgment regarding the environment in which the delegation is to take place and the individuals involved.

Delegation is an essential element of the directing phase of the management process because much of the work accomplished by managers (first-, middle-, and top-level managers) occurs not only through their own efforts but also through those of their subordinates. For the manager, delegation is not an option but a necessity. Frequently, there is too much work to be accomplished by one person. In these situations, delegation often becomes synonymous with productivity.

There are many good reasons for delegating. Sometimes, managers must delegate routine tasks so they are free to handle problems that are more complex or require a higher level of expertise. Managers may delegate work if someone else is better prepared or has greater expertise or knowledge about how to solve a problem. Delegation can also be used to provide learning or "stretching" opportunities for subordinates. Subordinates who are not delegated enough responsibility may become bored, nonproductive, and ineffective. Thus, in delegating, the leader–manager contributes

DISPLAY 20.1 Leadership Roles and Management Functions Associated With Delegation

Leadership Roles

1. Functions as a role model, supporter, and resource person in delegating tasks to subordinates
2. Encourages followers to use delegation as a time management strategy and team-building tool
3. Assists followers in identifying situations appropriate for delegation
4. Communicates clearly and assertively in delegating tasks
5. Maintains patient safety as a minimum criterion in determining the most appropriate person to carry out a delegated task
6. Is an informed and active participant in the development of local, state, and national guidelines for UAP scope of practice
7. Is sensitive to how cultural phenomena affect transcultural delegation

Management Functions

1. Creates job descriptions and scope of practice statements for all personnel, including UAP, that conform to national, state, and professional recommendations for ensuring safe patient care
2. Is knowledgeable regarding legal liabilities of subordinate supervision
3. Accurately assesses subordinates' capabilities and motivation when delegating
4. Delegates a level of authority necessary to complete delegated tasks
5. Develops and implements a periodic review process for all delegated tasks
6. Provides recognition or reward for the completion of delegated tasks

to employees' personal and professional development. The leadership roles and management functions inherent in delegation are shown in Display 20.1.

COMMON DELEGATION ERRORS

Delegation is a critical leadership skill that must be learned. Kleinman and Saccomano (2006) state that the nurse must be taught delegation skills, both in academic and clinical settings. Further, they maintain that the decision to delegate should be consistent with the steps of the nursing process and based on an analysis of patient's needs and circumstances. Frequent mistakes made by managers in delegating include underdelegating, overdelegating, and improper delegating (Display 20.2).

Underdelegating

Underdelegating frequently stems from the manager's false assumption that delegation may be interpreted as a lack of ability on his or her part to do the job correctly or completely. Delegation does not need to limit the manager's control, prestige, and power; rather, delegation can extend the manager's influence and capability by increasing what can be accomplished.

DISPLAY 20.2 **Common Delegating Errors**

Underdelegating
Overdelegating
Improper delegating

Another frequent cause of underdelegating is the manager's desire to complete the whole job personally due to a lack of trust in the subordinates; the manager believes that he or she needs the experience or that he or she can do it better and faster than anyone else. It is important to remember that time spent in training another to do a job can be repaid 10-fold in the future. In addition to increased productivity, delegation can also provide the opportunity for subordinates to experience feelings of accomplishment and enrichment. An additional cause of underdelegation is the fear that subordinates will resent having work delegated to them. Properly delegated work actually increases employee satisfaction and fosters a cooperative working relationship between managers and staff (Quallich, 2005).

 The right to delegate and the ability to provide formal rewards for successful completion of delegated tasks are a reflection of the legitimate authority inherent in the management role.

Managers also may underdelegate because they lack experience in the job or in delegation itself. Other managers refuse to delegate because they have an excessive need to control or be perfect. The manager who accepts nothing less than perfection limits the opportunities available for subordinate growth and often wastes time redoing delegated tasks.

Some novice managers emerging from the clinical nurse role underdelegate because they find it difficult to assume the manager role. This occurs, in part, because the nurses have been rewarded in the past for their clinical expertise and not their management skills. As managers come to understand and accept the need for the hierarchical responsibilities of delegation, they become more productive and develop more positive staff relationships.

Overdelegating

In contrast to underdelegating, which overburdens the manager, some managers *overdelegate*, burdening their subordinates. Some managers overdelegate because they are poor managers of time, spending most of it just trying to get organized. Others overdelegate because they feel insecure in their ability to perform a task. Managers also must be careful not to overdelegate to exceptionally competent employees, because they may become overworked and tired, which can decrease their productivity.

Improper Delegating

Improper delegation includes such things as delegating at the wrong time, to the wrong person, or for the wrong reason. It also may include delegating tasks and responsibilities that are beyond the capability of the person to whom they are being delegated or that should be done by the manager.

Delegating decision making without providing adequate information also is an example of improper delegation. If the manager requires a higher quality than *satisficing*, this must be made clear at the time of the delegation. Not everything that is delegated needs to be handled in a maximizing mode.

EFFECTIVE DELEGATING

Although some managers balk at the idea of sharing enough information or authority for delegation to be effective, a variety of strategies can be implemented to ensure effective delegation.

Plan Ahead

Plan ahead when identifying tasks to be accomplished. Assess the situation, and clearly delineate the desired outcomes.

Identify Necessary Skills and Levels

Identify the skill or educational level necessary to complete the job. Often, legal and licensing statutes determine this. Although, Quallich (2005) maintains that many state's nurse practice acts (NPAs) may address the issue of delegation vaguely, it is still essential for nurses to be aware of their state NPA essential elements regarding delegation, including the following:
- The state's NPA definition of delegation
- Items that cannot be delegated
- Items that cannot be routinely delegated
- Guidelines for RNs about tasks that can be delegated
- A description of professional nursing practice
- A description of LVN/LPN nursing practice and unlicensed nursing roles
- The degree of supervision required to complete a task
- The guidelines for lowering delegation risks
- Warnings about inappropriate delegation
- If there is a restricted use of the word "nurse" to licensed staff

The manager should know the official job description expectations for each worker classification in the organization, as they may be more restrictive than the state NPA.

Select Most Capable Personnel

Identify the qualified person best able to complete the job in terms of capability and time to do so. Managers should ask the individuals to whom they are delegating if they are capable of completing the delegated task but should also validate this perception by direct observation. It also is important that the person to whom the task is being delegated considers the task to be important.

Communicate Goal Clearly

Managers should encourage employees to attempt to solve problems themselves; however, employees often need to ask questions about the task or to clarify the desired outcome. When this happens, the manager should clearly communicate what is to be done, including the purpose for doing so, and verify comprehension. The manager should also include any limitations or qualifications that have been imposed. Although the desired end product should be specified, it is important to give the subordinate feedback and an appropriate degree of autonomy in deciding exactly how the work can be accomplished.

Empower the Delegate

Delegate the authority and the responsibility necessary to complete the task. Nothing is more frustrating to a creative and productive employee than not having the resources or authority to carry out a well-developed plan.

Responsibility is shared when a task is delegated.

Set Deadlines and Monitor Progress

Set time lines, and monitor how the task is being accomplished through informal but regularly scheduled meetings. This shows an interest on the part of the manager, provides for a periodic review of progress, and encourages ongoing communication to clarify any questions or misconceptions. Research by Kalisch (2006) suggests that adverse patient outcomes such as missed care occur when delegation is ineffective. The researcher found that (a) failure to obtain a buy-in to the delegated task by the individual being delegated to, (b) failure to retain accountability, and (c) lack of conflict management skills led to poor patient outcomes. Monitoring delegated tasks keeps the delegated task before the subordinate and the manager so that both share accountability for its completion. Although the final responsibility belongs to the manager, the subordinate doing the task accepts responsibility for completing it appropriately and is accountable to the manager.

Model the Role and Provide Guidance

If the subordinate is having difficulty carrying out the delegated task, the manager should be available as a role model and resource in helping to identify alternative solutions. The manager should also convey a feeling of confidence and encouragement. Reassuming the delegated task should be a manager's last resort, because this action fosters a sense of failure in the employee and demotivates rather than motivates. Delegation is useless if the manager is unwilling to allow divergence in problem solving and thus re-does all work that has been delegated. However, the manager may need to delegate work previously assigned to an employee so that the employee has time to do the newly assigned task.

Evaluate Performance

Evaluate the subordinate's performance after the task has been completed. Include positive and negative aspects of how the person has completed the task. Were the outcomes achieved? Quallich (2005) states that specific feedback can provide a chance for personal and professional growth. Without this feedback, delegators and subordinates are unable to have a mutually trusting and productive relationship.

DISPLAY 20.3   Steps to Successful Delegation

Understanding the principles of delegation:
Ability to communicate clearly
Capacity to see the value that delegation has in developing others
Building trust and self-esteem
Recognizing that different personalities and capabilities exist
Acknowledging the following:
- Right person
- Right task
- Right circumstances
- Right direction and communication
- Right supervision and evaluation

Source: Reprinted from *Urologic Nursing*, 2005, *25*(2), 121. Reprinted with permission of the publisher, the Society of Urologic Nurses and Associates, Inc. (SUNA), East Holly Avenue, Box 56, Pitman, NJ 08071–0056; (856) 256-2300; FAX (856) 589-7463; email: *uronsg@ajj.com*; website: *http:// www.suna.org/*.

Reward Accomplishment

Be sure to appropriately reward a successfully completed task. Leaders today are often measured by the successes of those on their teams. Therefore, the more recognition team members receive, the more recognition will be given to their leader.

> The mark of a great leader is when he or she can recognize the excellent performance of someone else and allow others to shine for their accomplishments.

LEARNING EXERCISE 20.1

Difficulty in Delegation
Is it difficult for you to delegate to others? If so, do you know why? Are you more apt to underdelegate, overdelegate, or delegate improperly? Think back to the last thing you delegated. Was this delegation successful? What safeguards can you build in to decrease this delegation error?

Delegation is a high-level skill essential to the manager; delegation improves with practice. As managers gain the maturity and self-confidence needed to delegate wisely, they increase their impact and power both within and outside the organization. Subordinates gain self-esteem and increased job satisfaction from the responsibility and authority given to them, and the organization moves a step closer toward achieving its goals. Display 20.3 lists steps to successful delegation.

DELEGATION AS A FUNCTION OF PROFESSIONAL NURSING

With the restructuring of care delivery models, RNs at all levels are increasingly being expected to make assignments for and supervise the work of different levels of employees. To increase the likelihood that increased delegation, which is required in today's restructured health care organizations, does not result in creating an unsafe work environment, organizations should take appropriate action. Huston (2006) suggests that (a) organizations have a clearly defined structure where RNs are recognized as leaders of the health care team, (b) job descriptions clearly define the roles and responsibilities of all, (c) educational programs are developed to help personnel learn roles and responsibilities of each others roles, and (d) adequate programs are developed to foster leadership and delegation.

RNs who are asked to assume the role of supervisor and delegator need preparation to assume these leadership tasks. Some RNs who supervise subordinates, especially those who practiced only in the 1980s, have experienced only total RN staffing or primary nursing systems of care delivery. Thus, they have received little or no instruction in personnel supervision and delegation principles. Repeated education programs on delegation principles and role clarity are necessary for RNs to demonstrate consistency in delegating appropriate role activities and to begin to feel confident in delegating because in many cases, nurses who are well prepared to provide care for patients may not be well prepared to be a delegator.

 The RN, although well trained in the role of direct care provider, is often inadequately prepared for the role of delegator.

In addition, nursing schools and health care organizations need to do a better job of preparing professional RNs for the delegator role. This includes educating professional nurses about the NPA governing the scope of practice in their state; basic principles of delegating to the right person, at the right time and for the right reason; and actions that must be undertaken when work is delegated in an inappropriate or unsafe manner.

LEARNING EXERCISE 20.2

Assessing Nurses' Comfort With Delegation
Informally survey nurses in the agency in which you work or do clinical practicums. How many of them have received formal education on delegation principles? How comfortable do these nurses feel in determining what should be delegated to whom? How comfortable do you feel in delegating work to other members of the health care team?

Delegating to Unlicensed Assistive Personnel

In an effort to contain spiraling health care costs, many health care providers in the 1990s chose to eliminate RN positions or to replace licensed professional nurses with *unlicensed assistive personnel* (UAP). The term *UAP* includes but is not limited to nurse extenders, care partners, nurse's aides, orderlies, assistants, attendants, and technicians (Huston, 2006).

Almost all RNs in acute-care institutions and long-term care facilities are currently involved in some capacity with the assignment, delegation, and supervision of the UAP in the delivery of nursing care. The primary argument for utilizing the UAP in acute-care settings is cost (although the current professional nursing shortage is a contributing factor). UAP can free professional nurses from tasks and assignments (specifically, non-nursing functions) that can be completed by less extensively trained personnel at a lower cost.

Assuming the role of delegator and supervisor to the UAP, however, increases the scope of liability for the RN. Although nurses are not automatically held liable for all acts of negligence on the part of those they supervise, they may be held liable if they were negligent in the supervision of those employees at the time they committed the negligent acts. Liability is based on a supervisor's failure to determine which patient needs could safely be assigned to a subordinate or for failing to closely monitor a subordinate who requires such supervision. In delegating, the RN needs to know well the skills of the person to whom work is delegated. The liability of supervision was discussed in Chapter 5.

 In assigning tasks to the UAP, the RN must be aware of the job description, knowledge base, and demonstrated skills of each person.

RNs should recognize that although the Omnibus Budget Reconciliation Act of 1987 established regulations for the education and certification of nurse's aides (minimum of 75 hours of theory and practice and successful completion of an examination in both areas), no federal or community standards have been established for training the more broadly defined UAP (Huston, 2006). Some standards and guidelines are now required for the preparation and use of UAP in certified home health agencies and skilled nursing facilities, but there are no required education standards or guidelines for the use of UAP in acute-care hospitals that cross state lines and jurisdictions.

This does not imply that all UAP are uneducated and unprepared for the roles they have been asked to fill. Indeed, UAP educational levels vary from less than a high school graduate to those holding advanced degrees (Case, 2004). It merely suggests that the RN, in delegating to a UAP, must carefully assess what skills and knowledge that each UAP has or risk increased personal liability for the failure to do so (Huston, 2006).

Unfortunately, many institutions do not have distinct job descriptions for the UAP that clearly define their scope of practice. While some institutions limit the scope of practice for the UAP to non-nursing functions, some organizations allow the UAP to perform many skills traditionally reserved for the licensed nurse. According to Kleinman and Soccamano (2006), "this model of practice is considered a viable alternative to care provided primarily by registered nurses and demand for UAP is only expected to grow" (p. 163).

UAP usually have little background in health care and only rudimentary training. Yet they may insert catheters, read electrocardiograms, suction tracheostomy tubes, change sterile dressings, and perform other traditional nursing functions. To keep patients from becoming unduly alarmed, some hospitals now prohibit employees from wearing name badges that identify their titles (Huston, 2006).

Some agencies interpret regulations broadly, allowing UAP a broader scope of practice than that advocated by professional nursing associations or state boards of nursing. In a 1998 survey of 53 state and territorial boards of nursing, a majority of states reported that they had regulations and guidelines for RNs who supervised the UAP and regulations that protected the use of the RN title (Huston, 2006). Few states used the ANA or NCSBN definitions for delegation, supervision, or assignment. Most states, however, reported no standardized curriculum in place for the UAP employed in acute-care hospitals, and more than half the states reported that no plans existed for developing such a curriculum (Huston, 2006).

Some state boards of nursing, in an effort to more clearly define the scope of practice for UAP, have issued task lists for UAP. Training of the UAP is not based on the notion that such individuals will be performing activities independently. Task lists, however, suggest no need for delegation,

EXAMINING THE EVIDENCE 20.1

Source: Potter, P., & Grant, E. (2004). Understanding RN and unlicensed assistive personnel working relationships in designing care delivery strategies. *Journal of Nursing Administration, 34*(1), 19–25.

This qualitative study investigated the relationship between RNs and UAP and the impact this had on patient care delivery. Twenty-two staff (13 RNs and 9 UAP) were asked to tell stories of "good" or "difficult" working relationships and the care delivery practices on their units.

Trust was found to be central for good relationships. The study also found that there was no standardized approach used by the RNs in proving shift reports to the UAP. The study concluded that successful partnering occurs when there is a shared patient care focus, ready access to one another during the course of the shift, and a *means for ongoing* and timely communication.

as the UAP already has a list of nursing activities that he or she may perform without waiting for the delegation process. But what happens when the condition of a client changes? Is the UAP with fewer than 75 hours of training astute enough to recognize that there has been a change in the client's condition and alert the RN?

Research by Potter and Grant (2004) highlights another concern for the RN in supervising the UAP. Their research examined the working relationships between the UAP and RNs. They found that there was no standardized approach used by RNs in providing beginning shift report to the UAP, and the UAP were often assigned to work with multiple RNs on a given shift. Examining the Evidence 20.1 describes the results of this study.

It is critical, then, that the RN never loses sight of his or her ultimate responsibility for ensuring that patients receive appropriate, high-quality care. This means that while the UAP may complete non-nursing functions such as bathing, vital signs, and the measurement and recording of intake and output, it is the RN who must analyze that information and then use the nursing process to see that desired patient outcomes are achieved. Only RNs have the formal authority to practice nursing, and activities that rely on the nursing process or require specialized skill, expert knowledge, or professional judgment should never be delegated (Kleinman & Saccomano, 2006).

The outcomes associated with the increased use of UAP are not yet known. An increasing number of studies suggest a direct link between decreased RN staffing and declines in patient outcomes. Some of these declines in patient outcomes noted in the literature include an increased incidence of patient falls, nosocomial infections, and medication errors (Huston, 2006). Hall, Doran, and Pink (2004) also found that the lower the proportion of professional nursing staff employed on a unit, the higher the number of medication errors and wound infections. Similarly, Dunton, Gajewski, Taunton, and Moore (2004) reported that higher fall rates were associated with fewer nursing hours per patient-day and a lower percentage of RNs.

Certainly, at some point, given the increasing complexity of health care and the increasing acuity of patient illnesses, there is a maximum representation of UAP in the staffing mix that should not be breached. Until those levels are determined, RNs can expect a continued increase in the utilization of UAP. To protect their patients and their professional license, RNs must continue to seek current information regarding national efforts to standardize scope of practice for UAP and professional guidelines regarding what can be safely delegated to the UAP.

Quallich (2005) developed a guide to assist nurses in determining situations where delegation can appropriately be instituted. Although this list was for a urological unit, it is an example of the type of guidelines that should be available on all units when delegating to UAP (Display 20.4). Most importantly, the guide gives examples of tasks that cannot be delegated. Some examples of professional responsibilities include patent assessment, care planning, patient teaching, patient outcome evaluation, and interpretation of test results.

DISPLAY 20.4 To Delegate or Not to Delegate: Is This Really the Question?

Various nursing tasks can be appropriately delegated, after considering:
- Patient condition, especially stability
- Patient capacity for self-care
- Complexity of the task
- Repetitive nature of the task
- Technical nature of the task
- Skills and experience of the UAP
- Medical technology involved
- Infection control/safety precautions involved
- Predictability of outcome
- RN supervision available
- Extent of interaction with the patient
- Environment (such as ICU vs. rehab unit)
- Potential for harm

Examples of tasks that can be delegated:
- Answering phones
- Cleaning up after procedures
- Patient transportation (stable patients)
- Ordering supplies and other clerical tasks
- Stocking procedure and exam rooms
- Assisting with procedures
- Data collection without analysis (such as vital signs, performing ECGs)

Examples of tasks that cannot be delegated:
- Any task that would involve nursing judgment or sophisticated application of the nursing process
- Initial assessment on new patients
- Assessing pain
- Teaching injections
- Evaluating success of a treatment
- Interpreting test results
- Establishing plans of care
- Identifying needs
- Triage
- Counseling and teaching

Source: Reprinted from *Urologic Nursing*, 2005, *25*(2), 122. Reprinted with permission of the publisher, the Society of Urologic Nurses and Associates, Inc. (SUNA), East Holly Avenue, Box 56, Pitman, NJ 08071-0056; (856) 256-2300; FAX (856) 589-7463; email: *uronsg@ajj.com*: website: *http://www.suna.org/*.

Subordinate Resistance to Delegation

Resistance is a common response by subordinates to delegation. One of the most common causes of subordinate resistance to, or refusal of, delegated tasks is the failure of the delegator to see the subordinate's perspective. Workloads assigned to the UAP are generally highly challenging, both physically and mentally. In addition, the UAP frequently must adapt rapidly to changing priorities, often imposed on him or her by more than one delegator. If the subordinate is truly overwhelmed, additional delegation of tasks is inappropriate, and the RN should reexamine the necessity of completing the delegated task personally or finding someone else who is able to complete the task.

Some subordinates resist delegation simply because they believe that they are incapable of completing the delegated task. If the employee is capable but lacks self-confidence, the astute leader may be able to use performance coaching to empower the subordinate and build self-confidence levels. If, however, the employee is truly at high risk for failure, the appropriateness of the delegation must be questioned and a task more appropriate to that employee's ability level should be delegated.

Another cause of subordinate resistance to delegation is an inherent resistance to authority. Some subordinates simply need to "test the water" and determine what the consequences are of not completing delegated tasks. In this case, the delegator must be calm but assertive about his or her expectations and provide explicit work guidelines, if necessary, to maintain an appropriate authority power gap. It is an ongoing leadership challenge to instill a team spirit between delegators and their subordinates.

Finally, resistance to delegation may be occurring because tasks are overdelegated in terms of specificity. All subordinates need to believe that there is some room for creativity and independent thinking in delegated tasks. Failure to allow for this human need results in disinterested subordinates who fail to internalize responsibility and accountability for the delegated task. When delegating to the UAP, the RN should try to mix routine and boring tasks with more challenging and rewarding assignments. An additional strategy is to provide the UAP with consistent, constructive feedback, both positive and negative, to foster growth and self-esteem.

When subordinates resist delegation, the delegator may be tempted to avoid confrontation and simply do the delegated task independently. This is seldom appropriate. Instead, the delegator must ascertain why the delegated task was not accomplished and take appropriate action to eliminate these restraining forces.

LEARNING EXERCISE 20.3

Dealing With Resistance to Delegation
You are the team leader for ten patients. An experienced LVN/LPN and nurse's aide are also assigned to the team. It is an extremely busy day, and there is a great deal of work to be done. Several times today, you have found the LVN/LPN taking long breaks in the lounge or chatting socially at the front desk, despite the unmet needs of many patients. On those occasions, you have clearly delegated work tasks and time lines to her. Several hours later, you follow up on the delegated tasks and find that they were not completed. When you seek out the LVN/LPN, you find that she went to lunch without telling you or the aide. You are furious at her apparent disregard for your authority.

● ASSIGNMENT: What are possible causes of the LVN/LPN's failure to follow up on delegated tasks? How will you deal with this LVN/LPN? What goal serves as the basis for your actions? Justify your choice with rationale.

Delegating to a Transcultural Work Team

Davidhizar and Shearer (2005) maintain that the diversity of the nursing population is steadily increasing. This increased diversity has ramifications in delegation. Challenges in delegation are seen both for the cultural diverse delegatee as well as the delegator. According to Giger and Davidhizar (2004), there are six cultural phenomena that must be considered when working with staff from a culturally diverse background: communication, space, social organization, time, environmental control, and biologic variations.

Communication, the first of the cultural phenomena, is greatly affected by cultural diversity in the workforce because dialect, volume, use of touch, context of speech, and kinesics such as gestures, stance, and eye movement all influence how messages are sent and received. For example, delegation delivered in a softer tone may be perceived as less important than delegation received in a loud tone, even if the delegated tasks have equal importance. Similarly, a manager may make an inappropriate assumption about a person's inability to carry out an important delegated task if that person represents a culture that values softer speech and more passive behavior.

Space is the second cultural phenomenon influencing delegation. Space refers to the distance and intimacy techniques that are used when relating verbally or nonverbally to others (Giger & Davidhizar, 2004). It is important, that the delegator recognizes the personal space needs of each staff member and acts accordingly. If these space needs are not recognized and respected, the likelihood that a delegated task will be heard and followed through on appropriately will be reduced.

The third cultural phenomenon, *social organization*, refers to the importance of a group or unit in providing social support in a person's life. For many cultures, the family unit is the most important social organization. In some cultures, the duty to family always takes precedence over the needs of the organization. In other cultures, this values ranking is less clear, and the employee may experience great intrapersonal conflict in prioritizing delegated work tasks and obligations to the family unit. It is important, then, that the delegator is aware that employees' values differ and is sensitive in delegating critical tasks to employees who are experiencing stress in the family unit.

Time is the fourth cultural phenomenon affecting delegation. Cultural groups can be past, present, or future oriented. *Past-oriented cultures* are interested in preserving the past and maintaining tradition. *Present-oriented cultures* focus on maintaining the *status quo* and on daily operations. *Future-oriented cultures focus* on goals to be achieved and are more visionary in their approach to problems. For example, strategic planning might best be delegated to a person from a future-oriented culture, although the leader–manager should always be alert for opportunities to create new insight and stretching opportunities for subordinates.

Environmental control, the fifth cultural phenomenon, refers to the person's perception of control over his or her environment (internal *locus of control*). Some cultures believe more strongly in fate, luck, or chance than other cultures, and this may affect how a person approaches and carries out a delegated task. The person who believes that he or she has an internal locus of control is more likely to be creative and autonomous in decision making.

The final phenomenon, *biological variations*, refers to the biopsychosocial differences between racial and ethnic groups, such as susceptibility to disease and physiological differences. Display 20.5 provides a summary of considerations when delegating to a transcultural work team.

All of these cultural phenomena have the potential to affect the relationship between the delegator and his or her subordinates as well as the understanding and implementation of the delegated task. However, Robb and Douglas (2004) warn that labeling others as different, for example in their

DISPLAY 20.5   Cultural Phenomena to Consider When Delegating to a
                Transcultural Team

Communication: Especially dialect, volume, use of touch and eye contact
Space: Interpersonal space differs between cultures
Social organization: Family unit of primary importance in some cultures
Time: Cultures tend to be past, present, or future oriented
Environmental control: Cultures often have either internal or external locus of control
Biological variations: Susceptability to diseases (e.g., Tay-Sachs) and physiological
    differences (e.g., height, color)

communication style, raises fundamental questions about the nature of cultural and other "differences." Labeling a group of people as "different" can be seen as an exercise in power, a way of putting people "in their place" and keeping them there. Therefore, recognizing that cultural diversity may be a significant factor in delegation is a critical first step. Applying transcultural sensitivity in delegation is, however, what is ultimately needed to create a productive, multicultural work team.

LEARNING EXERCISE 20.4

Cultural Considerations in Delegation

You are a new charge nurse working on a surgical unit and have one of the recently hired Filipino travel nurses working on your unit. This is the end of her second week of orientation on the unit. She also received a month of classroom orientation and enculturation when she was first hired. Today, you assign her as one of your team leaders, responsible for a team of LVN/LPNs and CNAs. She has been working with another team leader for more than a week, but this is her first day to have the team to herself.

   You check with her several times during the morning to see how things are going. She speaks shyly without making eye contact and says that "everything is okay." At about noon, one of the LVN/LPNs comes to you and says that the new nurse has not delegated tasks appropriately and is trying to do too much of the work herself. Additionally, some of the other members of the team find her unsmiling behavior and lack of eye contact unsettling.

● ASSIGNMENT: Do you feel that you made an appropriate assignment? Since things do not seem to be going well, what should you do now? In a small group, develop a plan of action with the following goals: (a) ensure that patient care is accomplished safely, (b) build self-esteem in the Filipino nurse, and (c) be a cultural bridge to staff.

INTEGRATING LEADERSHIP ROLES AND MANAGEMENT FUNCTIONS IN DELEGATION

The right to delegate and the ability to provide formal rewards for successful completion of delegated tasks reflect the legitimate authority inherent in the management role. Delegation provides a means of increasing unit productivity. It is also a managerial tool for subordinate accomplishment and enrichment. Delegation, however, is not easy. It requires high-level management skills. Novice managers often make delegation errors such as delegating too late, not delegating enough, delegating to the wrong person or for the wrong reason, and failing to provide appropriate supervision and guidance of delegated tasks. Delegation also requires highly developed leadership skills such as sensitivity to subordinates' capabilities and needs, the ability to communicate clearly and directly, the willingness to support and encourage subordinates in carrying out delegated tasks, and the vision to see how delegation might result in increased personal growth for subordinates as well as increased unit productivity.

With the increased use of the UAP in patient care, the need for nurses to have highly developed delegation skills has never been greater. The ability to use delegation skills appropriately will help to reduce the personal liability associated with supervising and delegating to the UAP. It will also ensure that clients' needs are met and their safety is not jeopardized.

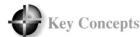 ## Key Concepts

* Professional nursing organizations and regulatory bodies are actively engaged in clarifying the scope of practice for unlicensed workers and delegation parameters for RNs.
* *Delegation* is not an option for the manager—it is a necessity.
* Delegation should be used for assigning routine tasks and tasks for which the manager does not have time. It also is appropriate as a tool for problem solving, changes in the manager's own job emphasis, and building capability in subordinates.
* In delegation, managers must clearly communicate what they want done, including the purpose for doing so. Limitations or qualifications that have been imposed should be delineated. Although the manager should specify the end product desired, it is important that the subordinate has an appropriate degree of autonomy in deciding how the work is to be accomplished.
* Managers must delegate the *authority* and the *responsibility* necessary to complete the task.
* RNs who are asked to assume the role of supervisor and delegator need preparation to assume these leadership tasks.
* Assuming the role of delegator and supervisor to the UAP increases the scope of liability for the RN.
* Although the Omnibus Budget Reconciliation Act of 1987 established regulations for the education and certification of "nurse's aides" (minimum of 75 hours of theory and practice and successful completion of an examination in both areas), no federal or community standards have been established for training the more broadly defined UAP.
* The RN always bears the ultimate responsibility for ensuring that the nursing care provided by his or her team members meets or exceeds minimum safety standards.
* When subordinates resist delegation, the delegator must ascertain why the delegated task was not accomplished and take appropriate action to remove these restraining forces.
* Transcultural sensitivity in delegation is needed to create a productive *multicultural work team.*

ADDITIONAL LEARNING EXERCISES AND APPLICATIONS

LEARNING EXERCISE 20.5

Need for Immediate Delegation

You are the charge nurse on the 7 AM to 3 PM shift in an oncology unit. Immediately after report in the morning, you are overwhelmed by the following information:

- The nursing aide reports that Mrs. Jones has become comatose and is moribund. Although this is not unexpected, her family members are not present, and you know that they would like to be notified immediately.
- There are three patients who need 0730 parenteral insulin administration. One of these patients had an 0600 blood sugar of 400.
- Mr. Johnson inadvertently pulled out his central line catheter when he was turning over in bed. His wife just notified the ward clerk by the call-light system and states that she is applying pressure to the site.
- The public toilet is overflowing, and urine and feces are pouring out rapidly.
- Breakfast trays arrived 15 minutes ago, and patients are using their call lights to ask why they do not yet have their breakfast.
- The medical director of the unit has just discovered that one of her patients has not been started on a chemotherapeutic drug that she ordered 3 days ago. She is furious and demands to speak to you immediately.

● ASSIGNMENT: The other RNs are all very busy with their patients, but you have the following people to whom you may delegate: yourself, a ward clerk, and an IV-certified LVN/LPN. Decide who should do what and in what priority. Justify your decision.

LEARNING EXERCISE 20.6

Issues with Delegating Discipline

You are the supervisor of the oncology unit. One of your closest friends and colleagues is Paula, the supervisor of the medical unit. Frequently, you cover for each other in the event of absence or emergency. Today, Paula stops at your office to let you know that she will be gone for 7 days to attend a management workshop on the East Coast. She asks that you check on the unit during her absence. She also asks that you pay particularly close attention to Mary Jones, an employee on her unit. She states that Mary, who has worked at the hospital for 4 years, has been counseled repeatedly about her unexcused absences from work and has recently received a written reprimand specifying that she will be terminated if there is another unexcused absence. Paula anticipates that Mary may attempt to break the rules during her absence. She asks that you follow through on this disciplinary plan in the event that Mary again takes an unexcused absence. Her instructions to you are to terminate Mary if she fails to show up for work this week for any reason.

When you arrive at work the next day, you find that Mary called in sick 20 minutes after the shift was to begin. The hospital's policy is that employees are to notify the staffing office of illness no less than 2 hours before the beginning of their shift. When you attempt to contact Mary by telephone at home, there is no answer.

Later in the day, you finally reach Mary and ask that she come in to your office early the next morning to speak about her inadequate notice of sick time. Mary arrives 45 minutes late the next morning. You are already agitated and angry with her. You inform her that she is to be terminated for any rule broken during Paula's absence and that this action is being taken in accord with the disciplinary contract that had been established earlier.

Mary is furious. She states that you have no right to fire her because you are not her "real boss" and that Paula should face her herself. She goes on to say that "Paula told me that the disciplinary contract was just a way of formalizing that we had talked and that I shouldn't take it too seriously." Mary also says, "Besides, I didn't get sick until I was getting ready for work. The hospital rules state that I have 12 sick days each year." Although you feel certain that Paula was very clear about her position in reviewing the disciplinary contract with Mary, you begin to feel uncomfortable with being placed in the position of having to take such serious corrective action without having been involved in prior disciplinary review sessions. You are, however, also aware that this employee has been breaking rules for some time and that this is just one in a succession of absences. You also know that Paula is counting on you to provide consistency of leadership in her absence.

● ASSIGNMENT: Discuss how you will handle the situation. Was it appropriate for Paula to delegate this responsibility to you? Is it appropriate for one manager to carry out another manager's disciplinary plan? Does it matter that a written disciplinary contract had already been established?

LEARNING EXERCISE 20.7

How Will You Plan This Busy Morning?
You are a staff nurse who functions as a modular leader on a general medical–surgical unit. The group for which you are responsible is assigned patients in Rooms 401 through 409, with a maximum capacity of 13 patients.

In your unit, a modular type of patient care organization is employed, using a combination of licensed and unlicensed staff. Each module consists of one RN, one LVN/LPN, and one UAP. The LVN/LPN is IV certified and can maintain and start IVs but cannot hang piggybacks or give IV push medications. The LVN/LPN may give all other medications except IV medications. The RN gives all IV medications. The UAP, with the assistance of his or her modular team members, generally bathes and feeds patients and provides other care that does not require a license.

The RN, as modular leader, divides up the workload at the beginning of the shift between the three modular team members. In addition, he or she acts as a teacher and resource person for the other members of the module.

Today is Wednesday. You have one LVN/LPN and one UAP assigned to work with you—LVN Franklin and UAP Martinez. LVN Franklin is 26 years old and the mother of four preschool children. Her husband is a city bus driver. UAP Martinez is 53 years old and a grandmother

(Learning Exercise continues on page 484)

with no children living at home. Her husband died 2 years ago. She says that work keeps her "happy." The patient roster this morning is as follows:

Room	Patient	Age	Diagnosis	Condition	Acuity Level
401	Mrs. Jones	33	Mastectomy for breast CA	2 days postop/fair	II
402	Mrs. Redford	55	Back pain—Pelvic	Good	I
403	Mrs. Worley	46	Cholecystectomy	2 days postop/ good	III
404-1	Mrs. Smith	83	Parkinson's, CVD, hypertension	Fair	II
404-2	Mrs. Dewey	26	PID	Good—home today	I
405-1	Mr. Arthur	71	Metastatic CA	Poor—semi- comatose/ chemotherapy	IV
405-2	Mr. Vines	34	Possible peptic ulcer	Good—UGI today	III
406-1	Vacant				
406-2	Miss Brown	24	Dilatation and curettage	To OR this AM	III
407-1	Mrs. West	41	Myocardial infarction Heparin lock from yesterday/telemetry	Fair/ ICU	III
408-1	Mr. Niles	21	Open reduction femur (MVA)	Fair/3 days postop	III
408-2	Mr. Ford	44	Gastrectomy	Fair/1 day postop	III
409	Mrs. Land	42	Depression	Fair/barium enema today	III

Additional information about patients:
- Mr. Niles is depressed because he believes that his football career is over.
- There have been problems with Mr. Ford's IV and his nasogastric tube. Both will need to be replaced today.
- Mrs. Worley requires frequent changes (every 2 to 3 hours) of the dressings at the laparoscopy site owing to a high volume of serous drainage.
- Mrs. Jones will need instructions regarding her postoperative activities and has begun to talk about her prognosis.
- Mrs. Land began to talk with you yesterday about her husband's recent death.
- The preparation for the barium enema will result in Mrs. Land's having frequent toileting needs today.
- Mrs. Smith requires assistance with feeding at mealtime.
- Mr. Arthur is no longer able to turn himself in bed.
- Mr. Vines states that being in the same room with a critically ill patient upsets him, and he has asked to be moved to a new room.

● ASSIGNMENT: How will you make out your assignments this morning? Assign these patients to the LVN/LPN, UAP, and yourself. Be sure to include assessments, procedures, and basic care needs. What will you do if a patient is admitted to your team? Explain the rationale for all your patient assignments. Refer to the sample acuity levels provided to assist in deter-mining patient needs and staffing.

LEARNING EXERCISE 20.8

Evaluating Staffing Safeguards

Interview a middle- or top-level manager of a local health care agency. Ascertain the staffing mix at his or her agency. Are there minimum hiring criteria for the UAP? Are there written guidelines for determining tasks appropriate for UAP delegation? What educational or training opportunities on delegation are made available to staff who must delegate work assignments on a regular basis?

On the basis of your interview results, write an essay evaluating whether you believe there are adequate safeguards in place at that agency to protect the licensed staff, unlicensed staff, and clients. Would you feel comfortable working in such a facility?

LEARNING EXERCISE 20.9

Deciding Delegation Using the Nurse Practice Act

Which of the following tasks would you be willing to delegate to a UAP? Use your state's NPA as a reference for this case. Discuss your answers in small groups. Did you all agree? If not, what factors were significant in your differences?

1. Uncomplicated wet-to-dry dressing change on a patient 3 days post–hip replacement
2. Every-2-hour checks on a patient with soft wrist restraints to assess circulation, movement, and comfort
3. Cooling measures for a patient with a temperature of 104°F
4. Calculation of IV credits, clearing IV pumps, and completing shift intake/output totals
5. Completing phlebotomy for daily drawing of blood
6. Holding pressure on the insertion site of a femoral line that has just been removed
7. Educating a patient about components of a soft diet
8. Conducting guaiac stool tests for occult blood
9. Performing electrocardiographic testing
10. Feeding a patient with swallowing precautions (high risk of choking post CVA)
11. Oral suctioning
12. Tracheostomy care
13. Ostomy care

Web Links

RN Utilization of Unlicensed Assistive Personnel
http://nursingworld.org/MainMenuCategories/HealthcareandPolicyIssues/ANAPositionStatements/uap.aspx
Position statement of the ANA regarding the utilization of UAP.

Delegation Tips
http://www.liraz.com/tdelegat.htm
Effective delegation will not only give you more time to work on your important opportunities, but you will also help others on your team learn new skills.

Delegation

http://www.see.ed.ac.uk/~gerard/MENG/ME96/Documents/Aspects/delegate.html
Delegation—A key aspect of leadership is delegation.

The Five Rights of Delegation

http://www.mass.gov/?pageID=eohhs2subtopic&L=8&L0=Home&L1=Provider&L2=Certification%
2C+Licensure%2C+and+Registration&L3=Occupational+and+Professional&L4=Nursing&L5=
Nursing+Practice&L6=Advisory+Rulings+on+Nursing+Practice&L7=Delegation+to+Unlicensed+
Assistive+Personnel&sid=Eeohhs2
*The Board of Registration in Nursing (Massachusetts) presents a framework for delegation decision mak-
ing and accountability based on a model that identifies the five key elements of any delegated act: the
right task, the right circumstances, the right person, the right direction/communication, and the right
supervision and evaluation.*

References

Barter, M. (2002). Follow the team leader. *Nursing Management,
33*(10), 55–59.

Case, B. (2004). Delegation skills. *Advance for Nurses, 1*(3),
20–26.

Davidhizar, R., & Shearer, R. (2005). When your nursing student
is culturally diverse. *Health Care Manager, 24*(4), 356–363.

Dunton, N., Gajewski, B., Taunton, R. L., & Moore, J. (2004).
Nurse staffing and patient falls on acute care hospital units.
Nursing Outlook, 52(1), 53–59.

Giger, J., & Davidhizar, R. (2004). *Transcultural nursing:
Assessment and intervention* (4th ed.). St Louis, MO:
Mosby–Year Book.

Hall, L. M., Doran, D., & Pink, G. H. (2004). Nurse staffing
models, nursing hours and patient safety. *Journal of Nursing
Administration, 34*(1), 41–45.

Huston, C. (2006). *Professional issues in nursing.* Philadelphia:
Lippincott Williams & Wilkins.

Kalisch, B. J. (2006). Missed nursing care. *Journal of Nursing
Care Quarterly, 21*(4), 306–313.

Kleinman, C. S., & Saccomano, S. J. (2006). Registered nurses
and unlicensed assistive personnel: An uneasy alliance. *Journal of Continuing Education in Nursing, 37*(4), 162–170.

Potter, P., & Grant, E. (2004). Understanding RN and unlicensed
assistive personnel working relationships in designing care
delivery strategies. *Journal of Nursing Administration, 34*(1),
19–25.

Quallich, S. A. (2005). A bond of trust: Delegation. *Urologic
Nusring, 25*(9), 120–123.

Robb, M., & Douglas, J. (2004). Continuing professional development. Managing diversity. *Nursing Management, 11*(1), 25–29.

Bibliography

Adlersberg, M. (2006). You asked. Is it within the scope of practice or is delegation? *Nursing BC, 38*(3), 19.

Anderson, I. (2006). Should health care assistants apply com-
pression bandages? *Nursing Times, 102*(4), 36–37.

Arford, P. M. (2005). Nurse-physician communication: An organizational accountability. *Nursing Economics, 23*(2), 72–77.

Boswell, A. (2005). Careers. How effective delegation can build
better teams. *Nursing Times, 101*(20), 60–61.

Cox, S. D. (2006). How to delegate to UAPs. *Nursing,* June Supplement: *Travel Nursing,* 10–11.

Curtis, E., & Nicholl, H. (2004). Delegation: A key function of
nursing. *Nursing Management, 11*(8), 26–31.

Henderson, D. (2005). Nursing EDGE: Evaluating delegation
guidelines in education. *International Journal of Nursing
Education Scholarship, 3*(1), 1–10.

Klein, T. A. (2005). Scope of practice and the nurse practitioner:
Regulation, competency, expansion and evolution. *Topics in
Advanced Practice Nursing, 5*(2), 1–8.

Lanier, J. K. (2006). Medication aides—What the laws and rules
say. *Ohio Nurses Review, 81*(2), 16–21, quiz 22–23.

Redman, R. W. (2006). Practice environments. The challenge of
interdisciplinary teams. *Research and Theory for Nursing
Practice, 20*(2), 105–107.

Sansom, C. (2005). To delegate or not to delegate? That is the
question. *Neveda RNformation, 14*(3), 4.

Starr, D. S. (2005). Legal advisor. The art of effective delegation.
Nurse Practitioners, 8(4), 86.

Storey, L. (2005). Delegation to health care assistants. *Practice
Nursing, 16*(6), 294–296.

Whitman, M. M. (2005). Professional development. Return and
report: Establishing accountability in delegation. *American
Journal of Nursing, 105*(3), 97.

Zehier, J. K. (2005). Delegation do's and don'ts. *Arkansas Nursing News, 2*(1), 14, 17, 19–20.

21

Managing Conflict

. . . peace is not the absence of conflict but the presence of creative alternatives for responding to conflict—alternatives to passive or aggressive responses, alternatives to violence.

—Dorothy Thompson

. . . it is important to remember that conflict is a natural and expected part of collaboration.

—Deborah B. Gardner

*C*onflict is generally defined as the internal or external discord that results from differences in ideas, values, or feelings between two or more people. Because managers have interpersonal relationships with people having a variety of different values, beliefs, backgrounds, and goals, conflict is an expected outcome. Conflict is also created when there are differences in economic and professional values and when there is competition among professionals. Scarce resources, restructuring, and poorly defined role expectations also are frequent sources of conflict in organizations.

Conflict is neither good nor bad, and it can produce growth or destruction, depending on how it is managed.

Openly acknowledging that conflict is a naturally occurring and expected phenomenon in organizations reflects a tremendous shift from how sociologists viewed conflict a century ago. The current sociological view is that organizational conflict should be neither avoided nor encouraged but managed. The manager's role is to create a work environment where conflict may be used as a conduit for growth, innovation, and productivity. When organizational conflict becomes dysfunctional, the manager must recognize it in its early stages and actively intervene so that subordinates' motivation and organizational productivity are not adversely affected.

Conflict resolution, or problem solving, appears to be learned less frequently through developmental experiences; rather, it requires a conscious learning effort. Indeed, recent incidents of violence among work groups have led corporations to develop programs to teach individuals how

DISPLAY 21.1 Leadership Roles and Management Functions Associated With Conflict Resolution

Leadership Roles

1. Is self-aware and conscientiously works to resolve intrapersonal conflict
2. Addresses conflict as soon as it is perceived and before it becomes felt or manifest
3. Seeks a win–win solution to conflict whenever feasible
4. Lessens the perceptual differences that exist between conflicting parties and broadens the parties' understanding about the problems
5. Assists subordinates in identifying alternative conflict resolutions
6. Recognizes and accepts the individual differences of staff
7. Uses assertive communication skills to increase persuasiveness and foster open communication
8. Role models honest and collaborative negotiation efforts

Management Functions

1. Creates a work environment that minimizes the antecedent conditions for conflict
2. Appropriately uses legitimate authority in a competing approach when a quick or unpopular decision needs to be made
3. When appropriate, formally facilitates conflict resolution involving subordinates
4. Accepts mutual responsibility for reaching predetermined supraordinate goals
5. Obtains needed unit resources through effective negotiation strategies
6. Compromises unit needs only when the need is not critical to unit functioning and when higher management gives up something of equal value
7. Is adequately prepared to negotiate for unit resources, including the advance determination of a bottom line and possible trade-offs
8. Addresses the need for closure and follow-up to negotiation
9. Pursues alternative dispute resolution when conflicts cannot be resolved by using traditional conflict management strategies

to deal with conflict (Hockley, 2006; Rew & Ferns, 2005). The efforts to reduce conflict violence lead one to believe that the skills necessary to manage conflict effectively can be learned.

This chapter presents an overview of growth-producing versus dysfunctional conflict in organizations. The history of conflict management, categories of conflict, the conflict process itself, and strategies for successful conflict resolution are discussed. Negotiation as a conflict resolution strategy is emphasized. Leadership skills and management functions necessary for conflict resolution at the unit level are outlined in Display 21.1.

THE HISTORY OF CONFLICT MANAGEMENT

Early in the 20th century, conflict was considered to be an indication of poor organizational management, was deemed destructive, and was avoided at all costs. When conflict occurred, it was ignored, denied, or dealt with immediately and harshly. The theorists of this era believed that conflict could be avoided if employees were taught the one right way to do things and if expressed employee dissatisfaction was met swiftly with disapproval.

In the mid-20th century, when organizations recognized that worker satisfaction and feedback were important, conflict was accepted passively and perceived as normal and expected. Attention centered on teaching managers how to resolve conflict rather than how to prevent it. Although conflict was considered to be primarily dysfunctional, it was believed that conflict and cooperation could happen simultaneously. The interactionist theorists of the 1970s, however, recognized conflict as a necessity and actively encouraged organizations to promote conflict as a means of producing growth. From this, one can infer that some conflict is desired, although its extent is difficult to know.

> **Some level of conflict in an organization appears desirable, although the optimum level for a specific person or unit at a given time is difficult to determine.**

Too little conflict results in organizational stasis. Too much conflict reduces the organization's effectiveness and eventually immobilizes its employees (Fig. 21.1). With few formal instruments to assess whether the level of conflict in an organization is too high or too low, the responsibility for determining and creating an appropriate level of conflict on the individual unit often falls to the manager.

Conflict also has a qualitative nature. A person may be totally overwhelmed in one conflict situation yet can handle several simultaneous conflicts at a later time. The difference is in the

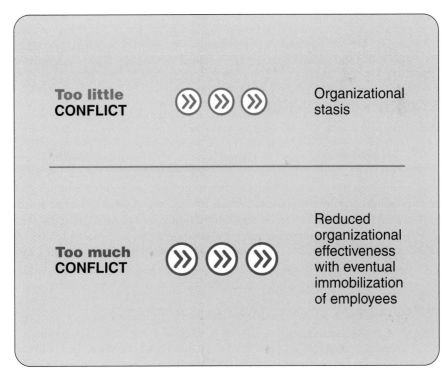

Figure 21.1 The relationship between organizational conflict and effectiveness.

quality or significance of that conflict to the person experiencing it. Although *quantitative* and *qualitative* conflicts produce distress at the time they occur, they can lead to growth, energy, and creativity by generating new ideas and solutions. If handled inappropriately, quantitative and qualitative conflicts can lead to demoralization, decreased motivation, and lowered productivity. Fulmano (2005) states, "Most people detest conflict and avoid it whenever possible. But as a leader, it's your job to manage it where it arises. If you can learn to transcend it, to embrace conflict as simply a part of your life experience, it becomes easier to manage. Conflict isn't a bad word. It's a difference of opinion or viewpoints, it's diversity in thinking" (p. 14).

LEARNING EXERCISE 21.1

Thinking and Writing About Conflict
Do you generally view conflict positively or negatively?
Does conflict affect you more cognitively, emotionally, or physically?
How was conflict expressed in the home in which you grew up?
Does the way that you handle conflict mirror that of your role models as a child?
Do you believe that you have too much or too little conflict in your life?
Do you feel like you have control over the issues that are now causing conflict in your life?

● ASSIGNMENT: Write a one-page essay, answering one of the questions above.

Nursing managers can no longer afford to respond to conflict traditionally (i.e., to avoid or suppress it), because this is nonproductive. In an era of shrinking health care dollars, it has become increasingly important for managers to confront and manage conflict appropriately. The ability to understand and deal with conflict appropriately is a critical leadership skill.

CATEGORIES OF CONFLICT

There are three primary categories of conflict: intergroup, intrapersonal, and interpersonal (Fig. 21.2).

Intergroup conflict occurs between two or more groups of people, departments, or organizations. An example of intergroup conflict might be two political affiliations with widely differing or contradictory beliefs. Nurses often experience intergroup conflict with family and work issues. Research by Grzywacz, Frone, Brewer, and Kovner (2006) revealed that nurses experience more work interference with family than conflict caused by family interfering with work. This finding held true for a significant number of nurses in the study.

Intrapersonal conflict occurs within the person. It involves an internal struggle to clarify contradictory values or wants. For managers, intrapersonal conflict may result from the multiple areas of responsibility associated with the management role. Managers' responsibilities to the organization, subordinates, consumers, the profession, and themselves may sometimes conflict, and that conflict may be internalized. Being self-aware and conscientiously working to resolve intrapersonal conflict as soon as it is first felt is essential to the leader's physical and mental health.

Interpersonal conflict, also known as "horizontal violence" or "bullying" happens between two or more people with differing values, goals, and beliefs (Hockley, 2006). Interpersonal conflict

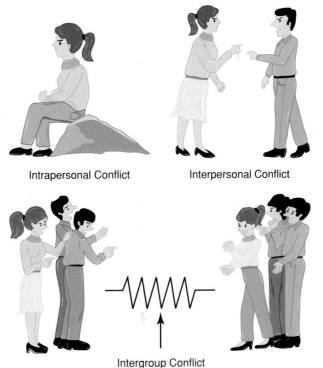

Intrapersonal Conflict   Interpersonal Conflict

Intergroup Conflict

Figure 21.2   Primary categories of conflict.

is a significant issue confronting the nursing profession, especially new graduates. Because this interpersonal conflict may not be reported or managed, it results in consequences such as absenteeism and turnover.

Violence and workplace aggression are increasingly being recognized as epidemic in the health care workplace.

Although there has been some difficulty in developing a consistent definition of *workplace violence,* Hockley (2006) maintains that in addition to physical violence, the term describes various antisocial behaviors and incidents that lead a person to believe that he or she has been harmed by the experience. It includes but is not limited to such behaviors as engaging in favoritism, being verbally abusive, sending abusive correspondence, bullying, pranks, and setting workers up for failure. It also includes economic aggression such as denying workers promotional opportunities.

Countless practice settings are hindered by maladaptive social behaviors that victimize nurses and impact patient care. She maintains that the responsibility for dealing with this type of conflict should initially lie with front-line staff, but the manager must become involved if the conflict is not resolved. According to Ramos (2006), "bullying and other behaviors have no role in the culture of the organization because all social interactions must be open and supportive" (p. 40).

THE CONFLICT PROCESS

Before managers can or should attempt to intervene in conflict, they must be able to assess its five stages accurately. The first stage in the conflict process, *latent conflict*, implies the existence of antecedent conditions such as short staffing and rapid change. In this stage, conditions are ripe for conflict, although no conflict has actually occurred and none may ever occur. Much unnecessary conflict could be prevented or reduced if managers examined the organization more closely for antecedent conditions. For example, change and budget cuts almost invariably create conflict. Such events, therefore, should be well thought out so that interventions can be made before the conflicts created by these events escalate.

If the conflict progresses, it may develop into the second stage: *perceived conflict.* Perceived or substantive conflict is intellectualized and often involves issues and roles. The person recognizes it logically and impersonally as occurring. Sometimes, conflict can be resolved at this stage before it is internalized or felt.

The third stage, *felt conflict*, occurs when the conflict is emotionalized. Felt emotions include hostility, fear, mistrust, and anger. It also is referred to as *affective conflict.* It is possible to perceive conflict and not feel it (e.g., no emotion is attached to the conflict, and the person views it only as a problem to be solved). A person also can feel the conflict but not perceive the problem (e.g., he or she is unable to identify the cause of the felt conflict).

In the fourth stage, *manifest conflict,* also called *overt conflict*, action is taken. The action may be to withdraw, compete, debate, or seek conflict resolution. Individuals are uncomfortable with or reluctant to address conflict for many reasons. These include fear of retaliation, fear of ridicule, fear of alienating others, a sense that they do not have the right to speak up, and past negative experiences with conflict situations. Indeed, people often learn patterns of dealing with manifest conflict early in their lives, and family background and experiences often directly affect how conflict is dealt with in adulthood. Sherman (2006) suggests that there are also generational differences in how individuals deal with conflict.

Gender also may play a role in how we respond to conflict (Gardner, 2005). Traditionally, men are socialized to respond more aggressively to conflict, while women are more apt to try to avoid conflicts or to pacify them. Power also plays a role in conflict resolution. Gardner maintains that often conflict resolution is focused on the single power concept of dominance with a victory of one side over another. Culture also plays a part in how we deal with conflict. Yu and Davidhizar (2004) state that "nurses and other health team members with diverse cultural background bring to the workplace different conflict behaviors that directly impact the outcomes of conflicts" (p. 46). Therefore, the action an individual takes to resolve conflict is often influenced by culture, gender, age, power position, and upbringing.

> The aftermath of conflict may be more significant than the original conflict if the conflict has not been handled constructively.

The final stage in the conflict process is *conflict aftermath.* There is always conflict aftermath—positive or negative. If the conflict is managed well, people involved in the conflict will believe that their position was given a fair hearing. If the conflict is managed poorly, the conflict issues frequently remain and may return later to cause more conflict. Figure 21.3 shows a schematic of this conflict process.

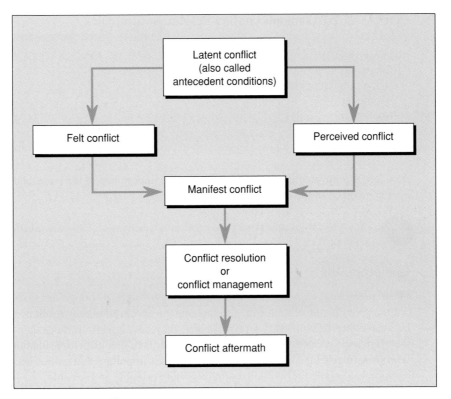

Figure 21.3 The conflict process.

LEARNING EXERCISE 21.2

Personal Conflict Solving
It is important for managers to be self-aware regarding how they view and deal with conflict. In your personal life, how do you solve conflict? Is it important for you to win? When was the last time you were able to solve conflict by reaching supraordinate goals with another person? Are you able to see the other person's position in conflict situations? In conflicts with family and friends, are you least likely to compromise values, scarcities, or role expectations?

CONFLICT MANAGEMENT

The optimal goal in resolving conflict is creating a win–win solution for all involved. This outcome is not possible in every situation, and often the manager's goal is to manage the conflict in a way that lessens the perceptual differences that exist between the involved parties. A leader recognizes which conflict management or resolution strategy is most appropriate for each situation. Common conflict management strategies are identified in Display 21.2. The choice of the most appropriate strategy depends on many variables, such as the situation itself, the urgency of the

DISPLAY 21.2   Common Conflict Resolution Strategies

Compromising
Competing
Cooperating/accommodating
Smoothing
Avoiding
Collaborating

decision, the power and status of the players, the importance of the issue, and the maturity of the people involved in the conflict.

 The optimal goal in resolving conflict is creating a win–win solution for all involved.

Compromising

In *compromising*, each party gives up something it wants. Although many see compromise as an optimum conflict resolution strategy, antagonistic cooperation may result in a lose–lose situation because either or both parties perceive that they have given up more than the other and may therefore feel defeated. For compromising not to result in a lose–lose situation, both parties must be willing to give up something of equal value. It is important that parties in conflict do not adopt compromise prematurely if collaboration is both possible and feasible.

Competing

The *competing* approach is used when one party pursues what it wants at the expense of the others. Because only one party wins, the competing party seeks to win regardless of the cost to others. Win–lose conflict resolution strategies leave the loser angry, frustrated, and wanting to get even in the future.

Managers may use competing when a quick or unpopular decision needs to be made. It is also appropriately used when one party has more information or knowledge about a situation than the other. Competing in the form of resistance is also appropriate when an individual needs to resist unsafe patient care policies or procedures, unfair treatment, abuse of power, or ethical concerns. Garon (2006) maintains that such action may actually be positive for both the staff nurse and the organization.

Cooperating/Accommodating

Cooperating is the opposite of competing. In the cooperating approach, one party sacrifices his or her beliefs and allows the other party to win. The actual problem is usually not solved in this win–lose situation. *Accommodating* is another term that may be used for this strategy. The person cooperating or accommodating often collects IOUs from the other party that can be used at a later date. Cooperating and accommodating are appropriate political strategies if the item in conflict is not of high value to the person doing the accommodating. Sullivan (2004) suggests that sometimes it is advisable to lose a battle if the payoff helps you to win the war. The battle is an individual incident, and the war is the long-term outcome.

Smoothing

Smoothing is used to manage a conflict situation. One person "smoothes" others involved in the conflict in an effort to reduce the emotional component of the conflict. Managers often use smoothing to get someone to accommodate or cooperate with another party. Smoothing occurs when one party in a conflict attempts to compliment the other party or to focus on agreements rather than differences. Although it may be appropriate for minor disagreements, smoothing rarely results in resolution of the actual conflict.

Avoiding

In the *avoiding* approach, the parties involved are aware of a conflict but choose not to acknowledge it or attempt to resolve it. Avoidance may be indicated in trivial disagreements, when the cost of dealing with the conflict exceeds the benefits of solving it, when the problem should be solved by people other than you, when one party is more powerful than the other, or when the problem will solve itself. The greatest problem in using avoidance is that the conflict remains, often only to reemerge at a later time in an even more exaggerated fashion.

Collaborating

Collaborating is an assertive and cooperative means of conflict resolution that results in a win–win solution. In collaboration, all parties set aside their original goals and work together to establish a *supraordinate* or priority common goal. In doing so, all parties accept mutual responsibility for reaching the supraordinate goal. Although it is very difficult for people truly to set aside original goals, collaboration cannot occur if this does not happen. For example, a couple experiencing serious conflict over whether to have a baby may first want to identify whether they share the supraordinate goal of keeping the marriage together. A nurse who is unhappy that she did not receive requested days off might meet with her supervisor and jointly establish the supraordinate goal that staffing will be adequate to meet patient safety criteria. If the new goal is truly a jointly set goal, each party will perceive that an important goal has been achieved and that the supraordinate goal is most important. In doing so, the focus remains on problem solving and not on defeating the other party.

Collaboration is rare when there is a wide difference in power between the groups or individuals involved. Many think of collaboration as a form of cooperation, but this is not an accurate definition. In collaboration, problem solving is a joint effort with no superior–subordinate, order-giving–order-taking relationships. True collaboration requires mutual respect; open and honest communication; and equitable, shared decision-making powers.

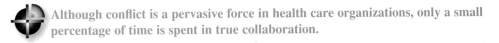 Although conflict is a pervasive force in health care organizations, only a small percentage of time is spent in true collaboration.

Gardner (2005) maintains that collaboration is both an outcome and a process whereby conflict is addressed by key stakeholders. For a leader to gain competence in facilitating collaboration, the following ten lessons must be learned.

1. *Know thyself.* As individuals come to the process of collaboration, they must be conscious of their own goals and values so that they may be more reflective.

2. *Learn to value and manage diversity.* Diverse perspectives assist with synthesis and improve quality of the collaboration process. Diversity includes both gender and cultural differences.

3. *Develop constructive conflict resolution skills.* Conflict resolution skills are essential for successful collaboration. These skills include an understanding of the conflict process, the nature of emotional versus task conflict, and effective conflict management.

4. *Use your power to create win–win situations.* While dominant power has no place in the collaboration process, the leader can use power to mediate, draw out others, show respect for members, demonstrate goodwill, share information, and use the power of position to facilitate the collaborative process.

5. *Master interpersonal and process skills.* Interpersonal skills such as flexibility and cooperation are important as well as the organizational skills of systems thinking, especially understanding organizational connections.

6. *Recognize that collaborating is a journey.* Establishing rapport, clarifying expectations, and requesting feedback takes time, and lack of time often limits opportunities for effective collaboration. But each successive collaborative effort is a step in the journey to establishing a climate of collaboration for future conflict.

7. *Leverage multidisciplinary forums to increase collaboration.* Shared decision making is a hallmark of the collaborative process. Use forums to both listen to others and to put forth your own position.

8. *Appreciate that collaboration can occur spontaneously.* Sometimes, the best collaboration may begin in a hallway conversation that results in people beginning to work together and share ideas to solve a conflict. Such exchanges can be exciting when a shared commitment for action is agreed upon.

9. *Balance autonomy and unity in collaborative relationships.* The leader must balance cooperation with the need to meet one's own needs to find integrative solutions.

10. *Remember that collaboration is not required for all decisions.* Autonomous decision making is still vital, and taking the time for the collaborative process is often not cost-effective for many conflict issues.

Lindeke and Sieckert (2005) maintain that emotional maturity is the foundation for effective collaboration. Collaboration enhances a person's participation in decision making to accomplish mutual goals and therefore is the best method to resolve conflict to achieve long-term benefits. Because it may involve others over whom the manager has no control and because its process is often lengthy, it may not be the best approach for all situations. However, collaboration often remains the best alternative for complex problem solving involving others.

LEARNING EXERCISE 21.3

Conflicting Personal, Professional, and Organizational Obligations

You are an RN. You have been working on the oncology unit since your graduation from the state college a year ago. Your supervisor, Mary, has complimented your performance. Lately, she has allowed you to be relief charge nurse on the 3 PM to 11 PM shift when the regular charge nurse is not there. Occasionally, you have been asked to work on the medical–surgical units when your department has a low census. Although you dislike leaving your own unit, you have cooperated because you felt that you could handle the other clinical assignments and wanted to show your flexibility.

On arriving at work tonight, the nursing office calls and requests that you help out in the busy delivery room. You protest that you do not know anything about obstetrics and that it is impossible for you to take the assignment. Carol, the supervisor from the nursing office, insists that you are the most qualified person; she says to "just go and do the best you can." Your own unit supervisor is not on duty, and the charge nurse says that she does not feel comfortable advising you in this conflict. You feel torn between professional, personal, and organizational obligations.

● ASSIGNMENT: What should you do? Select the most appropriate conflict resolution strategy. Give rationale for your selection and for your rejection of the others. After you have made your choice, read the analysis found in the Appendix.

MANAGING UNIT CONFLICT

Managing conflict effectively requires an understanding of its origin. Some of the sources of organizational conflict are shown in Display 21.3. Some common causes of unit conflict are unclear expectations, poor communication, lack of clear jurisdiction, incompatibilities or disagreements based on differences of temperament or attitudes, individual or group conflicts of interest, and operational or staffing changes.

Not only does diversity in gender, age, and culture influence conflict resolution, it may also create conflict itself. This occurs as a result of communication difficulties, including language and literacy issues and a growing recognition that some factors are beyond assimilation. In addition, people are currently more willing to celebrate their differences and are not as willing to assimilate into one homogeneous group.

All of these types of unit conflicts can disrupt working relationships and result in lower productivity. It is imperative, then, that the manager can identify the origin of unit conflicts and intervene as necessary to promote cooperative, if not collaborative, conflict resolution. Research by Hendel, Fish, and Galon (2005) found that leadership style and length of tenure influenced the strategy selected by managers to solve such conflicts. They also concluded that organizational leadership set the tone for conflict management. Examining the Evidence 21.1 reveals the results of their study.

DISPLAY 21.3   **Common Causes of Organizational Conflict**

- Poor communication
- Inadequately defined organizational structure
- Individual behavior (incompatibilities or disagreements based on differences of temperament or attitudes)
- Unclear expectations
- Individual or group conflicts of interest
- Operational or staffing changes
- Diversity in gender, culture, or age

EXAMINING THE EVIDENCE 21.1

Source: Hendel, T., Fish, M., & Galon, V. (2005). Leadership style and choice of strategy in conflict management among Israeli nurse managers in general hospitals. *Journal of Management, 13*, 137–146.

In this study, 60 nurse–managers were surveyed in five general Israeli hospitals to determine the relationship between leadership style and mode of choice in handling conflicts. Demographic characteristics were also studied.

The results found that head nurses perceive themselves significantly more as transformational leaders than as transactional leaders. However, compromise was found to be the most commonly used conflict management strategy used. Approximately half of the nurses used only one mode of conflict resolution to solve conflict issues. The subjects tended to choose a type of lose–lose strategy in solving conflict. The only demographic that was found to be significant was length of time as a head nurse.

At times, unit conflict requires that the manager facilitates conflict resolution between others. The following is a list of strategies that a manager may use to deal effectively with interpersonal, organizational, or unit conflict:

- *Confrontation.* Many times, subordinates inappropriately expect the manager to solve their interpersonal conflicts. Managers instead can urge subordinates to attempt to handle their own problems by using face-to-face communication to resolve conflicts, as emails, answering machine messages, and notes are too impersonal for the delicate nature of negative words.
- *Third-party consultation.* Sometimes, managers can be used as a neutral party to help others resolve conflicts constructively. This should be done only if all parties are motivated to solve the problem and if no differences exist in the status or power of the parties involved. If the conflict involves multiple parties and highly charged emotions, the manager may find outside experts helpful for facilitating communication and bringing issues to the forefront.
- *Behavior change.* This is reserved for serious cases of dysfunctional conflict. Educational modes, training development, or sensitivity training can be used to solve conflict by developing self-awareness and behavior change in the involved parties.
- *Responsibility charting.* When ambiguity results from unclear or new roles, it is often necessary to have the parties come together to delineate the function and responsibility of roles. If areas of joint responsibility exist, the manager must clearly define such areas as ultimate responsibility, approval mechanisms, support services, and responsibility for informing. This is a useful technique for elementary jurisdictional conflicts. An example of a potential jurisdictional conflict might arise between the house supervisor and unit manager in staffing or between an in-service educator and unit manager in determining and planning unit educational needs or programs.
- *Structure change.* Sometimes, managers need to intervene in unit conflict by transferring or discharging people. Other structure changes may be moving a department under another manager, adding an ombudsman, or putting a grievance procedure in place. Often,

increasing the boundaries of authority for one member of the conflict will act as an effective structure change to resolve unit conflict. Changing titles and creating policies also are effective techniques.

• *Soothing one party.* This is a temporary solution that should be used in a crisis when there is not time to handle the conflict effectively or when the parties are so enraged that immediate conflict resolution is unlikely. Waiting a few days allows most individuals to deal with their intense feelings and to be more objective about the issues. Regardless of how the parties are soothed, the manager must address the underlying problem later or this technique will become ineffective

NEGOTIATION

Negotiation in its most creative form is similar to collaboration and in its most poorly managed form may resemble a competing approach. Negotiation frequently resembles compromise when it is used as a conflict resolution strategy. During negotiation, each party gives up something, and the emphasis is on accommodating differences between the parties. People have conflicting needs, wants, and desires that must be constantly compromised. Few people are able to meet all of their needs or objectives. Most day-to-day conflict is resolved with negotiation. A nurse who says to another nurse "I'll answer that call light if you'll count narcotics" is practicing the art of negotiation.

Although negotiation implies winning and losing for both parties, there is no rule that each party must lose and win the same amount. Most negotiators want to win more than they lose, but negotiation becomes destructively competitive when the emphasis is on winning at all costs. A major goal of effective negotiation is to make the other party feel satisfied with the outcome. The focus in negotiation should be to create a *win–win* situation.

Many small negotiations take place every day spontaneously and succeed without any advance preparation. However, not all nurses are expert negotiators. If managers wish to succeed in important negotiations for unit resources, they must (a) be adequately prepared, (b) be able to use appropriate negotiation strategies, and (c) apply appropriate closure and follow-up. To become more successful at negotiating, managers need to do several things before, during, and after the negotiation (Display 21.4).

Before the Negotiation

For managers to be successful, they must systematically prepare for the negotiation. As the negotiator, the manager begins by gathering as much information as possible regarding the issue to be negotiated. Because knowledge is power, the more informed the negotiator is, the greater is his or her bargaining power. Adequate preparation prevents others in the negotiation from catching the negotiator off guard or making him or her appear uninformed.

Additionally, individuals must remember that few negotiations begin at the table; most have been going on behind the scenes for some time (Tate, 2005). This makes it especially important to know the who, what, when, where, and how of an issue. This is the area where strategies are prepared. However, another level of preparation is the emotional level, which is the human side of every negotiation and interaction. Remember that the "opponents" you face across the bargaining table are individuals like you. The way the other party perceives you as being fair and open to negotiate often plays a role in the decisions that will be reached in the negotiation.

DISPLAY 21.4 **Before, During, and After the Negotiation**

Before

1. Be prepared mentally by having done your homework.
2. Determine your starting point, trade-offs, and bottom line.
3. Look for hidden agendas, both your own and the parties with whom you are negotiating.

During

1. Maintain composure.
2. Role model good communication skills (speaking and listening), assertiveness, and flexibility.
3. Avoid using destructive negotiation techniques, but be prepared to counter them if they are used against you.

After

1. Restate what has been agreed upon, both verbally and in writing.
2. Recognize and thank all participants for their contributions to a successful negotiation.

It also is important for managers to decide where to start in the negotiation. Tate (2005) suggests that managers should initially focus on seeking a bigger pie instead of dividing the pie up. In other words, the negotiators add value to the package rather than seek concessions from each other. When this is not possible, the focus must shift to compromise and priority setting. Because managers must be willing to make compromises, they should choose a starting point that is high but not ridiculous. This selected starting point should be at the upper limits of their expectations, realizing that they may need to come down to a more realistic goal. For instance, let's say that you would really like four additional full-time RN positions and a full-time clerical position budgeted for your unit. You know that you could make do with three additional full-time RN positions and a part-time clerical assistant, but you begin by asking for what would be ideal.

It is almost impossible in any type of negotiation to escalate demands; therefore, the manager must start at an extreme but reasonable point. It also must be decided beforehand how much can be compromised and what is an acceptable *bottom line* (or the least acceptable resolution). Can the manager accept, at a minimum, one full-time RN position or two or three?

The very least for which a person will settle is often referred to as the bottom line.

The wise manager also has other options in mind when negotiating for important resources. An alternative option is another set of negotiating preferences that can be used so that managers do not need to use their bottom lines but still meet their overall goal. For instance, you have requested four full-time RN positions and one full-time clerical position. You could get by with three full-time RNs and one part-time clerk. However, you believe strongly that you cannot continue to provide safe patient care unless you are given two RNs and a part-time clerk—your bottom line. However, if the original negotiation is unsuccessful, reopen negotiations by saying that a second option that does not entail increasing the staff would be to float a ward clerk for 4 hours each day, implement a unit-dose system, require housekeeping to pass out linen, and have dietary pass all the patient meal trays. This way, the overall goal of providing more direct patient care by the nursing staff could still be met without adding nursing personnel.

The manager needs to consider other trade-offs that are possible in these situations. *Trade-offs* are secondary gains, often future-oriented, that may be realized as a result of conflict. For example, while attending college, a parent may feel intrapersonal conflict because he or she is unable to spend as much time as desired with his or her children. The parent is able to compromise by considering the trade-off: eventually, everyone's life will be better because of the present sacrifices. The wise manager will consider trading something today for something tomorrow as a means to reach satisfactory negotiations.

The manager also must look for and acknowledge *hidden agendas*—the covert intention of the negotiation. Usually, every negotiation has a covert and an overt agenda. For example, new managers may set up a meeting with their superior with the established agenda of discussing the lack of supplies on the unit. However, the hidden agenda may be that the manager feels insecure and is really seeking performance feedback during the discussion. Having a hidden agenda is not uncommon and is not wrong by any means. Everyone has them, and it is not necessary or even wise to share these hidden agendas. Managers, however, must be introspective enough to recognize their hidden agendas so that they are not paralyzed if the agenda is discovered and used against them during the negotiation. If the manager's hidden agenda is discovered, he or she should admit that it is a consideration but not the heart of the negotiation. For instance, although the hidden agenda for increasing unit staff might be to build the manager's esteem in the eyes of the staff, there may exist a legitimate need for additional staff. If, during the negotiations, the fiscal controller accuses the manager of wanting to increase staff just to gain power, the manager might respond by saying, "It is always important for a successful manager to be able to gain resources for the unit, but the real issue here is an inadequate staff." Managers who protest too strongly that they do not have a hidden agenda appear defensive and vulnerable.

During the Negotiation

Because negotiation may be a highly charged experience, the negotiator always wants to appear calm, collected, and self-assured. At least part of this self-assurance comes from having adequately prepared for the negotiation. Part of the preparation should have included learning about the people with whom the manager is negotiating. People come in a variety of personality types, and over the course of their careers, managers will come across most if not all of these personality types in various negotiations. Preparation, however, is not enough. In the end, the negotiator must have clarity in his or her communication, assertiveness, good listening skills, the ability to regroup quickly, and flexibility.

 Negotiation is psychological and verbal. The effective negotiator always appears calm and self-assured.

Strategies commonly used by leaders during negotiation to increase their persuasiveness and foster open communication include the following:
- Use only factual statements that have been gathered in research.
- Listen carefully, and watch nonverbal communication.

- Keep an open mind, because negotiation always provides the potential for learning. It is important not to prejudge. Instead, a cooperative (not competitive) climate should be established.
- Try to understand where the other party is coming from. It is probable that one person's perception is different from that of another. The negotiation needs to concentrate on understanding, not just on agreeing.
- Always discuss the conflict. It is important not to personalize the conflict by discussing the parties involved in the negotiation.
- Try not to belabor how the conflict occurred or to fix blame for the conflict. Instead, the focus must be on preventing its recurrence.
- Be honest.
- Start tough so that concessions are possible. It is much harder to escalate demands in the negotiation than to make concessions.
- Delay when confronted with something totally unexpected in negotiation. In such cases, the negotiator should respond, "I'm not prepared to discuss this right now" or "I'm sorry, this was not on our agenda; we can set up another appointment to discuss that." If asked a question about something that the negotiator does not know, he or she should simply say, "I don't have that information at this time."
- Never tell the other party what you are willing to negotiate totally. You may be giving up the ship too early.
- Know the bottom line, but try never to use it. If the bottom line is used, the negotiator must be ready to back it up or he or she will lose all credibility. Negotiations should always result in both sides improving their positions; however, in reality, people some-times have to walk away from the negotiating table if the situation cannot be improved because not every negotiation can result in terms that are agreeable to each party. If the bottom line is reached, the negotiator should tell the other party that an impasse has been reached and that further negotiation is not possible at this time. Then, the other party should be encouraged to sleep on it and reconsider. The door should always be left open for further negotiation. Another appointment can be made. Both parties should be allowed to save face.
- Take a break if either party becomes angry or tired during the negotiation. Go to the bath-room or make a telephone call. Remember that neither party can effectively negotiate if either is enraged or fatigued.

Destructive Negotiation Tactics

Some negotiators win by using specific intimidating or manipulative tactics. People using these tactics take a competing approach to negotiation rather than a collaborative approach. These tactics might be conscious or unconscious but are used repeatedly because they have been suc-cessful for that person. Successful managers do not use these types of tactics, but because oth-ers with whom they negotiate may do so, they must be prepared to counter such tactics.

One such tactic is *ridicule*. The goal in using ridicule is to intimidate others involved in the negotiation. If you are negotiating with someone who uses ridicule, maintain a relaxed body posture, steady gaze, and patient smile. Body language must also remain relaxed and non-threatening.

Another tactic some people use is *ambiguous* or *inappropriate questioning*. For example, in one negotiating situation, the ICU supervisor had requested additional staff to handle open-heart surgery patients. During her bargaining, the CEO suddenly said, "I never did understand the heart; can you tell me about the heart?" The supervisor did not fall into this trap and instead replied that the physiology of the heart was irrelevant to the issue. Because people tend to answer an authority figure, it is necessary to be on guard for this type of diversionary tactic.

Flattery is another technique that makes true collaboration in negotiation very difficult. The person who has been flattered may be more reluctant to disagree with the other party in the negotiation, and thus his or her attention and focus are diverted. One method that managers can use to discern flattery from other honest attempts to compliment is to be aware of how they feel about the comment. If they feel unduly flattered by a gesture or comment, it is a good indication that they were being flattered. For example, asking for advice or instruction may be a subtle form of flattery, or it may be an honest request. If the request for advice is about an area in which the manager has little expertise, it is undoubtedly flattery. However, exchanging positive opening comments with each other when beginning negotiation is an acceptable and enjoyable practice performed by both parties.

Nurses are also particularly sympathetic to gestures of *helplessness*. Because nursing is a helping profession, the tendency to nurture is high, and managers must be careful not to lose sight of the original intent of the negotiation—securing adequate resources to optimize unit functioning.

Some people win in negotiation simply by rapidly and *aggressively taking over* and controlling the negotiation before other members realize what is happening. If managers believe that this may be happening, they should call a halt to the negotiations before decisions are made. Saying simply, "I need to have time to think this over" is a good method of stopping an aggressive takeover. The manager needs to be aware of destructive negotiation tactics and develop strategies to overcome them because such tactics are antithetical to collaboration.

Destructive negotiation tactics are never a part of collaborative conflict resolution.

Leaders use an honest, straightforward approach and develop assertive skills for use in conflict negotiation. Maintaining human dignity and promoting communication require that all conflict interactions be assertive, direct, and open. Conflict must be focused on the issues and resolved through joint compromise.

Closure and Follow-Up to Negotiation

Just as it is important to start the formal negotiation with some pleasantries, it is also good to close on a friendly note. Once a compromise has been reached, restate it so that everyone is clear about what has been agreed upon. If managers win more in negotiation than they anticipated, they should try to hide their astonishment. At the end of any negotiation, whether it is a short 2-minute conflict negotiation in the hallway with another RN or an hour-long formal salary negotiation, the result should be satisfaction by all parties that each has won something. It is a good idea to follow up formal negotiation in writing by sending a letter or a memo stating what was agreed.

LEARNING EXERCISE 21.4

An Exercise in Negotiation Analysis
You are one of a group of staff nurses who believe that part of your job dissatisfaction results from being assigned different patients every day. Your unit uses a system of total patient care, and the head nurse makes assignments. Two staff nurses have gone to the head nurse and requested that each nurse be allowed to pick his or her own patients based on the previous day's assignment and the ability of the nurse. The head nurse believes that the staff nurses are being uncooperative because it is the head nurse's responsibility to see that all the patients get assigned and receive adequate care. Although continuity of care is the goal, many part-time nurses are used on the unit, and not all the nurses are able to care for every type of patient. At the end of the conference, the two nurses are angry, and the head nurse is irritated. However, the next day, the head nurse indicates willingness to meet with the staff nurses. The other nurses believe this is a sign that the head nurse is willing to negotiate a compromise. They plan to get together tonight to plan the strategy for tomorrow's meeting.

● ASSIGNMENT: What are the goals for each party? What could be a possible hidden agenda for each party? What could happen if the conflict escalates? Devise a workable plan that would accomplish the goals of both parties, and develop strategies for implementation (see the Appendix for an analysis of these problems).

ALTERNATIVE DISPUTE RESOLUTION

Sometimes, parties cannot reach agreement through negotiation. In these cases, *alternative dispute resolution* (ADR) may be indicated to keep some privacy in the dispute and to avoid expensive litigation. Types of ADR include mediation, fact finding, arbitration, and the use of ombudspersons (Epstein, 2003).

Mediation, which uses a neutral third party, is a confidential, legally nonbinding process designed to help bring the parties together to devise a solution to the conflict. As such, the mediator does not take sides and has no vested interest in the outcome (Epstein, 2003). The mediator's role, then, becomes one of asking questions to clarify the issues at hand (*fact finding*); listening to both parties; caucusing with parties privately as necessary; making suggestions for areas of improvement; and hopefully, drafting a settlement agreement for both parties to sign (Epstein, 2003).

There are times when mediators are unable to help conflicted parties come to agreement. When this occurs, formal *arbitration* may be used. Unlike mediation, which seeks to help conflicted parties come together to reach a decision themselves, arbitration is a binding conflict resolution process in which the facts of the case are heard by an individual who makes a final decision for the parties in conflict.

There are, however, several other types of arbitration. One type is *mediation–arbitration,* in which a third party joins the negotiation process before any serious disputes arise (Ellis & Hartley, 2004). This individual acts only as a mediator unless some deadlock is reached in the negotiation. Then, the mediator becomes an official arbitrator.

Another type of arbitration is the *final offer approach* (Ellis & Hartley, 2004). In this approach, the conflicted parties reach agreement on as many issues as possible. A final position for deadlocked issues from each side is then presented to the arbitrator, who is obligated to select only the most reasonable package. Arbitration may be requested from the American Arbitration Association or be available from state, public, and private mediation and conciliation services (Ellis & Hartley, 2004).

Another option for individuals experiencing conflict may be guidance from *ombudspersons*. Ombudspersons generally hold an official title as such within an organization. Their function is to investigate grievances filed by one party against another and to ensure that individuals involved in conflicts understand their rights as well as the process that should be used to report and resolve the conflict.

SEEKING CONSENSUS

Consensus means that negotiating parties reach an agreement that all parties can support, even it does not represent everyone's first priorities. Consensus decision making does not provide complete satisfaction for everyone involved in the negotiation as an initially unanimous decision would, but it does indicate willingness by all parties to accept the agreed-upon conditions.

In committees or groups working on shared goals, consensus is often used to resolve conflicts that may occur within the group. To reach consensus often requires the use of an experienced facilitator, and having consensus-building skills is a requirement of good leadership. Building consensus ensures that everyone within the group is heard but that the group will ultimately end up with one agreed-upon course of action. Consensual decisions are best used for decisions that relate to a core problem or need a deep level of group support to implement successfully.

Perhaps the greatest challenge in using consensus as a conflict resolution strategy is that like collaboration, it is time-consuming. It also requires all of the parties involved in the negotiation to have good communication skills and to be open-minded and flexible. It is also important for the leader to recognize when achieving consensus has become unrealistic. When this occurs, the best strategy is for the manager to receive group input and then make a unilateral decision (Lindeke & Sieckert, 2005),

INTEGRATING LEADERSHIP SKILLS AND MANAGEMENT FUNCTIONS IN MANAGING CONFLICT

The manager who creates a stable work environment that minimizes the antecedent conditions for conflict has more time and energy to focus on meeting organizational and human resource needs. When conflict does occur in the unit, managers must be able to discern constructive from destructive conflict. Conflict that is constructive will result in creativity, innovation, and growth for the unit. When conflict is deemed to be destructive, managers must deal appropriately with that conflict or risk an aftermath that may be even more destructive than the original conflict. Consistently using conflict resolution strategies with win–lose or lose–lose outcomes will create disharmony within the unit. Leaders who use optimal conflict resolution strategies with a win–win outcome promote increased employee satisfaction and organizational productivity.

Negotiation also requires both management functions and leadership skills. Well-prepared managers know with whom they will be negotiating and prepare their negotiation accordingly. They are prepared with trade-offs, multiple alternatives, and a clear bottom line to ensure that their unit acquires needed resources. Successful negotiation mandates the use of the leadership components of self-confidence and risk taking. If these attributes are not present, the leader–manager has little power in negotiation and thus compromises the unit's ability to secure desired resources. Other attributes that make leaders effective in negotiation are sensitivity to others and the environment and interpersonal communication skills. The leader's use of assertive communication skills, rather than destructive tactics, results in an acceptable level of satisfaction for all parties at the close of the negotiation.

Key Concepts

* *Conflict* can be defined as the internal discord that results from differences in ideas, values, or feelings of two or more people.
* Because managers have a variety of interpersonal relationships with people with different values, beliefs, backgrounds, and goals, conflict is an expected outcome.
* The most common sources of organizational conflict are communication problems, organizational structure, and individual behavior within the organization.
* Conflict theory has changed dramatically during the last 100 years. Currently, conflict is viewed as neither good nor bad because it can produce growth or be destructive, depending on how it is managed.
* Too little conflict results in organizational stasis, whereas too much conflict reduces the organization's effectiveness and eventually immobilizes its employees.
* The three categories of conflict are *intrapersonal*, *interpersonal*, and *intergroup*.
* The first stage in the conflict process is called *latent conflict*, which implies the existence of antecedent conditions. Latent conflict may proceed to *perceived conflict* or to *felt conflict. Manifest conflict* may also ensue. The last stage in the process is *conflict aftermath*.
* The optimal goal in conflict resolution is creating a *win–win* solution for everyone involved.
* Common conflict resolution strategies include *compromise, competing, accommodating, smoothing, a*voiding, and *collaboration.*
* As a negotiator, it is important to win as much as possible, lose as little as possible, and make the other party feel satisfied with the outcome of the negotiation.
* Because knowledge is power, the more informed the negotiator is, the greater is his or her bargaining power.
* The leader, while able to recognize and counter negotiation tactics, always strives to achieve an honest, collaborative approach to negotiation.
* The manager must know his or her *bottom line* but try never to use it.
* Closure and follow-up are important parts of the negotiation process.
* *Alternative dispute resolution* usually involves at least one of the elements of *mediation, fact finding, arbitration,* and the use of *ombudspersons.*
* Seeking *consensus,* a concord of opinion, although time-consuming, is an effective conflict resolution and negotiation strategy.

ADDITIONAL LEARNING EXERCISES AND APPLICATIONS

LEARNING EXERCISE 21.5

Choosing the Most Appropriate Resolution Approach
In the following situations, choose the most appropriate conflict resolution strategy (avoiding, smoothing, accommodating, competing, compromising, or collaborating). Support your decision with rationale, and explain why other methods of conflict management were not used.

Situation 1
You are a circulating nurse in the operating room. Usually, you are assigned to Room 3 for general surgery, but today you have been assigned to Room 4, the orthopedic room. You are unfamiliar with the orthopedic doctors' routines and attempt to brush up on them quickly by reading the doctors' preference cards before each case today. So far, you have managed to complete two cases without incident. The next case comes in the room, and you realize that everyone is especially tense; this patient is the wife of a local physician, and the doctors are performing a bone biopsy for possible malignancy. You prepare the biopsy area, and the surgeon, who has a reputation for a quick temper, enters the room. You suddenly realize that you have prepped the area with Betadine, and this surgeon prefers another solution. He sees what you have done and yells, "You are a stupid, stupid nurse."

Situation 2
You are the ICU charge nurse and have just finished an exhausting 8 hours on duty. Working with you today were two nurses who work 12-hour shifts. Each of you were assigned two patients, all with high acuity levels. You are glad that you are going out of town tonight to attend an important seminar, because you are certainly tired. You also are pleased that you scheduled yourself an 8-hour shift today and that your replacement is coming through the door. You will just have time to give report and catch your plane.

It is customary for 12-hour nurses to continue with their previous patients and for assignments not to be changed when 8-hour and 12-hour staff are working together. Therefore, you proceed to give report on your patients to the 8-hour nurse coming on duty. One of your patients is acutely ill with fever of unknown origin and is in the isolation room. It is suspected that he has meningitis. Your other patient is a multiple trauma victim. In the middle of your report, the oncoming nurse says that she has just learned that she is pregnant. She says, "I can't take care of a possible meningitis patient. I'll have to trade with one of the 12-hour nurses." You approach the 12-hour nurses, and they respond angrily, "We took care of all kinds of patients when we were pregnant, and we are not changing patients with just 4 hours left in our shift."

When you repeat this message to the oncoming nurse, she says, "Either they trade or I go home!" Your phone call to the nursing office reveals that because of a flu epidemic, there are absolutely no personnel to call in, and all the other units are already short staffed.

Situation 3
You are an RN graduate of a BSN nursing program. Since you graduated 6 months ago, you have been working at an outpatient emergency clinic and have just recently begun to feel more confident in your new role. However, one of the older, diploma-educated nurses working with you constantly belittles baccalaureate nursing education. Whenever you request assistance in problem solving or in learning a new skill, she says, "Didn't they teach you anything in nursing

(Learning Exercise continues on page 508)

school?" The clinic supervisor has given you satisfactory 3-month and 6-month evaluations, but you are becoming increasingly defensive regarding the comments of the other nurse.

Situation 4

You are the charge nurse on a step-down unit. It is your first day back from a 2-week vacation. The shift begins in 10 minutes, and you sit down to make staffing assignments. The central staffing office has noted that you must float one of your RNs to the oncology unit. When you check the floating roster, you note that Jenny, one of the RNs assigned to work on your unit today, was the last to float. (She floated yesterday.) That leaves you to choose from Mark and Lisa, your other two RNs. According to the float roster, Mark floated 10 days ago, and Lisa floated last 11 days ago. You tell Lisa that it is her turn to float.

Lisa states that she floated three times in a row while Mark was on vacation for 2 weeks last month. Mark says that vacations should not count and that he should not float because it is not his turn. Lisa says that Jenny should float, as she floated to oncology yesterday and already knows the patients. Jenny says that she agreed to come in and work today (on her day off) to help the unit, and she would not have agreed to do this if she had known that she would have to float. Mark says that it is the last day of a 6-day stretch, and he does not want to float. Jenny says that it is not her turn to float, and she does not want to float willingly.

LEARNING EXERCISE 21.6

Negotiating the Graduation Ceremony

Often, one group is more powerful or has greater status and refuses to relinquish this power position, thus making collaboration impossible. Therefore, negotiating a compromise to a win–win solution, rather than a lose–lose solution, becomes imperative. In the following situation, describe if you could, and how you would, go about negotiating a win–win solution to conflict.

You are a senior member of a traditional on-campus baccalaureate nursing class. Three years ago, your university implemented an online RN-BSN program. The first students from that program graduated last year, and they held a small, private end-of-program ceremony, separate from the on-campus BSN students.

This year, as a result of ongoing state budget cuts, the school of nursing can no longer subsidize two separate end-of-program ceremonies. This means that the 21 RN-BSN students and the 33 on-campus BSN students must now work together to plan a joint ceremony.

Resistance is high. The two groups of students have spent no time together and do not know each other. The on-campus students have been planning their ceremony since they started the nursing program and have collected additional money each semester to fund a formal dinner and dance reception in the evening and breakfast at one of the nicest hotels in town. Money from the school of nursing would be used to subsidize the cost of a live band and the reception hall. The online students would like to limit the evening reception to cake and punch at the college to reduce the cost because most of them will incur additional travel and lodging costs to attend graduation. However, they would like to have the school of nursing use the funds available to host a "picnic in the park" the following day, to which they can bring their families. Both groups perceive that the "other group is trying to control the situation and is not being sensitive to our needs or wants." Both groups have contacted University officials to complain about the situation, and a number of students are threatening not to attend the ceremony if the two groups must be merged.

You have been appointed as the unofficial spokesperson for the RN-BSN graduates. Joan is the unofficial spokesperson for the on-campus BSN students. You live only 30 miles from campus, so coming to campus to try to resolve the conflict is not a significant hardship.

The faculty member, Alice, who is the liaison for the end-of-program ceremony has become alarmed at the situation and has contacted both you and Joan. She states that she will cancel the ceremony if the conflict is not resolved. The faculty member agrees to work with you and Joan to mediate the conflict, but time is of the essence. The semester ends soon, and the on-campus students can get no refund on their reception hall deposit after the end of the current week. She wants the conflict resolved in a win–win situation so that no parties leave angry.

● ASSIGNMENT: Where will you begin? How will you get input from the group that you are representing? Would you plan a face-to-face meeting with Joan to attempt to resolve this conflict? What strategies might you use to help both groups win as much as possible and lose as little as possible? Explain your rationale. Remember, you wish to negotiate a compromise, and although you desire a win–win solution, you are limited in time and may not be able to facilitate a true collaboration. How will you deal with conflicted parties who perceive that they have lost more than they have won? What is your bottom line?

LEARNING EXERCISE 21.7

Behavioral Tactics—Appropriate or Not?

You are a woman who is a unit manager with a master's degree in health administration. You are about to present your proposed budget to the CEO, who is a man. You have thoroughly researched your budget and have adequate rationale to support your requests for increased funding. Because the CEO is often moody, predicting his response is difficult.

You also are aware that the CEO has some very traditional views about women's role in the workplace, and generally this does not include a major management role. Because he is fairly paternalistic, he is charmed and flattered when asked to assist "his" nurses with their jobs. Your predecessor, also a woman, was fired because she was perceived as brash, bossy, and disrespectful by the CEO. In fact, the former unit manager was one of a series of nursing managers who had been replaced in the last several years because of these characteristics. From what you have been told, the nursing staff did not share these perceptions.

You sit down and begin to plan your strategy for this meeting. You are aware that you are more likely to have your budgetary needs met if you dress conservatively, beseech the CEO's assistance and support throughout the presentation, and are fairly passive in your approach. In other words, you will be required to assume a traditionally feminine, helpless role. If you appear capable and articulate, you may not achieve your budgetary goals and may not even keep your job. It would probably not be necessary for you to continue to act this way, except in your interactions with the CEO.

● ASSIGNMENT: Are such behavioral tactics appropriate if the outcome is desirable? Are such tactics simply smart negotiation, or are they destructively manipulative? What would you do in this situation? Outline your strategy for your budget presentation, and present rationale for your choices.

LEARNING EXERCISE 21.8

Your First Budget Presentation

You are the unit manager of the new oncology unit. It is time for your first budget presentation to the administration. You have already presented your budget to the director of nurses, who had a few questions but expressed general agreement. However, it is the policy at Memorial Hospital that the unit manager's present budget be presented to the budget committee, consisting of the fiscal manager, the director of nurses, a member of the board of trustees, and the executive director. You know that money is scarce this year because of the new building, but you really believe that you need the increases you have requested in your budget. Basically, you have asked for the following:

- Replace the 22% aides on your unit with 10% LVNs/LPNs and 12% RNs.
- Increase educational time paid by 5% to allow for certification in chemotherapy.
- Provide a new position of clinical nurse specialist in oncology.
- Convert one room into a sitting room and mini-kitchen for patients' families.
- Add shelves and a locked medication box in each room to facilitate primary nursing.
- Provide no new equipment, but replace existing equipment that is broken or outdated.

● ASSIGNMENT: Outline your plan. Include your approach what is and what is not negotiable and what arguments you would use. Give a rationale for your plan.

LEARNING EXERCISE 21.9

Handling Staff–Patient Conflict

You are the supervisor of a rehabilitation unit. Two of your youngest female nursing assistants come to your office today to report that a young male paraplegic patient has been making lewd sexual comments and gestures when they provide basic care. When you question them about their response to the actions of the patient, they maintain that they normally simply look away and try to ignore him, although they are offended by his actions. They are reluctant to confront the patient directly.

Because it is anticipated that this patient may remain on your unit for at least a month, the nursing assistants have asked you to intervene in this conflict by either talking to the patient or by assigning other nurses responsibility for his care.

● ASSIGNMENT: How will you handle this staff–patient conflict? Is avoidance (assigning different staff to care for the patient) an appropriate conflict resolution strategy in this situation? Will you encourage the nursing assistants to confront the patient directly? What coaching or role playing might you use with them if you choose this approach? Will you confront the patient yourself? What might you say?

LEARNING EXERCISE 21.10

Handling Personal Issues in a Professional Manner

You are a male unit supervisor of a pediatric trauma unit at Children's Hospital. Three years ago, you ended a serious romantic relationship with a nurse named Susan, who was employed at a different hospital in the same city. The break up was not mutual, and Susan was hurt and angry.

Six months ago, Susan accepted a position as a unit supervisor at Children's Hospital. This has required you and Susan to interact formally at department head meetings and informally regarding staffing and personnel issues on a regular basis. Often, these interactions have been marked by either covert hostility on Susan's part, nonverbal aggression, or sniping comments. When you attempted to confront Susan about her behavior, she stated that "she didn't have a problem and that you shouldn't flatter yourself to think that she does."

The situation is becoming increasingly more difficult to "work around," and both staff and fellow unit supervisors have become aware of the ongoing tension. You love your position and do not want to leave Children's Hospital, but it is becoming increasingly apparent that the situation cannot continue as it is.

● ASSIGNMENT: Answer the following questions:
1. How might gender have influenced the latent conditions, perceived or felt conflict, manifest conflict, and conflict aftermath in this situation?
2. What conflict strategies might you use to try to resolve this conflict? Avoidance? Smoothing? Accommodation? Competing? Compromise? Collaboration?
3. Would the use of a mediator be helpful in this situation?

Web Links

College Recruiter.com—Suggested Salary Negotiation Guidelines for Recent College Graduates
http://www.adguide.com/pages/articles/article257.htm
Defines negotiation, explains the process, and provides interview and negotiation suggestions.

International Council of Nurses
http://www.icn.ch/sewworkplace.htm
Includes framework guidelines addressing workplace violence in the health sector as well as a state-of-the-art paper.

Teamwork Resolves Conflict (TRC)
http://www.ebl.org/trc.html
Emphasizes team building as essential to conflict management and includes a solved team-building case study.

References

Ellis, J. R., & Hartley, C. L. (2004). *Nursing in today's world* (8th ed.). Philadelphia: Lippincott Williams & Wilkins.

Epstein, D. G. (2003). Mediation, not litigation. *Nursing Management, 34*(10), 40–42.

Fulmano, J. (2005). Navigate through conflict, not around it. *Nursing Management, 36*(8), 14, 18.

Gardner, D. B. (2005). Ten lessons in collaboration. *Online Journal of Issues in Nursing, 10*(1), 1–15.

Garon, M. (2006). The positive face of resistance: Nurses relate their stories. *Journal of Nursing Administration, 36*(5), 249–258.

Grzywacz, J. G., Frone, M. R., Brewer, C. S., & Kovner, C. T. (2006). Quantifying work-family conflict among registered nurses. *Research in Nursing and Health, 29*(5), 414–426.

Hendel, T., Fish, M., & Galon, V. (2005). Leadership style and choice of strategy in conflict management among Israeli nurse managers in general hospitals. *Journal of Management, 13*, 137–146.

Hockley, C. (2006). Violence in nursing: The expectations and the reality. In C. J. Huston (Ed.), *Professional issues in nursing*. Philadelphia: Lippincott Williams & Wilkins.

Lindeke, L. L., & Sieckert, A. M. (2005). Nurse-physician workplace collaboration. *Online Journal of Issues in Nursing*, *10*(1), 10–11.

Rew, M., & Ferns, T. (2005). Conflict management: A balanced approach to dealing with violence and aggression at work. *British Journal of Nursing*, *14*(4), 227–232.

Ramos, M. C. (2006). Eliminate destructive behaviors through example and evidence. *Nursing Management*, *37*(9), 34, 37–38, 40–41.

Sherman, R. O. (2006). Leading a multigenerational nursing workforce: Issues, challenges and strategies. *Online Journal of Issues in Nursing*, *11*(2), 1–5.

Sullivan, E. J. (2004). *Becoming influential: A guide for nurses*. Upper Saddle River, NJ: Pearson/Prentice Hall.

Tate, C. W. (2005). Negotiate in style. *Nursing Standard*, *20*(6), 69.

Yu X., & Davidhizar, R. (2004). Conflict management styles of Asian and Asian American nurses. *Health Care Manager*, *23*(1), 46–55.

Bibliography

Bowers, L. (2006). On conflict, containment and the relationship between them. *Nursing Inquiry*, *13*(3), 172–180.

Briles, J. (2005). Zapping conflict builds better teams. *Hospital Nursing*, *35*(11), 32–38.

Cohen, S. (2005). To resolve or confront, that is the question. *Nursing Management*, *36*(6), 12.

Cox, S. (2005). Taking the "con" out of conflict. *Nursing Management*, *36*(12), 57.

Elchos, S. (2006). Conflict resolution: Communicate, communicate, communicate! *Critical Care Nurse*, *26*(2), S24.

Greene, J. (2006). Avoiding confrontation affects productivity. *OR Manager*, *22*(7), 22.

Hocking, B. A. (2006). Using reflection to resolve conflict. *AORN Journal*, *84*(2), 249–250, 253–259.

Hutton, S. (2006). Workplace incivility: State of the science. *Journal of Nursing Administration*, *36*(2), 22–27.

Kelly, J. (2006). An overview of conflict. *Dimensions of Critical Care Nursing*, *25*(1), 22–28.

McMillan, I. (2005). 750,000 staff to be trained in conflict management. *Learning Disability Practice*, *8*(9), 4.

Molloy, S., & Henderson, I. (2006). Education and practice: Conflict resolution training in the NHS. *Journal of Perioperative Practice*, *16*(7), 323–326.

Rowe, M., & Sherlock, H. (2005). Stress and verbal abuse in nursing: Do burned out nurses eat their young? *Journal of Nursing Management*, *13*, 242–248.

Smith, A., & Nelson, G. (2005). Excise the dysfunction from your executive team. *Nursing Management*, *36*(5), 18.

Sportsman, S. (2005). Build a framework for conflict assessment. *Nursing Management*, *36*(4), 32, 34–36, 38.

Vivar, C. G. (2006). Putting conflict management into practice: A nursing case study. *Journal of Nursing Management*, *14*(3), 201–206.

22

Understanding Collective Bargaining, Unionization, and Employment Laws

. . . without union representation and a negotiated procedure for appealing against management actions, nurses have no guarantee that their side of the story will ever be heard, and little hope that unfair personnel decisions will be overturned.

—Suzanne Gordon

. . . we are the last line of defense for patients against healthcare corporations that want to squeeze every last penny out of the system.

—Deborah Burger

Factors that have an impact on the directing aspects of management are collective bargaining, unionization, and employment laws. It is possible to make these factors positive rather than negative influences on management effectiveness. To accomplish this, task managers must first understand the interrelationship of unionization and management, the proliferation of legislation regarding employment practices, and the impact of both on the health care industry.

Managers must be able to see collective bargaining and employment legislation from four perspectives: the organization, the worker, general historical and societal, and personal. Managers who can gain this broad perspective will better understand how management and employees can work together cooperatively despite unionization and employment legislation. Many industrialized countries have adopted an attitude of acceptance and tolerance for the difficulties of managing under these influences. Indeed, Gordon (2004) states that "collective bargaining in most industrialized counties is well established and rarely challenged" (p. 8).

However, in the United States, many organizations view these forces with resentment and hostility. This chapter examines the leadership roles and management functions necessary to

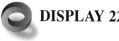

DISPLAY 22.1 Leadership Roles and Management Functions Associated With Understanding Collective Bargaining, Unionization, and Employment Laws

Leadership Roles

1. Is self-aware regarding personal attitudes and values regarding collective bargaining and employment laws
2. Recognizes and accepts reasons why people seek unionization
3. Creates a work environment that eliminates the need for unionization to meet employees' needs
4. Maintains an accommodating or cooperative approach when dealing with unions and employment legislation
5. Is a role model for fairness
6. Is nondiscriminatory in all personal and professional actions
7. Examines the work environment periodically to ensure that it is supportive for all members regardless of gender, race, age, disability, or sexual orientation
8. Actively seeks a culturally and ethnically diverse workforce to meet the needs of an increasingly diverse client population

Management Functions

1. Understands and appropriately implements union contracts
2. Administers personnel policies fairly and consistently
3. Works cooperatively with the personnel department and top-level administration when dealing with union activity
4. Understands and follows labor and employment laws that relate to the manager's sphere of influence
5. Ensures that the work environment is safe
6. Is alert for discriminatory employment practices in the workplace
7. Follows through on investigating any employee reports of discrimination
8. Ensures that the unit or department meets state licensing regulations
9. Immediately and fully investigates all complaints regarding violations of the collective bargaining contract and takes appropriate action

create a climate in which unionization and legislation are compatible with organizational goals. These leadership roles and management functions inherent in dealing with unions and employment laws are shown in Display 22.1.

UNIONS AND COLLECTIVE BARGAINING

Collective bargaining involves activities occurring between organized labor and management that concern employee relations. Such activities include negotiation of formal labor agreements and day-to-day interactions between unions and management. Huston (2006a) maintains that at the heart of the debate about collective bargaining and nursing is whether nursing, long recognized as a caring profession, should be a part of bargaining efforts to improve working conditions. Although this may seem to represent a dichotomy, it is also true that unions and collective bargaining are very much a part of many nurses' lived experience.

DISPLAY 22.2 **Collective Bargaining Terminology**

Agency shop: Also called an *open shop*. Employees are not required to join the union.

Arbitration: Terminal step in the grievance procedure, where a third party reviews the grievance, completes fact finding, and reaches a decision. Always indicates the involvement of a third party. Arbitration may be voluntary on the part of management and labor or imposed by the government in a compulsory arbitration.

Collective bargaining: Relations between employers, acting through their management representatives, and organized labor.

Conciliation and mediation: Synonymous terms that refer to the activity of a third party to help disputants reach an agreement. However, unlike an arbitrator, this person has no final power of decision making.

Fact finding: Rarely used in the private sector but used frequently in labor–management disputes that involve government-owned companies. In the private sector, fact finding is usually performed by a board of inquiry.

Free speech: Public Law 101, Section 8 states that "the expressing of any views, argument, or dissemination thereof, whether in written, printed, graphic, or visual form, shall not constitute or be evidence of an unfair labor practice under any provisions of this Act, if such expression contains no threat of reprisal or force or promise of benefit."

Grievance: Perception on the part of a union member that management has failed in some way to meet the terms of the labor agreement.

Lockout: Closing a place of business by management in the course of a labor dispute for the purpose of forcing employees to accept management terms.

National Labor Relations Board: Labor board formed to implement the Wagner Act. Its two major functions are to (a) determine who should be the official bargaining unit when a new unit is formed and who should be in the unit and (b) adjudicate unfair labor charges.

Professionals: Professionals have the right to be represented by a union but cannot belong to a union that represents nonprofessionals unless a majority of them vote for inclusion in the nonprofessional unit.

Strike: Concerted withholding of labor supply to bring about economic pressure on employers and cause them to grant employee demands.

Union shop: Also called a *closed shop*. All employees are required to join the union and pay dues.

Although first- and middle-level managers usually have little to do with negotiating the labor contract, they are greatly involved with the contract's daily implementation. The middle manager has the greatest impact on the quality of the relationship that develops between labor and management. Terminology associated with unions and collective bargaining is shown in Display 22.2.

HISTORICAL PERSPECTIVE OF UNIONIZATION IN AMERICA

Unions have been present in America since the 1790s. Skilled craftsmen formed early unions to protect themselves from wage cuts during the highly competitive era of industrialization. The history of unionization reveals that union membership and activity increase sharply during times of high employment and prosperity and decrease sharply during economic recessions and layoffs.

Union activity also tends to change in response to workforce excesses and shortages. For decades, employment demand for nurses has increased and decreased periodically. High demand for nurses is tied directly to a healthy national economy, and historically, this has been correlated with increased union activity. Similarly, when nursing vacancy rates are low, union membership and activity tends to decline.

Nurses' perceptions of the quality of their supervision have always had an impact on unionization rates. The rapid downsizing and restructuring of the 1990s left many nurses feeling that management did not listen to them or care about their needs. Bruno (2005) says that new restructuring models are being implemented daily, and some programs are being introduced that obviate RN professional judgment and assessment.

With restructuring comes expanded corporate health care, resulting in hospitals looking for areas to cut costs. One of the hardest-hit areas of benefits is health care. As well, grocery, airline, and other industries have seen such cuts. Health benefits were the main issue in 55% of all contract talks monitored by the federal mediation service in 2004 (Bruno, 2005). Bruno also reports that RNs are learning the bitter lessons of other workers as pensions and retiree health benefits become a major target for financial managers in hospitals. Other issues, such as mandatory overtime and staffing ratios, are factors in increased unionization among nurses. Research by Buerhaus, Donelan, Ulrich, Kirby, Normal, and Dittus (2005) showed that in 2002 and 2004, the majority of RNs surveyed found that unionization had a positive impact on patient care.

 Management that is perceived to be deaf to the workers' needs provides a fertile ground for union organizers, because unions thrive in a climate that perceives the organizational philosophy to be insensitive to the worker.

For many reasons, collective bargaining was slow in coming to the health care industry. Until labor laws were amended, unionization of health care workers was illegal. Nursing's long history as a service commodity further delayed labor organization in health care settings. Initial collective bargaining in the profession took place in organizations that were deemed government or public. This was made possible by *Executive Order 10988*, authored in 1962. This order lifted restrictions preventing public employees from organizing. Therefore, collective bargaining by nurses at city, county, and district hospitals and health care agencies began in the 1960s.

In 1974, Congress amended the Wagner Act, extending national labor laws to private, nonprofit hospitals; nursing homes; health clinics; health maintenance organizations; and other health care institutions. These amendments opened the doors to much union activity for professions and the public employee sector. Indeed, a review of union membership figures readily shows that since 1960, most collective bargaining activity in the United States occurred in the public and professional sectors of industry, most notably among faculty at institutions of higher education, teachers at primary and secondary levels, and physicians. There has been little growth of unionization in the private and blue-collar sectors since membership peaked in the 1950s.

From 1962 through 1989, slow but steady increases occurred in the numbers of nurses represented by collective bargaining agents. In 1989, the National Labor Relations Board (NLRB) ruled that nurses could form their own separate bargaining units, and union activity increased. However, the American Hospital Association (AHA) immediately sued the American Nurses Association (ANA), and the ruling was halted until 1991, when the Supreme Court upheld the 1989 *NLRB* decision. Table 22.1 outlines legislation that led to unionization in health care.

TABLE 22.1   **Labor Legislation**

Year	Legislation	Effect
1935	National Labor Act/Wagner Act	Gave unions many rights in organizing; resulted in rapid union growth
1947	Taft-Hartley Amendment	Returned some power to management; resulted in a more equal balance of power between unions and management
1962	Kennedy *Executive Order 10988*	Amended the 1935 Wagner Act to allow public employees to join unions
1974	Amendments to Wagner Act	Allowed nonprofit organizations to join unions
1989	National Labor Relations Board ruling	Allowed nurses to form their own separate bargaining units

Various unions represent nurses and other health care workers. The Service Employees International Union (SEIU) is the largest union in the health care industry, representing more than 870,000 health care workers, including 84,000 RNs in 23 states (SEIU, 2007). SEIU is also the largest union of nursing home workers in the United States, representing more than 145,000 employees. Some of the other unions that represent nurses include the ANA; the National Union of Hospital and Health Care Employees of Retail, Wholesale and Department Store Union; the American Federation of Labor–Congress of Industrial Organizations (AFL-CIO); the United Steelworkers of America (USWA); the American Federation of Government Employees, AFL-CIO; the American Federation of State, County, and Municipal Employees, AFL-CIO; the International Brotherhood of Teamsters; the American Federation of State, County, and Municipal Employees, which operates mostly in the public sector; and the United Auto Workers.

Union representation also varies by state. The states with the most union organizing for all industries, including health care, are New York, California, Pennsylvania, Michigan, and Illinois (Huston, 2006a). The actual total number of all nurses belonging to unions varies among reports, from 16% to 22%. The discrepancies have to do with how the numbers are calculated.

AMERICAN NURSES ASSOCIATION AND COLLECTIVE BARGAINING

One difficult union issue faced by nurse–managers that is not typically encountered in other disciplines stems from the dual role of their professional organization, the ANA. The NLRB recognizes the ANA, at most state levels, as a collective bargaining agent. The use of state associations as bargaining agents has been a divisive issue among American nurses. Some nurse–managers believe that they have been disenfranchised by their professional organization. Other managers recognize the conflicts inherent in attempting to sit on both sides of the bargaining table. For some members of the nursing profession, this issue presents no conflict. Regardless of individual values, there does appear to be some conflict in loyalty.

This conflict has manifested itself in recent splitting away of state nurses associations from the parent ANA organization. Bruno (2005) suggests that the ANA has not shown leadership in a time of professional nursing crisis and that the ANA has supported management interests over those of nurses. Since California RNs broke from the ANA, there have been other states, Massachusetts and Maine, that have disaffiliated. Additionally, two other states, New York and Pennsylvania, have declared their independence (Revolution, 2005). There are no easy solutions to the dilemma created by the dual role held by the ANA. Clarifying these issues begins with the manager examining the motivation of nurses to participate in collective bargaining. The manager must at least try to hear and understand employees' points of view.

LEARNING EXERCISE 22.1

The Role of the ANA as Collective Bargaining Agent
How do you feel about the ANA's certification as a collective bargaining agent? Do you belong to the state student nurses association? Why or why not? Do you plan to join your state ANA? What are the primary driving and restraining forces for your decision? Divide into two groups to debate the pros and cons of having the ANA, rather than other unions, represent nurses.

EMPLOYEE MOTIVATION TO JOIN OR REJECT UNIONS

Knowing that human behavior is goal directed, it is important to examine what personal goals a union membership fulfills. Nurse–managers often tell each other that health care institutions differ from other types of industrial organizations. This is really a myth, because most nurses work in large and impersonal organizations. The nurse frequently feels powerless and vulnerable as an individual alone in a complex institution.

Six primary motivations for joining a union exist (Display 22.3). The first is to increase the power of the individual. Employees know that singly, they are much more dispensable. Because a large group of employees is generally less dispensable, nurses greatly increase their bargaining power and reduce their vulnerability by joining a union. This is a particularly strong motivating force for nurses when jobs are scarce and they feel vulnerable. Indeed, during the massive downsizing and restructuring of the 1990s, collective bargaining priorities shifted from wages and benefits to job security.

> A feeling of powerlessness or the perception that administration does not care about employees is a major driving force for unionization.

When there are nursing shortages, nurses feel less vulnerable, and other reasons to join unions become motivating factors. A second motivator driving nurses toward unionization is the desire to communicate their aims, feelings, complaints, and ideas to others and to have input into organizational decision making.

Because unions emphasize equality and fairness, nurses also join them because they need to eliminate discrimination and favoritism. This might be an especially strong motivator for members of groups that have experienced discrimination, such as women and minorities.

DISPLAY 22.3   Union Membership: Pros and Cons

Reasons Why Nurses Join Unions

1. To increase the power of the individual
2. To increase their input into organizational decision making
3. To eliminate discrimination and favoritism
4. Because of a social need to be accepted
5. Because they are required to do so as part of employment (closed shop)
6. Because they believe it will improve patient outcomes and quality of care

Reasons Why Nurses Do Not Want to Join Unions

1. A belief that unions promote the welfare state and oppose the American system of free enterprise
2. A need to demonstrate individualism and promote social status
3. A belief that professionals should not unionize
4. An identification with management's viewpoint
5. Fear of employer reprisal
6. Fear of lost income associated with a strike or walkout

Many social factors also act as motivators to nurses regarding union activity. A fourth motivation for joining a union stems from the social need to be accepted. Sometimes, this social need results from family or peer pressure. Because many working-class families have a long history of strong union ties, children are frequently raised in a cultural milieu that promotes unionization.

A fifth reason why nurses sometimes join unions is because the union contract dictates that all nurses belong to the union. This has been a big driving force among blue-collar workers. However, the *closed shop*, or requirement that all employees belong to a union, has never prevailed in the health care industry. Most health care unions have *open shops*, allowing nurses to choose if they want to join the union.

Finally, some nurses join unions because they believe that patient outcomes are better in unionized organizations due to better staffing and supervised management practices. Bruno (2005) suggests a positive relationship between unionization and safe standards of care and effective patient advocacy. Twarog (2005) says that mandating safe needles, limiting mandatory overtime, and setting nurse-to-patient ratios have all been pushed first by unions and that accomplishing these results was not due to employer's benevolence or goodwill. These were union-driven accomplishments.

Bauer (2005) states that there is debate as to whether unionization leads to better working conditions but that there is no debate about union wages being higher. He states that unionized RNs on an average earn $6,100 more yearly than non-union nurses.

Just as there are many reasons to join unions, there also are reasons why nurses reject unions (Display 22.3). Perhaps the strongest are societal and cultural factors. Many people distrust unions because they believe that unions promote the welfare state and undermine the American system of free enterprise. Other reasons for rejecting unions might be a need to demonstrate that nurses can get ahead on their own merits.

Professional employees have been slow in forming unions for several reasons that deal with class and education. They argue that unions were appropriate for the blue-collar worker but not for the university professor, physician, or engineer. Nurses who reject unions on this basis usually are driven by a need to demonstrate their individualism and social status. Some employees identify with management and thus frequently adopt its viewpoint toward unions. Such nurses, therefore, would reject unions because their values more closely align with management than with workers. Although employees are protected under the *National Labor Relations Act* (NLRA), many reject unions because of fears of employer reprisal. Nurses who reject unions on this basis could be said to be motivated most of all by a need to keep their job.

Finally, some nurses reject unions out of the fear of lost income associated with a *strike* or *walkout*. Strikes and walkouts are a reality of unionization; however, they are regulated by law. The NLRA states in part that "employees shall have the right to engage in other concerted activities for the purpose of collective bargaining or other mutual aid or protection." The phrase *other concerted activities* refers to "working to rule," "blue flu" epidemics, work slowdowns, filing a barrage of grievances, participating in informational or recognition picketing, contracting government agencies such as the Department of Health or Occupational Safety and Health Administration, and striking (Forman & Powell, 2003). Unions must, however, give employers and the Federal Mediation and Conciliation Service (FMCS) 10 days notice of their intent to strike (Forman & Powell, 2003).

Once managers understand the drives and needs behind joining unions, they can begin to address those needs and possibly avert some staff needs for unionization. Organizations with unfair management policies are more likely to become unionized.

 It is within managerial power to eliminate some of the needs that staff have for joining unions.

Managers can encourage feelings of power by allowing subordinates to have input into decisions that will affect their work. Managers also can listen to ideas, complaints, and feelings and take steps to ensure that favoritism and discrimination are not part of their management style. Additionally, the manager can strengthen the drives and needs that make nurses reject unions. By building a team effort, sharing ideas and future plans from upper management with the staff, and encouraging individualism in employees, the manager can facilitate identification of the worker with management.

When nurses begin to show signs of job dissatisfaction, when they feel frustrated, stressed or powerless, they are sending a wake-up call to nursing management. Leaders must be alert to employment practices that are unfair or insensitive to employee needs and must intervene appropriately before such issues lead to unionization. However, organizations offering liberal benefit packages and fair management practices may still experience union activity if certain social and cultural factors are present. If union activity does occur, managers must be aware of specific employee and management rights so that the NLRA is not violated by managers or employees.

LEARNING EXERCISE 22.2

Discussing Pros and Cons of Unions

List the reasons why you would or would not join a union. Share this with others in your group, and examine the following questions. Would you feel differently about unions if you were a manager? What influences you the most in your desire to join or reject unions? Have you ever felt discriminated against or powerless in the workplace?

DISPLAY 22.4   **Some Union-Organizing Strategies**

1. Meetings (both group and one-on-one)
2. Leaflets and brochures
3. Pressure on the hospital corporation through media and community contacts
4. Political pressure of regional legislators and local lawmakers
5. Corporate campaign strategies
6. Activism of local employees
7. Using lawsuits
8. Bringing pressure from financiers
9. Technology

UNION-ORGANIZING STRATEGIES

Haugh (2006) suggests that unions use a variety of tactics when organizing health care workers. Among the strategies that he discusses are meetings—both group and one-on-one. Contacts are made by union representatives (Display 22.4). Other strategies used are providing literature about union benefits, writing letters, and otherwise contacting potential union members. However, Haugh feels that unions recently have added new methods of organizing—namely, community and corporate pressure. This pressure is usually directed at acute-care hospitals.

In corporate campaigns, the union uses public events, political connections, and the local media to bring into question a hospital's quality of care, level of charity work, its tax exempt status (if nonprofit), and nurse staffing. Haugh (2006) maintains that unions are very effective in involving influential power brokers, both financiers and lawmakers. Unions are designing corporate campaigns with allegations of discrimination, boycotts, rallies, and visits to board members' homes. Another strategy contributing to labor union successes is activism. Central labor councils, local labor unions, and state labor federations are reaching out to community groups, faith-based organizations, and elected officials in an effort to create unrest and change the community environment in which workers organize.

Unions often file lawsuits against the employer. Labor unions maintain the goal of breaking employer resolve and demonstrate their ability to protect employees by initiating legal action on behalf of employees against targeted employers. Other corporate strategies include union organizers establishing websites to enable them to keep tabs on the hospital system (Haugh, 2006). The Internet has made accessing information about how to organize a union very accessible to interested workers. Email has also proved to be an inexpensive and efficient means of mass communication regarding critical union issues.

MANAGERS' ROLE DURING UNION ORGANIZING

Because of the health care industry's movement toward unionization, most nurses will probably be involved with unions in some manner during their careers. Managers who are not employed in a unionized health care organization should anticipate that one or more unions will attempt to

DISPLAY 22.5 **Before the Union Comes**

1. Know and care about your employees.
2. Establish fair and well-communicated personnel policies.
3. Use an effective upward and downward system of communication.
4. Ensure that all managers are well trained and effective.
5. Establish a well-developed formal procedure for handling employee grievances.
6. Have a competitive compensation program of wages and benefits.
7. Have an effective performance appraisal system in place.
8. Use a fair and well-communicated system for promotions and transfers.
9. Use organizational actions to indicate that job security is based on job performance, adherence to rules and regulations, and availability of work.
10. Have an administrative policy on unionization.

organize nurses within the next few years. Display 22.5 lists practices that the organization should have in place that will discourage union activity. If the organization waits until the union arrives, it will be too late to perform these functions.

One way to remain abreast of employee potential concerns is to review current literature and research on nurse satisfaction and dissatisfaction. When managers are aware of national concerns of RNs, they are better able to assess their own staff's potential for the type of dissatisfaction that can lead to unionization. An example of such research is the ongoing surveys by Buerhaus and colleagues (2005) of nurses' perceptions of their work (Examining the Evidence 22.1).

 EXAMINING THE EVIDENCE 22.1

Source: Buerhaus, P. I., Donelan, K., Ulrich, B. T., Kirby, L., Norman, L., & Dittus, R. (2005). Registered nurses' perceptions of nursing. *Nursing Economics, 23*(3), 110–118, 143.

This research compared two surveys (2002 and 2004), and highlighted changes in nurses' perceptions of various aspects of nursing. In this Part II summary of the analysis, the findings focused on job satisfaction, comparing the two different survey periods. A total of 4,108 RNs completed the survey for a response rate of 55%.

Reports of being "very satisfied" with their job increased from 21% (2002) to 34% (2004) and was predicated on patient care, management recognition for personal lives, satisfaction with salary and benefits, job security, and positive relationship with other nurses and management.

From 2002 to 2004, among all respondents, the percentage of RNs who reported that they themselves and/or others in their workplace belonged to unions increased from 21% to 27%. More RNs perceived mostly or somewhat positive effects of unionization on the nursing profession than those who felt that the union's effects were mostly negative. In both surveys, the same percentage of nurses felt that unionization had a positive effect on patient care.

Nurse–managers, as legally defined hospital "supervisors," are legal spokespersons for the hospital. As such, the NLRB closely monitors what they may say and do. Until recently, only supervisors were considered managers and were the only ones prohibited from joining unions. However, a 2006 NLRB ruling has now deemed that charge nurses are also considered supervisors; even part-time charge nurses are so labeled. This finding is being fought by unions, and it remains to be seen if the NLRB will change its ruling at a later date (Burger, 2006).

Prohibited managerial activities include threatening employees, interrogating employees, promising employees rewards for cessation of union activity, and spying on employees. However, if the astute manager picks up early clues of union activity, the organization may be able to take steps that will discourage unionization of its employees.

 Employees have a right to participate in union organizing under the NLRA, and managers must not interfere with this right.

The first step in establishing a union is demonstrating an adequate level of desire for unionization by the employees. The NLRB requires that at least 30% of employees sign an interest card before an election for unionization can be held. Most unions, however, will require between 60% and 70% of the employees to sign interest cards before spending the time and money involved in an organizing campaign. Union representatives are generally careful to keep a campaign secret until they are ready to file a petition for election. They do this so that they can build momentum without interference from the employer. However, recent legislation has been introduced in the 2007 U.S. Congress, called the *Employee Free Choice Act* (HR 800). If passed, this will allow unions to request representation from the NLRB by the use of signed cards only. Therefore, it would eliminate the need for a secret ballot election to determine union representation. This bill has been supported by a bipartisan coalition in Congress (AFL-CIO, 2007).

Currently, after a designated number of cards have been generated, the organization is forced to have an election. At that time, all employees of the same classification, such as RNs, would vote on whether they desire unionization. A choice in every such election is *no representation*, which means that the voters do not want a union. During the election, 50% plus one of the petitioned unit must vote for unionization before the union can be recognized.

A process similar to that of certification can also decertify unions. *Decertification* may occur when at least 30% of the eligible employees in the bargaining unit initiate a petition asking to no longer be represented by the union (Forman & Kraus, 2003). By law, employers are not allowed to instigate or promote decertification but may provide employees with information regarding their rights to do so under the NLRA (Forman & Kraus, 2003).

It is important to remember that there are differences between organizing in a health care facility and other types of organizations. Generally, the solicitation and distribution of union literature is banned entirely in "immediate patient care areas." Managers should never, however, independently attempt to deal with union-organizing activity. They should always seek assistance and guidance from higher-level management and the personnel department.

The entire list of rights for management and labor during the organizing and establishment phases of unionization is beyond the scope of this book. Throughout the years, Congress has amended various labor acts and laws so that power is balanced between management and labor. At times, the balance of power has shifted to management or labor, but Congress wisely eventually enacts laws that restore the balance. The manager must ensure that the rights of management and employees are protected. The two most sensitive areas of any union contract, once wages have been agreed on, are discipline and the grievance process, which are discussed in Unit VII.

EFFECTIVE LABOR–MANAGEMENT RELATIONS

Before the 1950s, labor–management relations were turbulent. History books are filled with battles, strikes, mass-picketing scenes, and brutal treatment by management and employees. In the last 30 years, employers and unions have substantially improved their relationships. Although evidence is growing that contemporary management has come to accept the reality that unions are here to stay, businesses in the United States are still less comfortable with unions than their counterparts in many other countries. Likewise, unions have come to accept the fact that there are times when organizations are not healthy enough to survive aggressive union demands.

 Once management is faced with dealing with a bargaining agent, it has a choice of either accepting or opposing the union.

Faced with the reality of negotiations with a bargaining agent, management has choices. It may actively oppose the union by using various union-busting techniques, or it may more subtly oppose the union by attempting to discredit it and win employee trust. *Acceptance* also may run along a continuum. Management may accept the union with reluctance and suspicion. Although managers know that the union has legitimate rights, they often believe that they must continually guard against the union encroaching further into traditional management territory.

There also is the type of union acceptance known as *accommodation*. Increasingly common, accommodation is characterized by management's full acceptance of the union, with both union and management showing mutual respect. When these conditions exist, labor and management can establish mutual goals, especially in the areas of safety, cost reduction, efficiency, elimination of waste, and improved working conditions. This type of relationship has begun between unionized professional nurses and health care organizations, and hopefully, it will be a cooperative and new model of collective-bargaining relationship (Forman & Grimes, 2004). Such cooperation represents the most mature and advanced type of labor–management relations.

The attitudes and the philosophies of the leaders in management and the union determine the type of relationship that develops between the two parties in any given organization. When dealing with unions, managers must be flexible. It is critical that they do not ignore issues or try to overwhelm others with power. The rational approach to problem solving must be used.

Unionization in the health care industry will undoubtedly expand. It is important to learn how to deal with this potential constraint to effective management. Managers must learn to work with unions and develop the art of using unions to assist the organization in building a team effort to meet organizational goals.

LEARNING EXERCISE 22.3

List and Support Your Reasons For or Against Striking
You are a staff nurse in the ICU in one of your city's two hospitals. You have worked at this hospital for 5 years and transferred to the ICU 2 years ago. You love nursing but are sometimes frustrated in your job due to a short supply of nurses, excessive overtime demands, and the stress of working with such critically ill patients.

The hospital has a closed shop, so union dues are deducted from your pay even though you are not actively involved in the union. The present union contract is up for renegotiation, and union and management have been unable to agree on many issues. When management made its last offer, the new contract was rejected by the nurses. Now that the old contract has expired, nurses are free to strike if they vote to do so.

You had voted for accepting the management offer; you have two children to support, and it would be devastating to be without work for a long time. Last night, the nurses voted on whether to return to the bargaining table and try to renegotiate with management or to go out on strike. Again, you voted for no strike. You have just heard from your friend that the strike vote won. Now, you must decide if you are going to support your striking colleagues or cross the picket line and return to work tomorrow. Your friends are pressuring you to support their cause. You know that the union will provide some financial compensation during the strike but believe that it will not be adequate for you to support yourself and your children. You agree with union assertions that the organization has overworked and underpaid you and that it has been generally unresponsive to nursing needs. On the other hand, you believe that your first obligation is to your children.

● ASSIGNMENT: List all of the reasons for and against striking. Decide what you will do. Use appropriate rationale from outside readings to support your final decision. Share your thoughts with the class. Take a vote in class to determine how many would strike and how many would cross the picket line.

EMPLOYMENT LEGISLATION

Like unionization, the many legal issues involved in hiring and employment have an impact on the directing function. These potential constraints are present regardless of union presence. The American industrial relations system is regarded as one of the most legalistic in the Western world, and it continues to grow. Few aspects of the employment relationship are free from regulation by either state or federal law. Employment laws discussed here provide a cursory examination of such laws. Many of these regulations relate to specific aspects of personnel management, such as the laws that deal with collective bargaining or the equal employment laws that regulate hiring. Some personnel regulations are discussed in previous chapters and others are discussed later. The prudent manager will always work closely with human resource management when dealing with employment legislation issues.

Some observers believe that employment and labor–management laws have become so prescriptive that they preclude experimentation and creativity on the part of management. Others believe that like collective bargaining, the proliferation of employment laws must be viewed from a historical standpoint to understand their need. Regardless of whether one believes such laws and regulations are necessary, they are a fact of each manager's life.

> The feeling that the employer is fair to all will set the stage for the type of team building that is so important in effective management.

Being able to handle management's legal requirements effectively requires a comprehension of labor laws and their interpretation. The leader who embraces the intent of laws barring

TABLE 22.2 Employment and Labor Laws

Title of Legislation	Regulation
Fair Labor Standards Act (1938); has been amended many times since 1938	Sets minimum wage and maximum hours that can be worked before overtime is paid
Civil Rights Act of 1964	Sets equal employment practices
Executive Order 11246 (1965) and *Executive Order 11375* (1967)	Sets affirmative action guidelines
Age Discrimination Act (1967) and 1978 amendment	Protects against forced retirement
Rehabilitation Act (1973)	Protects the disabled
Vietnam Veterans Act (1973/1974)	Provides reemployment rights

discrimination and providing equal opportunity becomes a role model for fairness. Employment laws, summarized in Table 22.2, fall into one of five categories:

1. *Labor standards.* These laws establish minimum standards for working conditions regardless of the presence or absence of a union contract. Included in this set are minimum wage, health and safety, and equal pay laws.
2. *Labor relations.* These laws relate to the rights and duties of unions and employers in their relationship with each other.
3. *Equal employment.* The laws that deal with employment discrimination were introduced in Chapter 15.
4. *Civil and criminal laws.* These are statutory and judicial laws that proscribe certain kinds of conduct and establish penalties.
5. *Other legislation.* Nursing managers have some legal responsibilities that do not generally apply to industrial managers. For instance, licensed personnel are required to have a current, valid license from the state in which they practice. Additionally, most states require that employers of nurses report certain types of substance abuse to the state licensing boards. Confidentiality laws also have a significant impact on health care organizations.

Labor Standards

Labor standards are regulations dealing with the conditions of the employee's work, including physical conditions, financial aspects, and the amount of hours worked. Regulations may be issued by state and/or federal bodies. When the regulations overlap, the more stringent regulation is likely the one that applies.

 State and federal employment legislation often overlap; as a general rule, the employer must abide by the stricter of the two regulations.

Minimum Wages and Maximum Hours

More than 85% of all nonsupervisory employees are now covered by the *Fair Labor Standards Act* (FLSA). This law was enacted by Congress in 1938 and established an hourly minimum wage at that time of 25 cents. Since then, the law has been amended numerous times.

It is often said that in addition to putting a "floor under wages," the FLSA also puts a "ceiling over hours." The latter statement, however, is not quite accurate. The FLSA sets a maximum number of hours in any week beyond which a person may be employed only if he or she is paid an overtime rate. Some states have enacted a law that makes an exception to this weekly rule on overtime. The exception is an 80-hour, 2-week pay period ceiling, after which the employee must receive overtime pay. Overtime pay can be significant, so it is imperative that managers know which standard their organization is using.

Hours worked includes all the time that the employee is required to be on duty. Therefore, mandatory classes, orientation, conferences, and so on must be recorded as duty time and are subject to the overtime rules. The FLSA does not require time clocks but does require that some record be maintained of hours worked.

The FLSA also regulates the minimum amount of overtime pay, which is at least 1.5 times the basic rate. When state and federal laws differ on when overtime pay begins, the stricter rule usually applies. Some union contracts also have stricter overtime pay agreements than the FLSA.

Federal labor laws exempt certain employees from the minimum wage and overtime pay requirements. Executive employees, administrative employees, and professional employees are the three most notable white-collar exemptions. The functions of the position, rather than the title or the fact that employees are paid a monthly wage, differentiate an exempt employee. Certain students, apprentice learners, and other special circumstances also may qualify an employee for an exemption to FLSA regulations.

President Bush signed a $328 billion spending bill on January 23, 2004, that among other things enacted new regulations that allow companies to pay overtime to fewer white-collar workers, including nurses. Under the new regulations, low-income workers increased their eligibility for overtime compensation while workers earning more than $65,000 a year could be denied overtime pay if their employers classified them as administrators, professionals, or other exempt employees (Ray, 2004). The personnel department in any large organization is especially helpful to the manager in implementing these labor laws. Managers, however, should have a general understanding of how these laws restrict staffing and scheduling policies.

The Equal Pay Act of 1963 requires that men and women performing equal work receive equal compensation. Four equal pay tests exist: *equal skill, equal effort, equal responsibility,* and *similar working conditions.* This law had a great impact on nursing management when it was enacted. Before 1963, male "orderlies" were routinely paid a higher wage than female "aides" performing identical duties. Although this fact seems incredible today, at the time, many managers condoned this widespread practice of blatant wage discrimination. Most health care agencies now call these employees "nursing assistants," whether they are male or female, and all are paid the same wage.

LEARNING EXERCISE 22.4

Time Clocks

Until the 1950s, most health care organizations did not require that employees use a time clock when arriving at or leaving work for meal breaks. Now, time clocks are the norm for hospitals and some other, but not all, health care organizations.

● ASSIGNMENT: Survey several community hospitals, clinics, student health centers, home health care facilities, and other organizations that employ nurses. How many of them require nurses to use time clocks? How do you feel about professionals being required to punch or swipe in and out for meal breaks? Discuss this issue in class and with the nurses you know.

Labor Relations Laws

In addition to laws regarding collective bargaining, the manager needs to be aware of one section of the Wagner Act (1935) and the Taft-Hartley Amendment (1947), which deal with unfair labor practices by employers and unions. The original Wagner Act listed and prohibited five unfair labor practices:

1. To interfere with, restrain, or coerce employees in a manner that interfered with their rights as outlined under the act. Examples of these activities are spying on union gatherings, threatening employees with job loss, or threatening to close down a company if the union organizes.
2. To interfere with the formation of any labor organization or to give financial assistance to a labor organization. This provision was included to prohibit "employee representation plans" that were primarily controlled by management.
3. To discriminate with regard to hiring, tenure, and so on to discourage union membership.
4. To discharge or discriminate against an employee who filed charges or testified before the NLRB.
5. To refuse to bargain in good faith.

The original Wagner Act gave so much power to the unions that it was necessary in 1947 to pass additional federal legislation to restore a balance of power to labor–management relations. The Taft-Hartley Amendment retained the provisions under the Wagner Act that guaranteed employees the right to collective bargaining. However, the Taft-Hartley Amendment added the provision that employees have the right to refrain from taking part in unions. In addition to that provision, the Taft-Hartley Amendment added and prohibited the following six unfair labor practices of unions:

1. Requiring a self-employed person or an employer to join a union.
2. Forcing an employer to cease doing business with another person. This placed a ban on secondary boycotts, which were then prevalent in unions.
3. Forcing an employer to bargain with one union when another union has already been certified as the bargaining agent.
4. Forcing the employer to assign certain work to members of one union rather than another.
5. Charging excessive or discriminatory initiation fees.
6. Causing or attempting to cause an employer to pay for unnecessary services. This prohibited *featherbedding*, a term used to describe union practices that prevented the displacement of workers due to advances in technology.

Equal Employment Opportunity Laws

Under the American free enterprise system, employers have historically been able to hire whomever they desired. Today, a transplanted employer of the 1920s might be shocked to see that racial and ethnic minorities, women, the elderly, and the disabled have acquired substantial rights in the workplace. The first legislation in the area of employment hiring practices resulted from years of discrimination against minorities. More recent legislation has been aimed at eliminating discrimination that occurs for other reasons. The U.S. government's Equal Employment Opportunity Commission (EEOC) website lists the following types of discrimination: age, disability, equal pay, national origin, pregnancy, race, religion, retaliation, sex, and sexual harassment (USEEOC, 2007a).

Equal employment opportunities have fostered profound changes in the American workplace. Women, minorities, and the handicapped have had success in gaining jobs previously denied to them. However, only modest gains in achieving ethnic diversity have occurred in nursing (Huston, 2006b).

Although men are seen as a minority in nursing, there are those who feel that male minority status has led to advantages rather than discrimination, especially in hiring and promotion (Kleinman, 2004). Kleinman suggests that this may occur because traditional health care organizations were organized and managed along patricidal structures that favor male dominance.

Discrimination involving pregnant employees particularly interests nurse–managers because nursing is such a predominately female profession and because nurses are often exposed to hazardous chemical, radiation, and infectious organisms. Middaugh and Hester (2006) suggest that managers should understand the Pregnancy Discrimination Act, which requires that pregnant employees are treated the same as other employees who are temporarily disabled. Managers should use common sense as well as ethical and humane treatment when dealing with the pregnant employee.

Civil Rights Act of 1964

The *Civil Rights Act of 1964* laid the foundation for equal employment in the United States. The thrust of Title VII of the Civil Rights Act is twofold: It prohibits discrimination based on factors unrelated to job qualifications, and it promotes employment based on ability and merit. The areas of discrimination specifically mentioned are race, color, religion, sex, and national origin. This act was strengthened by President Lyndon Johnson's *Executive Order 11246* in 1965 and *Executive Order 11375* in 1967. These executive orders sought to correct past injustices. Because the government believed that some groups had a long history of being discriminated against, it wanted to build in a mechanism that would assist those groups in "catching up" with the rest of the American workforce. Therefore, it created an affirmative action component. *Affirmative action* plans are not specifically required by law but may be required by court order. In most states, affirmative action plans are voluntary unless government contracts are involved. Some states, such as California, have recently voted to eliminate affirmative action in the workplace, arguing that it actually resulted in reverse discrimination. Many organizations, however, have voluntarily put an affirmative action plan in place, if the plan does not conflict with state regulations.

Affirmative action differs from *equal opportunity*. The Equal Employment Opportunity legislation is aimed at preventing discrimination. Affirmative action plans are aimed at actively seeking to fill job vacancies with members from groups who are underrepresented, such as women, ethnic minorities, and the handicapped.

The EEOC is responsible for enforcing Title VII of the Civil Rights Act. The investigatory responsibility of the EEOC is broad. When it finds that a charge of discrimination is justified, the agency attempts to reach an agreement through persuasion and conciliation. When the EEOC is unable to reach an agreement, it has the power to bring civil action against the employer. When discrimination is found, the courts will order restoration of rightful economic status; this means that the employee may be ordered to receive back pay for up to 2 years. In health care organizations, when discrimination has been found (such as unequal pay for men and women in nursing assistant jobs), financial awards in class action suits have been extraordinarily high. Managers must be alert for any such discriminatory practices. Some states have fair employment legislation that is stricter than the federal act. Again, the stricter regulations always apply.

Age Discrimination and Employment Act

Enacted by Congress in 1967, the purpose of the *Age Discrimination and Employment Act* (ADEA) was to promote employment of older people based on their ability rather than age. In early 1978, the ADEA was amended to increase the protected age to 70. In 1987, Congress voted to remove even this age restriction except in certain job categories. Although some people are alarmed by the removal of mandatory age retirements, trends continue to be toward earlier retirement. However, reversal of this trend may have serious consequences for some organizations. In particular, it could have a significant impact on organizations that are labor intensive, especially if those labor-intensive organizations also have demanding physical requirements, such as those in nursing.

LEARNING EXERCISE 22.5

Addressing Mary's Failing Health

You are the manager of a well-baby newborn nursery. Among your staff is 73-year-old LVN/LPN Mary Jones, who has worked for the hospital for 50 years. No mandatory retirement age exists. This has not been a problem in the past, but Mary's general health is now making this a problem for your unit. Mary has grown physically fragile. Cataracts cloud her vision, and she suffers from hypertension. Last month, she began to prepare a little girl for circumcision because she did not read the armband properly.

Your staff has become increasingly upset over Mary's inability to fulfill her job duties. The physicians, however, support Mary and found the circumcision incident humorous. Last week, you requested that Mary have a physical examination, at hospital expense, to determine her physical ability to continue working.

You were not particularly surprised when she returned with medical approval. Her physician spoke sharply with you. Admitting privately that Mary's health was rapidly failing, the physician told you that working was her only reason for living and left you with these words: "Force Mary to retire, and she will die within the year."

● ASSIGNMENT: Using your knowledge of age discrimination, patient safety, employee rights, and management responsibilities, decide on an appropriate course of action for this case. Be creative and think beyond the obvious. Be able to support your decisions.

Sexual Harassment

Although job discrimination related to gender became illegal with the Civil Rights Act of 1964, it was not until 1977 that the federal appeals court upheld a claim that a supervisor's verbal and physical advances constituted sexual harassment in the workplace. Since then, sexual harassment has been recognized as a form of sex discrimination that violates Title VII of the Civil Rights Act.

The USEEOC (2007b) defines *sexual harassment* as unwelcome sexual advances, requests for sexual favors, and other verbal or physical conduct of a sexual nature when submission to or rejection of this conduct explicitly or implicitly affects an individual's employment; unreasonably interferes with an individual's work performance; or creates an intimidating, hostile, or offensive work environment. The EEOC states that sexual harassment can occur in a variety of circumstances, including but not limited to the following:

- The victim as well as the harasser may be a woman or a man. The victim does not have to be of the opposite sex.
- The harasser can be the victim's supervisor, an agent of the employer, a supervisor in another area, a co-worker, or a nonemployee.
- The victim does not have to be the person harassed but could be anyone affected by the offensive conduct.
- Unlawful sexual harassment may occur without economic injury to or discharge of the victim.
- The harasser's conduct must be unwelcome.

Since the 1977 ruling, allegations of sexual harassment and lawsuits have permeated virtually every type of industry, and the health care system is not immune. Legal Eagle Eye (2006) suggests that dealing effectively with sexual harassment requires taking prompt corrective action when the employer is first made aware of the complaint. This includes temporary steps to deal with the situation while it is determined whether the complaints are justified and permanent remedial steps taken by the employer once the investigation has been completed.

Neuson (2005) maintains that every employer should have in place clearly written, well-publicized, antiharassment policies that include directions on making a complaint. The policy should specify that violation may lead to discipline. Additionally, the policy should identify the person who has been designated to receive complaints (Neuson, 2005).

Last, nurses themselves must take appropriate action when they see harassment of others or when they themselves are targets of such offenses. When someone makes another uncomfortable in the workplace by the use of sexual innuendoes or jokes or invades another's personal space, the behavior can be clues for recognizing sexual harassment.

LEARNING EXERCISE 22.6

Confronting Sexual Harassment

You are a new female employee at Valley Medical Center's ICU and love your job. Although only 25 years old, you have been a nurse for 4 years, and the last two were spent in a small critical care unit in a rural hospital. You work the 3 PM to 11 PM shift. Ever since you came to work here, one of the male physicians (Dr. Jones) has been especially attentive to you. At first you were flattered, but more recently, you have become uncomfortable around him. He sometimes touches you and seems to be flirting with you. You have no romantic interest in him and know that he is married. Last night, he asked you to meet him for an after-work drink and you refused. He is a very powerful man in the unit and you do not want to alienate him, but you are becoming increasingly troubled by his behavior.

Today, you went to your shift charge nurse and explained how you felt. In response the nurse said, "Oh, he likes to flirt with all the new staff, but he is perfectly harmless." These comments did not make you feel better. About 7 PM, Dr. Jones came on the unit and again cornered you in a comatose patient's room and asked you out. You again said no, and you are feeling more anxious by his behavior.

● ASSIGNMENT: Outline an appropriate course of action. What options can you identify? What is your responsibility? What are the driving and restraining forces for action? What support systems for action can you identify? What responsibility does the organization have? Be creative and think beyond the obvious. Be able to support your decisions.

Legislation Affecting Americans With Disabilities

The *Rehabilitation Act of 1973* required all employers with government contracts of more than $25,000 to take affirmative action to recruit, hire, and advance disabled people who are qualified. Similar but less aggressive affirmative action steps were required for other companies doing business with the federal government, with specific requirements depending on the size of the company and the dollar amount of the contract. The Department of Labor was charged with enforcing this act. Although initially there was very slow progress in getting companies to hire those with disabilities, steady progress has been made.

In 1990, Congress passed the *Americans With Disabilities Act* to eliminate discrimination against Americans with physical or mental disabilities in the workplace and in social life. *Disability* is defined as "any physical or mental impairment that limits any major life activity." This includes people with obvious physical disabilities, but also those with cancer, diabetes, HIV, or AIDS and recovering substance users, among others.

Veterans Readjustment Assistance Act

The *Veterans Readjustment Act* provides employment rights and privileges for veterans with regard to positions that they held before they entered the armed forces. This act was used by some nurses after the Vietnam War and during the nursing surplus after the Persian Gulf War to gain reemployment after military service. There is a lesser need for nurses implementing this act when veterans return from war during a nursing shortage because jobs are readily available.

The Occupational Safety and Health Act

The manager needs to be especially cognizant of legislation imposed by the *Occupational Safety and Health Act* (OSHA) and state health licensing boards. OSHA speaks to the employer's requirements to provide a place of employment that is free from recognized hazards that may cause physical harm. The Department of Labor enforces this act. Because it is impossible for the Department of Labor to inspect physically all facilities, most inspections are brought about by employee complaint or employer request. The act allows fines to be levied if employers continue with unsafe conditions.

Since OSHA's inception, many organizations have vehemently criticized the act, specifically its administration. They have charged that the cost of meeting OSHA standards has excessively burdened American business. On the other hand, unions have asserted that the federal government has never staffed or funded OSHA adequately. They charge that OSHA has been negligent in setting standards for toxic substances, carcinogens, and other disease-producing agents.

Because the risk of discovery and the fine (if judged guilty) are both low, employers often choose to ignore unsafe working conditions. Nurse–managers are in a unique position to call attention to hazardous conditions in the workplace and should communicate such concerns to higher authority. Ongoing controversies regarding safety issues include the cost and effectiveness of universal precautions and immunizations for potential bioterrorism. Most states also have occupational and safety regulations. Again, the employer must comply with the more stringent regulation. Many state licensing boards have additional health regulations that differ from the federal regulations.

STATE HEALTH FACILITIES LICENSING BOARDS

In addition to health and safety requirements, many state boards have regulations regarding staffing requirements. It is the ultimate responsibility of top-level management to maintain the state license to operate. However, all managers are responsible for knowing and meeting the regulations that apply to their unit or department. For example, if the manager of an ICU has a state staffing level that mandates 12 hours of nursing care per patient per day and requires that the ratio of RNs to other staff be 2:1, then the supervisor is obligated to staff at that level or greater. If, during times of short staffing, supervisors are unable to meet this level of staffing, they must communicate this to upper-level management so that there can be joint resolution.

The variation in state licensing requirements makes a lengthy discussion of them inappropriate here. However, managers must be knowledgeable about state licensing regulations that pertain to their level of supervision.

INTEGRATING LEADERSHIP ROLES AND MANAGEMENT FUNCTIONS IN UNDERSTANDING COLLECTIVE BARGAINING, UNIONIZATION AND EMPLOYMENT LAWS

Unionization and legal constraints will seem less burdensome if managers remember that both primarily protect the rights of patients and employees. If managers perform their jobs well and work for organizations that desire to "do the right thing" by accepting their social responsibility, they do not need to fear unionization and legal constraints. If the organization is not unionized, the manager must use the leadership roles of communication, fairness, and shared decision making to ensure that employees do not feel unionization is necessary. The integrated leader–manager is a role model for fairness, knows unit employees well, and sincerely seeks to meet their needs.

When making decisions that deal with unions and employment legislation, the effective leader–manager always seeks to do what is just. Additionally, he or she seeks appropriate assistance before finalizing decisions that involve sensitive legal or contract issues. By incorporating the leadership role, the manager becomes fairer in personnel management. There is increased self-awareness and an understanding of an individual's need to seek unionization and of the necessity for employment legislation.

The effective manager maintains required staffing and ensures a safe working environment. Rights of the organization and the employee are protected as the manager uses personnel policies in a nondiscriminatory and consistent manner. The emphasis is on flexibility and accommodation of employment legislation and union contracts.

 Key Concepts

* Historically, union activity is greater during times of labor shortages and economic upswings.
* The ANA acts as a professional association for RNs and a *collective bargaining* agent. This dual purpose poses a conflict in loyalty to some nurses.
* People are motivated to join or reject unions as a result of many needs and values.
* Although all managers play an important role in establishing and maintaining effective *management–labor relationships*, the middle-level manager has the greatest influence on preventing unionization in a nonunion organization.

* Creating a climate in which labor and management can work together to accomplish mutual goals is possible.
* Labor relations laws concern the rights and duties of unions and employers in their relationship with each other.
* *Labor standards* are regulations dealing with the conditions of the employee's work, including physical conditions, financial aspects, and the number of hours worked.
* State and federal employment legislation often overlap; as a general rule, the employer must abide by the stricter of the two regulations.
* Much of the human rights legislation concerning employment practices resulted because of documented discrimination in the workplace.
* Although some legislation makes the job of managing people more difficult for managers, it has resulted in increased job fairness and opportunities for women, minorities, the elderly, and the disabled.

ADDITIONAL LEARNING EXERCISES AND APPLICATIONS

LEARNING EXERCISE 22.7

Writing About Employment Laws

Many employment laws generate emotion. Usually, people feel strongly about at least one of these issues. Select one of the following employment laws, and write a 250-word essay on why you support or disapprove of the law. Choose from the Equal Pay Act of 1963, equal opportunity laws, affirmative action, sexual harassment, or age discrimination.

LEARNING EXERCISE 22.8

Dilemma Involving an Expired Nursing License

At your long-term care facility, it is a policy that licensed employees have a current, valid license. This is in keeping with the state licensing code. It is always difficult to get people to bring their license in to verify that it is current.

You have just come from a meeting with the director, who reminded you that you must not have people performing duties that require a license if the license has expired. You decide to issue a memo stating that you will suspend all employees who have not verified their licenses with you.

Following this, all of the LVNs/LPNs brought their licenses in for verification. However, one of the LVNs/LPNs has an expired license. When questioned, the nurse admits that payment for relicensure was not made until after your memo was received. This nurse delayed payment because of a financial crisis. You call the licensing board, and learn that it will be 6 weeks before the employee will receive the license. Active license status cannot be verified over the telephone.

You consider the following facts. It is illegal to perform duties that require a license without one. The LVN/LPN had prior knowledge of the licensing laws and hospital policy. The LVN/LPN has been a good employee with no record of prior disciplinary action.

● ASSIGNMENT: Decide what you should do. What alternatives do you have? Provide rationale for your decision.

LEARNING EXERCISE 22.9

How Would You Handle This Petition?

Betty Smith, a unit clerk, has come to see you, the nurse–manager of the medical unit, to complain of flagrant discriminatory practices against female employees of University General Hospital. She alleges that women are denied promotional and training opportunities comparable to those made available to men. She shows you a petition with 35 signatures supporting her allegations. Ms. Smith has threatened to forward this petition to the administrator of the hospital, the press, and the Department of Labor unless corrective action is taken at once. Being a woman yourself, you have some sympathy for Ms. Smith's complaint. However, you believe overall that employees at University General are treated fairly regardless of their sex.

Ms. Smith, a fairly good employee, has worked on your unit for 4 years. However, she has been creating problems lately. She has been reprimanded for taking too much time for coffee breaks. Personnel evaluations that recommend pay raises and promotions are due next week.

● ASSIGNMENT: How should you handle this problem? Is the personnel evaluation an appropriate time to address the petition? Outline your plan, and give your rationale.

Web Links

American Nurses Association
http://www.nursingworld.org/
Website of the United American Nurses, a collective bargaining agent representing 100,000 nurses nationwide—and a full-fledged affiliate of both the ANA and the AFL-CIO. Site has membership information and news releases.

The U.S. Equal Employment Opportunity Commission—Facts About Sexual Harassment
http://www.eeoc.gov/facts/fs-sex.html
Provides facts about sexual harassment.

Advocates for Political Equality
http://www.equalrights.org/
A nonprofit law center that advocates for the economic and political equality of women, with online advice and topics such as affirmative action.

Equal Opportunity Publications, Inc.
http://www.eop.com/
Includes employment issues and statistics concerning ethnic minorities, women, and people with disabilities.

Pregnancy Leave Rights: What Are Your Rights?
http://www.momo.essortment.com/pregnancyleave_rubm.htm
Discusses health, safety, leave, and reinstatement issues related to pregnancy and employment.

References

AFL-CIO. (2007). *The employee free choice act*. Retrieved February 22, 2007, from *http://www.aflcio.org/joinaunioin/voiceatwork/efca/*.

Bauer, J. (2005). Earnings survey. *Registered Nurse, 68*(10), 46–53.

Bruno, E. (2005). Building a new national RN movement. *Revolution, 6*(1), 15–16, 18–21.

Buerhaus, P. I., Donelan, K., Ulrich, B. T., Kirby, L., Norman, L., & Dittus R. (2005). Registered nurses' perceptions of nursing. *Nursing Economics, 23*(3), 110–118, 143.

Burger, D. (2006). Letter from the president. *Registered Nurse, 10*(2), 2.

Forman H., & Grimes, T. C. (2004). Effective labor relations. The "New Age" of union organizing. *Journal of Nursing Administration, 23*(3), 120–124.

Forman, H., & Kraus, H. R. (2003). Decertification. Management's role when employees rethink unionization. *Journal of Nursing Administration, 33*(6), 313–316.

Forman, H., & Powell, T. A. (2003). Managing during an employee walkout. *Journal of Nursing Administration, 33*(9), 430–433.

Gordon, S. (2004). Collective thinking. *Nursing Management, 11*(2), 8.

Haugh, R. (2006). The new union strategy: Turning the community against you. *Hospitals and Health Networks, 80*(5), 32–37.

Huston, C. (2006a). Collective bargaining and the professional nurse. In C. Huston (Ed.), *Professional issues in nursing.* Philadelphia: Lippincott Williams & Wilkins.

Huston, C. (2006b). Diversity in the nursing workforce. In C. Huston (Ed.), *Professional issues in nursing.* Philadelphia: Lippincott Williams & Wilkins.

Kleinman, C. S. (2004). Understanding and capitalizing on men's advantages in nursing. *Journal of Nursing Administration, 34*(2), 78–82.

Middaugh, D., & Hester, C. (2006). Managing the pregnant employee. *MEDSURG Nursing, 15*(4), 238–240.

Neuson, B. (2005). Properly investigate harassment complaints. *Nursing Management, 36*(6), 14–16, 60.

Ray, R. (2004, February 9). New overtime legislation may exempt some nurses. *NurseWeek (California),* 2.

Breaking away. (2005). *Revolution: The Journal for RNS and Patient Advocacy, 6*(1), 19.

Service Employees International Union. (2007). *SEIU: America's largest and fastest growing union.* Retrieved February 22, 2007, from *http://www.seiu.org/health/nurses.*

Sexual harassment: Hospital fulfilled its obligations, nurse can still sue for retaliation. (2006). *Legal Eagle Eye Newsletter for the Nursing Profession, 14*(4), 6.

Twarog, J. (2005). Workplace benefits: Not the result of employee benevolence or goodwill. *Massachusetts Nurse, 76*(9), 6–7.

United States Equal Employment Opportunity Commission (USEEOC). (2007a). *Discrimination by type: Facts and guidance.* Retrieved February 22, 2007, from *http://www.eeoc.gov/.*

United States Equal Employment Opportunity Commission (USEEOC). (2007b). *Facts about sexual harassment.* Retrieved February 22, 2007, from *http://www.eeoc.gov/facts/fs-sex.html.*

Bibliography

Berney, B., Needleman, J., & Kovner, C. (2005). Factors influencing the use of registered nurse overtime in hospitals, 1995–2000. *Journal of Nursing Scholarship, 37*(2), 165–172.

Everitt, M. (2006). RNs rally for first major unionization. *Registered Nurse: Journal of Patient Advocacy, 102*(4), 10.

Kennedy, M. S. (2006). In the news. Nursing unions create a cooperative alliance: A way to represent more than 200,000 RNs. *American Journal of Nursing, 106*(4), 22.

King, S., Block, V. J., & Jamerson, P. A. (2005). Running a successful campaign against unionization. *Journal of Nursing Administration, 35*(4), 157.

Norton, E. (2005). Organizing and the law: Protecting your rights as a worker. *Massachusetts Nurse, 76*(7), 5, 7.

Parish, C. (2006). Unions call for real cost rise as government misses pay deadline. *Nursing Standard, 21*(4), 9.

Piknick, B. (2006). President's column. Question: What does Labor Day mean for nurses? *Massachusetts Nurse, 77*(7), 3.

Tammelleo, A. D. (2005). Supervisor refuses to make accommodation for pregnant employee. *Nursing Law's Regan Report, 45*(11), 1.

Twarog, J. (2005). The benefits of union membership: Numerous and measurable. *Massachusetts Nurse, 76*(4), 6.

Vonfrolio, L. G. (2006). Rise up (collectively). *Registered Nurse, 69*(2), 72.

23

Quality Control

> . . . public accountability looms large at U.S. institutions today, forcing a re-evaluation within many organizations of how, and how well, they are accomplishing their goals.
>
> —R. J. Bulger

> . . . because quality health care is a complex phenomenon, the factors contributing to quality in health care are as varied as the strategies needed to achieve this elusive goal.
>
> —Carol Huston

During the *controlling* phase of the management process, performance is measured against predetermined standards, and action is taken to correct discrepancies between these standards and actual performance. Employees who feel that they can influence the quality of outcomes in their work environment experience higher levels of motivation and job satisfaction. Organizations also need some control over productivity, innovation, and quality outcomes. Controlling, then, should not be viewed as a means of determining success or failure but as a way to learn and grow, both personally and professionally.

This unit explores controlling as the fifth and final step in the management process. Because the management process, like the nursing process, is cyclic, controlling is not an end in itself; it is implemented throughout all phases of management. Examples of management controlling functions include the periodic evaluation of unit philosophy, mission, goals, and objectives; the measurement of individual and group performance against pre-established standards; and the auditing of patient goals and outcomes.

DISPLAY 23.1   **Hallmarks of Effective Quality Control Programs**

1. Support from top-level administration
2. Commitment by the organization in terms of fiscal and human resources
3. Quality goals reflect search for excellence rather than minimums
4. Process is ongoing (continuous)

Quality control, a specific type of controlling, refers to activities that are used to evaluate, monitor, or regulate services rendered to consumers. For any quality control program to be effective, certain components need to be in place (Display 23.1). First, the program needs to be supported by top-level administration; a quality control program cannot merely be an exercise to satisfy various federal and state regulations. A sincere commitment by the institution, as evidenced by fiscal and human resource support, will be a deciding factor in determining and improving quality of services.

Although the organization must be realistic about the economics of rendering services, if nursing is to strive for excellence, then developed quality control criteria should be pushed to optimal levels rather than minimally acceptable levels. Finally, the process of quality control must be ongoing; that is, it must reflect a belief that the search for improvement in quality outcomes is continuous and that care can always be improved. Although controlling is generally defined as a management function, effective quality control requires managers to have skill in both leadership and management. Leadership roles and management functions inherent in quality control are delineated in Display 23.2.

To understand quality control, the manager must become familiar with the process and terminology used in quality measurement and improvement activities. This chapter introduces quality control as a specific and systematic process. Audits are presented as tools for assessing quality. In addition, the historical impact of external forces on the development and implementation of quality control programs in health care organizations is discussed. Quality control strategies, quality measurement tools, benchmarking, and clinical practice guidelines are introduced. Finally, strategies for creating a culture of safety are identified, as are the challenges of changing a system that all too often focuses on individual errors rather than on the need to make systemwide changes.

DEFINING QUALITY HEALTH CARE

Quality measurement and *outcomes accountability* have been buzzwords in health care since the 1980s and continue to be at the forefront of almost every health care agenda today (Huston, 2003). Defining and measuring quality of care are essential for health care providers to demonstrate accountability to insurers, patients, and legislative and regulatory bodies. However, achieving quality care is not just a matter of better training for providers or delivering more care. The problem is multidimensional, and its complexity begins with the very definition of quality care itself (Huston, 2003).

The Institute of Medicine (IOM) (1994) defines *health care quality* as "the degree to which health services for individuals and populations increase the likelihood of desired health

DISPLAY 23.2 Leadership Roles and Management Functions Associated with Quality Control

Leadership Roles

1. Encourages followers to be actively involved in the quality control process
2. Clearly communicates expected standards of care to subordinates
3. Encourages the setting of high standards to maximize quality instead of setting minimum safety standards
4. Embraces and champions quality improvement as an ongoing process
5. Uses control as a method of determining why goals were not met
6. Is active in communicating quality control findings and their implications to other health professionals and consumers
7. Acts as a role model for followers in accepting responsibility and accountability for nursing actions
8. Distinguishes between clinical standards and resource utilization standards, ensuring that patients receive at least minimally acceptable levels of quality care
9. Supports/actively participates in research efforts to identify and measure nursing-sensitive patient outcomes

Management Functions

1. In conjunction with other personnel in the organization, establishes clear-cut, measurable standards of care and determines the most appropriate method for measuring if those standards have been met
2. Selects and uses process, outcome, and structure audits appropriately as quality control tools
3. Accesses appropriate sources of information in data gathering for quality control
4. Determines discrepancies between care provided and unit standards and seeks further information regarding why standards were not met
5. Uses quality control findings in determining needed areas of staff education or coaching
6. Keeps abreast of current government, accrediting body, and licensing regulations that affect quality control
7. Actively participates in state and national benchmarking and "best practices" initiatives
8. Continually assesses the unit or organizational environment to identify and categorize errors that are occurring and proactively reworks the processes that led to the errors

outcomes and are consistent with current professional knowledge" (p. 3). While this definition is widely accepted, parts of it merit further examination. The first is the assertion that quality does not exist unless desired health outcomes are attained. Outcomes are only one indicator of quality. Sometimes, patients receive the best possible care with the information available and poor outcomes occur. At other times, poor care may still result in good outcomes. Using outcomes alone as a way to measure quality care is flawed (Huston, 2003).

 While outcomes are an important measure of quality care, it is dangerous to use them as the only criteria for quality measurement.

The second implication in the IOM definition that is questionable is that for care to be considered high quality, it must be consistent with current professional knowledge (Huston, 2003). Staying current in terms of professional knowledge in today's technological information firestorm is difficult for even the most dedicated providers. To complicate the issue even further, how quality of care is defined and measured often differs between providers and patients. Clearly, it is difficult to find a common definition of quality health care that represents the viewpoints of all stakeholders in the health care system. What is even more difficult, however, is identifying and elucidating the myriad factors that play a part in determining whether quality health care exists (Huston, 2003).

QUALITY CONTROL AS A PROCESS

If defining health care quality is problematic, then the measurement of health care quality is even more difficult. To make the process more effective and efficient, the collection of both quantitative and qualitative data is used as well as a specific and systematic process. This process, when viewed simplistically, can be broken down into three basic steps:

1. The criterion or standard is determined.
2. Information is collected to determine if the standard has been met.
3. Educational or corrective action is taken if the criterion has not been met.

The first step, as depicted in Figure 23.1, is the establishment of *control criteria* or *standards*. Measuring performance is impossible if standards have not been clearly established. Not only must standards exist, but leader–managers also must see that subordinates know and understand the standards. Because standards vary among institutions, employees must know the standard expected of them at their organization. Employees must be aware that their performance will be measured in terms of their ability to meet the established standard. For example, hospital nurses should provide postoperative patient care that meets standards specific to their institution. A nurse's performance can be measured only when it can be compared with a preexisting standard.

Many organizations have begun using *benchmarking*, the process of measuring products, practices, and services against best-performing organizations, as a tool for identifying desired standards of organizational performance. In doing so, organizations can determine how and why their performance differs from these exemplar organizations and use them as role models for standard development and performance improvement. Williams and Murphy (2005) suggest that in benchmarking, questions such as, "How did they do it?," "What tools did they use?," and "What were their lessons learned?" should be asked.

 Benchmarking is the process of measuring products, practices, and services against best-performing organizations.

Many states have initiated a best practices program that invites health care institutions to submit a description of a program or protocol relating to improvements in quality of life, quality of care, staff development, or cost-effectiveness practices. Experts review the submissions, examine outcomes, and then designate a *best practice*. The difference in performance between top-performing health care organizations and the national average is called the *quality gap* (National Committee for Quality Assurance [NCQA], 2004). While the quality gap is typically small in industries such as manufacturing, aviation, and banking, wide variation is the norm in health care, with the quality gap on many health care measures being 20% or more (NCQA, 2004).

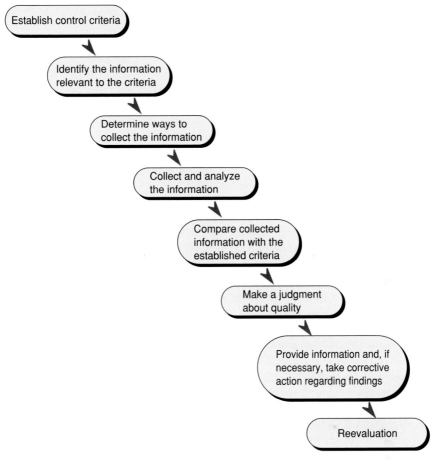

Figure 23.1 Steps in auditing quality control.

The second step in the quality control process includes identifying information relevant to the criteria. What information is needed to measure the criteria? In the example of postoperative patient care, this information might include the frequency of vital signs, dressing checks, and neurological or sensory checks. Often, such information is determined by reviewing current research or existing evidence.

Research by Heater, Becker, and Olson suggests that patients who receive care based on evidence from well-designed studies have nearly 30% better outcomes (Bennett, 2007). Bennett suggests that "evidence based practice, a problem solving approach to using best evidence in making decisions about patient care, is no longer an option for staff nurses. Patient care *must* be based on evidence of optimal outcomes" (p. 17). Similarly, Newhouse (2006) argues that "nursing's future in quality movement is dependent on the commitment of nurse leaders to incorporate evidence into all areas of nursing practice" (p. 337).

The third step is determining ways to collect information. As in all data gathering, the manager must be sure to use all appropriate sources. When assessing quality control of the postoperative patient, the manager could find much of the information in the patient chart. Postoperative flowsheets, the physician orders, and the nursing notes would probably be most helpful. Talking to the patient or nurse also could yield information.

The fourth step in auditing quality control is collecting and analyzing information. For example, if the standards specify that postoperative vital signs are to be checked every 30 minutes for 2 hours and every hour thereafter for 8 hours, it is necessary to look at how often vital signs were taken the first 10 hours after surgery. The frequency with which vital signs are assessed is listed on the postoperative flowsheet and then is compared with the standard set by the unit. The resulting discrepancy or congruency gives managers information with which they can make a judgment about the quality or appropriateness of the nursing care.

If vital signs were not taken frequently enough to satisfy the standard, the manager would need to obtain further information regarding why the standard was not met and counsel employees as needed. This is often done using a process known as *critical event analysis* (CEA) or *root cause analysis* (RCA). Both of these processes require data collection, investigation, determination and reporting of root causes, implementation of corrective actions, and monitoring for sustainability (Rooney & Vanden Heuvel, 2004). In other words, CEA and RCA help to identify not only what and how an event happened, but why it happened with the end goal being to ensure that a preventable negative outcome does not recur (McDonald & Leyhane, 2005).

In addition to evaluating individual employee performance, quality control provides a tool for evaluating unit goals. If unit goals are consistently unmet, the leader must reexamine those goals and determine if they are inappropriate or unrealistic. There is great danger here that the leader, in a desperate effort to meet unit goals, may lower standards to the point where quality is meaningless. This reinforces the need to determine standards first and then evaluate goals accordingly.

The last step in Figure 23.1 is reevaluation. If quality control is measured on 20 postoperative charts and a high rate of compliance with established standards is found, the need for short-term reevaluation is low. If standards are consistently unmet or met only partially, frequent reevaluation is indicated. However, quality control measures need to be ongoing, not put forth simply in response to a problem. Effective leaders ensure that quality control is proactive by pushing standards to maximal levels and by eliminating problems in early stages, before productivity or quality is compromised.

Quality control should not be implemented solely as a reaction to a problem.

LEARNING EXERCISE 23.1

Designing an Audit Tool

You are a public health nurse in a small, nonprofit visiting nurse clinic. The nursing director has requested that you chair the newly established quality improvement committee because of your experience with developing audit criteria. Because a review of the patient population indicates that maternal–child visits make up the greatest percentage of home visits, the committee chose to develop a retrospective-process audit tool to monitor the quality of initial postpartum visits. The criteria specified that the clients to be included in the audit had to have been discharged with infant from a birth center or obstetrical unit following uncomplicated vaginal delivery. The home visit would occur no later than 72 hours after the delivery.

● ASSIGNMENT: Design an audit tool appropriate for this diagnosis that would be convenient to use. Specify percentages of compliance, sources of information, and number of patients to be audited. Limit your process criteria to 20 items. Try solving this yourself before reading the possible solution that appears in the Appendix.

THE DEVELOPMENT OF STANDARDS

A *standard* is a predetermined level of excellence that serves as a guide for practice. Standards have distinguishing characteristics; they are predetermined, established by an authority, and communicated to and accepted by the people affected by them. Because standards are used as measurement tools, they must be objective, measurable, and achievable. There is no one set of standards. Each organization and profession must set standards and objectives to guide individual practitioners in performing safe and effective care. *Standards for practice* define the scope and dimensions of professional nursing. The American Nurses Association (ANA) has been instrumental in developing professional standards for almost 80 years.

In 1973, the ANA Congress first established standards for nursing practice, thereby providing a means of determining the quality of nursing that a patient receives, regardless of whether such services are provided by a professional nurse alone or in conjunction with nonprofessional assistants.

 The ANA has played a key role in developing standards for the profession.

Currently, the ANA cites 21 different standards for nursing practice that reflect different areas of specialty nursing practice (ANA, 2006). The *Standards of Clinical Nursing Practice*, originally published by ANA in 1991 and subsequently revised in both 1998 and 2004, provides a foundation for all RNs in clinical practice. These standards consist of *Standards of Care* and *Standards of Professional Performance* (Display 23.3).

The ANA publication *Scope and Standards for Nurse Administrators* may be of particular interest to nurse–managers. Other developed standards reflect such diverse fields of practice as diabetes nursing, forensic nursing practice, home health nursing practice, gerontological nursing, nursing practice in correctional facilities, parish nursing, oncology nursing, school nursing, psychiatric–mental health nursing practice, nursing informatics, and public health (ANA, 2006). All of these standards exemplify optimal performance expectations for the nursing profession and have provided a basis for the development of organizational and unit standards nationwide.

Organizational standards outline levels of acceptable practice within the institution. For example, each organization develops a policy and procedures manual that outlines its specific standards. These standards may be minimizing or maximizing in terms of the quality of service expected. Such standards of practice allow the organization to measure unit and individual performance more objectively.

One contemporary effort to establish standards for individual nursing practice has been the development of clinical practice guidelines. *Clinical practice guidelines* or *standardized clinical guidelines* provide diagnosis-based, step-by-step interventions for providers to follow in an effort to promote high-quality care while controlling resource utilization and costs. Clinical practice guidelines, such as those developed by the Agency for Health Care Research and Quality (AHRQ), are developed following an extensive review of the literature and suggest what interventions, in what order, will likely lead to the best possible patient outcomes. In other words, clinical practice guidelines are based on current research findings and best practices.

Clinical practice guidelines reflect evidence-based practice; that is, they should be based on cutting edge research and best practices.

DISPLAY 23.3 ANA Scope and Standards of Practice

Standards of Practice

1. ASSESSMENT—The registered nurse collects comprehensive data pertinent to the patient's health or the situation.
2. DIAGNOSIS—The registered nurse analyzes the assessment data to determine the diagnoses or issues.
3. OUTCOMES IDENTIFICATION—The registered nurse identifies expected outcomes for a plan individualized to the patient or the situation.
4. PLANNING—The registered nurse develops a plan that prescribes strategies and alternatives to attain expected outcomes.
5. IMPLEMENTATION—The registered nurse implements the identified plan.
6. EVALUATION—The registered nurse evaluates progress toward attainment of outcomes.

Standards of Professional Performance

7. QUALITY OF PRACTICE—The registered nurse systematically enhances the quality and effectiveness of nursing practice.
8. EDUCATION—The registered nurse attains knowledge and competency that reflects current nursing practice.
9. PROFESSIONAL PRACTICE EVALUATION—The registered nurse evaluates his/her own nursing practice in relation to professional practice standards and guidelines, relevant statutes, rules, and regulations.
10. COLLEGIALITY—The registered nurse interacts with and contributes to the professional development of peers and colleagues.
11. COLLABORATION—The registered nurse collaborates with the patient, family, and others in the conduct of nursing practice.
12. ETHICS—The registered nurse integrates ethical provisions in all areas of practice.
13. RESEARCH—The registered nurse integrates research findings in practice.
14. RESOURCE UTILIZATION—The registered nurse considers factors related to safety, effectiveness, cost, and impact on practice in planning and delivering nursing services.
15. LEADERSHIP—The registered nurse provides leadership in the professional practice setting and the profession.

Source: American Nurses Association (2004). *Nursing: Scope and standards of practice.* Washington, DC: Nursebooks.org.

In 1998, the AHRQ and the U.S. Department of Health, in partnership with the American Medical Association and American Association of Health Plans–Health Insurance Association of America, launched the *National Guideline Clearinghouse* (NGC). The NGC is a free, publicly available comprehensive database of evidence-based clinical practice guidelines and related documents in one easy-to-access location (NGC, 2007). The website for this clearinghouse and the key features of the NGC are shown in Display 23.4.

Some providers eschew clinical practice guidelines, arguing that they are "cookbook medicine"; however, the reality is that they likely serve as the best possible guide in caring for

DISPLAY 23.4   **The National Guideline Clearinghouse: Key Components**

1. Structured, standardized abstracts (summaries) about each guideline and its development
2. Links to full-text guidelines, where available, and/or ordering information for print copies
3. Palm-based PDA downloads of the complete NGC Summary for all guidelines represented in the database
4. A utility for comparing attributes of two or more guidelines in a side-by-side comparison
5. Syntheses of guidelines covering similar topics, highlighting areas of similarity and difference
6. An electronic forum for exchanging information on clinical practice guidelines, their development, implementation and use
7. Annotated bibliographies on guideline development methodology, structure, implementation, and evaluation

Source: National Guideline Clearinghouse. (2007). *About NGC*. Retrieved February 27, 2007, from *http://www.guideline.gov/about/about.aspx.*

specific patient populations that exists today. This does not mean that providers cannot deviate from evidence-based guidelines; they can and do. However, such deviations should be accompanied by the identification of the unique factors of the individual case that calls for that deviation.

AUDITS AS A QUALITY CONTROL TOOL

Whereas standards provide the yardstick for measuring quality care, audits are measurement tools. An *audit* is a systematic and official examination of a record, process, structure, environment, or account to evaluate performance. Auditing in health care organizations provides managers with a means of applying the control process to determine the quality of services rendered. Auditing can occur retrospectively, concurrently, or prospectively. *Retrospective audits* are performed after the patient receives the service. *Concurrent audits* are performed while the patient is receiving the service. *Prospective audits* attempt to identify how future performance will be affected by current interventions. The audits most frequently used in quality control include the outcome, process, and structure audits.

Outcome Audit

Outcomes can be defined as the end result of care. *Outcome audits* determine what results, if any, occurred as a result of specific nursing interventions for patients. These audits assume that the outcome accurately demonstrates the quality of care that was provided. Many experts consider outcome measures to be the most valid indicators of quality care, but until the past decade, most evaluations of hospital care have focused on structure and process.

 Outcomes reflect the end result of care, or how the patient's health status changed as a result of an intervention.

Outcome measurement, however, is not new; Florence Nightingale was advocating the evaluation of patient outcomes when she used mortality and morbidity statistics to publicize the poor quality of care during the Crimean War. In today's era of cost containment, outcome research is needed to determine whether managed care processes, restructuring, and other new clinical practices are producing the desired cost savings without compromising the quality of patient care.

Outcomes are complex, and it is important to recognize that many factors contribute to patient outcomes. There is growing recognition, however, that it is possible to separate out the contribution of nursing to the patient's outcome; this recognition of outcomes that are *nursing sensitive* creates accountability for nurses as professionals and is important in developing nursing as a profession.

Although outcomes traditionally used to measure quality of hospital care include mortality, morbidity, and length of hospital stay, these outcomes are not highly nursing sensitive. More nursing-sensitive outcome measures for the acute-care setting include patient fall rates, nosocomial infection rates, the prevalence of pressure sores, physical restraint use, and patient satisfaction rates. Haberfelde, Buffum, and Bedecarre (2005) suggest, however, that current databases of nursing-sensitive quality indicators, such as those developed by the ANA, the California Nursing Outcomes Coalition, and the Veterans Administration, still lack common definitions and standardized methods for comparison.

The need to standardize nursing languages cannot be overstated. A *standardized nursing language* provides a consistent terminology for nurses to describe and document their assessments, interventions, and the outcomes of their actions (McCloskey-Dochterman, & Bulechek, 2004). Currently, the ANA Nursing Information and Data Set Evaluation Center (NIDSEC) recognizes 13 standardized nursing languages (NIDSEC, 2007). One of the oldest is the *Nursing Minimum Data Set* (NMDS). The NMDS, developed by Werley and Lang, represents a decade-long effort to standardize the collection of nursing data. With the NMDS, a minimum set of items of information with uniform definitions and categories is collected to meet the needs of multiple data users. Thus, it creates a shared language that can be used by nurses in any care delivery setting as well as by other health professionals and researchers.

Although the NMDS is gaining recognition across the country, use and implementation have been limited. In 1990, however, the ANA House of Delegates recognized the NMDS as the minimum set of data elements to be included in any electronic patient record system. With it, nursing data can be used to compare nursing effectiveness, costs, and outcomes across clinical settings and nursing interventions.

Another tool that helps to link nursing interventions and patient outcomes is the *Nursing Interventions Classification* (NIC) developed by the Iowa Interventions Project, College of Nursing, Iowa City, Iowa. The NIC is a research-based classification system that provides a common, standardized language for nurses; it consists of independent and collaborative interventions of nurses in all specialty areas and in all settings. With 30 diverse classes of care, such as drug management, child bearing, community health promotion, physical comfort promotion, and perfusion management and multiple domains of interventions, the NIC can be linked with the *North American Nursing Diagnosis Association taxonomy*, the NMDS, and nursing outcomes to improve patient outcomes.

Finally, the International Council of Nurses (ICN) has developed the *International Classification for Nursing Practice* (ICNP), a compositional terminology for nursing practice that is applicable globally (Simpson, 2007). ICNP elements include nursing phenomena (diagnoses), actions, and outcomes (ICN, 2007) that can "serve as a system of nursing terminology for countries that have none and a unifying framework for countries that do" (Simpson, 2007, p. 15).

Process Audit

Process audits measure how nursing care is provided. The audit assumes a connection between process and quality of care. Critical pathways and standardized clinical guidelines are examples of efforts to standardize the process of care. They also provide a tool to measure deviations from accepted best practice process standards.

> Process audits are used to measure the process of care or how the care was carried out and assume that a relationship exists between the process used by the nurse and the quality of care provided.

Process audits tend to be task oriented and focus on whether practice standards are being fulfilled. Process standards may be documented in patient care plans, procedure manuals, or nursing protocol statements. A process audit might be used to establish whether fetal heart tones or blood pressures were checked according to an established policy. In a community health agency, a process audit could be used to determine if a parent received instruction about a newborn during the first postpartum visit.

Structure Audit

Structure audits assume that a relationship exists between quality care and appropriate structure. A structure audit includes resource inputs, such as the environment in which health care is delivered. It also includes all those elements that exist prior to and separate from the interaction between the patient and the health care worker. For example, staffing ratios, staffing mix, emergency department wait times, and the availability of fire extinguishers in patient care areas would all be structural measures of quality of care.

Structural standards, which are often set by licensing and accrediting bodies, ensure a safe and effective environment, but they do not address the actual care provided. An example of a structural audit might include checking to see if patient call lights are in place or if patients can reach their water pitchers. It also might examine staffing patterns to ensure that adequate resources are available to meet changing patient needs.

LEARNING EXERCISE 23.2

Identifying Structure, Process, and Outcome Measures
You are a charge nurse on a postsurgical unit. Retrospective survey data reveals that many patients report high levels of postoperative pain in the first 72 hours after surgery. You decide to make a list of possible structure, process, and outcome variables that may be impacting the situation. One of the structure measures you identify is that the narcotic medication carts are located some distance from the patient rooms, and that may be contributing to a delay in pain medication administration. One of the process measures you identify is that licensed staff are inconsistent in terms of how soon they make their initial pain assessments on postoperative patients as well as the tools they use to assess pain levels. An outcome measure might be the average wait time from the time a patient requests pain medication until it is administered.

● ASSIGNMENT: Identify at least three additional structure, process, and outcome measures for which you might collect data in an effort to resolve this problem. Select at least one of these measures, and specifically identify how you would collect the data. Then, describe how you would use your findings to increase the likelihood that future practice on the unit will be evidence based.

QUALITY IMPROVEMENT MODELS

Over the past several decades, the American health care system has moved from a *quality assurance* (QA) model to one focused on *quality improvement* (QI). The difference between the two concepts is that QA models target currently existing quality; QI models target ongoing and always improving quality. Two models that emphasize the ongoing nature of QI include *total quality management* (TQM) and the *Toyota Production System* (TPS).

 Quality assurance models seek to assure that quality currently exists, whereas quality improvement models assume that the process is ongoing and quality can always be improved.

Total Quality Management

TQM, also referred to as *continuous quality improvement* (CQI), is a philosophy developed by Dr. W. Edward Deming. TQM is one of the hallmarks of Japanese management systems. It assumes that production and service focus on the individual and that quality can always be better. Thus, identifying and doing the right things, the right way, the first time, and problem-prevention planning—not inspection and reactive problem solving—lead to quality outcomes.

 TQM is based on the premise that the individual is the focal element on which production and service depend (i.e., it must be a customer-responsive environment) and that the quest for quality is an ongoing process.

Because TQM is a never-ending process, everything and everyone in the organization are subject to continuous improvement efforts. No matter how good the product or service is, the TQM philosophy says that there is always room for improvement. Customer needs and experiences with the product are constantly evaluated. Workers—not a central QA/QI department—do this data collection, thus providing a feedback loop between administrators, workers, and consumers. Any problems encountered are approached in a preventive or proactive mode so that crisis management becomes unnecessary.

Another critical component of TQM is the empowerment of employees by providing positive feedback and reinforcing attitudes and behaviors that support quality and productivity. Based on the premise that employees have an in-depth understanding of their jobs, believe they are valued, and feel encouraged to improve product or service quality through risk taking and creativity, TQM trusts the employees to be knowledgeable, accountable, and responsible and provides education and training for employees at all levels. Although the philosophy of TQM emphasizes that quality is more important than profit, the resultant increase in quality of a well-implemented TQM program attracts more customers, resulting in increased profit margins and a financially healthier organization. The 14 quality management principles of TQM as outlined by Deming (1986) are summarized in Display 23.5.

LEARNING EXERCISE 23.3

Deming's Fourteen Total Quality Management Principles
Think back to the organization for which you have worked the longest. How many of Deming's 14 principles for TQM are used in that organization? Do you believe some of the 14 principles are more important than others? Why or why not? Could an organization have a successful quality management program if only some of the principles are used?

DISPLAY 23.5 Total Quality Management Principles

1. Create a constancy of purpose for the improvement of products and service.
2. Adopt a philosophy of continual improvement.
3. Focus on improving processes, not on inspection of product.
4. End the practice of awarding business on price alone; instead, minimize total cost by working with a single supplier.
5. Constantly improve every process for planning, production, and service.
6. Institute job training and retraining.
7. Develop the leadership in the organization.
8. Drive out fear by encouraging employees to participate actively in the process.
9. Foster interdepartmental cooperation, and break down barriers between departments.
10. Eliminate slogans, exhortations, and targets for the workforce.
11. Focus on quality and not just quantity; eliminate quota systems if they are in place.
12. Promote teamwork rather than individual accomplishments. Eliminate the annual rating or merit system.
13. Educate/train employees to maximize personal development.
14. Charge all employees with carrying out the total quality management package.

Source: Deming, W. E. (1986). *Out of the crisis.* Cambridge, MA: MIT Press.

The Toyota Production System

Another more contemporary, customer-focused quality improvement model is the TPS. According to Thompson, Wolf, and Spear (2003), this system is a "method of managing people engaged in work that emphasizes frequent rapid problem solving and work redesign that has become the global archetype for productivity and performance" (p. 585). Using TPS, the caregiver closest to the patient with an unmet need has the responsibility, resources, teaching, and managerial support to correct it, by determining the root cause and redesigning work to eliminate its recurrence (Thompson, Wolf, & Spear, 2003). TPS argues that solving individual problems this way, one at a time and where, when, and with whom they occur, prevents larger problems. Thus, management decisions are based on a long-term philosophy, even at the expense of short-term financial goals.

Implementing TPS, however, is not easy. It usually requires a change in organizational culture, values, and roles. Because every problem, big or small, must be addressed immediately, first-, middle-, and top-level managers must deal with far more requests for problem solving and involvement than managers in organizations where at least small problems are encouraged to be solved more independently (Thompson, Wolf, & Spear, 2003). Eliminating problems at their root is far different from solving an immediate problem at hand. Thus, adopting TPS in an organization requires a substantial commitment of leadership time and resources. It also requires a tremendous amount of staff preparation and involvement. However, Thompson, Wolf, and Spear (2003) argue that these efforts are offset by "greater quality of care, improved patient safety, lower costs, and increased job satisfaction" (p. 592).

WHO SHOULD BE INVOLVED IN QUALITY CONTROL?

Ideally, everyone in the organization should participate in quality control, because each individual is a recipient of the benefits. Quality control gives employees feedback about their current quality of care and how the care they provide can be improved. Many contemporary organizations, instead, designate an individual (frequently a nurse) to be their *patient safety officer* and charge them with quality data collection and the creation of a patient safety plan (Jessee, 2006). This strategy, however, is risky, as it may create the impression that the responsibility for quality care is not shared. It may also be perceived as an attempt to shift the ultimate responsibility for patient safety from the organization's leaders, both clinical and administrative (Jessee, 2006). Therefore, although it is impractical to expect full staff involvement throughout the quality control process, as many staff as possible should be involved in determining criteria or standards, reviewing standards, collecting data, or reporting.

Quality control requires evaluating the performance of all members of the multidisciplinary team. Professionals such as physicians, respiratory therapists, dietitians, and physical therapists contribute to patient outcomes and therefore must be considered in the audit process. Patients also should be actively involved in the determination of an organization's quality of care. It is important to remember, however, that quality care does not always equate with patient satisfaction.

 Patient satisfaction often has little to do with whether a patient's health improved during a hospital stay.

For example, the quality of food, provision of privacy, satisfaction with a roommate, or noisiness of the nursing station may play into a patient's satisfaction with a hospital admission. Patient satisfaction may be adversely affected by long waits for call lights to be answered and for transport to ancillary services such as the radiology department. Although these factors are an important component of patient comfort, and therefore quality of care, quality is more encompassing and must always include an examination of whether the patient received the most appropriate treatment from the most appropriate provider in a timely fashion. Ervin (2006) argues that "satisfaction in or of itself does not necessarily result in better patient outcomes [since it] does not inform nurses about how to improve the quality of care" (p. 127). It merely reflects whether the nurse was able to provide care that met the patient's preferences.

QUALITY MEASUREMENT AS AN ORGANIZATIONAL MANDATE

Organizational accountability for the internal monitoring of cost containment and quality has increased during the last 30 years. Most health care organizations today have complete QI programs and are actively involved in cost containment. Changing government regulations regarding quality control, however, continue to influence management decisions strongly. Managers must be cognizant of changing government and licensing regulations that affect their unit's quality control and standard setting. This awareness allows the manager to implement proactive rather than reactive quality control.

External Impacts on Quality Control

Although few organizations would debate the significant benefits of well-developed and implemented quality control programs, quality control in health care organizations has evolved primarily from external influences and not as a voluntary monitoring effort. When Medicare and Medicaid (government reimbursement for the elderly, disabled, and indigent) were implemented in the early 1960s, health care organizations had little need to justify costs or prove that the services provided met patients' needs. Reimbursement was based on the costs incurred in providing the service, and no real ceilings were placed on the amount that could be charged for services. Only when the cost of these programs skyrocketed did the government establish regulations requiring organizations to justify the need for services and to monitor the quality of services.

Professional Standards Review Organizations

Professional Standards Review Board legislation (PL 92-603), established in 1972, was among the first of the federal government's efforts to examine cost and quality. *Professional standards review organizations* (PSROs) mandated certification of need for the patient's admission and continued review of care; evaluation of medical care; and analysis of the patient profile, the hospital, and the practitioners.

This new kind of surveillance and the existence of external controls had a huge effect on the industry. Health care organizations began to question basic values and were forced to establish new methods for collecting data, keeping records, providing services, and accounting in general. Because government programs, such as Medicare and Medicaid, represent such a large group of today's patients, organizations that were unwilling or unable to meet these changing needs did not survive financially.

The Prospective Payment System

The advent of *diagnosis-related groups* (DRGs) in the early 1980s added to the ever-increasing need for organizations to monitor cost containment yet guarantee a minimum level of quality (Chapter 10). As a result of DRGs, hospitals became part of the *prospective payment system* (PPS), whereby providers are paid a fixed amount per patient admission regardless of the actual cost to provide the care. This system has been criticized as promoting abbreviated hospital stays and services leading to a reduced quality of care. Clearly, DRGs have resulted in increased acuity levels of hospitalized patients, a decrease in the length of patient stay, and a perception by many health care providers that patients are being discharged prematurely. All of these factors have contributed to growing levels of dissatisfaction by nurses regarding the quality of care they provide.

 Critics of the PPS argue that although DRGs may have helped to contain rising health care costs, the associated rapid declines in length of hospital stay and services provided have resulted in declines in quality of care.

LEARNING EXERCISE 23.4

Quality of Patient Care
How do you define quality of care? Is the quality of your care always what you would like it to be? If not, why not? What factors can you control in terms of providing high-quality care? (Which are internal and which are external?) In your clinical experience, have DRGs affected the quality of care provided? If so, how? Do you see differences in the quality of care provided to clients based on their ability to pay for that care? Or the type of insurance that they have?

The Joint Commission

The *Joint Commission* (formerly known as the Joint Commission for Accreditation of Healthcare Organizations [JCAHO]), an independent, not-for-profit organization that accredits more than 15,000 health care organizations and programs in the United States (Joint Commission, 2007), has historically had a tremendous impact on planning for quality control in acute-care hospitals. The Joint Commission was the first to mandate that all hospitals have a QA program in place by 1981. These QA programs were to include a review of the care provided by all clinical departments, disciplines, and practitioners; the coordination and integration of the findings of quality control activities; and the development of specific plans for known or suspected patient problems. Again, in 1982, the Joint Commission began to require quarterly evaluations of standards for nursing care as measured against written criteria.

In the late 1990s, the Joint Commission instituted its *Agenda for Change*, a multiphase, multidimensional set of initiatives directed at modernizing the accreditation process by shifting the focus of accreditation from organizational structure to organizational performance, or outcomes. This required the development of clinical indicators to measure the quality of care provided. To further this goal, the Joint Commission approved a milestone initiative, known as *ORYX*, in February 1997. This initiative integrates outcomes and other performance measures into the accreditation process.

Under ORYX, all organizations accredited by the Joint Commission were required to select at least one of 60 acceptable performance measurement systems and to enroll in that system by June 30, 1998. Data collection of two clinical measures was to begin by third quarter 1998. Two additional clinical measures were added for implementation in first quarter 1999. Two more clinical measures (a total of six) were added by the end of first quarter 2000. Organizations could also volunteer for *ORYX Plus*, an effort by the Joint Commission to create a national standardized database of 32 performance measures. In addition, the Joint Commission began collecting data on outcome measures including as the number of *sentinel events* overall error rate, number of reports on possible errors or near misses, hospital readmission rates, and rate of hospital-acquired infections in an effort to better measure quality of care.

Finally, the Joint Commission implemented its *core measures* program (also called *Hospital Quality Measures*) as part of ORYX in 2002 in an effort to better standardize its valid, reliable, and evidence-based data sets. The four areas targeted for implementation were acute myocardial infarction (nine measures), heart failure (four measures), pneumonia (six measures) and pregnancy (three measures) (Data Advantage Corporation, 2007). Hospitals were required to select up to three of these areas and begin reporting data as of 2002, with increased data reporting requirements in 2008.

It remains to be seen, however, whether compliance with core measures actually improves patient outcomes. Early research findings are mixed, with some hospitals reporting improved patient outcomes associated with core measures implementation and others finding no difference (Leighty, 2007). For example, VanSuch, Naessens, Stroebel, Huddleston, and Williams (2006) found that cardiac patients who received all discharge instructions, as advised in the heart failure core guidelines, were significantly less likely to be readmitted for heart failure than those who missed at least one type of instruction. However, there was no association between documentation of discharge instructions and mortality (Examining the Evidence 23.1). Another study by the University of Pennsylvania School of Medicine found that hospitals with high and low performance on the core measures had little difference in the death rates for heart attack, heart

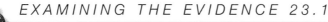

EXAMINING THE EVIDENCE 23.1

Source: VanSuch, M., Naessens, J. M., Stroebel, R. J., Huddleston, J. M., & Williams, A. R. (2006). Effect of discharge instructions on readmission of hospitalised patients with heart failure: Do all of the Joint Commission on Accreditation of Healthcare Organizations heart failure core measures reflect better care? *Quality and Safety in Health Care*, *15*(6), 414–417.

This retrospective study of a single tertiary-care hospital was conducted on a random sample of patients hospitalized between July 2002 and September 2003, with the diagnosis of heart failure. The researchers sought to determine if applying the Joint Commission core measures on heart failure, which include six required discharge instructions, had an impact on three patient outcomes: (a) time to death, (b) time to readmission for heart failure, and (c) readmission for any cause and time to death.

Study findings noted that 68% of patients received all instructions, and 6% received no instructions. Patients who received all instructions were significantly less likely to be readmitted for any cause ($p = 0.003$) and for heart failure ($p = 0.035$) than those who missed at least one type of instruction. Documentation of discharge instructions then was correlated with reduced readmission rates. However, there was no association between documentation of discharge instructions and mortality ($p = 0.521$).

failure, and pneumonia (Penn Medicine, 2006). The researchers concluded that further research should focus on developing measures more tightly linked to the clinical outcomes that patients care about.

Centers for Medicare and Medicaid Services

The *Centers for Medicare and Medicaid Services* (CMS), formerly the Health Care Financing Administration (HCFA), play an active role in setting standards for and measuring quality in health care. With the introduction of the *Medicare Quality Initiative* (MQI), in November 2001, health outcomes were targeted as the data source.

Harris (2003) describes the four-pronged approach inherent in the Quality Initiative. First, the state survey agencies and CMS conduct regulation and enforcement activities as usual. Second, information is made available to all consumers via a variety of media on the quality of care in target settings. Third, there are ongoing community-based improvement programs for the agencies that report outcomes data for the various quality initiatives. Finally, there is collaboration and partnership among all stakeholders, including QI organizations, state survey organizations, and providers of services. This initiative may become the new benchmark in terms of measuring health outcomes and making quality reports readily available to the consumer.

National Committee for Quality Assurance

Another external force affecting quality control in health care organizations is the *National Committee for Quality Assurance* (NCQA). The NCQA, a private nonprofit organization that accredits managed care organizations, has developed the *Health Plan Employer Data and*

Information Set (HEDIS) to compare quality of care in managed care organizations. Version 3.0/1998 of HEDIS contains 56 measures in the reporting set and 30 measures in the testing set that provide numerical and descriptive information about the quality of care, patient outcomes, access and availability of services, utilization, premiums, and the plan's financial stability and operating policies. Future versions are expected to have an even greater number of performance indicators as the growing Medicaid and Medicare segment of the population enrolled in managed care add more specific performance indicators. Version 3.0/1998 of HEDIS, with data gathered from more than 300 commercial health maintenance organizations (HMOs) and point-of-service products from across the United States, along with national and regional performance benchmarks, has been compiled into a national database known as *Quality Compass* (NCQA, 2006).

One of the most significant weaknesses of NCQA accreditation is that such accreditation is voluntary. Since 1999, however, Medicare and Medicaid have contracted their managed care plans only with health plans that are accredited by the NCQA. More employers are also adopting this policy, with the result that most managed care organizations will need this accreditation in the future to survive fiscally.

Maryland Hospital Association Quality Indicator Project

Another major initiative to measure quality in acute-care settings is the *Maryland Hospital Association Quality Indicator Project* (QI Project). The QI Project, a research project that began in 1985 with seven acute-care hospitals in Maryland, currently has more than 1,000 acute-care hospitals and other health care facilities participating (QI Project, 2004). It is important to remember that the QI Project is still considered a research project, and as such, the project is not intended to be used to establish performance thresholds or standards of care; however, its benchmark work in indicator identification and measurement is invaluable.

Quality indicators have been identified in the QI Project for inpatient data collection, psychiatric care, long-term care, and home care (QI Project, 2004). Indicators under study are shown in Display 23.6.

Participants collect data on any or all of the measures in an indicator set and submit these data to the Project on a quarterly basis. The Project, in turn, provides quarterly comparative feedback to participants in the form of quarterly reports and data analysis (QI Project, 2004). In addition, participants have access to a wide range of educational and analytical tools and services that are designed to improve their ability to put the data to work. All data submitted to the project are confidential, and participants must agree to maintain the confidentiality of the aggregate rates and related statistical data.

LEARNING EXERCISE 23.5

Classifying Quality Indicator Project Indicators
Look at the inpatient, ambulatory care, psychiatric, and long-term care indicators in use with the QI Project. Which ones would be classified as process indicators? Outcome indicators? Structure indicators? Which indicators do you believe would be most difficult to measure?

DISPLAY 23.6   Maryland Hospital Association Quality Indicator Project

Acute-Care Indicators

- Device-associated infections in ICUs
- Device use in ICUs
- Surgical-site infections
- Prophylaxis for surgical procedures
- Inpatient mortality
- Neonatal mortality
- Perioperative mortality
- Management of labor
- Unscheduled readmissions
- Unscheduled admissions following ambulatory procedures
- Unscheduled returns to an ICU
- Unscheduled returns to the operating room
- Isolated coronary artery bypass graft (CABG) perioperative mortality
- Physical restraint use
- Falls
- Complications following sedation and analgesia in ICUs, cardiac catheter labs, radiology suites, endoscopy suites, and emergency departments (EDs)
- Unscheduled returns to the ED
- Length of stay in the ED
- ED discrepancies and patient management
- Patients leaving the ED before treatment is complete
- Cancellation of ambulatory procedures

Source: Maryland Quality Indicator Project. *Quality Indicator Project: Acute care measures.* Retrieved February 26, 2007, from *http://www.qiproject.org/pdf/Acute_Care_Indicators.pdf*.

Psychiatric Care Indicators

- Injurious behaviors (adult and adolescent units)
- Unplanned departures resulting in discharge (adult and adolescent units)
- Transfers/discharges to inpatient acute care (adult units)
- Readmissions to inpatient psychiatric care (adult and adolescent units)
- Use of involuntary restraint (adult and adolescent units)
- Use of seclusion (adult and adolescent units)
- Partial hospitalization (adult units)
- Adult documented falls (adult units)
- Adolescent residential treatment center (RTC) injurious behaviors
- Adolescent RTC unplanned departures resulting in discharge
- Adolescent RTC readmissions
- Adolescent RTC use of involuntary restraint
- Adolescent RTC use of seclusion

Source: Maryland Quality Indicator Project. *Quality Indicator Project: Psychiatric care indicators.* Retrieved February 26, 2007, from *http://www.qiproject.org/pdf/Psych_Indicators.pdf*.

(continued)

DISPLAY 23.6   **Maryland Hospital Association Quality Indicator Project** (continued)

Long-Term Care Indicators

- Unplanned weight change
- Pressure ulcer prevalence
- Falls
- Transfers/discharges to inpatient acute care
- Nosocomial infections
- Use of physical restraint

Source: Maryland Quality Indicator Project. *QI Project indicator sets and measures.* Retrieved February 26, 2007, from *http://www.qiproject.org/pdf/QI_Indicator_List.pdf.*

Home Care Indicators

- Unscheduled transfers to inpatient acute care
- Use of emergent care services
- Discharges to nursing home care
- Acquired infections

Source: Maryland Quality Indicator Project. *QI Project indicator sets and measures.* Retrieved February 26, 2007, from *http://www.qiproject.org/pdf/QI_Indicator_List.pdf.*

Multistate Nursing Home Case Mix and Quality Demonstration

There also has been a major move to develop quality indicators in long-term care settings. One of the most significant efforts has been the *Multistate Nursing Home Case Mix and Quality demonstration,* funded by CMS. This demonstration seeks to develop and implement both a case mix classification system to serve as the basis for Medicare and Medicaid payment and a quality-monitoring system to assess the impact of case mix payment on quality and to provide better information to the nursing home survey process.

Report Cards

In response to the demand for objective measures of quality, a number of health plans, health care providers, employer purchasing groups, consumer information organizations, and state governments have begun to formulate health care quality report cards. Most states have laws requiring providers to report some type of data. In fact, Gearon (2006) reports that more than half of all states in the United States have developed their own HMO report cards or list complaint-related information to help consumers compare the performance of competing health plans in their area. AHRQ has also been exploring the development of a report card for the nation's health care delivery system.

However, it is important to remember that currently, most report cards do not contain information about the quality of care rendered by specific clinics, group practices, or physicians in a health plan's network. In addition, some critics of health care report cards point out that health plans may receive conflicting ratings on different report cards. This is a result of using different performance measures and how each report card chooses to pool and evaluate individual factors. Report cards may also not be readily accessible or may be difficult for the average consumer to understand.

MEDICAL ERRORS: AN ONGOING THREAT TO QUALITY OF CARE

Many studies across the past 2 decades suggest medical errors are rampant in the health care system. The most well known of these was likely the 1999 report of the IOM called *To Err Is Human*. This report found that between 44,000 and 98,000 Americans die each year as a result of medical errors, making medical errors the eighth leading cause of death in this country, even when the lower estimate was used (Kohn, Corrigan, & Donaldson, 2000).

The IOM study also looked at the type of errors that were happening. Medication errors stood out as a particularly high risk. Stumpf (2007) suggests that four types of medication errors (*prescribing errors, transcription and verification errors, pharmacy dispensing and delivery errors,* and *administration errors*) can lead to patient injuries, often called *adverse drug events* (ADEs). ADEs occur in about 6% of hospitalized patients and are to blame for about 20% of all disabling patient injuries due to medication errors (Stumpf, 2007).

Perhaps the most significant contribution of the IOM report, however, was the conclusion that most of these errors did not occur from individual recklessness. Instead, they occurred because of basic flaws in the way that the health delivery system is organized and delivered. The current focus in medical error research, then, is on fixing these flaws and creating and/or fostering environments that minimize the likelihood of errors occurring. Strategies to create such environments include better reporting of the errors that do occur, the Leapfrog initiatives, reform of the medical liability system, and other point-of-care strategies such as bar coding, smart IV pumps, and medication reconciliation.

Reporting and Analyzing Errors

At the institution level, there must be more mandatory reporting of medical errors as well as voluntary efforts. To achieve this goal, the *Patient Safety and Quality Improvement Act* was signed into law in 2005 (White House, 2005). This bill protects medical-error information voluntarily submitted to new private organizations (*patient safety organizations*) from being subpoenaed or used in legal discovery and generally requires that the information is treated as confidential.

Health care organizations also need to do a better job of identifying what errors are occurring, categorizing those errors, and examining and reworking the processes that led to the errors. Ignoring the problem, denying their existence, or blaming the individuals involved in the processes does nothing to eliminate the preventable morbidity, mortality, and waste of resources that poor processes generate each day (Chaiken, 2001). The reality is that research has already given us great insights as to why errors occur. According to Patterson, as cited in Kosnick, Brown, and Maund (2007), "Common human factors identified during adverse event or root cause analyses include extraordinary complexity of the work, deviations from usual workflow—often due to distractions or high workload demands, poor coordination across and between roles and job functions, poor dynamic task reallocation, lack of adequate handoff briefings, missed side effects of change, and compromised observability of situations, which limits the ability to detect and mitigate problems" (p. 27). It is the leader–manager who bears the responsibility for proactively creating a work environment that minimizes these risks.

The Leapfrog Group

To help minimize risks, the standards and expectations of oversight groups, insurers, and professional groups must be raised. One such effort is the *Leapfrog Group*, a growing conglomeration of non–health care Fortune 500 company leaders who are committed to modernizing the current health care system (Leapfrog Group, 2006). Based upon current research, the Leapfrog Group identified four evidence-based standards that they believe will provide the greatest impact on reducing medical errors: *computerized physician–provider order entry* (CPOE), *evidence-based hospital referral* (EHR), *ICU physician staffing* (IPS), and the use of *Leapfrog Safe Practices* scores (Leapfrog Group, 2006). These strategies and the evidence supporting their use are described more fully in Display 23.7

Scientific evidence indicates that these initiatives will reduce preventable medical errors. Their implementation is already under way or feasible in the short term; consumers can appreciate their value; and health plans, purchasers, or consumers can easily ascertain their presence or absence in selecting among health care providers (Leapfrog, 2007). According to the Leapfrog Group, "these leaps are a practical first step in using purchasing power to improve hospital safety and quality" (para. 11).

DISPLAY 23.7 **Leapfrog Initiatives**

Computerized Physician–Provider Order Entry

Requires primary care providers to enter orders into a computer instead of handwriting them. This reduces medication errors based on inaccurate transcription. Also gives providers vital *clinical decision support* via access to information tools that support a health care provider in decisions related to diagnosis, therapy, and care planning of individual patients.
Evidence: CPOE has been shown to reduce serious prescribing errors in hospitals by more than 50%, eliminating 522,000 serious medication errors each year.

Evidence-Based Hospital Referral

Suggests that patients with high-risk conditions should be treated at hospitals with characteristics shown to be associated with better outcomes.
Evidence: EHR can reduce a patient's risk of dying by 40%.

Intensive Care Unit Physician Staffing

Examines the level of training of ICU medical personnel and suggests that quality of care in hospital ICUs is strongly influenced by (a) whether *intensivists* (doctors with special training in critical-care medicine) are providing care and (b) the staff organization in the ICU.
Evidence: IPS has been shown to reduce the risk of patients dying in the ICU by 40%.

Leapfrog Safe Practices Scores

The *National Quality Forum* (NQF) endorsed 30 *safe practices*, which if utilized would reduce the risk of harm in certain processes, systems, or environments of care. Included in the 30 practices are the three initiatives noted above. This fourth initiative assesses a hospital's progress on the remaining 27 NQF safe practices.

Source: Collated from Leapfrog Group. (2006). *The Leapfrog Group fact sheet.* Retrieved February 26, 2007, from *http://www.leapfroggroup.org/about_us/leapfrog-factsheet*; and Huston, C. (2006). Chapter 14. Medical errors: An ongoing threat to quality health care. In C. Huston (Ed.), *Professional issues in nursing: Challenges and opportunities* (pp. 268–291). Philadelphia: Lippincott Williams & Wilkins.

Leapfrog also has endorsed the use of *bar coding* to reduce point-of-care medication errors. As set forth by the U.S. Food and Drug Administration's (FDA) 2004 rule, all prescription and over-the-counter medications used in hospitals must contain a *national drug code* (NDC) number (Dohnaleket al., 2004), which "uniquely identifies the drug, its strength, and its dosage forms" (Roark, 2004, p. 63). The FDA has suggested that a bar code system that is coupled with a computerized order entry system would greatly enhance the ability of all health care workers to follow the "five rights" of medication administration; that the right person receive the right amount of the drug at the right time by the right route.

Other Strategies for Error Reduction

Pratt, Thomas, and Atkins (2005) identify a four-pronged approach used by a hospital in Southern California to improve patient safety. First, educational efforts were implemented and a nonpunitive response was established so that a culture of patient safety could be created. Second, technology was implemented that reduced the likelihood of errors occurring. Such technology included "smart IV pumps with download of alarm information" and bar coding for lab specimens, blood bank, and medications (p. 17). Third, the organization adopted a *six sigma approach* (limiting defects to 3.4 errors per million opportunities or a 99.9996% success rate) as its performance improvement methodology. Finally, a team-training curriculum was implemented to improve *hand-offs* (end of shift reports) and team coordination.

Reforming the Medical Liability System

Finally, if quality health care is to be achieved, the medical liability system and our litigious society must be recognized as potential barriers to systematic efforts to uncover and learn from mistakes that are made in health care (Huston, 2003). Organizational cultures need to change for employees and patients to be comfortable in reporting hazards that can affect patient safety without fear of personal risk. Potlycki, Kimmel, Ritter, and Capuano (2006) reported that the primary barrier to reporting medication errors was a staff perception that this action carried a risk of disciplinary action. Indeed, "authoritarian attempts to improve patient safety and a resistance to change" have historically permeated health care organizations (p. 375).

Many experts have argued that the culture in health care organizations must shift from one of blame to one in which errors are identified and responded to in a timely manner. Stumpf (2007) states that safety aspects of care should be discussed at every opportunity: "on rounds, at department meetings, in discussions with administrators, and in teaching residents and medical students" (p. 61). Stumpf suggests also that creating or supporting protocols and guidelines and improving communication among all members of the health care team will reduce the chance of errors occurring. Similarly, Jessee (2006) suggests that an organizational climate must be created in which safety is an integral part of day-to-day operations, that adequate resources must be devoted to patient safety, and that organizational policies must be in place to support patient safety.

Looking to the Future

The IOM (2001) has published several major reports in follow up to *To Err Is Human*, including *Crossing the Quality Chasm: A New Health System for the 21st Century*. This study found large gaps between the preventive, acute, and chronic care that people should get and what they actually received. More important, perhaps, was the report's urgent call for fundamental change to quality gap problems and the identification of strategies to improve the quality of health care over the next 10 years (Stevens & Staley, 2006). These strategies included creating an environment that supports evidence-based practice, facilitating the use of information technology, and preparing a better-educated workforce to provide health care in a changing world.

The *Institute for Health Improvement* (IHI) also launched a campaign to close the quality gap and save patient lives with its *100,000 Lives* campaign. Dr. Donald Berwick, a Harvard professor and president of the Massachusetts-based nonprofit IHI, issued a challenge to hospital officials nationwide in December 2004 to implement six types of changes, including activating rapid-response teams, ensuring that heart-attack patients receive correct care, preventing medication errors, preventing central line infections, preventing surgical site infections, and preventing pneumonia in patients on ventilators, by 2007 (American Society for Quality, 2005). The *5 Million Lives Campaign* was a separate IHI initiative to protect patients from 5 million incidents of medical harm between December 2006 and December 2008 (IHI, 2007).

Preliminary reports suggest that the IHI 100,000 Lives campaign saved 122,342 lives in the first 18 months of implementation alone (Tanne, 2006), and this occurred with just over 3,100 hospitals joining the campaign. In fact, only about one third of the hospitals reported diligence in all six interventions (Healthblog, 2006). This leads one to wonder what improvement would be possible if 100% participation and compliance were assured. At Healthblog (2006), Bill Crounce suggests the following:

> Imagine how many unnecessary deaths we could prevent if physicians always had the best evidence-based guidelines at their disposal. That is the promise of knowledge-driven health care; giving exactly the most appropriate and personalized care to a patient based on genetics, scientific evidence, and proven research (para. 2).

Similarly Ulrich (2005) suggests that "nursing needs to follow the example of the 100,000 Lives campaign and set clear goals for what we will do and when we will do it for the things we know will improve the morbidity and mortality of our patients" (p. 473).

INTEGRATING LEADERSHIP ROLES AND MANAGEMENT FUNCTIONS IN QUALITY CONTROL

Quality control provides managers with the opportunity to evaluate organizational performance from a systematic, scientific, and objective viewpoint. To do so, managers must determine what standards will be used to measure quality care on their units and then develop and implement quality control programs that measure results against those standards. All managers are responsible for monitoring the quality of the product that their units produce; in health care organizations, that product is patient care. Managers also must assess and promote patient satisfaction whenever possible.

The manager, however, cannot operate in a vacuum in determining what quality is and how it should be measured. Demands for hard data on quality have increased as regulatory bodies, patients, payers, and hospital managers have required justification of services provided. Managers must be cognizant of rapidly changing quality control regulations and proactively adjust unit standards to meet these changing needs. Limited attention to quality measurement in health care occurred, however, up until the past 2 decades. As we enter the 21st century, however, there is an ever-increasing focus on the quality of care and the standardization of quality data collection and an increased accountability for outcomes from the system level to the individual provider.

Inspiring subordinates to establish and achieve high standards of care is a leadership skill. Leaders role model high standards in their own nursing care and encourage subordinates to seek maximum rather than minimum standards. One way that this can be accomplished is by involving subordinates in the quality control process. By studying direct cause–effect relationships, subordinates learn to modify individual and group performance to improve the quality of care provided.

Vision is another leadership skill inherent in quality control. The visionary leader looks at what is and determines what should be. This future focus allows leaders to shape unit goals proactively and improve the quality of care. Moreover, the integrated leader–manager in quality control must be willing to be a risk taker and to be accountable. In an era of limited resources and cost containment, there is great pressure to sacrifice quality in an effort to contain costs. The self-aware leader–manager recognizes this risk and seeks to achieve a balance between quality and cost containment that does not violate professional obligations to patients and subordinates.

Winning the war on quality will require sustained public interest to create the momentum to systematically change the health care system in a way that improves quality. Increasing consumer knowledge and participation in health care will be imperative in this effort (Huston, 2003). In addition, change agents must be able to successfully address the disconnection that still exists between consumers' perceptions of the quality of their own care and the actual quality provided. This dialogue has only just begun.

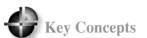 **Key Concepts**

* *Controlling* is implemented throughout all phases of management.
* *Quality control* refers to activities that are used to evaluate, monitor, or regulate services rendered to consumers.
* A *standard* is a predetermined baseline condition or level of excellence that constitutes a model to be followed and practiced.
* Because there is no one set of standards, each organization and profession must set standards and objectives to guide individual practitioners in performing safe and effective care.
* *Clinical practice guidelines* provide diagnosis-based, step-by-step interventions for nurses to follow in an effort to promote evidence-based, high-quality care and yet control resource utilization and costs.
* *Benchmarking* is the process of measuring products, practices, and services against those of best-performing organizations.
* The difference in performance between top performing health care organizations and the national average is called the *quality gap*. While the quality gap is typically small in industries such as manufacturing, aviation, and banking, wide variation is the norm in health care.
* *Critical event analysis* and *root cause analysis* help to identify not only what and how an event happened but why it happened, with the end goal being to ensure that a preventable negative outcome does not recur.
* *Outcome audits* determine what results, if any, followed from specific nursing interventions for patients.
* *Process audits* are used to measure the process of care or how the care was carried out.

* *Structure audits* monitor the structure or setting in which patient care occurs (such as the finances, nursing service structure, medical records, and environmental structure).
* There is growing recognition that it is possible to separate out the contribution of nursing to the patient's outcome; this recognition of outcomes that are *nursing sensitive* creates accountability for nurses as professionals and is important in developing nursing as a profession.
* *Standardized nursing languages* provide a consistent terminology for nurses to describe and document their assessments, interventions, and the outcomes of their actions.
* *Quality assurance* models seek to assure that quality currently exists whereas *quality improvement* models assume that the process is ongoing and that quality can always be improved.
* Quality control in health care organizations has evolved primarily from external forces and not as a voluntary effort to monitor the quality of services provided.
* Critics of the *Prospective Payment System* argue that although *diagnosis-related groups* may have helped to contain rising health care costs, the associated rapid declines in length of hospital stay and services provided have resulted in declines in quality of care.
* The *Joint Commission* (formerly known as Joint Commission for Accreditation of Healthcare Organizations) is the major accrediting body for health care organizations and programs in the United States. It also administers the *ORYX* initiative and collects data on four *core measures* in an effort to better standardize data collection across acute-care hospitals.
* The *National Committee for Quality Assurance*, a private nonprofit organization that accredits managed care organizations, also developed the *Health Plan Employer Data and Information Set* to compare quality of care in managed care organizations.
* Ideally, everyone in an organization should participate in quality control activities.
* In response to the demand for objective measures of quality, a number of health plans, health care providers, employer purchasing groups, consumer information organizations, and state governments have begun to formulate health care quality report cards.
* A plethora of studies across the past 2 decades suggests that medical errors are rampant in the health care system.
* *Adverse drug events* occur in about 6% of hospitalized patients and are to blame for about 20% of all disabling patient injuries due to medical errors.
* The *Patient Safety and Quality Improvement Act*, signed into law in 2005, protects medical-error information that is voluntarily submitted to new private organizations (*patient safety organizations*) from being subpoenaed or used in legal discovery and generally requires that the information is treated as confidential.
* The *Leapfrog Group* identified four evidence-based standards that they believe will provide the greatest impact on reducing medical errors: *computerized physician–provider order entry, evidence-based hospital referral, ICU physician staffing*, and the use of *Leapfrog Safe Practices scores*.
* The U.S. Food and Drug Administration has suggested that a *drug bar code* system coupled with a computerized order entry system would greatly decrease the risk of medication errors.
* As direct caregivers, staff nurses are in an excellent position to monitor nursing practice by identifying problems and implementing corrective actions that have the greatest impact on patient care.
* Initiatives such as the *100,000 Lives campaign* provide new hope for the standardization of quality improvement efforts that lead to improved patient outcomes.

ADDITIONAL LEARNING EXERCISES AND APPLICATIONS

LEARNING EXERCISE 23.6

Identifying Nursing-Sensitive Outcome Criteria

Some ill patients get better despite nursing care, not as a result of it. However, the quality of nursing care can affect patient outcomes tremendously. Do you believe that quality nursing care makes a difference in patients' lives? Identify five criteria that you would use to define *quality nursing care*. These criteria should reflect what you believe nurses do (nursing sensitive) that makes the difference in patient outcomes. Are the criteria you listed measurable? How?

LEARNING EXERCISE 23.7

Working Short Staffed—Again

You are a staff nurse at Mercy Hospital. The hospital's patient census and acuity have been very high for the last 6 months. Many of the nursing staff have resigned; a coordinated recruitment effort to refill these positions has been largely unsuccessful. The nursing staff is demoralized, and staff frequently call in sick or fail to show up for work. Today, you arrive at work and find that you are again being asked to work short handed. You will be the only RN on a unit with 30 patients. Although you have two LPNs/LVNs and two CNAs assigned to work with you, you are concerned that patient safety could be compromised. A check with the central nursing office ascertains that no additional help can be obtained.

You feel that you have reached the end of your rope. The administration at Mercy Hospital has been receptive to employee feedback about the acute staffing shortage, and you believe that they have made some efforts to try to alleviate the problem. You also believe, however, that the efforts have not been at the level they should have been and that the hospital will continue to expect nurses to work short handed until some major force changes things. Although you have thought about quitting, you really enjoy the work that you do and feel morally obligated to your co-workers, the patients, and even your superiors. Today, it occurs to you that you could anonymously phone the state licensing bureau and turn in Mercy Hospital for consistent understaffing of nursing personnel, leading to unsafe patient care. You believe that this could be the impetus needed to improve the quality of care. You also are aware of the action's political risks.

● ASSIGNMENT: Discuss whether you would take this action. What is your responsibility to the organization, to yourself, and to patients? How do you make decisions such as this one, which have conflicting moral obligations?

LEARNING EXERCISE 23.8

Examining Mortality Rates

You have been the nursing coordinator of cardiac services at a medium-sized urban hospital for the last 6 months. Among the hospital's cardiac services are open-heart surgery, invasive and noninvasive diagnostic testing, and a comprehensive rehabilitation program. The open-heart surgery program was implemented a little over a year ago. During the last 3 months, you have begun to feel uneasy about the mortality rate of postoperative cardiac patients at your facility. An audit of medical records shows a unit mortality rate that is approximately 30% above national norms. You approach the unit medical director with your findings. He becomes defensive and states that there have been a few freakish situations to skew the results but that the open-heart program is one of the best in the state. When you question him about examining the statistics further, he becomes very angry and turns to leave the room. At the door, he stops and says, "Remember that these patients are leaving the operating room alive. They are dying on your unit. If you stir up trouble, you are going to be sorry."

● ASSIGNMENT: Outline your plan. Identify areas in your data gathering that may have been misleading or that may have skewed your findings. If you believe action is still warranted, what are the personal and professional risks involved? How well developed is your power base to undertake these risks? To whom do you have the greatest responsibility?

LEARNING EXERCISE 23.9

Weighing Conflicting Obligations

You are the director of a private baccalaureate nursing program. In the past, your school averaged approximately 200 applicants for the 50 student openings each semester. This resulted in the school being very selective about which students would enter the program. Because entering students traditionally had high grade-point averages and had completed almost all non-nursing requirements, the attrition and dropout rate was fairly low, and academic failure was rare.

Three years ago, a less expensive program opened at a local public university. As a result, you saw a sharp decline in the number of students applying to your program. Students meeting only minimal grade-point average requirements and many who hadn't completed general studies course requirements were accepted into the program. You have seen the attrition and dropout rate quadruple in the last 3 years, with much of this attrition attributable to academic failure.

Recently, the faculty members have begun discussing changing the academic failure policy in an effort to increase student retention. The current policy results in automatic dismissal from the program if students fail two courses in the major. Faculty members are concerned that teaching positions will be cut as a result of the decreased enrollment and high attrition. You are aware that the university administration believes that nursing is an expensive major, that this situation is not going to improve in the near future, and that budget cuts may soon be mandated.

You, however, have grave concerns about eliminating or altering the academic failure policy because you believe you are in effect lowering program standards and thus the quality of its end product. You do not believe that students failing two courses in the major would be safe practitioners. You also believe that students in academic difficulty are taking a disproportionate amount of faculty time and energy at the expense of better students.

● ASSIGNMENT: What options are available to you? What obligations do you have to your faculty, to the students, to the public as consumers of health care, and to the university administration? How do you determine an appropriate course of action when these duties conflict?

LEARNING EXERCISE 23.10

Avoiding Adverse Events and Medication Errors

● ASSIGNMENT: Interview the patient safety officer or the manager of the risk management department at your local hospital. Use the following questions as a guide to begin the interview. Present a report to your peers regarding your findings.

1. What are the most common causes of medication errors in this facility?
2. Which medications are more commonly involved in medication errors? What factors has this agency identified that cause these errors to occur?
3. What are the most common adverse events affecting patients? What precipitating factors have been identified as increasing the possibility of these adverse events?
4. What new technologies have been adopted to increase patient safety? Examples might be IV smart pumps, bar coding of medications, computerized physician–provider order entry, and the like.
5. How are medication errors or adverse events reported? What safeguards have been built in to encourage voluntary reporting of errors? Do disincentives exist that would discourage someone from reporting such an error?
6. Are staff included in the quality control process? If so, how?
7. For which of The Joint Commission core measures are data being collected? What is the process for this data collection?

(Web Links)

Agency for Healthcare Research and Quality
http://www.ahrq.gov/
Practical health care information, research findings, and data to help consumers, health providers, health insurers, researchers, and policy makers make informed decisions about health care.

National Committee for Quality Assurance
http://www.ncqa.org
Independent, nonprofit organization that assesses and reports on the quality of care delivered by managed care organizations.

The Nursing Information and Data Set Evaluation Center
http://www.nursingworld.org/MainMenuCategories/ThePracticeofProfessionalNursing/DocInfo/
NursingTerminologies/NIDSEC.aspx
Funded by the ANA, this center develops standards and reviews standardized nursing languages that support the documentation of nursing care.

State-by-State List of HMO Report Cards Online
http://www.aarp.org/bulletin/yourhealth/a2003-08-07-hmoreport.html
A web exclusive by AARP that lists the status of report card development for each state in the United States.

References

American Nurses Association. (1998). *Standards of clinical nursing practice* (2nd ed.). Washington, DC: Author.

American Nurses Association. (2006). *ANA nursing standards.* Retrieved February 11, 2007, from *http://nursingworld.org/books/pdescr.cfm?CNUM=15.*

American Society for Quality. (2005). *Rapid response teams big part of 100,000 Lives campaign.* Retrieved February 27, 2007, from *http://www.asq.org/qualitynews/qnt/execute/ displaySetup? newsID=221.*

Bennett, C. (2007, February 19). Evidence-based practice. *Advance for Nurses, 4*(5), 15–18.

Chaiken, B. P. (2001). Patient safety: Is it really a problem? *Nursing Economics, 19*(4), 176–177.

Data Advantage Corporation. (2007). *Core measures component information.* Retrieved February 26, 2007, from *http://www.data-advantage.com/products/oryx/#CoreRequirements.*

Deming, W. E. (1986). *Out of the crisis.* Cambridge, MA: MIT Press.

Dohnalek, L. J., Cusaac, L., Westcott, J., Langeberg, A., & Sandler, S. G. (2004). The code to safer transfusions. *Nursing Management, 35*(6), 33–36.

Ervin, N. E. (2006). Does patient satisfaction contribute to nursing care quality? *Journal of Nursing Administration, 36*(3), 126–130.

Gearon, C. (January 2006). State-by-state list of HMO report cards online. *AARP Bulletin.* Retrieved 9/15/07 from *http://www. aarp. org/bulletin/yourhealth/a2003-08-07-hmoreport.html*

Haberfelde, M., Buffum, M., & Bedecarre, D. (2005). Nurse-sensitive patient outcomes. *Journal of Nursing Administration, 35*(6), 293–299.

Harris, M. J. (2003). Medicare quality initiative. *Policy, Politics and Nursing Practice, 4*(4), 263–265.

Healthblog. (2006, June 14). *Evidence-based medicine saves more than 100,000 lives!* Retrieved February 27, 2007, from *http://blogs.msdn.com/healthblog/archive/2006/06/14/631127. aspx.*

Huston, C. (2003). Quality health care in an era of diminished resources: Challenges and opportunities. *Journal of Nursing Care Quality, 18*(4), 295–301.

Institute for Health Improvement. (2007). *Protecting 5 million lives.* Retrieved February 27, 2007, from *http://www.ihi.org/ IHI/Programs/Campaign/.*

Institute of Medicine. (1994). *America's health in transition: Protecting and improving quality.* Washington, DC: National Academy Press.

Institute of Medicine. (2001). *Crossing the quality chasm: A new health system for the 21st century.* Committee on Quality of Health Care in America. Retrieved November 4, 2004, from *http://books.nap.edu/books/0309072808/html/ index.html.*

International Council of Nurses. (2007). *International classification for nursing practice (ICNP).* Retrieved February 28, 2007, from *http://www.icn.ch/icnp_def.htm.*

Jessee, W. (2006). What patient safety looks like. Six steps that mark an organization that really cares about medical errors. *Modern Healthcare, 36*(42), 18.

Joint Commission. (2007). *Facts about the Joint Commission.* Retrieved February 11, 2007, from *http://www.jointcommission.org/AboutUs/joint_commission_facts.htm.*

Kohn, L. T., Corrigan, J. M., & Donaldson, M. S. (Eds.). (2000). *To err is human: Building a safer health system.* Institute of Medicine, Committee on Quality of Health Care in America. Executive Summary, 1–14.

Kosnik, L. K., Brown, J., & Maund, T. (2007). Patient safety: Learning from the aviation industry. *Nursing Management, 38*(1), 25–31.

Leapfrog Group. (2006). *The Leapfrog Group fact sheet.* Retrieved February 26, 2007, from *http://www.leapfrog-group.org/about_us/leapfrog-factsheet.*

Leighty, J. (2007, February 12). *'Core measures' help RNs ensure top cardiac care.* Retrieved February 27, 2007, from *http://news. nurse.com/apps/pbcs.dll/article?AID=/20070212/ CA09/70210003.*

McCloskey-Dochterman, J., & Bulechek, G. (2004). *Nursing interventions classification (NIC).* Philadelphia: CV Mosby.

McDonald, A., & Leyhane, T. (2005, October). Drill down with root cause analysis. *Nursing Management, 36*(10), 27–32.

National Committee for Quality Assurance. (2004). *The state of health care quality: 2004.* Washington, DC: Author.

National Committee for Quality Assurance. (2006). *Quality compass.* Retrieved February 27, 2007, from *http://www.ncqa.org/ Info/QualityCompass/index.htm.*

National Guideline Clearinghouse. (2007). *About NGC.* Retrieved February 27, 2007, from *http://www.guideline.gov/about/ about.aspx.*

Newhouse, R. P. (2006). Examining the support for evidence-based nursing practice. *Journal of Nursing Administration, 36*(7–8), 337–340.

Nursing Information and Data Set Evaluation Center. (2007). *About NIDSEC.* Nursing World. Retrieved February 21, 2007, from *http://www.nursingworld.org/MainMenuCategories/ ThePracticeofProfessionalNursing/DocInfo/ NursingTerminologies/NIDSEC.aspx.*

Penn Medicine. (2006, December 12). *Hospital performance measures may not make much difference when it comes to mortality.* Retrieved February 26, 2007, from *http://www.uphs.upenn.edu/news/News_Releases/dec06/ medicare-quality-measures.htm.*

Potlycki, M. J., Kimmel, S. R., Ritter, M., & Capuano, T. (2006). Nonpunitive medication error reporting. *Journal of Nursing Administration, 36*(7–8), 370–376.

Pratt, N., Thomas, L., & Atkins, P. (2005). Measure patient harm in real time. *Nursing Management, 36*(11), 16–19.

Quality Indicator Project. (2004). *It's not the data . . . It's what you do with it.* Retrieved February 27, 2007, from *http://www.qiproject.org/index.asp?cmd5general_info.*

Roark, D. C. (2004). Bar codes and drug administration. *American Journal of Nursing, 104*(1), 63–66.

Rooney, J., & Vanden Heuvel, L. (2004). Root cause analysis for beginners. *Quality Progress, 37*(7), 45–53. Milwaukee, WI: American Society for Quality. Retrieved February 27, 2007, from *http://www.asq.org/pub/qualityprogress/past/0704/qp0704rooney.pdf.*

Simpson, R. L. (2007, February). ICNP: The language of worldwide nursing. *Nursing Management, 38*(2), 15, 18.

Stevens, K. R., & Staley, J. M. (2006). The Quality Chasm reports, evidence-based practice, and nursing's response to improve healthcare. *Nursing Outlook, 54*(2), 94–101.

Stumpf, P. G. (2007). Taking aim at the top 3 patient safety errors in ob/gyn. *Contemporary OB/GYN, 52*(1), 58–62.

Tanne, J. H. (2006, June 24). *U.S. campaign to save 100 000 lives exceeds its target. British Medical Journal,* 332:1468. Retrieved February 27, 2007, from *http://www.bmj.com/cgi/content/extract/332/7556/1468-b.*

Thompson, D. N., Wolf, G. A., & Spear, S. J. (2003). Driving improvements in patient care: Lessons from Toyota. *Journal of Nursing Administration, 33*(11), 585–595.

Ulrich, B. T. (2005, November). Some is not a number. Soon is not a time. *Journal of Nursing Administration, 35*(11), 473.

VanSuch, M., Naessens, J. M., Stroebel, R. J., Huddleston, J. M., & Williams, A. R. (2006). Effect of discharge instructions on readmission of hospitalised patients with heart failure: Do all of the Joint Commission on Accreditation of Healthcare Organizations heart failure core measures reflect better care? *Quality and Safety in Health Care, 15*(6), 414–417.

White House. (2005). *President signs Patient Safety and Quality Improvement Act of 2005.* Retrieved February 27, 2007, from *http://www.whitehouse.gov/news/releases/2005/07/20050729.html.*

Williams, J., & Murphy, P. (2005). Better project management. Better patient outcomes. *Nursing Management, 36*(11), 41–47.

Bibliography

Allen, D. E., Bockenhauer, B., Egan, C., & Kinnaird, L. S. (2006). Relating outcomes to excellent nursing practice. *Journal of Nursing Administration, 36*(3), 140–147.

Avery, J., Beyea, S. C., & Campion, P. (2005). Active error management. Use of a web-based reporting system to support patient safety initiatives. *Journal of Nursing Administration, 35*(2), 81–85.

Bergman S., Feldman L. S., & Barkun, J. S. (2006). Evaluating surgical outcomes. *Surgical Clinics of North America, 86*(1), 129–149.

Brush, J., Hill, A., O'Connor, R. E., & Ornato, J. P. (2007). One-third of EDs may fail to meet 90-minute target for heart attack patients. *ED Management, 19*(1), 1–3.

Buckley, T., Burns, S. M., & Black, T. (2005). A process improvement project. Achieving quality outcomes. *Journal of Nursing Administration, 35*(2), 94–99.

Clancy, T. R., Delaney, C. W., Morrison, B., & Gunn, J. K. (2006). The benefits of standardized nursing languages in complex adaptive systems such as hospitals. *Journal of Nursing Administration, 36*(9), 426–434.

Classen, D. C., Avery, A. J., & Bates, D. W. (2007). Evaluation and certification of computerized provider order entry systems. *Journal of the American Medical Informatics Association, 14*(1), 48–55.

Comeau, E., & Adkinson, K. (2007). Promoting quality patient care-reducing inpatient mortality. *Journal of Nursing Care Quality, 22*(1), 43–49.

Gelfand, E. W., Colice, G. L., Fromer, L., Bunn, W. B. III, & Davies, T. J. (2006). Use of the health plan employer data and information set for measuring and improving the quality of asthma care. *Annals of Allergy, Asthma and Immunology, 97*(3), 298–305.

Gingerich, B. S. (2007). Exploring access to and satisfaction with health services. Accreditation action. Quality improvement/quality of care center initiatives. *Home Health Care Management and Practice, 19*(2), 143–145.

Godleski, M., Jha, A., & Coll, J. (2007). Exploring access to and satisfaction with health services. *Topics in Spinal Cord Injury Rehabilitation, 12*(3), 56–65.

Grissinger, M. (2006). Medication errors. "Smart" infusion pumps join CPOE and bar coding as ways to prevent medication errors. *P&T: Journal for Formulary Management, 31*(10), 562.

Gross, P. A., & Bates, D. W. (2007). A pragmatic approach to implementing best practices for clinical decision support systems in computerized provider order entry systems. *Journal of the American Medical Informatics Association, 14*(1), 25–28.

Huston, C. (2006). Chapter 14. Medical errors: An ongoing threat to quality health care. In C. Huston (Ed.), *Professional issues in nursing: Challenges and opportunities* (pp. 268–291). Philadelphia: Lippincott Williams & Wilkins.

Improving performance through core measures: How one hospital uses clinical pathways to meet ORYX requirements. (2006). *Joint Commission Benchmark, 8*(2), 4–5.

Joint Commission focus: Redesigned ORYX performance measure reports updated four times a year. (2006). *Joint Commission Benchmark, 8*(3), 6–8.

Jones, S., & Moss, J. (2006). Computerized provider order entry. *Journal of Nursing Administration, 36*(3), 136–139.

Kaissi, A. (2006). An organizational approach to understanding patient safety and medical errors. *Health Care Manager, 25*(4), 292–305.

Keatings, M., Martin, M., McCallum, A., & Lewis, J. (2006). Medical errors: Understanding the patient's perspective. *Pediatric Clinics of North America, 53*(6), 1079–1089.

Landon, B. E., Normand, S. T., Lessler, A., O'Malley, A. J., Schmaltz, S., Loeb, J. M., & McNeil. B. J. (2006). Quality of care for the treatment of acute medical conditions in US hospitals. *Archives of Internal Medicine, 166*(22), 2511–2517.

Lundqvist, M. J., & Axelsson, A. U. E. (2007). Nurses' perceptions of quality assurance. *Journal of Nursing Management, 15*(1), 51–58.

Measuring performance for treating heart attacks and heart failure: The case for outcomes measurement. (2007). *Health Affairs, 26*(1), 75–85.

Ramsey, G. (2007). Nurses, medical errors, and the culture of blame . . . reprinted from the Hastings Center Report, March–April 2005. *Neonatal Intensive Care, 20*(1), 53–54.

Rangachari, P., & Hutchinson, D. M. (2006). A. systems approach to improving core measure outcomes in a small rural facility. *Journal for Healthcare Quality: Promoting Excellence in Healthcare, 28*(5), 37–43.

Shendell-Falik, N., Feinson, M., & Mohr, B. J. (2007). Enhancing patient safety. Improving the patient handoff process through appreciative inquiry. *Journal of Nursing Administration, 37*(2), 95–104.

Strategies for improving safety through patient and family involvement in care: Institutions create ways to achieve latest National Patient Safety Goals. (2007). *Patient Education Management, 14*(3), 25–29.

Upenieks, V. V., & Abelew, S. (2006). The Magnet designation process: A qualitative approach using Donabedian's conceptual framework. *Health Care Manager, 25*(3), 243–253.

Waring, J. J. (2007). Doctors' thinking about 'the system' as a threat to patient safety. *Health: An Interdisciplinary Journal for the Social Study of Health, Illness and Medicine, 11*(1), 29–46.

Weir, V. L. (2005). Preventing adverse drug events. *Nursing Management, 36*(9), 24–30.

24

Performance Appraisal

. . . it is a paradoxical but profoundly true and important principle of life that the most likely way to reach a goal is to be aiming not at that goal itself but at some more ambitious goal beyond it.

—*Arnold Toynbee*

. . . an effective appraisal process rewards productive employees and assists the professional growth and development of inexperienced and unproductive individuals.

—*Mable H. Smith (2003)*

An important managerial controlling responsibility is determining how well employees carry out the duties of their assigned jobs. This is done through *performance appraisals*, in which work performance is reviewed. Performance appraisals let employees know the level of their job performance as well as any expectations that the organization may have of them. Performance appraisals also generate information for salary adjustments, promotions, transfers, disciplinary actions, and terminations.

In performance appraisals, actual performance, not intent, is evaluated.

None of the manager's actions is as personal as appraising the work performance of others. Because work is an important part of one's identity, people are very sensitive to opinions about how they perform. For this reason, performance appraisal becomes one of the greatest tools an organization has to develop and motivate staff. When used correctly, performance appraisal can encourage staff and increase retention and productivity; in the hands of an inept or inexperienced manager, the appraisal process may discourage and demotivate staff. Because a manager's opinions and judgments are used for far-reaching decisions regarding the employee's work life, they must be determined in an objective, systematic, and formalized manner. Using a formal system of performance review also reduces the appraisal's subjectivity. The more professional a group

DISPLAY 24.1 **Leadership Roles and Management Functions Associated With Performance Appraisal**

Leadership Roles

1. Uses the appraisal process to motivate employees and promote growth
2. Uses appropriate techniques to reduce the anxiety inherent in the appraisal process
3. Involves employees in all aspects of performance appraisal
4. Is self-aware of own biases and prejudices
5. Develops employee trust by being honest and fair when evaluating performance
6. Encourages the peer review process among professional staff
7. Uses appraisal interviews to facilitate two-way communication
8. Provides ongoing support to employees who are attempting to correct performance deficiencies
9. Uses coaching techniques that promote employee growth in work performance
10. Individualizes performance goals and the appraisal interview as needed to meet the unique needs of a culturally diverse staff

Management Functions

1. Uses a formalized system of performance appraisal
2. Gathers data for performance appraisals that are fair and objective
3. Uses the appraisal process to determine staff education and training needs
4. Bases performance appraisal on documented standards
5. Is as objective as possible in performance appraisal
6. Maintains appropriate documentation of the appraisal process
7. Follows up on identified performance deficiencies
8. Conducts the appraisal interview in a manner that promotes a positive outcome
9. Provides frequent informal feedback on work performance

of employees is, the more complex and sensitive the evaluation process becomes. The skilled leader–manager who uses a formalized system appropriately builds a team approach to patient care.

This chapter focuses on the relationship between performance appraisal and motivation and discusses how performance appraisals can be used to determine developmental needs of staff. Emphasis is given to appropriate data gathering and the types of performance appraisal tools available. The performance appraisal interview is explored, and strategies are presented for reducing appraiser bias and increasing the likelihood that the appraisal itself will be growth producing. Finally, performance management is introduced as an alternative to the traditional annual performance appraisal. The leadership roles and management functions inherent in performance appraisal are shown in Display 24.1.

USING THE PERFORMANCE APPRAISAL TO MOTIVATE EMPLOYEES

Although systematic employee appraisals have been used in management since the 1920s, using the appraisal as a tool to promote employee growth did not begin until the 1950s.

This evolution of performance appraisals is reflected in its changing terminology. At one time, the appraisal was called a *merit rating* and was tied fairly closely to salary increases. More recently, it was termed *performance evaluation*, but because the term *evaluation* implies that personal values are being placed on the performance review, that term is used infrequently. Some organizations continue to use both of these terms or others, such as *competency assessment*, *effectiveness report*, or *service rating*. Most health care organizations, however, use the term *performance appraisal* because this term implies an appraisal of how well employees perform the duties of their job as delineated by the job description. An important point to consider, if the appraisal is to have a positive outcome, is how the employee views the appraisal.

 If employees believe that the appraisal is based on their job description rather than on whether the manager approves of them, they are more likely to view the appraisal as relevant.

Management research has shown that various factors influence whether the appraisal ultimately results in increased motivation and productivity. Some of these factors follow:

- The employee must believe that the appraisal is based on a standard to which other employees in the same classification are held accountable. This standard must be communicated clearly to employees at the time they are hired and may be a job description or an individual goal set by staff for the purpose of performance appraisal.
- The employee should have some input into developing the standards or goals on which his or her performance is judged. This is imperative for the professional employee.
- The employee must know in advance what happens if the expected performance standards are not met.
- The employee needs to know how information will be obtained to determine performance. The appraisal tends to be more accurate if various sources and types of information are solicited. Sources could include peers, coworkers, nursing care plans, patients, and personal observation. Employees should be told which sources will be used and how such information will be weighted.
- The appraiser should be one of the employee's direct supervisors. For example, the charge nurse who works directly with the staff nurse should be involved in the appraisal process and interview. It is appropriate and advisable in most instances for the head nurse and supervisor also to be involved. However, employees must believe that the person doing the major portion of the review has actually observed their work.
- The performance appraisal is more likely to have a positive outcome if the appraiser is viewed with trust and professional respect. This increases the chance that the employee will view the appraisal as a fair and accurate assessment of work performance. A summary of the factors influencing effectiveness of appraisals can be seen in Display 24.2.

DISPLAY 24.2 Factors Influencing Effective Performance Appraisal

Appraisal should be based on a standard.
Employee should have input into development of the standard.
Employee must know the standard in advance.
Employee must know the sources of data gathered for the appraisal.
Appraiser should be someone who has observed employee's work.
Appraiser should be someone who the employee trusts and respects.

LEARNING EXERCISE 24.1

Writing About Performance Appraisals
During your lifetime, you probably have had many performance appraisals. These may have been evaluations of your clinical performance during nursing school or as a paid employee. Reflect on these appraisals. How many of them encompassed the six recommendations listed in Display 24.2? How did the inclusion or exclusion of these recommendations influence your acceptance of the results?

● ASSIGNMENT: Select one of the above six recommendations about which you feel strongly. Write a three-paragraph essay on your personal experience involving this recommendation.

STRATEGIES TO ENSURE ACCURACY AND FAIRNESS IN THE PERFORMANCE APPRAISAL

If the goal of the performance appraisal is to satisfy requirements of the organization, then it is a time waster. On the other hand, if the employee views the appraisal as valuable and valid and growth producing, it can have many positive effects. Information obtained during the performance appraisal can be used to develop the employee's potential, to assist the employee in overcoming difficulties that he or she has in fulfilling the job's role, to point out strengths of which the employee may not be aware, and to aid the employee in setting goals.

> A performance appraisal wastes time if it is merely an excuse to satisfy regulations and the goal is not employee growth.

Because inaccurate and unfair appraisals are negative and can demotivate, it is critical that the manager use strategies that increase the likelihood of a fair and accurate appraisal. Although some subjectivity is inescapable, the following strategies will assist the manager in arriving at a fairer and more accurate assessment:

1. *The appraiser should develop an awareness of his or her own biases and prejudices.* This helps to guard against subjective attitudes and values influencing the appraisal.
2. *Consultation should be sought frequently.* Another manager should be consulted when a question about personal bias exists and in many other situations. For example, it is very important that new managers solicit assistance and consultation when they complete their first performance appraisals. Even experienced managers may need to consult with others when an employee is having great difficulty fulfilling the duties of the job. Consultation also must be used when employees work several shifts so that information can be obtained from all of the shift supervisors.
3. *Data should be gathered appropriately.* Many different sources should be consulted about employee performance, and the data gathered needs to reflect the entire time period of the appraisal. Frequently, managers gather data and observe an employee just before completing the appraisal, which gives an inaccurate picture of performance. Because all employees have periods when they are less productive and motivated, data should be gathered systematically and regularly.

4. *Accurate record keeping is another critical part of ensuring accuracy and fairness in the performance appraisal.* Information about subordinate performance (both positive and negative) should be recorded and not trusted to memory. The manager should make a habit of keeping notes about observations, others' comments, and his or her periodic review of charts and nursing care plans. Taking regular notes on employee performance is a way to avoid the *recency effect*, which favors appraisal of recent performance over less recent performance during the evaluation period.

 When ongoing anecdotal notes are not maintained throughout the evaluation period, the appraiser is more apt to experience the recency effect, where recent issues are weighed more heavily than past performance.

5. *Collected assessments should contain positive examples of growth and achievement and areas where development is needed.* Fuimano (2005) states, "When a nurse does her job well, it can go unnoticed because it's expected that she'll meet the requirements of her job description. But if she makes a mistake, we're sure to let her know about it" (p. 8). Nothing delights employees more than discovering that their immediate supervisor is aware of their growth and accomplishments and can cite specific instances in which good clinical judgment was used. Too frequently, collected data concentrate on negative aspects of performance. In the HBR Breakthrough Ideas for 2007, Hutson and Perry (2007) suggest that leader–managers should always be mindful of asking whether something they are about to do or say may be destructive or take away someone's hope. If so, it should be reframed in a more positive light.

6. *Some effort must be made to include the employee's own appraisal of his or her work.* Self-appraisal may be performed in several appropriate ways. Employees can be instructed to come to the appraisal interview with some informal thoughts about their performance, or they can work with their managers in completing a joint assessment. One advantage of *management by objectives* (MBO)—the use of personalized goals to measure individual performance—is the manner in which it involves the employee in assessing his or her work performance and in goal setting.

7. *The appraiser needs to guard against three common pitfalls of assessment: the halo effect, the horns effect, and central tendency.* The *halo effect* occurs when the appraiser lets one or two positive aspects of the assessment or behavior of the employee unduly influence all other aspects of the employee's performance. The *horns effect* occurs when the appraiser allows some negative aspects of the employee's performance to influence the assessment to such an extent that other levels of job performance are not accurately recorded. The manager who falls into the *central tendency* trap is hesitant to risk true assessment and therefore rates all employees as average. These appraiser behaviors lead employees to discount the entire assessment of their work.

8. *Finally, reviewers need to guard against a bias known as the Matthew effect.* In the Archer North Performance Appraisal System (2006), Gabris and Mitchell state, "The *Matthew Effect* is said to occur when employees receive the same appraisal results, year in and year out. That is, their appraisal results tend to become self-fulfilling: if they have done well, they will continue to do well; if they have done poorly, they will

EXAMINING THE EVIDENCE 24.1

Source: Archer North Performance Appraisal System. (2006). *Performance appraisal. Bias effects.* Retrieved February 28, 2007, from *http://www.performance-appraisal.com/bias.htm.*

In a study of an organization with the Archer North Performance Appraisal System (2006), a quarterly performance appraisal system, Gabris and Mitchell compared frustration levels in employees who consistently had high appraisal scores with those who consistently had low scores. When asked if the appraisal system was fair and equitable, 63% of the high performers agreed, compared with only 5% of the lower performers. Similarly, the groups were asked if their supervisors listened to them. Sixty-nine percent of the high performers said yes, whereas 95% of the low performers said no. Finally, almost half of the high performers felt that their supervisors were supportive, whereas none of the lower performers agreed.

The researchers concluded that while not everyone who received a poor appraisal was a victim of supervisory bias, to some extent, certain employees may be unfairly advantaged or disadvantaged by the Matthew effect. They concluded that employees should always have the opportunity to improve their appraisal results and that the process of performance appraisal is seriously flawed when this principle is denied in practice.

continue to do poorly" (para 3). Thus, past appraisals prejudice an employee's future attempts to improve. The Matthew effect is discussed further in Examining the Evidence 24.1. Display 24.3 provides a summary of performance appraisal strategies.

LEARNING EXERCISE 24.2

Planning an Employee's First Performance Appraisal

Mrs. Jones is a new LVN/LPN and has been working the 3 PM to 11 PM shift on the long-term care unit where you are the evening charge nurse. It is time for her 3-month performance appraisal. In your facility, each employee's job description is used as the standard of measure for performance appraisal. Essentially, you believe that Mrs. Jones is performing her job well, but you are somewhat concerned because she still relies on the RNs even for minor patient care decisions. Although you are glad that she does not act completely on her own, you would like to see her become more independent. The patients have commented favorably to you on Mrs. Jones's compassion and on her follow-through on all their requests and needs.

Mrs. Jones gets along well with the other LVNs/LPNs, and you sometimes believe that they take advantage of her hard-working and pleasant nature. On a few occasions, you believe that they inappropriately delegated some of their work to her. When preparing for Mrs. Jones's upcoming evaluation, what can you do to make the appraisal as objective as possible? You want Mrs. Jones's first evaluation to be growth producing.

● ASSIGNMENT: Plan how you will proceed. What positive forces are already present in this scenario? What negative forces will you have to overcome? Support your plan with readings from the Bibliography at the end of this chapter.

DISPLAY 24.3 Strategies to Ensure Performance Appraisal Accuracy

Develop self-awareness regarding own biases and prejudices.
Use appropriate consultation.
Gather data adequately over a period of time.
Keep accurate anecdotal records for the length of appraisal period.
Collect positive data and areas where improvement is needed.
Include employee's own appraisal of his or her performance.
Guard against the halo effect, horns effect, central tendency trap, and Matthew effect.

PERFORMANCE APPRAISAL TOOLS

Since the 1920s, many appraisal tools have been developed, all of which have been popular at different times. Since the early 1990s, the Joint Commission (formerly known as the Joint Commission on Accreditation of Healthcare Organizations [JCAHO]) has been advocating the use of an employee's job description as the standard for performance appraisal. The Joint Commission also suggests that employers must be able to demonstrate that employees know how to plan, implement, and evaluate care specific to the ages of the patients they care for. This continual refinement of critical *competencies* for professional nursing practice has a tremendous impact on the tools used in the appraisal process. It is important to remember, however, that competence assessments are not the same as performance evaluations. A *competence assessment* evaluates skill and knowledge; a *performance evaluation* evaluates execution of a task or tasks.

 A competence assessment evaluates whether an individual has the knowledge, education, skills, or experience to perform the task whereas a performance evaluation examines how well that individual actually completes that task.

The effectiveness of a performance appraisal system is only as good as the tools used to create those assessments. An effective competence assessment tool should allow the manager to focus on priority measures of performance. The following is an overview of some of the appraisal tools commonly used in health care organizations.

Trait Rating Scales

A *trait rating scale* is a method of rating a person against a set standard, which may be the job description, desired behaviors, or personal traits. The trait rating scale has been one of the most widely used of the many available appraisal methods. Rating personal traits and behaviors is the oldest type of rating scale. Many experts argue, however, that the quality or quantity of the work performed is a more accurate performance appraisal method than the employee's personal traits and that trait evaluation invites subjectivity. Rating scales also are subject to central tendency and halo- and horns-effect errors and thus are not used as often today as they were in the past. Instead, many organizations use two other rating methods, namely the job dimension scale and the *behaviorally anchored rating scale* (BARS). Display 24.4 shows a portion of a trait rating scale with examples of traits that might be expected in an RN.

DISPLAY 24.4   **Sample Trait Rating Scale**

Job Knowledge

Serious gaps in essential knowledge	Satisfactory knowledge of routine	Adequately informed on most phases of job	Good knowledge of all phases of job	Excellent under-standing of the job
1	2	3	4	5

Judgment

Decisions are often wrong on issues	Makes some decision errors	Good decisions	Sound and logical thinker	Makes good, complex decisions
1	2	3	4	5

Attitude

Resents suggestions, no enthusiasm, new ideas accepted reluctantly	Apathetic but cooperative and accepting	Generally cooperative and accepting of new ideas	Openly cooper-ates and accepts new ideas	Consistently helpful and offers new ideas
1	2	3	4	5

Job Dimension Scales

Job dimension scales require that a rating scale be constructed for each job classification. The rating factors are taken from the context of the written job description. Although job dimension scales share some of the same weaknesses as trait scales, they do focus on job requirements rather than on ambiguous terms such as "quantity of work." Display 24.5 shows an example of a job dimension scale for an industrial nurse.

Behaviorally Anchored Rating Scales

BARS, sometimes called *behavioral expectation scales*, overcome some of the weaknesses inherent in other rating systems. As in the job dimension method, the BARS technique requires

DISPLAY 24.5   **Sample Job Dimension Rating Scale for an Industrial Nurse**

Job Dimension	5	4	3	2	1
Renders first aid and treats job-related injuries and illnesses					
Holds fitness classes for workers					
Teaches health and nutrition classes					
Performs yearly physicals on workers					
Keeps equipment in good working order and maintains inventory					
Keeps appropriate records					
Dispenses medication and treatment for minor injuries					

(5 = Excellent; 4 = Good; 3 = Satisfactory; 2 = Fair; 1 = Poor)

that a separate rating form be developed for each job classification. Then, as in the job dimension rating scales, employees in specific positions work with management to delineate key areas of responsibility. However, in BARS, many specific examples are defined for each area of responsibility; these examples are given various degrees of importance by ranking them from 1 to 9. If the highest-ranked example of a job dimension is being met, it is less important than a lower-ranked example that is not.

Appraisal tools firmly grounded in desired behaviors can be used to improve performance and keep employees focused on the vision and mission of the organization. However, because separate BARS are needed for each job, the greatest disadvantage in using this tool with large numbers of employees is the time and expense. BARS also are primarily applicable to physically observable skills rather than to conceptual skills. Yet, this is an effective tool because it focuses on specific behaviors, allows employees to know exactly what is expected of them, and reduces rating errors.

Although all rating scales are prone to weaknesses and interpersonal bias, they do have some advantages. Many may be purchased, and although they must be individualized to the organization, there is little need for expensive worker hours to develop them. Rating scales also force the rater to look at more than one dimension of work performance, which eliminates some bias.

Checklists

There are several types of *checklist* appraisal tools. The *weighted scale*, the most frequently used checklist, is composed of many behavioral statements that represent desirable job behaviors. Each of these behavior statements has a weighted score attached to it. Employees receive an overall performance appraisal score based on behaviors or attributes. Often, merit raises are tied to the total point score (i.e., the employee needs to reach a certain score to receive an increase in pay).

Another type of checklist, the *forced checklist*, requires the supervisor to select an undesirable and a desirable behavior for each employee. Both desirable and undesirable behaviors have quantitative values, and the employee again ends up with a total score on which certain employment decisions are made.

Another type of checklist is the *simple checklist*. The simple checklist is composed of numerous words or phrases describing various employee behaviors or traits. These descriptors are often clustered to represent different aspects of one dimension of behavior, such as assertiveness or interpersonal skills. The rater is asked to check all those that describe the employee on each checklist. A major weakness of all checklists is that there are no set performance standards. In addition, specific components of behavior are not addressed. Checklists do, however, focus on a variety of job-related behaviors and avoid some of the bias inherent in the trait rating scales.

Essays

The *essay appraisal method* is often referred to as the *free-form review*. The appraiser describes in narrative form an employee's strengths and areas where improvement or growth is needed. Although this method can be unstructured, it usually calls for certain items to be addressed. This technique does appropriately force the appraiser to focus on positive aspects of the employee's performance. However, a greater opportunity for personal bias undoubtedly exists.

Many organizations combine various types of appraisals to improve the quality of their review processes. Because the essay method does not require exhaustive development, it can quickly be adapted as an adjunct to any type of structured format. This gives the organization the ability to decrease bias and focus on employee strengths.

Self-Appraisals

Employees are increasingly being asked to submit written summaries or *portfolios* of their work-related accomplishments and productivity as part of the *self-appraisal* process. Portfolios often provide examples of continuing education, professional certifications, awards, and recognitions. The portfolio also generally includes the employee's goals and an action plan for accomplishing these goals.

There are advantages and disadvantages to using self-appraisal as a method of performance review. Although introspection and self-appraisal result in growth when the person is self-aware, even mature people require external feedback and performance validation. Some employees look forward to their annual performance review in anticipation of positive feedback. Asking these employees to perform their own performance appraisal would probably be viewed negatively rather than positively. Indeed, Fuimano (2005) shares the story of a staff nurse who began crying during her annual performance review, despite her work being exceptional. When pressed as to why she was crying, she stated that it was because no one has ever told her how great she was and how much her work was appreciated.

 Some employees look on their annual performance review as an opportunity to receive positive feedback from their supervisor, especially if the employee receives infrequent praise on a day-to-day basis.

Some employees undervalue their own accomplishments or feel uncomfortable giving themselves high marks in many areas. In an effort to avoid this potential influence on their rating, managers may wish to complete the performance appraisal tool before reading the employee's self-analysis, or they should view the self-appraisal as only one of a number of data sources that should be collected when evaluating worker performance. When self-appraisal is not congruent with other data available, the manager may wish to pursue the reasons for this discrepancy during the appraisal conference. Such an exchange may provide valuable insight regarding the worker's self-awareness and ability to view himself or herself objectively.

Management by Objectives

Management by objectives (MBO) is an excellent tool for determining an individual employee's progress because it incorporates both the employee's assessments as well as the organization. The focus in this chapter, however, is on how these concepts are used as an effective performance appraisal method rather than on their use as a planning technique.

Although seldom used in health care, MBO is an excellent method to appraise the performance of the employee in a manner that promotes individual growth and excellence. The following steps delineate how MBO can be used effectively in performance appraisal:

1. The employee and supervisor meet and agree on the principal duties and responsibilities of the employee's job. (The job description serves as a guide only.) This is done as soon as possible after beginning employment.
2. The employee sets short-term goals and target dates in cooperation with the supervisor or manager. The manager guides the process so that it relates to the position's duties. The subordinate's goals must not be in conflict with the goals of the organization. In setting goals, it is important that the manager remember that one's values and beliefs simply reflect a single set of options among many. This is especially true in working with a multicultural staff.

Professional expectations and values can vary greatly among cultures, and the manager must be careful to resist judgmental reactions and allow for cultural differences in goal setting.

3. Both parties agree on the criteria that will be used for measuring and evaluating the accomplishment of goals. In addition, a time frame is set for completing the objectives, which depends on the nature of the work being planned. Common time frames used in health care organizations vary from 1 month to 1 year.

4. Regularly, but more than once a year, the employee and supervisor meet to discuss progress. At these meetings, some modifications can be made to the original goals if both parties agree. Major obstacles that block completion of objectives within the time frame are identified. In addition, the resources and support needed from others are identified.

5. The manager's role is supportive, assisting the employee to reach goals by coaching and counseling.

6. During the appraisal process, the manager determines whether the employee has met the goals.

7. The entire process focuses on outcomes and results and not on personal traits.

One of the many advantages of MBO is that the method creates a vested interest in the employee to accomplish goals because employees are able to set their own goals. Additionally, defensive feelings are minimized, and a spirit of teamwork prevails. MBO as a performance appraisal method also has its disadvantages. Highly directive and authoritarian managers find it difficult to lead employees in this manner. Also, the marginal employee frequently attempts to set easily attainable goals. However, research has shown that MBO, when used correctly, is a very effective method of performance appraisal.

LEARNING EXERCISE 24.3

Using Management by Objective as a Part of Performance Appraisal

It is time for Nancy Irwin's annual performance appraisal. She is an RN on a postsurgical unit, dealing with complex trauma patients requiring high-level nursing intensity. You are the evening charge nurse and have worked with Ms. Irwin for the 2 years since she graduated from nursing school. Last year, in addition to the regular 1 to 5 rating scale for job expectations, all of the charge nurses added an MBO component to the performance appraisal form. In collaboration with his or her charge nurse, each employee developed five goals that were supposed to have been carried out over a 1-year period.

In reviewing Ms. Irwin's performance, you use several sources, including your written notes and her charting, and your conclusion is that with her strengths and weaknesses, overall she is a better-than-average nurse. However, you believe that she has not grown much as an employee over the past 6 months. This observation is confirmed by a review of the following:

Objective	Result
1. Conduct a mini in-service or patient care conference twice monthly for the next 12 months.	Met goal first 2 months. Last 10 months conducted only six conferences.

(Learning Exercise continues on page 580)

2. Will attend five educational classes related to work area; at least one of these will be given by an outside agency.	Attended one surgical nursing wound conference in the city and one in-house conference on TPN.
3. Will become an active member of a nursing committee at the hospital.	Has become an active member of the Policies and Procedures Committee and regularly attends meetings.
4. Reduce the number of late arrivals at work by 50% (from 24 per year to 12).	First 3 months: not late. Second 3 months: three late arrivals. Third 3 months: six late arrivals. Last 3 months: six late arrivals.
5. Ensure that all patients discharged have discharge instructions documented in their charts.	Anecdotal notes show that Ms. Irwin still frequently forgets to document these nursing actions.

● ASSIGNMENT: As Ms. Irwin's charge nurse, what can you do to ensure that the current appraisal results in greater growth for her? What went wrong with last year's MBO plan? Devise a plan for the performance appraisal. Try solving this yourself before reading the possible solution that appears in the Appendix.

Peer Review

When peers rather than supervisors carry out monitoring and assessing work performance, it is referred to as *peer review*. Most likely, the manager's review of the employee is not complete unless some type of peer review data is gathered. Peer review provides feedback that can promote growth. It also can provide learning opportunities for the peer reviewers.

 The concept of collegial evaluation of nursing practice is closely related to maintaining professional standards.

Although the prevailing practice in most organizations is to have managers evaluate employee performance, there is much to be said for collegial review. Peer review is widely used in medicine and academe; however, health care organizations have been slow to adopt peer review for the following five reasons:

1. Staff are poorly oriented to the peer review method. Peer review is viewed as very threatening when inadequate time is spent orienting employees to the process and when necessary support is not provided throughout the process.
2. Peers feel uncomfortable sharing feedback with people with whom they work closely, so they omit needed suggestions for improving the employee's performance. Thus, the review becomes more advocacy than evaluation.
3. Peer review is viewed by many as more time-consuming than traditional superior–subordinate performance appraisals.
4. Because much socialization takes place in the workplace, friendships often result in inflated evaluations, or interpersonal conflict may result in unfair appraisals.

5. Because peer review shifts the authority away from management, the insecure manager may feel threatened.

Peer review has its shortcomings, as evidenced by some university teachers receiving unjustified tenure or the failure of physicians to maintain adequate quality control among some individuals in their profession. Additionally, peer review involves much risk taking, is time-consuming, and requires a great deal of energy. However, nursing as a profession should be responsible for setting the standards and then monitoring its own performance. Because performance appraisal may be viewed as a type of quality control, it seems reasonable to expect that nurses should have some input into the performance evaluation process of their profession's members.

Peer review can be carried out in several ways. The process may require the reviewers to share the results only with the person being reviewed, or the results may be shared with the employee's supervisor and the employee. The review would never be shared only with the employee's supervisor. The results may or may not be used for personnel decisions. The number of observations, number of reviewers, qualification and classification of the peer reviewer, and procedure need to be developed for each organization. If peer review is to succeed, the organization must overcome its inherent difficulties by doing the following before implementing a peer review program:

- Peer review appraisal tools must reflect standards to be measured, such as the job description.
- Staff must receive a thorough orientation to the process before its implementation. The role of the manager should be clearly defined.
- Ongoing support, resources, and information must be made available to the staff during the process.
- Data for peer review need to be obtained from predetermined sources, such as observations, charts, and patient care plans.
- A decision must be made about whether anonymous feedback will be allowed. This is controversial and needs to be addressed in the procedure.
- Decisions must be reached on whether the peer review will affect personnel decisions and, if so, in what manner.

Peer review has the potential to increase the accuracy of performance appraisal. It also can provide many opportunities for increased professionalism and learning. The use of peer review in nursing should continue to expand as nursing increases its autonomy and professional status. Display 24.6 provides a summary of types of performance appraisal tools.

DISPLAY 24.6 Summary of Performance Appraisal Tools

Trait rating scales: Rates an individual against some standard.

Job dimension scales: Rates the performance on job requirements.

Behaviorally anchored rating scales (BARS): Rates desired job expectations on a scale of importance to the position.

Checklists: Rates the performance against a set list of desirable job behaviors.

Essays: A narrative appraisal of job performance.

Self-appraisals: An appraisal of performance by the employee.

Management by objectives: Employee and management agree upon goals of performance to be reached.

Peer review: Assessment of work performance carried out by peers.

LEARNING EXERCISE 24.4

Addressing Mary's Change in Behavior

Even in organizations that have no formal peer review process, professionals must take some responsibility for colleagues' work performance, even if informally. The following scenario illustrates the need for peer involvement.

You have worked at Memorial Hospital since your graduation from nursing school. Your school roommate, Mary, also has worked at Memorial since her graduation. For the first year, you and Mary were assigned to different units, but you both were transferred to the oncology unit 6 months ago. You both work the 3 PM to 11 PM shift, and it is the policy for the charge nurse duties to alternate among three RNs assigned to the unit on a full-time basis. Both you and Mary are among the nurses assigned to rotate to the charge position. You have noticed lately that when Mary is in charge, her personality seems to change; she barks orders and seems tense and anxious.

Mary is an excellent clinical nurse, and many of the staff seek her out in consultation about patient care problems. You have, however, heard several of the staff grumbling about Mary's behavior when she is in charge. As Mary's good friend, you do not want to hurt her feelings, but as her colleague, you feel a need to be honest and open with her.

● ASSIGNMENT: A very difficult situation occurs when personal and working relationships are combined. Describe what, if anything, you would do. Use the readings from the Bibliography to assist you in making a plan.

The 360-Degree Evaluation

An adaptation of peer review, and a relatively new addition to performance appraisal tools, the *360-degree evaluation* includes an assessment by all individuals within the sphere of influence of the individual being appraised (Davidson, 2007). Getting feedback from multiple individuals provides a broader, more accurate perspective on the employee's work performance. For example, a 360-degree evaluation of a ward clerk or unit secretary might include feedback from the nursing staff, patients, and from staff from other departments who interact with that individual on a regular basis.

Heathfield (2007) suggests that in most 360-degree evaluations, an employee receives performance feedback from his or her supervisor and four to eight others, including staff members, co-workers and customers. According to Heathfield, this allows each individual "to understand how his effectiveness as an employee, coworker, or staff member is viewed by others" (para. 6). In addition, most 360-degree feedback tools include a self-assessment.

PLANNING THE APPRAISAL INTERVIEW

The most accurate and thorough appraisal will fail to produce growth in employees if the information gathered is not used appropriately. Many appraisal interviews have negative outcomes because the manager views them as a time to instruct employees only on what they are doing wrong rather than looking at strengths as well.

Managers often dislike the appraisal interview more than the actual data gathering. One of the reasons why managers dislike the appraisal interview is because of their own negative experiences when they have been judged unfairly or criticized personally. Both parties in the appraisal process tend to be anxious before the interview; thus, the appraisal interview remains an emotionally charged event. For many employees, past appraisals have been traumatizing. Although little can be done to eliminate the often-negative emotions created by past experiences, the leader–manager can manage the interview in such a manner that people will not be traumatized further.

OVERCOMING APPRAISAL INTERVIEW DIFFICULTIES

Feedback, perhaps the greatest tool a manager has for changing behavior, must be given in an appropriate manner. There is a greater chance that the performance appraisal will have a positive outcome if certain conditions are present before, during, and after the interview.

Before the Interview

- Make sure that the conditions mentioned previously have been met (e.g., the employee knows the standard by which his or her work will be evaluated), and he or she has a copy of the appraisal form.
- Select an appropriate time for the appraisal conference. Do not choose a time when the employee has just had a traumatic personal event or is too busy at work to take the time needed for a meaningful conference.
- Give the employee 2- to 3-days advance notice of the scheduled appraisal conference so that he or she can be prepared mentally and emotionally for the interview.
- Be prepared mentally and emotionally for the conference yourself. If something should happen to interfere with your readiness for the interview, it should be canceled and rescheduled.
- Schedule uninterrupted interview time. Hold the interview in a private, quiet, and comfortable place. Forward your telephone calls to another line, and ask another manager to answer any pages that you may have during the performance appraisal.
- Plan a seating arrangement that reflects collegiality rather than power. Having the person seated across a large desk from the appraiser denotes a power–status position; placing the chairs side by side denotes collegiality.

During the Interview

- Greet the employee warmly, showing that the manager and the organization have a sincere interest in his or her growth.
- Begin the conference on a pleasant, informal note.
- Ask the employee to comment on his or her progress since the last performance appraisal.
- Avoid surprises in the appraisal conference. The effective leader coaches and communicates informally with staff on a continual basis, so there should be little new information at an appraisal conference.
- Use coaching techniques throughout the conference.
- When dealing with an employee who has several problems—either new or long-standing—do not overwhelm him or her at the conference. If there are too many problems to be

addressed, select the major ones. Fuimano states that "often, people are so hard on themselves, that they don't need leaders to be hard on them as well" (p. 8).

- Conduct the conference in a nondirective and participatory manner. Input from the employee should be solicited throughout the interview; however, the manager must recognize that employees from some cultures may be hesitant to provide this type of input. In this situation, the manager must continually reassure the employee that such input is not only acceptable but also is desired.
- Focus on the employee's performance and not on his or her personal characteristics.
- Avoid vague generalities, either positive or negative, such as "your skills need a little work" or "your performance is fine." Be prepared with explicit performance examples. Be liberal in the positive examples of employee performance; use examples of poor perform-ance sparingly. Use several examples only if the employee has difficulty with self-awareness and requests specific instances of a problem area.
- When delivering performance feedback, be straightforward and state concerns directly so as not to retard communication or cloud the message.

 Indirectness and ambiguity are more likely to inhibit communication than enhance it, and the employee is left unsure about the significance of the message.

- Never threaten, intimidate, or use status in any manner. Holder and Schenthal (2007) discuss *professional boundaries* (the space between the professional's power and the client's vulnera-bility) and *power differentials* (the inequalities that exist between professionals and clients) that interfere with the ability of professionals to form meaningful relationships with their clients. These same issues can occur between managers and subordinates, as both may prevent the establishment of a meaningful and constructive relationship. This is not to say that man-agers should not maintain an appropriate authority power gap with their employees; it simply suggests that power and status issues should be minimized as much as possible so that the performance appraisal can appropriately focus on the subordinate's performance and needs.
- Let the employee know that the organization and the manager are aware of his or her uniqueness, special interests, and valuable contributions to the unit. Remember that all employees make some special contribution to the workplace.
- Make every effort to ensure that there are no interruptions during the conference.
- Use terms and language that are clearly understood and carry the same meaning for both parties. Avoid words that have a negative connotation. Do not talk down to employees or use language that is inappropriate for their level of education.
- Mutually set goals for further growth or improvement in the employee's performance. Decide how goals will be accomplished and evaluated and what support is needed.
- Plan on being available for employees to return retrospectively to discuss the appraisal review further. There is frequently a need for the employee to return for elaboration if the conference did not go well or if the employee was given unexpected new information. This is especially true for the new employee.

After the Interview

- Both the manager and employee need to sign the appraisal form to document that the con-ference was held and that the employee received the appraisal information. This does not

DISPLAY 24.7 **Performance Appraisal Documentation Form**

Performance appraisal for:
Name: _____
Unit: _____
Prepared by: _____
Reason: _____
(Merit, terminal, end of probation, general reviews)
Date of appraisal conference: _____
Comments by employee:

Employee's signature: _____
(Signature of employee denotes that the appraisal has been read. It *does not* signify
acceptance or agreement. Space is provided for any comments the employee wishes to
make.) Comments by appraiser.

(These comments are to be written at the time of the appraisal conference and in the
presence of the employee.)

_____   _____
Employee's signature (Date)   Evaluator's signature (Date)

mean that the employee is agreeing to the information in the appraisal; it merely means
that the employee has read the appraisal. An example of such a form is shown in
Display 24.7. There should be a place for comments by both the manager and the
employee.

• End the interview on a pleasant note.
• Document the goals for further development that have been agreed on by both parties. The
documentation should include target dates for accomplishment, support needed, and when
goals are to be reviewed. This documentation is often part of the appraisal form.
• If the interview reveals specific long-term coaching needs, the manager should develop a
method of follow-up to ensure that such coaching takes place.

PERFORMANCE MANAGEMENT

Some experts in human resource management have suggested that annual performance
appraisals should be replaced by ongoing *performance management*. In performance management, appraisals are eliminated and the manager places his or her efforts into ongoing coaching,
mutual goal setting, and the leadership training of subordinates. This focus requires the manager
to spend more regularly scheduled face-to-face time with subordinates.

In contrast to the annual performance review, which is often linked to an employee's hire date, the performance management calendar is generally linked to the organization's business calendar. This way, performance planning is coordinated throughout the entire organization, as strategic goals for the year can be identified and subordinates' roles to achieve those goals can be openly discussed and planned. Typically, performance-managed organizations identify role-based competency expectations for every employee, regardless of job description. Then, employees can determine how these qualities translate into performance in specific jobs.

COACHING: A MECHANISM FOR INFORMAL PERFORMANCE APPRAISAL

The word *coaching* has become a contemporary term to convey the spirit of leaders' and managers' roles in informal day-to-day performance appraisals, which promote improved work performance and team building. Coaching can guide others into increased competence, commitment, and confidence as well as help them to anticipate options for making vital connections between their present and future plans. In addition, Ponte and Gross (2006) also suggest that coaches can help individuals think through "challenging work environments or issues related to complex roles or relationships" (p. 320). While typically defined as a one-on-one relationship, coaching can also be done by dyads and teams (Ponte & Gross, 2006).

 Day-to-day feedback regarding performance is one of the best methods for improving work performance and building a team approach.

Manthey (2001) uses the terms *reflective practice* and *clinical coaching* to describe a management strategy that fuses both performance coaching and performance management. In clinical coaching, the manager or mentor meets with an employee regularly to discuss aspects of his or her work. Both individuals determine the agenda jointly with the goal of an environment of learning that can span the personal and professional aspects of the employee's experience. During clinical coaching, employees can discuss things that have made them feel angry or discouraged. They can also get new ideas and information about how to deal with situations from someone who often has experienced the same problems and issues. This shared connection between the manager and employee makes the employee feel validated and part of a larger team. When coaching is combined with informal performance appraisal, the outcome is usually a positive modification of behavior. For this to occur, however, the leader must establish a climate in which there is a free exchange of ideas.

Forman (2006) suggests that an additional part of day-to-day coaching is being a *cheerleader*. Cheerleaders are capable, high-profile individuals who "draw others to them with a smile, a look of approval, and even a broad sweeping gesture" (p. 346). By recognizing the good work of others, even when done informally in walking rounds, cheerleaders empower subordinates and encourage them to continue the desired behaviors.

BECOMING AN EFFECTIVE COACH

Ponte and Gross (2006) suggest that coaches require certain managerial skills to be successful, including a grounding in the behavioral sciences such as psychology and organizational development.

They must also have strong communication skills, an ability to reflect back, and be able to serve as a "mirror" for those being coached, in an "authentic, skillful, and compassionate way" (p. 322)

The following tactics will assist managers in becoming more effective coaches:

• Be specific, not general, in describing behavior that needs improvement.
• Be descriptive, not evaluative, when describing what was wrong with the work performance.
• Be certain that the feedback is not self-serving but meets the needs of the employee.
• Direct the feedback toward behavior that can be changed.
• Use sensitivity in timing the feedback.
• Make sure that the employee has clearly understood the feedback and that the employee's communication also has been clearly heard.

When employees believe that their manager is interested in their performance and personal growth, they will have less fear of the work performance appraisal. When that anxiety is reduced, the formal performance interview process can be used to set mutual performance goals.

INTEGRATING LEADERSHIP ROLES AND MANAGEMENT FUNCTIONS IN CONDUCTING PERFORMANCE APPRAISALS

Performance appraisal is a major responsibility in the controlling function of management. The ability to conduct meaningful, effective performance appraisals requires an investment of time, effort, and practice on the part of the manager. Although performance appraisal is never easy, if used appropriately, it produces growth in the employee and increases productivity in the organization.

To increase the likelihood of successful performance appraisal, managers should use a formalized system of appraisal and gather data about employee performance in a systematic manner, using many sources. The manager also should attempt to be as objective as possible, using established standards for the appraisal. The result of the appraisal process should provide the manager with information for meeting training and educational needs of employees. By following up conscientiously on identified performance deficiencies, employees' work problems can be corrected before they become habits.

Integrating leadership into this part of the controlling phase of the management process provides an opportunity for sharing, communicating, and growing. The integrated leader–manager is self-aware regarding his or her biases and prejudices. This self-awareness leads to fairness and honesty in evaluating performance. This, in turn, increases trust in the manager and promotes a team spirit among employees.

The leader also uses day-to-day coaching techniques to improve work performance and reduce the anxiety of performance appraisal. When anxiety is reduced during the appraisal interview, the leader–manager is able to establish a relationship of mutual goal setting, which has a greater potential to result in increased motivation and corrected deficiencies. The result of the integration of leadership and management is a performance appraisal that facilitates employee growth and increases organizational productivity.

 Key Concepts

❋ The employee *performance appraisal* is a sensitive and important part of the management process, requiring much skill.

* When accurate and appropriate appraisal assessments are performed, outcomes can be very positive.
* Performance appraisals are used to determine how well employees are performing their job. Therefore, appraisals measure actual behavior and not intent.
* *Job descriptions* often produce objective criteria for use in the performance appraisal.
* There are many different types of appraisal tools and methods, and the most appropriate one to use varies with the type of appraisal to be done and the criteria to be measured.
* The employee must be involved in the appraisal process and must view the appraisal as accurate and fair.
* *MBO* has been proved to increase productivity and commitment in employees.
* *Peer review* has great potential for developing professional accountability but is often difficult to implement.
* Unless the appraisal interview is carried out in an appropriate and effective manner, the appraisal data will be useless.
* Due to past experiences, performance appraisal interviews are highly charged, emotional events for most employees.
* Showing a genuine interest in the employee's growth and seeking his or her input at the interview will increase the likelihood of a positive outcome from the appraisal process.
* Performance appraisals should be signed to show that feedback was given to the employee.
* Informal work performance appraisals are an important management function.
* Leaders should routinely use *day-to-day* coaching to empower subordinates and improve work performance.
* In *performance management,* appraisals are eliminated. Instead, the manager places his or her efforts into ongoing coaching, mutual goal setting, and the leadership training of subordinates.

ADDITIONAL LEARNING EXERCISES AND APPLICATIONS

LEARNING EXERCISE 24.5

Requesting Feedback From Employees

You are the director of a home health agency. You have just returned from a management course and have been inspired by the idea of requesting input from your subordinates about your performance as a manager. You realize that there are some risks involved but believe that the potential benefits from the feedback outweigh the risks. However, you want to provide some structure for the evaluation, so you spend some time designing your appraisal tool and developing your plan.

● ASSIGNMENT: What type of tool will you use? What is your overall goal? Will you share the results of the appraisal with anyone else? How will you use the information obtained? Would you have the appraisal forms signed or have them be anonymous? Who would you include in the group that is evaluating you? Be able to support your ideas with appropriate rationale.

LEARNING EXERCISE 24.6

Making Appraisal Interviews Less Traumatic

You are the new night-shift charge nurse in a large ICU composed of an all-RN staff. When you were appointed to the position, your supervisor told you that there had been some complaints regarding the manner in which the previous charge nurse had handled evaluation sessions. Not wanting to repeat the mistakes, you draw up a list of things that you could do to make the evaluation interviews less traumatic. Because the evaluation tool appears adequate, you believe that the problems must lie with the interview itself. At the top of your list, you write that you will make sure each employee has advance notice of the evaluation.

● ASSIGNMENT: How much advance notice should you give? What additional criteria would you add to the list to help eliminate much of the trauma that frequently accompanies performance appraisal (even when the appraisal is very good)? Add six to nine items to the list. Explain why you think that each of these would assist in alleviating some of the anxiety associated with performance appraisals. Do not just repeat the guidelines listed in this chapter. You may make the guidelines more specific or use the Bibliography for assistance in developing your own list.

LEARNING EXERCISE 24.7

Helping a Seasoned Employee to Grow

Patty Brown is an LVN/LPN who has been employed on your unit for 10 years. She is an older woman and is very sensitive to criticism. Her work is generally of high quality, but in reviewing her past performance appraisals, you notice that during the last 10 years, at least seven times she has been rated unsatisfactory for not being on duty promptly and eight times for not attending staff development programs. Because you are the new charge nurse, you would like to help Patty grow in these two areas. You have given Patty a copy of the evaluation tool and her job description and have scheduled her appraisal conference for a time when the unit will be quiet. You can conduct the appraisal in the conference room.

● ASSIGNMENT: How would you conduct this performance appraisal? Outline your plan. Include how you would begin. What innovative or creative way would you attempt to provide direction or improvement in the areas mentioned? How would you terminate the session? Be able to give rationale for your decisions.

LEARNING EXERCISE 24.8

Could This Conflict Have Been Prevented?

Mr. Jones, a 49-year-old automobile salesman, was admitted with severe back pain. As his primary care nurse, you have established a rapport with Mr. Jones. He has a type A personality and has been very critical of much of his hospitalization. He also was very upset by the quality and quantity of his pain following his laminectomy. You agreed to ambulate him on your shift three times (at 4:00 PM, 7:00 PM, and 10:30 PM) so that he would need to be ambulated only

(Learning Exercise continues on page 590)

once during the day shift. He does not care for many of the day staff and feels that you help to ambulate him better than anyone else. You noted the ambulating routine on his nursing orders.

Yesterday, Joan Martin, a day nurse, believed that his bowel sounds were somewhat diminished. She urged him to ambulate more on the day shift, but he refused to do so. (The doctor had ordered ambulation q.i.d.) When Mr. Jones's physician visited, Nurse Martin told him that Mr. Jones ambulated only once on the shift. She did not elaborate further to the doctor. The physician proceeded to talk very sternly with Mr. Jones, telling him to get out of bed three times today. Nurse Martin did not mention this incident to you in report.

By the time that you arrived on duty and received report, Mr. Jones was very angry. He threatened to sign himself out against medical advice. You talked with his doctor, got the order changed, and finally managed to calm Mr. Jones down. You then wrote a nursing order that read, "Nurse Martin is not to be assigned to Mr. Jones again." When Joan Martin came on duty this morning, the night shift pointed out your notation. She was very angry and went to see the head nurse.

● ASSIGNMENT: Should you have done anything differently? If so, what? Could the evaluation of clinical performance by you and Nurse Martin have been done in a manner that would not have resulted in conflict? If you were Nurse Martin, what could you have done to prevent the conflict? Be able to discuss this case in relation to professional trust, peer review, and assertive communication.

LEARNING EXERCISE 24.9

Addressing Sally's Errors in Judgment

You are a senior baccalaureate nursing student. This is your sixth week of a medical–surgical advanced practicum. Your instructor assigns two students to work together in caring for four to six patients. The students alternate fulfilling leader and follower roles and providing total patient care. This is the second full day that you have worked as a team with Sally Brown.

Last week, when you were assigned with Sally, she was the leader and made numerous errors in judgment. She got a patient up who was on strict bed rest. She made an IV medication error by giving a medication to the wrong patient. She gave morphine too soon because she forgot to record the time in the medication record, and she frequently did not seem to know what was wrong with her patients.

Today, you have been the leader and have observed her contaminate a dressing and forget to check armbands twice when she was giving medications. When you asked her about checking placement of the nasogastric tube, she did not know how to perform this skill. You have heard some of the other students complain about Sally.

● ASSIGNMENT: What is your obligation to your patients, your fellow students, the clinical agency, and your instructor? Outline what you would do. Give rationale for your decisions.

(Web Links)———————————————————————

Coaching the Caterpillar to Fly: A Program for Development
http://www.squarewheels.com/coaching/coachcat.html
Interactive "square wheels" exercise and butterfly metaphor that emphasize coaching as a technique for creating trust and team building in organizations.

Performance Appraisal

http://www.performance-appraisal.com/intro.htm

Outlines basic purposes, methods, benefits, reward issues, conflict and confrontation, common mistakes, and bias effects associated with performance appraisal.

Employee's Self-Appraisal Form

http://www.uhv.edu/fin/forms/emp_self_appraisal.htm

This form was developed by the University of Houston–Victoria for individuals to use as part of a self-appraisal for performance review.

Performance Appraisals

http://www.businessballs.com/performanceappraisals.htm

This site by businessballs.com includes an appraisal guide as well as templates for appraisal forms. In addition, it includes strategies for implementing 360-degree reviews.

References

Archer North Performance Appraisal System. (2006). *Performance appraisal. Bias effects.* Retrieved February 28, 2007, from *http://www.performance-appraisal.com/bias.htm.*

Davidson, M. L. (2007). The 360 degree evaluation. *Clinics in Podiatric Medicine and Surgery, 24*(1), 65–94.

Forman, H. (2006). From cheerleader to patent processor. *Journal of Nursing Administration, 36* (7–8), 346–350.

Fuimano, J. (2005). Harness the power of praise. *Nursing Management, 36*(1), 8–9.

HBR Breakthrough Ideas for 2007. (2007, February). *The leader from hope.* From Hutson, H., & Perry, B. (2006). Putting hope to work: Five principles to activate your organization's most powerful resource. Co-presented by Harvard Business Review and the World Economic Forum. Retrieved February 28, 2007, from *http://harvardbusinessonline.hbsp.harvard.edu/hbrol/en/search/saSearchResults.jhtml?Ntt=the+leader+from+hope&searchCategory=hbr&N=0&hbr=%2Fhbrol%2Fen%2Fsearch%2FsaSearchResults.jhtml&hbo*

=%2Fb02%2Fen%2Fsearch%2FsearchResults.jhtml&referral=&Ntk=hbrsa&Ntx=mode%2Bmatchallpartial&x=11 &y=9.

Heathfield, S. M. (2007). *360 degree feedback: The good, the bad, and the ugly.* About.com: Human Resources. Retrieved February 28, 2007, from *http://humanresources.about.com/od/360feedback/a/360feedback.htm.*

Holder, K. V., & Schenthal, S. J. (2007). Watch your step: Nursing and professional boundaries. *Nursing Management, 38*(2), 24–30.

Manthey, M. (2001). Reflective practice. *Creative Nursing, 7*(2), 3–5.

Ponte, P. R., & Gross, A. H. (2006). Using an executive coach to increase leadership effectiveness. *Journal of Nursing Administration, 36*(6), 319–324.

Smith, M. H. (2003). Empower staff with praiseworthy appraisals. *Nursing Management, 34*(1), 15–18.

Bibliography

Chella, G. (2006, March 16). *Appraisal 2006—Let's do it differently!* The Hindu Business Line. Retrieved February 25, 2007, from *http://www.thehindubusinessline.com/2006/03/13/stories/2006031301360900.htm.*

Crumbie, A., & Kyle L. (2006). Leadership. Nurse partnership: The challenge of appraisal. *Primary Health Care, 16*(8), 14–16.

Doherty, L. (2006). Should bosses have more say on who is fit to nurse? *Nursing Times, 102*(47), 9.

Edwards, P. A., & Davis, C. R. (2006). Internationally educated nurses' perceptions of their clinical competence. *Journal of Continuing Education in Nursing, 37*(6), 265–269.

Esmail, A., & Abel, P. (2006). The impact of ethnicity and diversity on doctors' performance and appraisal. *British Journal of Health Care Management, 12*(10), 303–307.

Hawksley, B. (2007). Work-related stress, work/life balance and personal life coaching. *British Journal of Community Nursing, 12*(1), 34–36.

Heathfield, S. M. (2007). *Performance management is NOT an annual appraisal.* About.com: Human Resources. Retrieved February 2, 2007, from *http://humanresources.about.com/od/performanceevals/a/performancemgmt.htm.*

Heathfield, S. M. (2007). *Performance appraisals don't work.* About.com: Human Resources. Retrieved February 25, 2007, from *http://humanresources.about.com/od/performanceevals/a/perf_appraisal.htm.*

Jenkins, A. (2005, March). *Performance appraisal research: A critical review of work on "The Social Context and Politics of Appraisal."* ESSEC Research Center, ESSEC Business School in its series ESSEC Working Papers with number DR 05004. Retrieved February 25, 2007, from *http://www .performance-appraisals.org/cgi-bin/links/jump.cgi?ID=10527.*

Johnson, C. H. (2007). Competencies as an evaluation tool. *Clinics in Podiatric Medicine and Surgery, 24*(1), 103–117.

Keenan, R. (2006). Understanding the competence review process. *Kai Tiaki Nursing New Zealand, 12*(9), 26–27.

'Negative' feedback proves to be positive . . . 'Dilemma' (NT opinion, 7 November, p. 11). (2006, November 21–27). *Nursing Times, 102*(47), 14.

Sines, D., Harris, D., Firth, J., & Boden, L. E. (2006). Ensuring fitness for practice. *Nursing Management—UK, 13*(8), 28–31.

25

Problem Employees:
Rule Breakers, Marginal Employees, and the Chemically or Psychologically Impaired

> *. . . as patient advocates, nurse leaders must help ensure fitness for duty.*
>
> —*Richard Hader*

> *. . . difficult employees can make you question why you became a manager in the first place.*
>
> —*Mark Pipkin*

Employees' perceptions vary as to what they owe the organization and what they owe themselves. At times, organizational and individual needs, wants, and responsibilities are in conflict. The coordination and cooperation needed to meet organizational goals require leader–managers to control individual subordinates' urges that are counterproductive to these goals. Subordinates do this by self-control. Managers meet organizational goals by enforcing established rules, policies, and procedures. Leaders do this by creating a supportive and motivating climate and by coaching.

When employees are unsuccessful in meeting organizational goals, managers must attempt to identify reasons for this failure and counsel employees accordingly. If employees fail because they are unwilling to follow rules or established policies and procedures, or they are unable to perform their duties adequately despite assistance and encouragement, the manager has an obligation to take disciplinary action. However, progressive discipline is inappropriate for employees who are impaired as a result of disease or degree of ability. These employees have special problems and needs that require active coaching; support; and, often, professional counseling to maintain productivity. So that employees can be managed most appropriately, managers must be able to distinguish between employees in need of discipline and those who are impaired.

Regardless of the cause, however, supervisors should be quick to recognize and address inappropriate conduct and poor work performance (Hader, 2005). Delay only exacerbates such situations. Many employees are confronted by co-workers' below par performance on a daily basis (Martin, 2005). Martin says that the inability of managers to deal with poor performance results in diminished productivity, quality, and morale. When someone is not performing well, everyone knows it. And when management refuses to act, employees may perceive that their leaders lack the resolve necessary to make the organization successful.

 Not disciplining an employee who should be disciplined jeopardizes an organization's morale.

This chapter focuses on discipline, coaching, and referral as tools in promoting subordinates' growth and meeting organizational goals. The normal progression of steps taken in disciplinary action and strategies for administering discipline fairly and effectively are delineated. Formal and informal grievances are discussed. The chapter also focuses on two types of employees with special needs: the marginal employee and the impaired employee. *Marginal employees* are those employees who disrupt unit functioning because the quantity or quality of their work consistently meets only minimal standards. This chapter identifies the challenges inherent in working with marginal employees and presents managerial strategies for dealing with these problem employees.

For purposes of this discussion, *impairment* refers to employees who are unable to accomplish their work at the expected level as a result of chemical or psychological disease. While the emphasis in this chapter is on *chemical impairment* (impairment resulting from drug or alcohol addiction), *psychological impairment* is increasingly recognized as a significant problem for employees. The strategies used to deal with both types of impairment typically overlap. This chapter profiles chemical addiction among nurses as well as behaviors common to chemically impaired nurses. Steps in the recovery process and the reentry of the recovering chemically impaired nurse into the workforce are also discussed. Leadership roles and management functions appropriate for use with problem employees are shown in Display 25.1.

CONSTRUCTIVE VERSUS DESTRUCTIVE DISCIPLINE

Discipline involves training or molding of the mind or character to bring about desired behaviors. Discipline is often considered a form of punishment but is not the same thing as punishment. *Punishment* is an undesirable event that follows unacceptable behavior. Although discipline can have negative consequences, it can be a powerful motivator for positive change (Corrective Discipline, 2007). Moreover, discipline has an educational component as well as a corrective one.

Scientific management theory viewed discipline as a necessary means for controlling an unmotivated and self-centered workforce. Because of this traditional philosophy, managers primarily used threats and fear to control behavior. This "big stick" approach to management focused on eliminating all behaviors that could be considered to conflict with organizational goals. Although this approach may succeed on a short-term basis, it is usually demotivating and reduces long-term productivity because people will achieve only at the level that they believe is necessary to avoid punishment. This approach also is destructive because discipline is often

DISPLAY 25.1 Leadership Roles and Management Functions in Dealing With Problem Employees

Leadership Roles

1. Recognizes and reinforces the intrinsic self-worth of each employee and the role of successful work performance in maintaining a positive self-image
2. Encourages employees to be self-disciplined in conforming to established rules and regulations
3. Assists employees to identify with organizational goals, thus increasing the likelihood that the standards of conduct deemed acceptable by the organization will be accepted by its employees
4. Is self-aware regarding the power and responsibility inherent in having formal authority to set rules and discipline employees
5. Serves in the role of coach in performance deficiency coaching
6. Is self-aware regarding values, biases, and beliefs about chemical abuse
7. Uses active listening as a support tool in working with chemically and psychologically impaired subordinates but recognizes own limitations in counseling and refers impaired employees to outside experts for appropriate counseling
8. Examines the work environment for stressors that contribute to substance abuse and eliminates those stressors whenever possible

Management Functions

1. Clearly identifies performance expectations for all employees and confronts employees when those expectations are not met
2. Assigns employees to work roles and situations that successfully challenge or intermittently "stretch" the employee; does not allow employees to fail repeatedly
3. Seeks out and completes extensive education about chemical abuse in the work setting; provides these same opportunities to staff
4. Acts as a resource to chemically or psychologically impaired employees regarding professional services or agencies that provide counseling and support services
5. Collects and records adequate objective data when suspicious of employee chemical impairment
6. Focuses employee confrontations on performance deficits and not on the cause of the underlying problem or addiction
7. Works with the rule breaker, chemically impaired, and/or marginal employee to develop a remedial plan for action; ensures that the employee understands the performance expectations of the organization and the consequences of not meeting these expectations

arbitrarily administered and is unfair either in the application of rules or in the resulting punishment. The *Encyclopedia of Business* (2007) concurs, stating that a more effective approach being used currently by many businesses encourages employee commitment by showing workers the discrepancy between actual and expected performance and putting the burden on the employee to change. Leaders should seek to establish *commitment models* of leadership.

In contrast to punishment, discipline is called *constructive discipline* when it assists employee growth. Punishment is frequently inferred when defining discipline, but discipline also can be defined as training, educating, or molding. In fact, the word *discipline* comes from the Latin term *disciplina*, which means teaching, learning, and growing. In constructive discipline, punishment may be applied for improper behavior, but it is carried out in a supportive, corrective manner. Employees are reassured that the punishment given is because of their actions and not because of who they are.

 Constructive discipline uses discipline as a means of helping the employee grow, not as a punitive measure.

LEARNING EXERCISE 25.1

Thinking About Growth-Producing Versus Destructive Discipline
Think back to when someone in authority such as a parent, teacher, or boss set limits or enforced rules in such a way that you became a better child, student, or employee. What made this disciplinary action growth producing instead of destructive? What was the most destructive disciplinary action that you ever experienced? Did it modify your behavior in any way?

SELF-DISCIPLINE AND GROUP NORMS

The highest level and most effective form of discipline is *self-discipline*. When employees feel secure, validated, and affirmed in their essential worth, identity, and integrity, self-discipline is encouraged. Ideally, all employees would have adequate self-control and be self-directed in their pursuit of organizational goals. However, this is not always the case. Instead, group norms often influence individual behavior and make self-discipline difficult. *Group norms* are group-established standards of expected behavior that are enforced by social pressure. The leader, who understands group norms, is able to work within those norms to mold group behavior. This modification of group norms, in turn, affects individual behavior and thus self-discipline.

Although self-discipline is internalized, the leader plays an active role in developing an environment that promotes self-discipline in employees. It is impossible for employees to have self-control if they do not understand the acceptable boundaries for their behavior, nor can they be self-directed if they do not understand what is expected of them. Therefore, managers must discuss clearly all written rules and policies with subordinates, explain the rationale for the existence of the rules and policies, and encourage questions.

 Self-discipline is possible only if subordinates know the rules and accept them as valid.

Self-discipline also requires an atmosphere of mutual trust. Managers must believe that employees are capable of and actively seek self-discipline. Likewise, employees must respect their managers and perceive them as honest and trustworthy. Employees lack the security to have self-discipline if they do not trust their managers' motives. Finally, for self-discipline to develop, formal authority must be used judiciously. If formal discipline is quickly and widely used, subordinates do not have the opportunity to invoke self-discipline.

FAIR AND EFFECTIVE RULES

Several guidelines must be followed if discipline is to be perceived by subordinates as growth producing. This does not imply that subordinates enjoy being disciplined or that discipline should be a regular means of promoting employee growth. However, discipline, if implemented correctly, should not permanently alienate or demoralize subordinates. McGregor (1967) developed four rules to make discipline as fair and growth producing as possible (Display 25.2). These rules are called "hot stove" rules because they can be applied to someone touching a hot stove.

Most rule breaking is not enforced using McGregor's rules. For example, many people exceed the speed limit when driving. Generally, people are aware of speed limit regulations, and signs are posted along the roadway as reminders of the rules; thus, there is *forewarning*. There is not, however, *immediacy*, *consistency*, or *impartiality*. Many people exceed the speed limit for long periods before they are stopped and disciplined, or they may never be disciplined at all. Likewise, a person may be stopped and disciplined one day and not the next even though the same rule is broken. Finally, the punishment is inconsistent because some people are punished for their rule breaking, but others are not. Even the penalty varies among people.

DISPLAY 25.2   **McGregor's Hot Stove Rules for Fair and Effective Discipline**

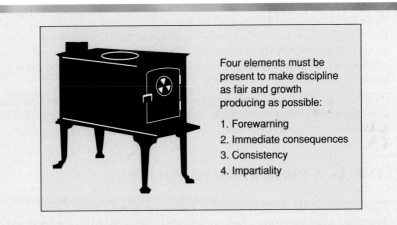

Four elements must be present to make discipline as fair and growth producing as possible:

1. Forewarning
2. Immediate consequences
3. Consistency
4. Impartiality

1. All employees must be *forewarned* that if they touch the hot stove (break a rule), they will be burned (punished or disciplined). They must know the rule beforehand and be aware of the punishment.
2. If the person touches the stove (breaks a rule), there will be *immediate consequences* (getting burned). All discipline should be administered immediately after rules are broken.
3. If the person touches the stove again, he or she will again be burned. Therefore, there is *consistency*; each time the rule is broken, there are immediate and consistent consequences.
4. If any other person touches the hot stove, he or she also will get burned. Discipline must be *impartial*, and everyone must be treated in the same manner when the rule is broken.

Imagine if automobiles had been developed that required drivers to place a built-in electronic sensor on the end of their fingers before the automobile would operate. The purpose of this sensor would be to deliver a low-charge but painful electrical shock every time the car exceeded the posted speed limit. The driver would be forewarned of the consequences of breaking the speed limit rule. If each time the rule was broken, the driver immediately received an electrical shock, and if all automobiles included this feature, speeding would probably be eliminated.

If a rule or regulation is worth having, it should be enforced. When rule breaking is allowed to go unpunished, other people tend to replicate the behavior of the rule breaker. Likewise, the average worker's natural inclination to obey rules can be dissipated by lax or inept enforcement policies because employees develop contempt for managers who allow rules to be disregarded. The enforcement of rules using McGregor's hot stove rules keeps morale from breaking down and allows structure within the organization.

An organization should, however, have as few rules and regulations as possible. A leadership role involves regularly reviewing all rules, regulations, and policies to see if they should be discarded or modified in some way. If managers find themselves spending much of their time enforcing one particular rule, it would be wise to reexamine the rule and consider whether there is something wrong with the rule or how it is communicated.

LEARNING EXERCISE 25.2

Rule Breakers and Outdated Rules
Part 1: Think back to "rule breakers" you have known. Were they a majority or minority in the group? How great was their impact on group behavior? What characteristics did they have in common? Did the group modify the rule breaker's behavior, or did the rule breaker modify group behavior?

Part 2: Rules quickly become outdated and need to be deleted or changed in some way. Think of a policy or rule that needs to be updated. Why is the rule no longer appropriate? What could you do to update this rule? Does the rule need to be replaced with a new one?

DISCIPLINE AS A PROGRESSIVE PROCESS

Managers have the formal authority and responsibility to take progressively stronger forms of discipline when employees fail to meet expected standards of achievement. However, inappropriate discipline (too much or too little) can undermine the morale of the whole team. Determining appropriate disciplinary action, then, is often difficult, and many factors must be considered. Discipline is generally administered by using a progressive model. Union contracts include provision for disciplinary procedures, which are usually based upon some sort of *progressive discipline* process (Encyclopedia of Business, 2007). However, even in non-union organizations, managers should have a disciplinary procedure that is written and well communicated.

 Action must be taken when employees continue undesirable conduct, either by breaking rules or by not performing their job duties adequately.

Generally, the first step of the disciplinary process is an *informal reprimand* or *verbal admonishment*. This reprimand includes an informal meeting between the employee and manager to discuss the broken rule or performance deficiency. The manager suggests ways in which the employee's behavior might be altered to keep the rule from being broken again. Often, an informal reprimand is all that is needed for behavior modification.

The second step is a *formal reprimand* or *written admonishment*. If rule breaking recurs after verbal admonishment, the manager again meets with the employee and issues a written warning about the behaviors that must be corrected. This written warning is very specific about what rules or policies have been violated, the potential consequences if behavior is not altered to meet organizational expectations, and the plan of action that the employee is expected to take to achieve expected change. Both the employee and the manager should sign the warning to signify that the problem or incident was discussed. The employee's signature does not imply that the employee agrees with everything on the report, only that it has been discussed. The employee must be allowed to respond in writing to the reprimand, either on the form itself or by attaching comments to the disciplinary report; this allows the employee to air any differences in perception between the manager and the employee. One copy of the written admonishment is then given to the employee, and another copy is retained in the employee's personnel file. Display 25.3 presents a sample written reprimand form.

The third step in progressive discipline is usually a *suspension from work*, either with or without pay. If the employee continues the undesired behavior despite verbal and written warnings, the manager should remove the employee from his or her job for a brief time, generally a few

DISPLAY 25.3   Sample Written Reprimand Form

Employee name
_____

Position _____ Date of hire _____
Person completing report _____
Position _____ Date report completed _____
Date of incident(s) _____ Time _____
Description of incident(s):

Prior attempts to counsel employee regarding this behavior (cite date and results of disciplinary conferences):

Disciplinary contract (plan for correction) and time lines:

Consequences of future repetition:

Employee comments (additional documentation or rebuttal may be attached):

_____   _____
Signature of individual making the report   Employee signature

Date _____   Date _____

Date and time of follow-up appointment to review disciplinary contract:

days to several weeks. Such a suspension gives the employee the opportunity to reflect on the behavior and to plan how he or she might modify the behavior in the future.

The last step in progressive discipline is *involuntary termination* or *dismissal*. In reality, many people terminate their employment voluntarily before reaching this step, but the manager cannot count on this happening. Termination should always be the last resort when dealing with poor performance. However, if the manager has given repeated warnings and rule breaking or policy violations continue, then the employee should be dismissed. Although this is difficult and traumatic for the employee, the manager, and the unit, the cost in terms of managerial and employee time and unit morale of keeping such an employee is enormous.

When using progressive discipline, the steps are followed only for repeated infractions of the same rule. At the end of a predesignated time period, the slate is wiped clean. For example, although an employee may have previously received a formal reprimand for unexcused absences, discipline for a first-time offense of tardiness should begin at the first step of the process. Also remember that although discipline is generally administered progressively, some rule breaking is so serious that the employee may be suspended or dismissed with the first infraction. Table 25.1 presents a progressive discipline guide for managers.

 When using progressive discipline in all but the most serious infractions, the slate should be wiped clean at the conclusion of a predesignated period.

LEARNING EXERCISE 25.3

Deciding Upon Disciplinary Action

You are a supervisor in a neurological care unit. One morning, you receive a report from the night-shift RNs, Nurse Caldwell and Nurse Jones. Neither of the nurses reports anything out of the ordinary, except that a young head-injury patient has been particularly belligerent and offensive in his language. This young man was especially annoying because he appeared rational and then would suddenly become abusive. His language was particularly vulgar. You recognize that this is fairly normal behavior in a patient with a head injury, but yesterday morning, his behavior was so offensive to his neurosurgeons that one of them threatened to wash his mouth out with soap.

After both night nurses leave the unit, you receive a phone call from the house night supervisor who relates the following information: When the supervisor made the usual rounds to the neuro unit, Nurse Caldwell was on a coffee break and Nurse Jones was in the unit with two LVNs/LPNs. Nurse Jones reported that Nurse Caldwell became very upset with the head-injury patient because of his abusive and vulgar language and had taped his mouth shut with a four-inch piece of adhesive tape. Nurse Jones had observed the behavior and had gone to the patient's bedside and removed the piece of tape and suggested that Nurse Caldwell go get a cup of coffee.

The supervisor observed the unit several times following this, and nothing else appeared to be remiss. Stating that no harm had come to the patient, Nurse Jones was reluctant to report the incident but believed that perhaps one of the supervisors should counsel Nurse Caldwell. You thank the night supervisor and consider the following facts in this case:

- Nurse Caldwell has been an excellent nurse but is occasionally judgmental.
- Nurse Caldwell is a very religious young woman and has led a rather sheltered life.
- Taping a patient's mouth with a four-inch piece of adhesive tape is very dangerous, especially for someone with questionable chest and abdominal injuries and neurological injuries.
- Nurse Caldwell has never been reprimanded before.

You call the physician and explain what happened. The physician believes that no harm was done and agrees with you that it is up to you whether to discipline the employee and to what degree. However, the physician believes that most of the medical staff would want the nurse fired.

You phone the nurse and arrange for a conference with her. She tearfully admits what she did. She states that she lost control. She asks you not to fire her, although she agrees this is a dischargeable offense. You consult with the administration, and everyone agrees that you should be the one to decide the disciplinary action in this case.

● ASSIGNMENT: Decide what you would do. You have a duty to your patients, the hospital, and your staff. List at least four possible courses of action. Select from among these choices, and justify your decision.

TABLE 25.1 Guide to Progressive Discipline

Offense	First Infraction	Second Infraction	Third Infraction	Fourth Infraction
Gross mistreatment of a patient	Dismissal			
Discourtesy to a patient	Verbal admonishment	Written admonishment	Suspension	Dismissal
Insubordination	Written admonishment	Suspension	Dismissal	
Intoxication while on duty (this offense is difficult to prove)	Verbal admonishment	Written admonishment	Dismissal	
Use of intoxicants while on duty	Dismissal			
Neglect of duty	Verbal admonishment	Written admonishment	Suspension	Dismissal
Theft or willful damage of property	Written admonishment	Dismissal		
Falsehood	Verbal admonishment	Written admonishment	Dismissal	
Unauthorized absence	Verbal admonishment	Written admonishment	Dismissal	
Abuse of leave	Verbal admonishment	Written admonishment	Suspension	Dismissal
Deliberate violation of instruction	Verbal admonishment	Written admonishment	Suspension	Dismissal
Violation of safety rules	Verbal admonishment	Written admonishment	Dismissal	
Fighting	Verbal admonishment	Written admonishment	Suspension	Dismissal
Inability to maintain work standards	Verbal admonishment	Written admonishment	Suspension	Dismissal
Excessive unexcused tardiness*	Verbal admonishment	Written admonishment	Dismissal	

*The first, second, and third infractions do not mean the first, second, and third time an employee is late but the first, second, and third time that unexcused tardiness becomes excessive as determined by the manager.

DISCIPLINARY STRATEGIES FOR THE NURSE–MANAGER

It is vital that managers recognize their power in evaluating and correcting employees' behavior. Because a person's job is very important to him or her—often as a part of self-esteem and as a means of livelihood—disciplining or taking away a person's job is a very serious action and should not be undertaken lightly. The manager can implement several strategies to increase the likelihood that discipline will be fair and produce growth.

The first strategy that the manager must use is to investigate thoroughly the situation that has prompted the employee discipline. A supervisor must investigate all allegations of misconduct even if the misconduct is anonymously reported or appears initially to have no basis. To determine the appropriate level of discipline, the manager must investigate, document, examine the employee's record, and look at the severity of the problem (Corrective Discipline, 2007).

The manager might ask the following questions: Was the rule clear? Did this employee know that he or she was breaking a rule? Is cultural diversity a factor in this rule breaking? Has this employee been involved in a situation like this before? Was he or she disciplined for this behavior? What was his or her response to the corrective action? How serious or potentially serious is the current problem or infraction? Who else was involved in the situation? Does this employee have a history of other types of disciplinary problems? What is the quality of this employee's performance in the work setting? Have other employees in the organization also experienced the problem? How were they disciplined? Could there be a problem with the rule or policy? Were there any special circumstances that could have contributed to the problem in this situation? What disciplinary action is suggested by organizational policies for this type of offense? Has precedent been established? Will this type of disciplinary action keep the infraction from recurring? The wise manager will ask all these questions so that a fair decision can be reached regarding an appropriate course of action.

Another strategy that the manager should use is always to consult with either a superior or the human resources department before dismissing an employee. Most organizations have very clear policies about which actions constitute grounds for dismissal and how that dismissal should be handled. To protect themselves from charges of willful or discriminatory termination, managers should carefully document the behavior that occurred and any attempts to counsel the employee. Managers also must be careful not to discuss with one employee the reasons for discharging another employee or to make negative comments about past employees, which may discourage other employees or reduce their trust in the manager.

Performance Deficiency Coaching

Performance deficiency coaching is another strategy that the manager can use to create a disciplined work environment. This type of coaching may be ongoing or problem centered. *Problem-centered coaching* is less spontaneous and requires more managerial planning than *ongoing coaching*. In performance deficiency coaching, the manager actively brings areas of unacceptable behavior or performance to the attention of the employee and works with him or her to establish a plan to correct deficiencies. Because the role of coach is less threatening than that of enforcer, the manager becomes a supporter and helper. Performance deficiency coaching helps employees, over time, to improve their performance to the highest level of which they are capable. As such, the development, use, and mastery of performance deficiency coaching should result in improved performance for all. The scenario depicted in Display 25.4 is an example of performance deficiency coaching.

LEARNING EXERCISE 25.4

Writing a Performance Deficiency Coaching Plan

You are the professional staff coordinator of a small emergency-care clinic. Historically, the clinic is busiest on weekend evenings, when most drunk-driving injuries, stabbings, and gunshot wounds occur. Many also come to the clinic on weekends to take care of nonemergency medical needs that were not addressed during regular physician office hours. Jane has been an RN at the clinic since it opened 2 years ago. She is well liked by all the employees and provides a sense of humor and lightheartedness in what usually is a highly stressful environment.

Jane has a reputation for being a "party animal." She is known to begin partying after work on Friday night and close down the bars Saturday morning. During the last 3 months, Jane has called in sick five of the seven Saturday evenings that she was scheduled to work. The other employees have worked understaffed on what is generally the busiest night of the week, and they are becoming angry. They have asked you to talk to Jane or to staff an additional employee on those Saturday evenings that Jane is assigned to work.

● ASSIGNMENT: You have decided to begin performance deficiency coaching with Jane. Write a possible coaching scenario that includes the following:
   • The problem stated in behavioral terms
   • An explanation to the employee of how the problem is related to organizational functioning
   • A clear statement of possible consequences of the unwanted behavior
   • A request for input from the employee
   • Employee participation in the problem solving
   • A plan for follow-up on the problem

DISPLAY 25.4 Performance Deficiency Coaching Scenario

Coach: I am concerned that you have been regularly coming into report late. This interrupts the other employees who are trying to hear report and creates overtime because the night shifts must stay and repeat report on the patients you missed. It also makes it difficult for your modular team members to prioritize their plan of care for the day if the entire team is not there and ready to begin at 0700. Why is this problem occurring?

Employee: I've been having problems lately with an unreliable babysitter and my car not starting. It seems like it's always one thing or another, and I'm upset about not getting to work on time, too. I hate starting my day off behind the eight ball.

Coach: This hospital has a long-standing policy on attendance, and it is one of the criteria used to judge work performance on your performance appraisal.

Employee: Yes, I know. I'm just not sure what I can do about it right now.

Coach: What approaches have you tried in solving these problems?

Employee: Well, I'm buying a new car, so that should take care of my transportation problems. I'm not sure about my babysitter, though. She's young and not very responsible, so she'll call me at the last minute and tell me she's not coming. I keep her, though, because she's willing to work the flexible hours and days that this job requires, and she doesn't charge as much as a formal day care center would.

(continued)

DISPLAY 25.4   **Performance Deficiency Coaching Scenario** (continued)

> *Coach:* Do you have family in the area or close friends you can count on to help with child care on short notice?
> *Employee:* Yes, my mother lives a few blocks away and is always glad to help, but I couldn't count on her on a regular basis.
> *Coach:* There are employment registry lists at the local college for students interested in providing child care. Have you thought about trying this option? Often, students can work flexible hours and charge less than formal day care centers.
> *Employee:* That's a good idea. In fact, I just heard about a child care referral service that also could give me a few ideas. I'll stop there after work. I realize that my behavior has affected unit functioning, and I promise to try to work this out as soon as possible.
> *Coach:* I'm sure these problems can be corrected. Let's have a follow-up visit in 2 weeks to see how things are going.

The Disciplinary Conference

When coaching is unsuccessful in modifying problem behavior, the manager must take more aggressive steps and use more formal measures, such as a *disciplinary conference*. After thoroughly investigating an employee's offenses, managers must confront the employee with their findings. This occurs in the form of a disciplinary conference. The following steps are generally part of the disciplinary conference.

 Disciplinary problems, if unrecognized or ignored, generally do not go away, they only get worse.

Reason for Disciplinary Action

Begin by clearly specifying why the employee is being disciplined. The manager must not be hesitant or apologetic. The role of the manager includes authority. Despite the assignment of authority, novice managers often feel uncomfortable with the disciplinary process and may provide unclear or mixed messages to the employee regarding the nature or seriousness of a disciplinary problem. A major responsibility in this role is evaluating employee performance and suggesting appropriate action for improved or acceptable performance.

 In the disciplinary conference, managers must assume the authority given to them by their role.

Employee's Response to Action

Give the employee the opportunity to explain why the rule was not followed. Allowing employees feedback in the disciplinary process ensures them recognition as human beings. It also reassures them that your ultimate goal is to be fair and promote their growth.

Rationale for Disciplinary Action

Explain the disciplinary action that you are going to take and why you are going to take it. Although the manager must keep an open mind to new information that may be gathered in the second step, preliminary assessments regarding the appropriate disciplinary action should already have been made. This discipline should be communicated to the employee. The employee who has been counseled at previous disciplinary conferences should not be surprised at the punishment, as it should have been discussed at the last conference.

Clarification of Expectations for Change

Describe the expected behavioral change, and list the steps needed to achieve this change. Explain the consequences of failure to change. Again, do not be apologetic or hesitant; otherwise, the employee will be confused about the seriousness of the issue. Because they may lack self-control, employees who have repeatedly broken rules need firm direction. It must be very clear to the employee that timely follow-up will occur.

Agreement and Acceptance of Action Plan

Get agreement and acceptance of the plan. Give support, and let the employee know that you are interested in him or her as a person. Remember too that the leader–manager administers discipline to promote employee growth rather than to impose punishment. Although the expected standards must be very clear, the leader imparts a sense of genuine concern for and desire to help the employee grow. This approach helps the employee to recognize that the discipline is directed at the offensive behavior and not at the individual. The leader must be cautious, however, not to relinquish the management role in an effort to nurture and counsel. The leadership role is to provide a supportive environment and structure so that the employee can make the necessary changes.

Besides understanding what should be covered in the disciplinary conference, the leader must be sensitive to the environment in which discipline is given. Although the employee must receive feedback about his or her rule breaking or inappropriate behavior as soon as possible after it has occurred, the manager should implement discipline privately, never in front of patients or peers. If more than an informal admonishment is required, the manager should inform the employee of the unacceptable action and then schedule a formal disciplinary conference later.

All discipline, even informal admonishments, should be conducted in private.

All formal disciplinary conferences should be scheduled in advance at a time agreeable to both the employee and manager. Both will want time to reflect on the situation that has occurred. Allowing time for reflection should reduce the situation's emotionalism and promote employee self-discipline, because employees often identify their own plan for keeping the behavior from recurring.

In addition to privacy and advance scheduling, the length of the disciplinary conference is important. It should not be so long that it degenerates into a debate, nor so short that both the employee and manager cannot provide input. If the employee seems overly emotional or if great discrepancies exist between the manager and employee's perceptions, an additional conference can be scheduled. Employees often need time to absorb what they have been told and to develop a plan that is not defensive.

The Termination Conference

At times, the disciplinary conference must be a termination conference. Although many of the principles are the same, the termination conference differs from a disciplinary conference in that planning for future improvement is eliminated. The following steps should be followed in the termination conference:

1. *Calmly state the reasons for dismissal.* The manager must not appear angry or defensive. Although managers may express regret that the outcome is termination of employment, they must not dwell on this or give the employee reason to think that the decision is not final. The manager should be prepared to give examples of the behavior in question.
2. *Explain the employment termination process.* State the date on which employment is terminated as well as the employee's and organization's role in the process.
3. *Ask for employee input.* Termination conferences are always tense; raw, spontaneous emotional reactions are common. Listen to the employee, but do not allow yourself to be drawn emotionally into his or her anger or sorrow. Always stay focused on the facts of the case and attempt to respond without reacting.
4. *End the meeting on a positive note, if possible.* The manager should also inform the employee what, if any, references will be supplied to prospective employers. Finally, it is usually best to allow the employee who has been dismissed to leave the organization immediately. If the employee continues to work on the unit after dismissal has been discussed, it can be demoralizing for all the employees who work on that unit.

GRIEVANCE PROCEDURES

Growth can occur only when employees perceive that feedback and discipline are fair and just. When employees and managers perceive "fair" and "just" differently, the discrepancy can usually be resolved by a more formal means called a *grievance procedure*. The grievance procedure is essentially a statement of wrongdoing or a procedure to follow when one believes that a wrong has been committed. This procedure is not limited to resolving discipline discrepancies; employees can use it any time they believe that they have not been treated fairly by management. This chapter, however, focuses specifically on grievances that result from the disciplinary process. Most grievances or conflicts between employees and management can be resolved informally through communication, negotiation, compromise, and collaboration. Generally though, even informal resolution has well-defined steps that should be followed.

Formal Process

If the employee and management cannot resolve their differences informally, a formal grievance process begins. The steps of the formal grievance process are generally outlined in all union contracts or administrative policy and procedure manuals. Generally, these steps include the progressive lodging of formal complaints up the chain of command. If resolution does not occur at any of these levels, a formal hearing is usually held. Several people or a small group is impaneled, much in the same way as a jury, to make a determination of what should be done. Such groups are often at risk of favoring the individual employee over the all-powerful institution. This tendency reinforces the need for the manager to have clear, objective, and comprehensive written records regarding the problem employee's behavior and attempts to counsel.

Arbitration

If the differences cannot be settled through a formal grievance process, the matter may finally be resolved in a process known as arbitration. In *arbitration*, both sides agree on the selection of a *professional mediator* who will review the grievance, complete fact-finding, and interview witnesses before coming to a decision.

Although grievance procedures extract a great deal of time and energy from both employees and managers, they serve several valuable purposes. Grievance procedures can settle some problems before they escalate into even larger ones. The procedures also are a source of data to focus attention on ambiguous contract language for labor–management negotiation at a later date.

 Perhaps the most important outcome of a grievance is the legitimate opportunity that it provides for employees to resolve conflicts with their superiors.

Employees who are not given an outlet for resolving work conflicts become demoralized, angry, and dissatisfied. These emotions affect unit functioning and productivity. Even if the outcome is not in the favor of the person filing the grievance, the employee will know that the opportunity was given to present the case to an objective third party, and the chances of constructive conflict resolution are greatly increased. In addition, managers tend to be fairer and more consistent when they know that employees have a method of redress for arbitrary managerial action.

Rights and Responsibilities in Grievance Resolution

Employees and managers have some separate and distinct rights and responsibilities in grievance resolution, but many rights and responsibilities overlap. Although it is easy to be drawn into the emotionalism of a grievance that focuses on one's perceived rights, the manager and employee must remember that they both have rights and that these rights have concomitant responsibilities. For example, although both parties have the right to be heard, both parties are equally responsible to listen without interrupting. The employee has the right to a positive work environment but has the responsibility to communicate needs and discontent to the manager. The manager has the right to expect a certain level of productivity from the employee but has the responsibility to provide a work environment that makes this possible. The manager has the right to expect employees to follow rules but has the responsibility to see that these rules are clearly communicated and fairly enforced.

Both the manager and the employee must show goodwill in resolving grievances. This means that both parties must be open to discussing, negotiating, and compromising and must attempt to resolve grievances as soon as possible. The ultimate goal of the grievance should not be to win but to seek a resolution that satisfies both the person and the organization.

In many cases, the manager can eliminate or reduce his or her risk of being involved in a grievance by fostering a work environment that emphasizes clear communication and fair, constructive discipline. Employees also can eliminate or reduce their risk of being involved in a grievance by being well informed about the labor contract, policies and procedures, and organizational rules. If both employee and employer recognize their rights and responsibilities, the incidence of grievances in the workplace should decrease. When mutual problem solving, negotiation, and compromise are ineffective at resolving conflicts, the grievance process can provide a positive and growth-producing resolution to disciplinary conflict.

DISCIPLINING THE UNIONIZED EMPLOYEE

It is essential that all managers be fair and consistent in disciplining employees regardless of whether a union is present. The presence of a union does, however, usually entail more procedural, legalistic safeguards in administering discipline and a well-defined grievance process for employees who believe that they have been disciplined unfairly. Usually, the manager of nonunionized employees has greater latitude in selecting which disciplinary measure is appropriate for a specific infraction. Although this gives the manager more flexibility, discipline among employees may be inconsistent.

On the other hand, unionized employees generally must be disciplined according to specific, preestablished steps and penalties within an established time frame. For example, the union contract may be very clear that excessive unexcused absences from work must be disciplined first by a written reprimand, then a 3-day work suspension, and then termination. This type of discipline structure is generally fairer to the employee but allows the manager less flexibility in evaluating each case's extenuating circumstances.

Another aspect of discipline that may differ between unionized and nonunionized employees is following due process in disciplining union employees. *Due process* means that management must provide union employees with a written statement outlining disciplinary charges, the resulting penalty, and the reasons for the penalty. Employees then have the right to defend themselves against such charges and to settle any disagreement through formal grievance hearings.

Another difference between unionized and nonunionized employee discipline lies in the *burden of proof*, which is the responsibility of the employee without union membership, but is the responsibility of the manager of the employee who belongs to a union. This means that managers who discipline union employees must keep detailed records regarding misconduct and counseling attempts.

 In disciplinary situations with nonunionized employees, the burden of proof typically falls on the employee. With union employees, the burden of proof for the wrongdoing and need for subsequent discipline falls on management.

Another common difference between unionized and nonunionized employees is that most nonunion employees are classified as *at will*, meaning that they are subject to dismissal "at the will" of the employer. The *at-will doctrine*, which is applicable in many states, permits an employer to terminate employment for any or no reason and at the discretion of the supervisor. In states that do not subscribe to the employment-at-will doctrine, or in organizations that have union representation for employees, employers must have good and legal cause to dismiss an employee.

It must be noted, however, that even when the employment-at-will doctrine is applicable, there are numerous exceptions, and an employer must be knowledgeable of each exception. Such exceptions where at-will dismissal would not apply might include when employment is being terminated based on membership in a protected legal group such as race, sex, pregnancy, national origin, religion, disability, age, or military status.

The contract language used by unions regarding discipline may be quite specific or quite general. Most contracts recognize the right of management to discipline, suspend, or dismiss employees for just cause. *Just cause* can be defined as having appropriate rationale for the actions taken. For just cause to exist, the manager must be able to prove that the employee violated established rules, that corrective action or penalty was warranted, and that the penalty was appropriate for the offense. These contracts also generally recognize the right of the employee to submit grievances when he or she believes that these actions have been taken unfairly or are discriminatory in some way.

Managers are responsible for knowing all union contract provisions that affect how discipline is administered on their units. Managers also should work closely with others employed in human resources or personnel positions in the organization. These professionals generally prove to be invaluable resources in dealings with union employees.

THE MARGINAL EMPLOYEE

Marginal employees are another type of problem employee; however, traditional discipline is generally not constructive in modifying their behavior. This is because marginal employees often make tremendous efforts to meet competencies yet usually manage to meet only minimal standards at best. White (2006) refers to marginal employees as "C" players and says that they are painful for managers because they lower the bar for everyone. All organizations have at least a few such employees. Managing these employees then is often a frustrating and tiring task.

 Marginal employees usually do not warrant dismissal, but they contribute very little to overall organizational efficiency.

Managers typically try multiple strategies to deal with marginal employees. One common strategy is simply to transfer the employee to another department, section, or unit. Although some marginal employees may be more successful on one unit than another, more commonly, the problem is simply transferred from one unit to another and the marginal employee experiences yet another failure.

Other managers choose to dismiss marginal employees or attempt to talk them into early retirement or resignation. Again, this does little to help the marginal employee succeed. Other managers simply choose to ignore the problem and attempt to "work around" the employee. This is not always possible, however, and the end result is frequently resentment from co-workers who have to carry the burden of finishing work the marginal employee was unable to accomplish. Beasley (2006) suggests that termination should be the last resort, and an attempt should be made to find the right intervention to assist the employee.

The most time-intensive option in dealing with marginal employees is *coaching*. With this strategy, the manager attempts to improve the marginal employee's performance through active coaching and counseling. While this strategy holds the greatest promise for personal growth in the marginal employee, there is no guarantee that the employee's performance will improve or that the end results will justify the time and energy costs to the manager. The strategy chosen for dealing with the marginal employee often varies with the level of the manager. Ignoring the problem is a passive response and is more frequently used by lower-level managers. Higher-level managers tend to employ the more active measures of coaching, transferring, and dismissal.

The nature of the organization also plays a role in determining what strategy is used to deal with the marginal employee. Government-controlled organizations are more likely to use passive measures, whereas managers in nongovernmental organizations are more likely to use active measures. The size of the organization also influences how managers deal with the marginally productive employee. In larger organizations, the trend has been toward passive managerial coping strategies with marginal employees.

It is important for the manager to remember that each person and situation is different and that the most appropriate strategy depends on many variables. Looking at past performance will help to determine if the employee is merely burnt out, needs educational or training opportunities, is unmotivated, or just has very little energy and only marginal skills for the job. If the latter is true, then the employee may never become more than a marginal employee, no matter what management functions and leadership skills are brought into play.

White (2006) suggests a four-pronged approach to deal with these employees: (a) identify who they are; (b) develop an explicit action plan; (c) use fairness and respect to deliver candid feedback and instructive coaching; and (d) when necessary, support them in making a decision to leave the organization. Learning Exercise 25.5, which has been solved for the reader (see the Appendix), depicts alternatives that managers may consider in dealing with the marginal employee.

LEARNING EXERCISE 25.5

The Marginal Employee

You are the oncology supervisor in a 400-bed hospital. There are 35 beds on your unit that usually are full. It is an extremely busy unit, and your nursing staff needs high-level assessment and communication skills in providing patient care. Because the nursing care needs on this floor are unique and because you use primary nursing, it has been very difficult in the past to float staff from other units when additional staffing has been required. Although you have been able to keep the unit adequately staffed on a day-to-day basis, there are two open positions for RNs on your unit that have been unfilled for almost 3 months.

Historically, your staff members have been excellent employees. They enjoy their work and are highly productive. Unit morale has been exceptionally good. However, in the last 3 months, the staff has begun complaining about Judy, a full-time employee who has been on the unit for about 4 months. Judy has been an RN for about 15 years and has worked in oncology units at other facilities. References from former employers identified Judy's work as competent, although little other information was given. At Judy's 6-week and 3-month performance appraisals, you coached her regarding her barely adequate work habits, assessment and communication skills, and decision making. Judy responded that she would attempt to work on improving her performance in these areas because working on this unit was one of her highest career goals.

Although Judy has been receptive to your coaching and has verbalized to you her efforts to improve her performance, there has been little observable difference in her behavior. You have slowly concluded that Judy is probably currently working at the highest level of which she is capable and that she is a marginal employee at best. The other nurses believe that Judy is not carrying her share of the workload and have asked that you remove her from the unit.

● ASSIGNMENT: Use the traditional problem-solving process to help you resolve this issue. Compare your solution to the one in the Appendix.

THE CHEMICALLY IMPAIRED EMPLOYEE

Substance misuse involves maladaptive patterns of psychoactive substance abuse, with the substance user continuing use in the face of recurrent occupational, social, psychological or physical problems, and/or dangerous situations. Effective management demands that the organization takes an active role in ensuring patient safety by immediately removing these employees from the work setting. However, managers also have a responsibility to help these employees deal with their disease so that they can return to the workforce in the future as productive employees.

 Nursing administrators may face no management problem more costly or emotionally draining than that of nurses whose practice is impaired by substance abuse or psychological dysfunction.

Modlin and Montes (1964) first documented chemical dependency in the health professions in studies in the late 1940s, although there is little doubt that chemical dependency has been around for as long as alcohol and drugs. The exact magnitude of chemical impairment within nursing is not known and estimates vary widely, but a review of the literature suggests that somewhere between 6% and 14% of all nurses are chemically impaired. In addition, the chemical impairment rate of health professionals is generally acknowledged as being greater than that of the general public.

One difference, however, between chemically impaired health professionals and other addicts is that chemically impaired nurses and physicians tend to obtain their drugs of choice through channels such as legitimate prescriptions that were written for them or diversionary measures on the job rather than purchasing them illegally on the street (Darbro, 2005). Despite narcotic-dispensing machines, introduced to reduce the diversion of these drugs, workplace theft has been identified as the most frequent source of illegally obtained narcotics. In fact, the majority of disciplinary actions by licensing boards are related to misconduct resulting from chemical impairment, including the misappropriation of drugs for personal use and the sale of drugs and drug paraphernalia to support an addiction (Lillibridge, 2006).

Although alcohol is the most frequently abused substance, meperidine (Demerol) is a drug of choice, while oxycodone (OxyContin) and clonazepam (Klonopin) are increasing in popularity (National Institute on Drug Abuse, n.d.). Other frequently abused chemicals include such benzodiazepines as diazepam (Valium) and narcotic drugs such as morphine and pentazocine (Talwin). Barbiturates may replace alcohol in the workplace so that the employee may feel a similar effect without having alcohol detectable on their breath.

Recognizing the Chemically Impaired Employee

Although most nurses have finely tuned assessment skills for identifying patient problems, they generally are less sensitive to behaviors and actions that may signify chemical impairment of an employee or colleague (Dunn, 2005). Sensitivity to others and to the environment is a leadership skill. The profile of the impaired nurse may vary greatly, although several behavior patterns and changes are noted frequently. These behavior changes can be grouped into three primary areas: personality/behavior changes, job performance changes, and time and attendance changes. Display 25.5 shows characteristics of these categories.

As the employee progresses into chemical dependency, managers can more easily recognize these behaviors. Typically, in the earliest stages of chemical dependency, the employee uses the addictive substance primarily for pleasure, and although the alcohol or drug use is excessive, it is primarily recreational and social. Thus, substance use usually does not occur during work hours, although some secondary effects of its use may be apparent.

As chemical dependency deepens, the employee develops tolerance to the chemical and must use greater quantities more frequently to achieve the same effect. At this point, the person has

DISPLAY 25.5 Characteristic Changes in Chemically Impaired Employees

Changes in Personality or Behaviors

- Increased irritability with patients and colleagues, often followed by extreme calm
- Social isolation; eats alone, avoids unit social functions
- Extreme and rapid mood swings
- Euphoric recall of events or elaborate excuses for behaviors
- Unusually strong interest in narcotics or the narcotic cabinet
- Sudden dramatic change in personal grooming or any other area
- Forgetfulness ranging from simple short-term memory loss to blackouts
- Change in physical appearance, which may include weight loss, flushed face, red or bleary eyes, unsteady gait, slurred speech, tremors, restlessness, diaphoresis, bruises and cigarette burns, jaundice, and ascites
- Extreme defensiveness regarding medication errors

Changes in Job Performance

- Difficulty meeting schedules and deadlines
- Illogical or sloppy charting
- High frequency of medication errors or errors in judgment affecting patient care
- Frequently volunteers to be medication nurse
- Has a high number of assigned patients who complain that their pain medication is ineffective in relieving their pain
- Consistently meeting work performance requirements at minimal levels or doing the minimum amount of work necessary
- Judgment errors
- Sleeping or dozing on duty
- Complaints from other staff members about the quality and quantity of the employee's work

Changes in Attendance and Use of Time

- Increasingly absent from work without adequate explanation or notification; most frequent absence on a Monday or Friday
- Long lunch hours
- Excessive use of sick leave or requests for sick leave after days off
- Frequent calling in to request compensatory time
- Arriving at work early or staying late for no apparent reason
- Consistent lateness
- Frequent disappearances from the unit without explanation

made a conscious lifestyle decision to use chemicals. There is a high use of defense mechanisms, such as justifying, denying, and bargaining about the drug. Often, the employee in this stage begins to use the chemical substance both at and away from work. At this stage, work performance generally declines in the areas of attendance, judgment, quality, and interpersonal relationships. An appreciable decline in unit morale, resulting from an unreliable and unproductive worker, becomes apparent.

In the final stages of chemical dependency, the employee must continually use the chemical substance, even though he or she no longer gains pleasure or gratification. Physically and psychologically addicted, the employee generally harbors a total disregard for self and others. Because the need for the substance is so great, the employee's personal and professional lives focus on the need for drugs, and the employee becomes unpredictable and undependable in the work area. Assignments are incomplete or not done at all, charting may be sloppy or illegible, and frequent judgment errors occur. Because the employee in this stage must use drugs frequently, signs of drug use during work hours may be seen. Narcotic vials are missing. The employee may be absent from the unit for brief periods with no plausible excuse. Mood swings are excessive, and the employee often looks physically ill.

The bottom line is that chemically impaired employees should be removed from the work setting long before they reach this stage. The reality, however, is that the identification of chemical impairment is often very difficult. Even when chemical impairment is suspected, managers may not be aware of nurses who are at risk nor may they know how to proceed (Dunn, 2005). Nursing school courses generally focus on the physiological effects of alcohol and other drugs, dealing little with the psychological process of addiction and even less with chemical dependency in nurses. Because of this limited knowledge about chemical impairment, many nurses are ill prepared to deal with chemical impairment.

Confronting the Chemically Impaired Employee

Unlike most alcoholics or IV narcotic users, health care professionals do not achieve tacit peer acceptance of their addictive behavior. Indeed, research by Lillibridge, Cox, and Cross (2006) suggests that the fear of discovery as well as the subsequent loss of livelihood and identity associated with being a nurse were central to the lived experience of substance-impaired nurses. Thus, physicians and nurses are much less likely to admit, even to colleagues, that they are using, much less that they are addicted to, a controlled substance. Frequently, they deny their chemical impairment even to themselves.

This self-denial is perpetuated because nurses and managers traditionally have been slow to recognize and reluctant to help these colleagues. This is changing. All but a few state boards of nursing now have treatment programs for nurses (discussed later in this chapter), and as managers gain more information about chemical impairment, how to recognize it, and how to intervene, more employees are being confronted with their impairment.

The first step in dealing with the chemically impaired employee actually occurs before the confrontation process. In the data- or evidence-gathering phase, the manager collects as much hard evidence as possible to document suspicions of chemical impairment in the employee. All behavior, work performance, and time and attendance changes presented in the displays in this chapter should be noted objectively and recorded in writing. If possible, a second person should be asked to validate the manager's observations. In suspected drug addiction, the manager also may examine unit narcotic records for inconsistencies and check to see that the amount of narcotic the nurse signed out for each patient is the same as the amount ordered for that patient.

Because few nurses drink alcohol while on duty, managers have to observe for more subtle clues, such as the smell of alcohol on the employee's breath. If the organization's policy allows for it, the manager may wish to require an employee suspected of alcohol impairment while on duty to have a serum alcohol analysis. If the employee refuses to cooperate, the organization's policy for documenting and reporting this incident should be followed.

> Proving alcohol impairment is more difficult than detecting drug impairment, as an employee can generally hide alcoholism more easily than drug addiction.

If at any time the manager suspects that an employee is chemically influenced and thus presents a potential hazard to patient safety, the employee must be immediately removed from the work environment and privately confronted with the manager's perceptions (Blair, 2005). The manager should decisively and unemotionally tell the employee that he or she will not be allowed to return to the work area because of the manager's perception that the employee is chemically impaired. The manager should arrange for the employee to be taken home so that he or she does not drive while impaired. A formal meeting to discuss this incident should be scheduled within the next 24 hours.

This type of direct confrontation between the manager and the employee is the second phase in dealing with the employee suspected of chemical impairment. Although some employees admit their problem when directly confronted, many use defense mechanisms (including denial) because they may not have admitted the problem to themselves. Denial and anger should be expected in the confrontation. If the employee denies having a problem, documented evidence demonstrating a decline in work performance should be shared. The manager must be careful to keep the confrontation focused on the employee's performance deficits and not allow the discussion to be directed to the cause of the underlying problem or addiction. These are issues and concerns that the manager is unable to address. The manager also must be careful not to preach, moralize, scold, or blame.

Confrontation always should occur before the problem escalates too far. However, in some situations, the manager may have only limited direct evidence but still may believe that the employee should be confronted because of rapidly declining employee performance or unit morale. There is, however, a greater risk that confrontation at this point may be unsuccessful in terms of helping the employee. If direct confrontation is unsuccessful, it may have been too early; the employee may not have been desperate enough or may still be in denial. In these situations, job performance will probably continue to be marginal or unsatisfactory, and progressive discipline may be necessary. If the employee continues to deny chemical impairment and work performance continues to be unsatisfactory despite repeated constructive confrontation, dismissal may be necessary.

The last phase of the confrontation process is outlining the organization's plan or expectations for the employee in overcoming the chemical impairment. This plan is similar to the disciplinary contract in that it is usually written and outlines clearly the rehabilitative measures that should be undertaken by the employee and consequences if remedial action is not sought. Although the employee is generally referred informally by the manager to outside sources to help deal with the impairment, the employee is responsible for correcting his or her work deficiencies. Time lines are included in the plan, and the manager and employee must agree on and sign a copy of the contract.

LEARNING EXERCISE 25.6

The Chemically Impaired Colleague

Write a two-page essay that speaks to the following: Has your personal or professional life been affected by a chemically impaired person? In what ways have you been affected? Has it colored the way that you view chemical abuse and chemical impairment? Do you believe that you can separate your personal feelings about chemical abuse from the actions that you must take as a manager in working with chemically impaired employees? Have you ever suspected a work colleague of chemical abuse? What, if anything, did you do about it? If you did suspect a colleague, would you approach him or her with your suspicions before talking to the unit manager? Describe the risks involved in this situation.

The Manager's Role in Assisting the Chemically Impaired Employee

Clearly, the incidence of chemical impairment in health professionals is substantial. On a personal level, a person suffers from an illness that may go undetected and untreated for many years. On a professional level, the chemically impaired employee affects the entire health care system. Nurses with impaired skills and judgment jeopardize patient care. The chemically impaired nurse also compromises teamwork and continuity as colleagues attempt to pick up the slack for their impaired team member. The personal and professional cost of chemical impairment demands that nursing leaders and managers recognize the chemically impaired employee as early as possible and intervene.

Because of the general nature of nursing, many managers find themselves wanting to nurture the impaired employee, much as they would any other person who is sick. However, this nurturing can quickly become enabling. The employee who already has a greatly diminished sense of self-esteem and a perceived loss of self-control may ask the manager to participate actively in his or her recovery. This is one of the most difficult aspects of working with the impaired employee. Others who have greater expertise and objectivity should assume this role.

 The manager must be very careful not to assume the role of counselor or treatment provider for the impaired nurse.

The manager also must be careful not to feel the need to diagnose the cause of the chemical addiction or to justify its existence. Protecting patients must be the top priority, taking precedence over any tendency to protect or excuse subordinates. The manager's role is to identify clearly performance expectations for the employee and to confront the employee when those expectations are not met. This is not to say that the manager should not be humanistic in recognizing the problem as a disease and not a disciplinary problem or that he or she should be unwilling to refer the employee for needed help. Although the manager may suggest appropriate help or refer the impaired employee to someone, a manager's primary responsibility is to see that the employee becomes functional again and can meet organizational expectations before returning to work.

The manager can play a vital role in creating an environment that decreases the chances of chemical impairment in the work setting. This may be done by controlling or reducing work-related stressors whenever possible and by providing mechanisms for employee stress management. The manager also should control drug accessibility by implementing, enforcing, and monitoring policies and procedures related to medication distribution. Finally, the manager should provide opportunities for the staff to learn about substance abuse, its detection, and available resources to help those who are impaired.

LEARNING EXERCISE 25.7

Working Under the Influence
There have been rumors for some time that Mrs. Clark, one of the night nurses on the unit you supervise, has been coming to work under the influence of alcohol. Fellow staff have reported the odor of alcohol on her breath, and one staff member stated that her speech is often slurred. The night supervisor states that she believes "this is not my problem," and your night charge nurse has never been on duty when Mrs. Clark has shown this behavior. This morning, one of the patients whispered to you that he thought Mrs. Clark had been drinking when she came to work last night. When you question the patient further, he states, "Mrs. Clark seemed to perform her nursing duties okay, but she made me nervous." You have decided that you must talk with Mrs. Clark. You call her at her home and ask her to come to your office at 3 PM.

● ASSIGNMENT: Determine how you are going to approach Mrs. Clark. Outline your plan, and give rationale for your choices. What flexibility have you built into your plan? How much of your documentation will be shared with Mrs. Clark?

The Recovery Process

Although most authorities disagree on the name or number of steps in the recovery process, they do agree that certain phases or progressive observable behaviors suggest that the person is recovering from the chemical impairment. In the first phase, the impaired employee continues to deny the significance or severity of the chemical impairment but does reduce or suspend chemical use to appease family, peers, or managers. These employees hope to reestablish their substance use in the future.

In the second phase, as denial subsides, the impaired employee begins to see that the chemical addiction is having a negative impact on his or her life and begins to want to change. Frequently, people in this phase are buoyant with hope and commitment but lack maturity about the struggles they will face. This phase generally lasts for about 3 months.

During the third phase, the person examines his or her values and coping skills and works to develop more effective coping skills. Frequently, this is done by aligning himself or herself with support groups that reinforce a chemical-free lifestyle. In this stage, the person realizes how sick he or she was in the active stage of the disease and is often fraught with feelings of humiliation and shame.

In the last phase, people gain self-awareness regarding why they became chemically addicted, and they develop coping skills that will help them deal more effectively with stressors. As a result of this, self-awareness, self-esteem, and self-respect increase. When this happens, the person can decide consciously whether he or she wishes to or should return to the workplace.

State Board of Nursing Treatment Programs

Although chemical dependency can impair nurses' physical, psychological, social, and professional functioning, the problem was largely ignored until the late 1970s, when the American Nurses Association (ANA) began efforts to secure assistance for chemically and mentally impaired nurses (Clark & Farnsworth, 2006). This assistance occurred primarily in the form of *diversion programs* (also called *intervention* or *peer assistance* programs). A diversion program is a voluntary, confidential program for nurses whose practice may be impaired due to chemical dependency or mental illness.

The goal of a diversion program is to protect the public by early identification of impaired nurses and by providing these nurses access to appropriate intervention programs and treatment services. Public safety is protected by immediate suspension of practice, when needed, and by ongoing careful monitoring of the nurse. Many state programs allow the nurse to resume work, often on a limited license, while in recovery (Blair, 2005). In addition to rehabilitating nurses with chemical dependence, most diversion programs also serve nurses impaired by certain mental illnesses such as anxiety, depression, bipolar disorder, and schizophrenia. Some programs cover nurses with physical disabilities as well. As of 2007, only ten states did not have some type of diversion program (ANA, 2007). Other countries are also developing diversion programs (Support for Nurses, 2006).

Several factors have led state boards to adopt diversion programs. First, a punitive system creates barriers to reporting and keeps impaired nurses from getting help. Nurse colleagues or practitioners who are treating an impaired nurse may well hesitate to report something that could cost a nurse his or her job and license. From an employer's standpoint, the fear of litigation often makes it easier to dismiss a nurse without charges of misconduct. But this practice leaves the nurse, who is at risk for self-harm and for harming patients, free to seek work elsewhere. Even if a nurse is reported to the state board, a purely disciplinary approach to impairment shows not only a lack of compassion but also inadequate protection of the public (Dunn, 2005). A board investigation can take months to 2 years, during which time the nurse in question can continue working without restraint. If the nurse is licensed in another state, he or she can simply move away to avoid disciplinary action altogether.

Diversion programs are voluntary and confidential. Besides helping the nurse with recovery, the programs offer assistance to the employers and staff in coping with employee substance abuse. Impaired nurses who refuse participation in diversion programs are subject to disciplinary review by their state board of nursing and possible license revocation. The ANA maintains that nurses should advocate for those who are impaired so that they receive appropriate assistance, treatment, and access to fair institutional and legal processes (ANA, 2007). Indeed, Darbro (2005) suggests that fear of being ostracized by their colleagues has kept some nurses from seeking help even though they knew they were addicted to drugs.

Diversion programs have a good success rate (Darbro, 2005). Her research also found other positive aspects of a diversion program, including improved nursing practice and learning to be more tolerant and compassionate. Examining the Evidence 25.1 describes the findings of Darbro's study of impaired nurses in a diversion program.

 EXAMINING THE EVIDENCE 25.1

Source: Darbro, N. (2005). Alternative diversion programs for nurses with impaired practice: Completers and non-completers. *Journal of Addictions Nursing, 16*(169), 169–185.

Sixteen nurses who participated in an alternative diversion program for chemically dependent nurses were interviewed. Fourteen nurses completed a second interview. Many of the nurses worked in critical care, noted stressful working conditions, and diverted medications from the workplace for their own use.

Most of the nurses identified a pivotal event as being the leverage to move them into a lifestyle of recovery. Positive aspects of their recovery included learning to use support systems that led them from isolation, shame, and guilt to involvement and disclosure. Although only half of the nurses completed the program, all but one of the sixteen remained in recovery.

LEARNING EXERCISE 25.8

Researching Your State Board of Nursing's Recovery Program
Determine if your state board of nursing offers some type of recovery program for chemically impaired nurses and for mentally ill nurses. You may either call the board or use the Internet. Research the following questions:
- Is the program voluntary and confidential?
- What is the rate of *recidivism*?
- What types of monitoring mechanisms are in place?
- What is the duration of the program?
- Are nurses allowed to continue practicing while completing the treatment program?
- Are there practice restrictions?

● ASSIGNMENT: Write a one-page report of your findings.

The Chemically Impaired Employee's Reentry to the Workplace

Because chemically impaired nurses recover at varying rates, predicting how long this process will take is difficult. Many experts believe that impaired employees must devote at least 1 year to their recovery without the stresses of drug availability, overtime, and shift rotation. Success in reentering the workforce depends on factors such as the extent of the recovery process and individual circumstances. Again, although managers must show a genuine personal interest in their employee's rehabilitation, their primary role is to be sure that the employee understands the organization's right to insist on unimpaired performance in the workplace. The following are generally accepted reentry guidelines for the recovering nurse:
- No psychoactive drug use will be tolerated.
- The employee should be assigned to day shift for the first year.
- The employee should be paired with a successfully recovering nurse whenever possible.
- The employee should be willing to consent to random urine screening with toxicology or alcohol screens.
- The employee must give evidence of continuing involvement with support groups such as Alcoholics Anonymous or Narcotics Anonymous. Employees should be encouraged to attend meetings several times each week.
- The employee should be encouraged to participate in a structured aftercare program.
- The employee should be encouraged to seek individual counseling or therapy as needed.

These guidelines should be a part of the employee's return to work contract. Mandatory drug testing, however, invokes questions about privacy rights and generally should not be implemented without advice from human resources personnel or legal counsel. Humanistic leaders recognize the intrinsic self-worth of each individual employee and strive to understand the unique needs these workers have. If the leader genuinely cares about and shows interest in each employee, employees learn to trust and the helping relationship has a chance to begin.

Managers have the responsibility to be proactive in identifying and confronting chemically impaired employees. Prompt and appropriate intervention by managers is essential for positive outcomes. Organizations have an ethical responsibility to actively assist these employees to return as productive members of the workforce.

INTEGRATING LEADERSHIP ROLES AND MANAGEMENT FUNCTIONS THROUGH DEALING WITH PROBLEM EMPLOYEES

The leader recognizes that all employees have intrinsic worth and assists them in reaching their maximal potential. Because individual abilities, achievement drives, and situations vary, the leader recognizes each employee as an individual with unique needs and intervenes according to those specific needs. In some situations, such as frequent rule breaking, discipline may be the most effective tool for ensuring that employees succeed. In the case of the chemically impaired, psychologically impaired, or marginal employee, coaching and assisting the employee to get the treatment needed is the primary management responsibility.

Both roles require leadership and management skills. In administering discipline, the leader actively shapes group norms and promotes self-discipline. The leader also is a supporter, motivator, enabler, and coach. The humanistic attributes of the leadership role make employees want to follow the rules of the leader and thus the organization. In dealing with the employee with special needs (the marginal employee, those who are psychologically or chemically impaired), the leader serves more as a coach and resource person than as a counselor, disciplinarian, or authority figure.

The manager, however, must enforce established rules, policies, and procedures, and although good managerial practice greatly reduces the need for discipline, some employees still need external direction and discipline to accomplish organizational goals. Discipline allows employees to understand clearly the expectations of the organization and the penalty for failing to meet those expectations. The manager's primary obligation is to see that patient safety is assured and that productivity is adequate to meet unit goals. The manager uses the authority inherent in his or her position to provide positive and negative sanctions for employee behavior in an effort to meet these goals.

The integrated leader–manager blends these unit productivity needs and human resource needs; however, selecting and implementing appropriate strategies to meet both goals is difficult. The leader–manager believes that each employee has the potential to be a successful and valuable member of the unit and intervenes accordingly to meet each employee's special needs.

Key Concepts

* It is essential that managers are able to distinguish between employees who need *progressive discipline* and those who are *chemically impaired, psychologically impaired,* or *marginal employees* so that the employee can be managed in the most appropriate manner.
* *Discipline* is a necessary and positive tool in promoting subordinate growth.
* The optimal goal in *constructive discipline* is assisting employees to behave in a manner that allows them to be self-directed in meeting organizational goals.
* To ensure fairness, rules should include McGregor's "hot stove" components of *forewarning, immediate application, consistency,* and *impartiality.*
* If a *rule* or *regulation* is worth having, it should be enforced. When rule breaking is allowed to go unpunished, groups generally adjust to and replicate the low-level performance of the rule breaker.
* As few rules and regulations as possible should exist in the organization. All rules, regulations, and policies should be regularly reviewed to see if they should be deleted or modified in some way.

* Except for the most serious infractions, discipline should be administered in progressive steps, which include *verbal admonishment*, *written admonishment*, *suspension*, and *dismissal*.

* In *performance deficiency coaching*, the manager actively brings areas of unacceptable behavior or performance to the attention of the employee and works with him or her to establish a short-term plan to correct deficiencies.

* The *grievance procedure* is essentially a statement of wrongdoing or a procedure to follow when one believes that a wrong has been committed. All employees should have the right to file grievances about disciplinary action that they believe has been arbitrary or unfair in some way.

* The presence of a union generally entails more procedural, legalistic safeguards for administering discipline and a well-defined grievance process for employees who believe that they have been disciplined unfairly.

* Because *chemical* and *psychological impairment* are diseases, traditional progressive discipline is inappropriate because it cannot result in employee growth.

* The profile of the impaired nurse may vary greatly, although typically behavior changes are seen in three areas: personality/behavior changes, job performance changes, and time and attendance changes.

* Nurses and managers traditionally have been slow to recognize and respond to chemically impaired colleagues.

* Confronting an employee who is suspected of chemical impairment should always occur before the problem escalates and before patient safety is jeopardized.

* The manager should not assume the role of counselor or treatment provider or feel the need to diagnose the cause of the chemical addiction. The manager's role is to identify clearly performance expectations for the employee and to confront the employee when those expectations are not met.

* Strategies for dealing with *marginal employees* vary with management level, the nature of the health care organization, and the current prevailing attitude toward passive or active intervention.

ADDITIONAL LEARNING EXERCISES AND APPLICATIONS

LEARNING EXERCISE 25.9

Determining an Appropriate Action When Proof Is Unavailable

You are the supervisor of a pediatric acute-care unit. One of your patients, Joey, is a 5-year-old boy who sustained 30% third-degree burns, which have been grafted and are now healing. He has been a patient in the unit for approximately 2 months. His mother stays with him nearly all the waking hours and generally is supportive of both him and the staff.

In the last few weeks, Joey has begun expressing increasing frustration with basic nursing tasks, has frequently been uncooperative, and in your staff's opinion has become very manipulative. His mother is frustrated with Joey's behavior but believes that it is understandable given the trauma he has experienced. She has begun working with the staff on a mutually acceptable behavior modification program.

Although you have attempted to assign the same nurses to care for Joey as often as possible, it is not possible today. This lack of continuity is especially frustrating because the night shift has reported frequent tantrums and uncooperative behavior. The nurse who you have assigned to Joey is Monica. She is a good nurse but has lacked patience in the past with uncooperative patients. During the morning, you are aware that Joey is continuing to act out. Although Monica begins to look more and more harried, she states that she is handling the situation appropriately.

When you return from lunch, Joey's mother is waiting at your office. She furiously reports that Joey told her that Monica hit him and told him he was "a very bad boy" after his mother had gone to lunch. His mother believes that physical punishment was totally inappropriate, and she wants this nurse to be fired. She also states that she has contacted Joey's physician and that he is on his way over.

You call Monica to your office, where she emphatically denies all the allegations. Monica states that during the lunch hour, Joey refused to allow her to check his dressings and that she followed the behavior modification plan and discontinued his television privileges. She believes that his accusations further reflect his manipulative behavior. You then approach Joey, who tearfully and emphatically repeats the story that he told to his mother. He is consistent about the details and swears to his mother that he is telling the truth. None of your staff was within hearing range of Joey's room at the time of the alleged incident. When Joey's doctor arrives, he demands that Monica be fired.

● ASSIGNMENT: Determine your action. You do not have proof to substantiate either Monica or Joey's story. You believe that Monica is capable of the charges but are reluctant to implement any type of discipline without proof. What factors contribute the most to your decision?

LEARNING EXERCISE 25.10

What Type of Discipline Is Appropriate?

Susie has been an RN on your medical–surgical unit for 18 months. During that time, she has been competent in terms of her assessment and organizational skills and her skills mastery. Her work habits, however, need improvement. She frequently arrives 5 to 10 minutes late for work and disrupts report when she arrives. She also frequently extends her lunch break 10 minutes beyond the allotted 30 minutes. Her absence rate is twice that of most of your other employees. You have informally counseled Susie about her work habits on numerous past occasions. Last month, you issued a written reprimand about these work deficiencies and placed it in Susie's personnel file. Susie acknowledged at that time that she needed to work on these areas but that her responsibilities as a single parent were overwhelming at times and that she felt demotivated at work. Every day this week, Susie has arrived 15 minutes late. The staff are complaining about Susie's poor attitude and have asked that you take action.

You contemplate what additional action you might take. The next step in progressive discipline would be a suspension without pay. You believe that this action could be supported given the previous attempts to counsel the employee without improvement. You also realize that many of your staff are closely watching your actions to see how you will handle this situation. You also recognize that suspending Susie would leave her with no other means of financial support and that this penalty is somewhat uncommon for the offenses described. In addition, you are unsure if this penalty will make any difference in modifying Susie's behavior.

● ASSIGNMENT: Decide what type of discipline, if any, is appropriate for Susie. Support your decision with appropriate rationale. Discuss your actions in terms of the effects on you, Susie, and the department.

LEARNING EXERCISE 25.11

Discipline and Insubordination

You are the coordinator of a small, specialized respiratory rehabilitation unit. Two other nurses work with you. Because all of the staff are professionals, you have used a very democratic approach to management and leadership. This approach has worked well, and productivity has always been high. The nurses work out schedules so that there are always two nurses on duty during the week, and they take turns covering the weekends, at which time there is only one RN on duty. With this arrangement, it is possible for three nurses to be on duty 1 day during the week, if there is no holiday or other time off scheduled by either of the other two RNs.

Several months ago, you told the other RNs that the state licensing board was arriving on Wednesday, October 16, to review the unit. It would, therefore, be necessary for both of them to be on duty because you would be staying with the inspectors all day. You have reminded them several times since that time.

Today is Monday, October 14, and you are staying late preparing files for the impending inspection. Suddenly, you notice that only one of the RNs is scheduled to work on Wednesday. Alarmed, you phone Mike, the RN who is scheduled to be off. You remind him about the inspection and state that it will be necessary for him to come to work. He says that he is sorry that he forgot about the inspection but that he has scheduled a 3-day cruise and has paid a large, nonrefundable deposit. After a long talk, it becomes obvious to you that Mike is unwilling to change his plans. You say to him, "Mike, I feel this borders on insubordination. I really need you on the 16th, and I am requesting that you come in. If you do not come to work, I will need to take appropriate action." Mike replies, "I'm sorry to let you down. Do what you have to do. I need to take this trip, and I will not cancel my plans."

● ASSIGNMENT: What action could you take? What action should you take? Outline some alternatives. Assume that it is not possible to float in additional staff because of the specialty expertise required to work in this department. Decide what you should do. Give rationale for your decision. Did ego play a part in your decision?

(Web Links)────────────────────────────────

Addiction Recovery Resources for the Professional
http://www.lapage.com/arr/
Identifies resources for chemically impaired health care professionals.

Employee Relations: Positive Discipline
http://www.bizmove.com/personnel/m4i4.htm
Defines positive discipline and proposes guidelines for establishing a climate of positive discipline as well as outlines strategies.

Employee Discipline and Termination Checklist
http://www.workplaceissues.com/freereports.htm
This checklist provides questions that are designed to be a guide for use in the proper discipline or dismissal of an employee.

References

American Nurses Association. (2007). *Impaired nurses resource center*. Retrieved March 23, 2007, from *http://www.nursing-world.org/impaired/*.

Beasley, C. (2006). Guidance on under-performing staff. *UK Nursing Management, 13*(8), 5.

Blair, P. (2005). Spot the signs of drug impairment. *Nursing Management, 36*(2), 20–21, 52.

Clark, C., & Farnsworth, J. (2006). Research for practice: Program for recovering nurses—An evaluation. *MEDSURG Nursing, 15*(4), 223–230.

Corrective discipline and discharge. (2007). HR Human Resources. Retrieved March 23, 2007, from *http://www.hr. arizona.edu/05_prf/coaching/corr.php*.

Darbro, N. (2005). Alternative diversion programs for nurses with impaired practice: Completers and non-completers. *Journal of Addictions Nursing, 16*(4), 169–185.

Dunn, D. (2005). Home study program: Substance abuse among nurses-Intercession and intervention. *AORN Journal, 82*(5), 777–799.

Encyclopedia of Business. (2007). *Employee discipline*. Retrieved March 23, 2007, from *http://www.answers.com/ main/ntquery?tname=employee%2Ddiscipline*.

Hader, R. (2005). How do you measure workforce integrity? *Nursing Management, 36*(9), 32–37.

Lillibridge, J. (2006). The chemically impaired nurse: Discipline or treatment? In C. Huston (Ed.), *Professional issues in nursing*. Philadelphia: Lippincott Williams & Wilkins.

Lillibridge, J., Cox, M., & Cross, W. (2002). Uncovering the secret: Giving voice to the experiences of nurses who misuse substances. In C. Huston (Ed.), *Professional issues in nursing*. Philadelphia: Lippincott Williams & Wilkins.

Martin, C. A. (2005). Leadership: Make it H.O.T. *Nursing Management, 36*(9), 38–45.

McGregor, D. (1967). *The professional manager*. New York: McGraw-Hill.

Modlin, H. C., & Montes, A. (1964). Narcotics addiction in physicians. *American Journal of Psychiatry, 121*, 358–363.

National Institute on Drug Abuse (NIDA). (n.d.). *NIDA InfoFacts: Prescription pain and other medications*. Retrieved March 23, 2007, from *http://www.drugabuse.gov/infofax/painmed.html*.

Support for nurses a welcome first. (2006). *Australian Nursing Journal, 13*(9), 9.

White, K. M. (2006). Better manage your human capital. *Nursing Management, 37*(1), 16–19.

Bibliography

Beesley, J. (2005). Making sense of grievance procedures. *British Journal of Perioperative Nursing, 15*(8), 337–338, 340–341.

Collins, S. E., & Mikos, C. A (2006). Legal checkpoints. Nursing practice violations: What's your response? *Nursing Management, 37*(2), 23–24.

Haidinyak, C., & Walker, G. C. (2005). Don't let the grievance process cause grief. *Nurse Educator, 30*(2), 73–75.

Johnson, A. (2006). Grievance 101: Understanding the process and purpose of the grievance procedure. *Chart, 103*(2), 6.

Kenner, C., & Pressler, J. L. (2006). Rx for deans. Addressing the underperformance of faculty and staff. *Nurse Educator, 31*(6), 233–234.

Larson, N. J. (2006). Nurses practicing while under impairment: It's more common than you think! *Iowa Nurse Reporter, 19*(2), 7.

Mace, K. A. (2005). Is employee discipline the solution for patient safety? *Nursing Management, 36*(12), 57–59.

Pipkiin, M. (2006). How to deal with difficult employees. *Nursing and Residential Care, 8*(6), 278–280.

Pistone, C. (2006). Hiring, firing, and everything between: How to manage employees. *Gastroenterology Nursing, 29*(2), 167.

Rosenstein, A. H., & O'Daniel, M. (2005). Disruptive behavior & clinical outcomes: Perceptions of nurses & physicians. *American Journal of Nursing, 105*(1), 54–65.

Salladay, S. A. (2006). Suspected drug diversion. *Nursing2006, 36*(12), 28.

Shumaker, R., & Hickey, P. (2006). Patient safety first. Medication diversion in the perioperative setting. *AORN Journal, 83*(3), 745–746, 748–749.

Somnier, I. O. (2005). Drunk in charge? *Occupational Health, 57*(9), 10–11.

Staines, R. (2006). Will guidance address the problems over suspension? *Nursing Times, 102*(46), 9.

Appendix

Solutions to Selected Learning Exercises

The following are possible solutions for challenging situations presented in various Learning Exercises in this textbook.

LEARNING EXERCISE 5.6

This is how the staff nurse solved the problem of a patient's family member (Mrs. Brown's husband) reading the patient's chart. The chart was accidentally left in the patient's room.

Confidentiality of Charts

The nurse needs to determine the most important goal in this situation. Possible goals include (a) getting the chart away from Mr. Brown as soon as possible, (b) protecting the privacy of Mrs. Brown, (c) gathering more information, or (d) becoming an advocate for the Browns.

In solving the case, it is apparent that not enough information has been gathered. Mr. Brown now has the chart, and it seems pointless to take it away from him. Usually, the danger in patients' families reading the chart lies in the direction of their not understanding the chart and thereby obtaining confusing information or the patient's privacy being invaded because the patient has not consented to family members' access to the chart.

Using this as the basis for rationale, the nurse should use the following approach:

- Clarify that Mr. Brown has Mrs. Brown's permission to read the chart by asking her directly.
- Ask Mr. Brown if there is anything in the chart that he did not understand or anything that he questions. You may even ask him to summarize what he has read. Clarify the things that are appropriate for the nurse to address, such as terminology, procedures, or nursing care.
- Refer questions that are inappropriate for the nurse to answer to the physician, and let Mr. Brown know that you will help him in talking with the physician regarding the medical plan and prognosis.
- When finished talking with Mr. Brown, the nurse should request the chart and place it in the proper location. The incident should be reported to the immediate supervisor.
- The nurse should follow through by talking with the physician about the incident and Mr. Brown's concerns and by assisting the Browns to obtain the information they have requested.

Conclusion

The nurse first gathered more information before becoming the adversary or advocate. It is possible that the Browns had only simple questions to ask and that the problem was a lack of communication between staff and their patients rather than a physician–patient communication deficit. Legally, patients have a right to understand what is happening to them, and that should be the basis for the decisions in this case.

LEARNING EXERCISE 12.3

Cultures and Hierarchies

Below is an analysis of how one might approach a problem involving a non-nursing department but affecting the nurses' work and the nursing staff.

Analysis: Data Assessment

1. A copy of the organization chart was given to you when you were hired. The formal structure is a line-and-staff organization. The housekeeping department head is below the nursing director and the nursing section supervisor but at the same level as the immediate clinic supervisor. The housekeeping department head reports directly to the maintenance and engineering department head.
2. The county administrator has stated she has an open door policy. You do not know if this means that bypassing department heads is acceptable or merely that the administrator is interested in the employees. An important reason for not skipping intermediate supervisors when communicating is that they must know what is going on in their departments. A manager's position, value, and status are strengthened if he or she serves as a vital and essential link in the vertical chain of command.
3. You have twice attempted to talk with your immediate supervisor; however, whether you followed up regarding your supervisor's action on the complaint is unclear.
4. You are a new employee and therefore probably do not know how the formal or informal structure works. This newness might render the complaints less credible.
5. Possible risks include creating trouble for the housekeeping staff or their immediate supervisor, being labeled a troublemaker by others in the organization, and alienating your immediate supervisor.
6. Before proceeding, you need to assess your own values and determine what is motivating you to pursue this issue.

Alternatives for Action

Many choices are available to you:

1. You can do nothing. This is often a wise choice and should always be an alternative for any problem. Some problems solve themselves if left alone. Sometimes, the time is not right to solve the problem.
2. You can talk with the county health administrator. Although this involves some risk, the possibility exists that the administrator will be able to take action. At the very least, you will have unburdened your problem on someone.
3. You can talk directly with the individual housekeepers by using "I" messages, such as, "I get angry when the housekeeping staff take naps and the bathrooms are dirty." Perhaps if feelings and frustrations were shared, you would learn more about the problem.

(Learning Exercise continues on page 626)

Maybe there is a reason for their behavior; maybe they only socialize during their breaks. This alternative involves some risk: The housekeepers might look on you as a troublemaker.

4. Have all of the evening staff sign a petition, and give it to the immediate supervisor. Forming a coalition often produces results. However, the supervisor could view this action as overreacting or meddlesome and might feel threatened.

5. Go to the housekeeping staff's department head and report them. In this way, you are saving some time and going right to the person who is in charge. However, this might be unfair to the housekeepers and certainly will create some enemies for you.

6. Follow up with the immediate supervisor. You could request permission to take action yourself and ask for the best way to proceed. This would involve your immediate supervisor and keep her informed. However, it also shows that you are willing to take risks and devote some personal time and energy to solving the problem.

Selecting an Alternative

This problem has no right answer. Under certain conditions, various solutions could be used. Under most circumstances, it is more fair to others and more efficient for you to select the third alternative listed. However, because you are new and have little knowledge of the formal and informal organizational structure, your wisest choice would be alternative 6. New employees need to seek guidance from their immediate supervisors. For this follow-up session with the supervisor to be successful, you need to do the following:

1. Talk with the supervisor during a quiet time.
2. Admit to personally "owning" the problem without involving colleagues.
3. Acknowledge that legitimate reasons for the housekeepers' actions may exist.
4. Request permission to talk directly with the housekeepers. Role-play an appropriate approach with the supervisor.

You must accept the consequences of your actions. However, your attempt to correct the problem may motivate your supervisor to pursue the problem directly with the housekeeping staff's supervisor. If this is the action that your supervisor takes, you should ask to speak with the housekeeping staff directly first. If, after talking with the housekeeping staff, you decide that a problem still exists and you elect to address that problem, then you should return to your immediate supervisor before proceeding.

Analysis of the Problem Solving

Would you have solved this problem differently? What are some other alternatives that could have been generated? Have you ever gone outside the chain of command and had a positive experience as a result?

LEARNING EXERCISE 13.5

Turning Lemons Into Lemonade

This is the strategy that Sally Jones used to solve the conflict with Bob Black. In analyzing this case, one must forego feelings of resentment regarding Bob's obvious play for control and power. In reality, what real danger does his empire building pose for the director of nursing? Isn't Sally really just ridding herself and her staff of clerical duties and interruptions?

A certain amount of power is inherent in the ability to hire. Employees develop a loyalty for the person who actually hires them. Because Sally Jones or her designee will still actually make the final selection, Bob's proposal should result in little loss of loyalty or power.

Let's look at what the real Sally Jones did to solve this conflict. When she was able to see that Bob was not stripping her of any power, Sally was capable of using some very proactive strategies. Here was a chance for her to appear compromising, thereby increasing her esteem in the CEO's eyes and gaining political clout in the organization. When she met with Jane Smith and Bob, Sally began by complimenting Bob on his ideas. Then, she suggested that because nurses were in the habit of coming to the nursing department to apply for positions and because human resources offices were rather cold and formal places, stationing the new personnel clerk in the nursing office would be more convenient and inviting. Sally knew that the human resources department lacked adequate space and that the nursing office had some extra room. She went on to say that because some of her unit clerks were very knowledgeable about the hospital organization, Bob might want to interview several of them for the new position. Although an experienced unit clerk would be difficult to replace, Sally said that she was willing to make this sacrifice for the new plan to succeed.

The CEO, very impressed with Sally's generous offer, turned to Bob and said, "I think Sally has an excellent idea. Why don't you hire one of her clerks and station her in the nursing office?" Jane then said to Sally, "Now, do we understand that the clerk will be Bob's employee and will work under him?"

Sally agreed with this because she felt that she had just pulled off a great power play. Let's examine what Sally won in this political maneuver.

1. She gained by not competing with Bob, therefore not making him her enemy.
2. She gained by impressing the CEO with her flexibility and initiative.
3. She gained a new employee.

Although the new employee would be working for Bob with the salary charged to his cost center, the clerk would be Sally's former employee. Because the clerk would be working in the nursing office, she would have some allegiance to Sally. In addition, the clerk would be doing all the work that Sally and her assistants had been doing and at no cost to the nursing department.

When Sally first received Bob's memo, she was angry; her initial reaction was to talk to the CEO privately and complain about Bob. Fortunately, she did not do this. It is nearly always a political mistake for one manager to talk about another behind his or her back and without his or her knowledge. This generally reflects unfavorably on the employee, with a loss of respect from the supervisor.

Another option that Sally had was to compete with Bob and be uncooperative. Although this might have delayed centralizing the personnel department, in the end, Bob undoubtedly would have accomplished his goal, and Sally would not have been able to reap such a great political victory.

The later effects of this political maneuver were even more rewarding. The personnel clerk remained loyal to Sally. Bob became less adversarial and more cooperative with Sally on other issues. The CEO gave her a sly grin later in the week and said, "Great move with Bob Black." This case might be concluded by saying that this is an example of someone being given a lemon and then making lemonade.

LEARNING EXERCISE 21.3

Conflicting Personal, Professional, and Organizational Obligations

The following is conflict resolution strategy used by you when the nursing office supervisor (Carol), who considers you to be competent and responsible, asked you to help cover the workload in the delivery room. Although this supervisor believes that you can do the job, you think that you do not know enough about labor and delivery nursing to be effective. Here are some strategies that you can use to resolve the conflict.

Analysis: You need to examine your goal, the supervisor's goal, and a goal on which you can both agree. Your goal might be protection of your license and doing nothing that would bring harm to a patient. Carol's goal might be to provide assistance to an understaffed unit. A possible supraordinate goal would be for neither you nor Carol to do anything that would bring risk or harm to the organization.

The following conflict resolution strategies were among your choices:

Accommodating. Accommodating is the most obvious wrong choice. If you really believe that you are unqualified to work in the delivery room, this strategy could be harmful to patients and your career. Such a decision would not meet with your goal or the supraordinate goal.

Smoothing or Avoiding. Because you have little power and no one is available to intervene on your behalf, you are unable to choose either of these solutions. The problem cannot be avoided nor will you be able to smooth the conflict away.

Compromising. In similar situations, you might be able to negotiate a compromise. For instance, you might say, "I cannot go to the delivery room, but I will float to another medical–surgical area if there is someone on another medical–surgical unit who has OB experience." Alternatively, you could compromise by stating, "I feel comfortable working postpartum and will work in that area if you have a qualified nurse from postpartum that can be sent to the delivery room." It is possible that either solution could end the conflict, depending on the availability of other personnel and how comfortable you would feel in the postpartum area. Often, someone attempting to problem solve, such as the supervisor in this case, becomes so overburdened and stressed that other alternatives are not apparent.

Collaborating. If time allows and the other party is willing to adopt a common goal, this is the preferred method of dealing with conflict. However, the power holder must view the other as having something important to contribute if this method of conflict management is to be successful. Perhaps you could convince Carol that both she and the hospital could be at risk if an unqualified RN was assigned to an area requiring special skills. Once the supraordinate goal is adopted, you and Carol would be able to find alternative solutions to the problem. There are always many more ways to solve a problem than any one person can generate.

Competing. Normally, competing is not an attractive alternative for resolving conflict, but sometimes, it is the only recourse. Before using competition as a method to manage this conflict, you need to examine your motives. Are you truly unqualified for work in the delivery room, or are you using your lack of experience as an excuse not to float to an unfamiliar area that would cause you anxiety? If you are truly convinced that you are unqualified, then you possess information that the supervisor does not have (a criterion necessary for the use of competing as a method of conflict resolution). Therefore, if other methods for solving the conflict are not effective, you must use competition to solve the conflict. You must win at the expense of the supervisor's losing. You risk much when using this type of resolution. The supervisor might fire you for insubordination or, at best, may view you as uncooperative. The most appropriate method for using competition in this situation is an assertive approach. An example would be repeating firmly but nonaggressively, "I cannot go to the delivery room to work because I would be putting patients at risk. I am unqualified to work in that area." This approach is usually effective. You must not work in an area where patient safety would be at risk. It would be morally, ethically, and legally wrong for you to do so. (*Note:* The legal implications of this case are discussed in Chapter 5.)

LEARNING EXERCISE 21.4

An Exercise in Negotiation Analysis

Analysis: A head nurse's goal is to be sure that all patients receive safe and adequate care. However, some hidden agendas may exist. One might be that the head nurse does not want to relinquish any authority or does not want to devote energy to the change that has been proposed. The staff nurses have goals of job satisfaction and providing more continuity of care; however, their hidden agenda is probably the need for more autonomy and control of the work setting.

If the conflict is allowed to escalate, the staff nurses could begin to disrupt the unit because of their dissatisfaction, and the head nurse could transfer some of the "ringleaders" or punish them in some other way. The head nurse is wise in reconsidering these nurses' request. By demonstrating a willingness to talk and negotiate the conflict, the staff will view the head nurse as cooperative and interested in their job satisfaction.

The staff nurses must realize that they are not going to obtain everything they want in this conflict resolution nor should they expect that result. To demonstrate their interest, they should develop some sort of workable policy and procedure for patient care assignments, recognizing that the head nurse will want to modify their procedure. Once the plan is developed, the nurses need to plan their strategy for the coming meeting. The following may be their outline:

1. Select as a spokesperson a member of the group who has the best assertive skills but whose approach is not abrasive or aggressive. This keeps the group from appearing overpowering to the head nurse. The other group members will be at the meeting lending their support but will speak only when called on by the group leader. Preferably, the spokesperson should be someone who the head nurse knows well and whose opinion is respected.
2. The designated leader of the group should begin by thanking the head nurse for agreeing to the meeting. In this way, the group acknowledges the authority of the head nurse.
3. There should be a sincere effort by the group to listen to the head nurse and to follow modifications to their plan. They must be willing to give up something as well, perhaps some modification in the staffing pattern.
4. As the meeting progresses, the leader of the group should continue to express the goal of the group—to provide greater continuity of patient care—rather than focus on how unhappy the group is with the present system.
5. At some point, the nurses should show their willingness to compromise and offer to evaluate the new plan periodically.

Ideally, the outcome of the meeting would be some sort of negotiated compromise in patient care assignment, which would result in more autonomy and job satisfaction for the nurses, enough authority for the head nurse to satisfy ongoing responsibilities, and increased continuity of patient care assignment.

LEARNING EXERCISE 23.1

Designing an Audit Tool

When writing audit criteria, define the patient population as clearly as possible first so that information can be retrieved quickly. In this case, eliminate patients who had complicated births, births of abnormal newborns, cesarean section births, and home births because these patients will need more assessment and teaching. The performance expectations should be set at 100% compliance with an allowance made for reasonable exceptions. One hundred percent is recommended because if any of these criteria are not recorded in the patient's record, remedial actions should be taken.

Select the patient's record as the most objective source of information. It should be assumed that if criteria were not charted, they were not met. Audit 30 charts to give the agency enough data to make some assumptions but not too many as to make it economically burdensome to review records. An audit form that could be developed follows:

NURSING AUDIT FORM FOR VISITING NURSES

Nursing Diagnosis: Initial home visit within 72 hours after uncomplicated vaginal delivery, with normal newborn, occurring in a birth center or obstetrical facility
Source of Information: Patient's record
Expected Compliance: 100%, unless specific exceptions are noted
Number of Records to Be Audited: 30

After the audit committee reviews the records, a summary should be made of the findings. A summary could look like this:

SUMMARY OF AUDIT FINDINGS

Nursing Diagnosis: Initial home visit, within 72 hours after uncomplicated delivery, with normal newborn, occurring in a birth center or obstetrical facility
Number of Records Audited: 30
Date of Audit: 7/6/08
Summary of Findings: 100% compliance in all areas except recording of mother's temperature (50% compliance) and of newborn's temperature (70% compliance)
Suggestions for Improving Compliance: Remind nurses to record temperature of mother and infant in record, even if normal. Time might be a factor in initial home visit because temperatures for both were generally recorded on subsequent visits. Committee agrees that temperatures on mother and baby should be taken during first home visit and suggests an in-service and staff meeting regarding this area of noncompliance.

Signed, Chair of the Committee _____

The summaries should be forwarded to the individual responsible for quality improvement, in this case the director of the agency. At no time should individual public health nurses be identified as not having met the criteria. Quality improvement must always be separate from performance appraisal.

LEARNING EXERCISE 24.3

Using Management by Objectives as a Part of Performance Appraisal

Analysis: This case could have several different approaches, depending on whether motivation or change theory or another rationale was being implemented to support the decisions. In reality, a manager may employ several different theories to increase productivity. However, this case will be solved by using only performance appraisal techniques to demonstrate that they can also serve as an effective method to control productivity.

There are several aspects that seem to stand out in the information presented in this case. First, it appears that Ms. Irwin is a person who needs to be reminded. She functions well in Objective 3 because she received monthly reminders of the meetings, and since she worked with a group of people, she was able to make a real contribution to this committee. The similarities among the other four objectives are that (a) they all required Ms. Irwin to work alone to accomplish them and (b) there were no built-in reminders.

Rather than viewing this performance appraisal critically, the charge nurse should expend her energy in developing a plan to help Ms. Irwin succeed in the coming months. Nothing is as depressing or demotivating to an employee as failure. The following plan concentrates only on the MBO portion of Ms. Irwin's performance appraisal and does not center on the rating scale of job performance.

Prior to the Interview

1. Ask Ms. Irwin to review her objectives from last year and to come prepared to discuss them.
2. Set a convenient time for you and Ms. Irwin and allow adequate time and privacy.

Rationale

1. Gives the employee opportunity for individual problem solving and personal introspection.
2. Shows interest in and respect for the employee.

At the Interview

1. Begin by complimenting Ms. Irwin on meeting Objective #3. Ask her about her work on the committee, what procedures she is working on, and so forth.
2. Review each of the other four objectives and ask for Ms. Irwin's input. Withhold any evidence or criticism at this point.
3. Ask Ms. Irwin if she sees a pattern.
4. Tell Ms. Irwin that MBO often works better if objectives are reviewed on a more timely basis, and ask how she feels about this.
5. Suggest that she keeps her unmet four objectives, and add one new one.

Rationale

1. Shows interest in and support of employee.

2. Allows the employee to make her own judgments about her performance.

3. Guide the employee into problem solving on her own.
4. This is an offer to assist the employee in achieving improved performance and is not a punitive measure. It allows the employee to have input.
5. Employees should be encouraged to meet objectives unless they were stated poorly or were unrealistic.

(Learning Exercise continues on page 632)

6. Work with Ms. Irwin in developing a reminder or check point system that will assist her in meeting her objectives.

6. Again, this helps the employee to succeed. Do not simply tell employees that they should do better; help them to identify how to do better.

7. Do not sympathize or excuse her for not meeting objectives.

7. The focus should remain on growth and not on the status quo.

8. End on a note of encouragement and support: "I know that you are capable of meeting these objectives."

8. Employees often live up to their manager's expectations of them, and if those expectations are for growth, then the chances are greater that it will occur.

LEARNING EXERCISE 25.5

The Marginal Employee

As the nursing supervisor of a 35-bed oncology unit in a 400-bed hospital, this is how you may solve the problems posed by a marginal employee (Judy) on your staff.

1. *Identify the problem.* The marginal performance of one employee is affecting unit morale.
2. *Gather data to analyze the causes and consequences of the problem.* The following information should be gathered and considered:
   - Judy has been an RN for 15 years and probably has always been a marginal employee.
   - Judy states that she is highly motivated to be an oncology nurse.
   - Judy has been coached on several occasions regarding how she might improve her performance, and no improvement is evident.
   - It is difficult to recruit and retain staff nurses for this unit.
   - The unit is already short two full-time RN positions.
   - Judy's performance is not unsatisfactory; it is marginal.
   - The other nurses on the floor considered Judy's performance to be disruptive enough to ask you to remove her from the floor.
3. *Identify alternative solutions.*
   Alternative 1. Terminate Judy's employment.
   Alternative 2. Transfer Judy to another floor.
   Alternative 3. Continue coaching Judy, and help her to identify specific and realistic goals about her performance.
   Alternative 4. Do nothing and hope that the problem resolves itself.
   Alternative 5. Work with the other staff nurses to create a work environment that will make Judy want to be transferred from the unit.
4. *Evaluate the alternatives.*
   Alternative 1. Although this would provide a rapid solution to the problem, there are many negative aspects to this alternative. Judy, although performing at a marginal level, has not done anything that warrants discipline or termination. Although some staff have requested her removal from the unit, this action could be viewed as arbitrary and grossly unfair by a silent minority. Thus, employees' sense of security and unit morale could decrease even more. In addition, it would be difficult to fill Judy's position.

Alternative 2. This alternative would immediately remove the problem from the supervisor and would probably please the staff. This alternative merely transfers the problem to a different unit, which is counterproductive to organizational goals. This might be an appropriate alternative if the supervisor could show that Judy could be expected to perform at a higher level on another unit. It is difficult to predict how Judy would feel about this alternative. Judy is probably aware of the other staff's frustration with her, and a transfer would provide at least temporary shelter from her colleagues' hostility. Although Judy would be pleased that she was not dismissed, she would appropriately view the transfer as her failure. This recognition is demoralizing, and the opportunity for her to fulfill a long-term career goal would be denied.

Alternative 3. This alternative requires a long-term and time-consuming commitment on the part of the manager. There is inadequate information in the case to determine whether the supervisor can make this type of commitment. In addition, there is no guarantee that setting short-term, specific, and realistic goals will improve Judy's work performance. It should, however, increase Judy's self-esteem and reinforce her supervisor's interest in her as a person. It also retains an RN who is difficult to replace. This alternative does not address the staff's dissatisfaction.

Alternative 4. There are few positive aspects to this alternative other than that the supervisor would not have to expend energy at this point. The problem, however, will probably snowball, and unit morale will likely become worse.

Alternative 5. Although most would agree that this alternative is morally corrupt, there are some advantages. Judy would voluntarily leave the unit, and the supervisor and staff would not have to deal with the problem. The disadvantages are similar to those cited in Alternative 1.

5. *Select the appropriate solution.* As in most decisions with an ethical component, there is no one right answer, and all the alternatives have desirable facets. Alternative 3 probably presents the least number of undesirable attributes. The cost to the supervisor is in time and effort. There is really little to lose in attempting this plan to increase employee productivity, because there are no replacements to fill the position anyway. Losing Judy by dismissal or transfer merely increases the workload on the other employees due to short staffing. It also cannot help the employee.

6. *Implement the solution.* In implementing Alternative 3, the supervisor should be very clear with Judy about her motives. She also must be sure that the goals they set are specific and realistic. Although the staff may continue to verbalize their unhappiness with Judy's performance, the supervisor should be careful not to discuss confidential information about Judy's coaching plan with them. The manager should, however, reassure the staff that she is aware of their concerns and that she will follow the situation closely.

7. *Evaluate the results.* The supervisor elected to review her problem solving 6 months after the plan was implemented. She found that although Judy was satisfied with her performance and appreciative of her supervisor's efforts, her performance had not improved appreciably. Judy continued to be a marginal employee but was meeting minimal competency levels. The supervisor did find, however, that the staff seemed to be more accepting of Judy's level of ability and rarely verbalized their dissatisfaction with her anymore. In general, unit morale increased again.

Index

Page numbers followed by *d* indicate displays, those followed by *f* indicate figures, and those followed by *t* indicate tables.

A

Accommodation, union, 524
Accomplishment, rewarding, 473
Accountability, 278
    ethical and fiscal, for staffing, 412–413
    organizational, 550–556 (*See also* Quality control)
    outcomes, 538
Accounting. *See also* Fiscal planning
    responsibility, 210
Achievement-oriented people, 427
Achievement pathway, 432, 432*d*
Acuity index, 212*d*
Acute care case management, 323–324
Ad hoc design, 274
Administrative agencies, 95–96, 95*d*
Administrative cases, 96–97, 96*t*
Administrative decision making, 19
Administrative man, 19–20, 19*t*
Administrative simplification plan, 111
Admonishment
    verbal, 598–599
    written, 599, 599*d*
Adult learning theory, 373, 373*d*, 374*t*
Adverse drug events (ADEs), 557. *See also* Medical
        errors
Advisory (staff) positions, 268
Advocacy, 119–133
    definitions in, 119–120
    leadership roles and management functions in, 120*d*,
        133
    learning of, 120–121
    media and, 131–132, 132*d*
    professional, 127–128
    subordinate, 124–125
    whistle-blowing as, 125–126
Advocacy, nursing, 119–120
    in legislation and public policy, 128–131, 130*d*
    values central to, 121, 121*d*
Advocacy, patient, 121–123, 122*d*, 124*d*
Affective conflict, 492
Affiliation-oriented people, 427
Affirmative action, 529
Affirming consequences, 13
Age Discrimination and Employment Act (ADEA), 530
Agency nurses, 403
Agency shop, 515
Agenda for Change, 552

Agendas, hidden, 501
Aggression, workplace, 491
Aggressive people, 454
Aging
    organizational, 179
    of workforce, 148, 338–339, 341, 341*d*
Alcohol abuse, 611. *See also* Chemically impaired
        employee
Alternative dispute resolution (ADR), 504–505
Alternatives, generating many, 12–13
Ambiguous questioning, 503
American Nurses Credentialing Center (ANCC), 248
Americans with Disabilities Act, 532
Analogy, arguing from, 13
Analysis tools, 13–14
Androgogy, 373, 374*t*
Anticipatory socialization, 384
Appearance, in communication, 453
Applied ethics, 69
Appraisal
    performance, 569–587 (*See also* Performance appraisal)
    self-, 573, 578
Arbitration, 504, 515, 606–607
Archer North Performance Appraisal System,
        573–574
Arguing from analogy, 13
Argyris, Chris, 36
Aristotle, 37
Aspirational ethics, 84
Assault, 104
Assertive behavior, 454–455
Assessment
    competency, 247–248, 571
    employee, 244
    of staff development needs, 376–377
Attitudes
    learning new roles and, 382
    of managers, 433–434
At-will doctrine, 608
Audits, 538, 545–547
Aukerman, M., 42, 43
Authentic leadership, 57–59, 58*d*
Authoritarian leadership, 38
Authority, 278, 293, 296. *See also* Power
    interdependence of response to, 298, 298*f*
    leadership roles and management functions in,
        integrating, 309–310

Authority dependence, 298
Authority figures, 297
Authority–power gap, 297–301
Autonomy, 74, 74*d*
Avoiding, 495
Avoliio, B.J., 43

B
Balanced Budget Act (BBA) of 1997, 223–224, 226
Barbiturate abuse, 611. *See also* Chemically impaired
    employee
Bar coding, 559
Bargaining agent, 524
Baseline data, 212*d*
Bass, B.M., 43
Battery, 104–105
Behavior change, 498
Behavioral expectation scales, 576–577
Behavioral theories of leadership, 38–39
Behaviorally anchored rating scales (BARS), 576–577
Benchmarking, 540
Beneficence, 74, 74*d*
Benefit time, 216
Bennis, W., 43
Benzodiazepine abuse, 611. *See also* Chemically
    impaired employee
Best practice, 540
Biases, confirmation, 24
"Big stick" approach, 594
Bill of rights, 123, 124*d*
Biometrics, 148
Blake, 40
Blanchard, K., 40
Body language, 450
Boland, S., 42, 43
Boom generation, 410, 411*t*
Bottom line, 500
Boundaries
    for practice, 98
    professional, 584
Brain hemisphere dominance, thinking styles and, 16–17
Brainstorming, 12
Brandt, M.A., 41–42
Breach of duty, 99
Break-even point, 212*d*
Budget, workforce, 214–217
Budget busters, 218*d*
Budgetary process, 211, 214
Budgets, 211, 214–221
    budget busters in, 218*d*
    capital, 218
    fixed, 212*d*
    flexible, 220–221
    incremental, 219
    new performance, 220

    operating, 217–218
    perpetual, 214
    personnel, 214–217 (*See also* Personnel budgets)
    zero-based, 219–220, 219*d*
Bullying, 490–491, 491*f*
Burden of proof, 608
Bureaucratic organizational designs, 34, 275
Burnout, avoiding, 433–434
Burns, F., 41
Burns, J.M., 42
Business letter, formal, 452
Butterfly effect, 174

C
Capital budget, 218
Capitation, 212*d*, 224
Care-centered organizations, 275
Career coaching, 244–245, 246*d*
Career development, 239–257
    career coaching in, 244–245, 246*d*
    competency assessment in, 247–248, 571
    components of, 241*d*
    definition of, 239
    employee transfers in, 249–251
    justifications for, 240–243, 241*d*
    leadership roles and management functions in, 240*d*,
        257
    management development in, 253–254
    organization's responsibility for, 243–244
    planning *vs.* management in, 241*d*
    professional portfolio in, 256–257
    professional specialty certification in, 248–249, 248*d*
    promotions in, 251–253
    résumé preparation in, 254–256, 256*d*
Career information dissemination, 243
Career paths, 243
Care pairs, 321
Care pathways, 221, 222
Case management, 323–325
Case method of assignment, 317, 318*f*
Case mix, 212*d*
Case study learning, 3
Cash flow, 212*d*
Centers for Medicare and Medicaid Services (CMS),
        553
Central tendency, 573
Centrality, 271–273
Centralized decision making, 276
Centralized staffing, 398–399
Certification, 248
    professional specialty, 248–249, 248*d*
Certification programs, 113
Chain of command, 268
    examining people in, 271
    in reporting inadequate care, 105

Change, 166
  planned (*See* Planned change)
Change agent, 167, 169
Change strategies, classic, 174–175
Change theory, 167–169, 170*d*
  driving and restraining forces in, 170–171, 172*f*
Chaos theory, 173–174
Charismatic power, 297
Charitable immunity, doctrine of, 103
Chart, organizational. *See* Organizational charts
Charting, responsibility, 498
Checklist appraisal tools, 577
Chemically impaired employee, 610–618, 612*d*
  confrontation of, 613–615
  diversion programs for, 616–618
  drugs used by, 611
  history of, 611
  manager's role in assisting of, 615–616
  recognition of, 611–613, 612*d*
  recovery process for, 616
  reentry to workplace of, 618
  State Board of Nursing treatment programs for, 616–618
  toll of, 611
Chief executive officer (CEO), 270
Chief nurse officer (CNO), 270
Chief operations officer (COO), 270
Chunking, 376
Civil cases, 96, 96*t*
Civil laws, 526
Civil Rights Act of 1964, 529
Clinical coaching, 586
Clinical nurse–leader, 329
Clinical pathways, 221, 222
Clinical practice guidelines, 543–545, 544*d*, 545*d*
Clonazepam abuse, 611. *See also* Chemically impaired employee
Closed shop, 515
Closed-unit staffing, 411
Closure, of group communication, 456
Coaching, 586–587
  career, 244–245, 246*d*
  of marginal employees, 609
  ongoing, 602
  performance deficiency, 602, 603*d*–604*d*
  problem-centered, 602
  as teaching strategy, 388–389
Coalitions, developing, 308
Code of Ethics for Nurses, ANA, 77, 78*d*
Coercive power, 296
Cognitive dissonance, between personal and organizational values, 155
Collaboration, 495–497
Collaborative practice matrix, 42
Collective bargaining, 514–515, 515*d*
  ANA and, 517–518

definition of, 515
  historical perspective of, 515–517, 517*t*
Commitment models, 595
Committees
  responsibilities and opportunities in, 285–286
  structure of, 284–285, 285*d*
Communication, 441–461
  aggressive, 454, 455
  assertive, 454–455
  channels of, 448–449
  confidentiality in, 459–460
  culture and, 479
  definitions of, 443–444
  diagonal, 449
  downward, 449
  effective, 442, 445
  expert handling of, 307
  face-to-face, 450
  on financial performance, 442
  gender in, 445–446
  grapevine, 277, 449
  group dynamics in, 456–459, 458*d* (*See also* Group dynamics)
  horizontal, 449
  internal and external climate in, 444
  leadership roles and management functions in, 442, 443*d*, 461
  listening skills in, 456
  modes of, 449–450
  nonverbal, 450, 452–454
  passive, 454
  process of, 443–445, 444*f*
  telecommunication and e-mail in, 447–448
  telephone, 450
  upward, 448
  verbal skills for, 454–455
  written, 450–452
Communication, organizational, 441–442
  strategies of, 446–447, 447*d*
  technology on, 447–448
  variables in, 445–446
  written, 450–452
Competence, 376
Competency assessment, 247–248, 571
Competency model, of differentiated nursing practice, 327, 327*d*
Complex adaptive systems theory, 172–173, 173*d*
Complexity science, 172
Compromising, 494
Conciliation, 515
Conference
  disciplinary, 604
  termination, 605–606
Confidentiality, 74*d*, 76, 459–460

Confirmation biases, 24
Conflict, 487
    affective, 492
    definition and nature of, 487
    felt, 492
    intergroup, 490, 491*f*
    interpersonal, 490–491, 491*f*
    intrapersonal, 490, 491*f*
    latent, 492
    manifest, 492
    overt, 492
    perceived, 492
    qualitative, 489–490
    quantitative, 489–490
Conflict aftermath, 492
Conflict management, 493–506
    alternative dispute resolution in, 504–505
    avoiding in, 495
    collaborating in, 495–497
    competing in, 494
    compromising in, 494
    conflict resolution in, 487–488
    consensus in, 505
    cooperating/accommodating in, 494
    gender in, 492
    goal of, 493–494
    history of, 488–490, 489*f*
    leadership roles and management functions in, 488*d*,
        505–506
    negotiation in, 499–504, 500*d* (*See also* Negotiation)
    smoothing in, 495
    strategies for, 493–494, 494*d*
    in units, 497–499, 497*d*
Conflict process, 492–493, 493*f*
Conflict resolution, 487–488
Confrontation, 498
Connections pathway, 431, 432*d*
Consensus, 505
Consent
    express, 107
    implied, 106–107
    informed, 106, 106*d*
Consequences, affirming, 13
Consequence tables, 22–23, 23*t*
Consequential ethics, 84
Consequentialist theory, 72–73, 73*t*
Consistency, 597, 597*d*
Constitution, 95, 95*d*
Constructive discipline, 596
Contingency leadership theory, 39
Continuous health improvement, 325–327, 326*d*
Continuous quality improvement (CQI), 548
Contracting, selective, 224
Control criteria, establishing, 540, 541*f*
Controllable costs, 212*d*

Controllable expenses, 211
Controlling, in management process, 35, 35*f*
Cooperating, 494
Coordinating, 421
Core measures program, 552–553
Cost
    controllable, 212*d*
    direct, 212*d*
    fixed, 212*d*
    full, 212*d*
    indirect, 213*d*
    noncontrollable, 211, 213*d*
    vs. quality, 210
Cost-benefit ratio, 212*d*
Cost center, 212*d*
Cost drivers, 325
Cost-effectiveness
    definition of, 210
    of staff development programs, 378
Counsel, seeking, 304
Court decisions, 95*d*, 96
Courts, types of, 96–97, 96*t*
Cover letter, résumé, 255–256
C players, 609
Credential requirements, 354
Criminal cases, 96, 96*t*
Criminal laws, 526
Critical event analysis (CEA), 542
Critical indicator patient classification system, 405
Critical pathways, 221, 222, 324
Critical thinker, 3*d*
Critical thinking
    components of, 2–3
    definition of, 2–3
    experiential learning, 5
    Marquis-Huston critical thinking teaching model for,
        3–5, 4*f*
Cross-training, 411
Crusaders, 176
Cultivation, 381
Cultural bridging, 61–62
Cultural diversity, 61
    in committees, 286
    conflict from, 497
    staff education and, 389–390
    in staff management, 399–400
    workforce, legal considerations in, 111–112
Cultural diversity enhancement group (CDEG), 385
Culture, organizational, 278–280, 281*d*–282*d*
Cycle time reduction, 324
Cyclical staffing, 402, 402*f*d

D

Daily planning actions, 193
Data gathering, careful, 10–11, 10*d*

Day-to-day feedback, 586
Decentralized decision making, 276
Decentralized staffing, 398–399
Decision grid, 20, 20*f*
Decision making, 1–28
  centralized, 276
  critical elements, 9–14, 9*d*
    choose and act decisively, 14
    define objectives clearly, 10
    gather data carefully, 10–11, 10*d*
    generate many alternatives, 12–13
    think logically, 13–14
    use evidence-based approach, 11–12, 12*d*
  decentralized, 276
  definition of, 2
  ethical, 77–84
  ethical frameworks for, 72–73, 73*t* (*See also* Ethical
    issues)
  individual variations in, 14–17
    brain hemisphere dominance, 16
    life experience, 15–17
    preference, 16–18
    thinking styles, 16–18
    values, 15, 17
  individual vulnerability in, overcoming, 17–18
  intuitive models of, 8–9
  managerial models of, 6
  MORAL, 82–84
  naturalistic, 8
  organizational, 18–24
    consequence tables, 22–23, 23*t*
    decision trees, 21–22
    grids, 20, 20*f*
    logic models, 23
    organizational power on, 18–19
    payoff tables, 21
    program evaluation and review technique, 23–24,
      24*f*
    rational and administrative, 19–20, 19*t*
    tools, 20
  participative, 36
  proactive, 307
  rational and administrative, 19–20, 19*t*
  theoretical approaches to, 5–9
    heuristics, 5
    IDEALS model, 8
    intuitive model, 8–9
    managerial models, 6
    nursing process, 7–8, 7*f*, 7*t*
    structured approach, 5–6
    traditional problem-solving process, 6
  tools in, 20, 25
Decision making hierarchy/pyramid, 275–276
Decision package, 219–220
Decision trees, 21–22

Decisive choices and actions, 14
Defamation, 105
Defendant, 98
Delegation, 468–481
  common errors in, 469–471, 471*d*
  communicating goal clearly in, 471–472
  definitions of, 468
  difficulty in, 473
  effective, 471–473
  empowerment in, 472
  as function of professional nursing, 473–480
    leadership roles and management functions in,
      integrating, 480–481
    preparation for role of, 474
    steps in, 473*d*
    subordinate resistance to, 478
    task-based guide to, 477, 477*d*
    to transcultural work team, 479–480, 480*d*
    to unlicensed assistive personnel, 474–476
  improper, 470–471
  leadership roles and management functions in,
    469*d*
  necessary skills and levels in, identifying, 471
  overdelegating in, 470
  performance evaluation in, 472
  planning ahead in, 471
  rewarding accomplishment in, 473
  role modeling and guidance in, 472
  selecting capable personnel in, 471
  setting deadlines and monitoring progress in, 472
  underdelegating in, 469–470
Democratic leadership, 38–39
Deontological ethics, 73, 73*t*, 84
Destructive discipline, 594–595
Destructive negotiation tactics, 502–503
Diagnosis-related groups (DRGs), 212*d*, 223, 551
Diagonal communication, 449
Diazepam abuse, 611. *See also* Chemically impaired
    employee
Differentiated nursing practice, 327–328, 327*d*
Direct costs, 212*d*
Directing, 35, 35*f*, 421
Director of nursing, 270
Disciplinary conference, 604
Disciplinary strategies, 602–606
  agreement and acceptance of action plan, 605
  clarification of expectations for change, 605
  disciplinary conference, 604
  employee's response to action, 604
  overview, 602
  performance deficiency coaching, 602,
    603*d*–604*d*
  rationale for action, 604–605
  reasons for disciplinary action, 604
  termination conference, 605–606

Discipline, 593–619
  for chemically impaired employee, 610–618, 612d
    (*See also* Chemically impaired employee)
  constructive *vs.* destructive, 594–596
  definition and origin of, 594, 596
  enforcement of, 594
  fair and effective rules for, 597–598, 597d
  grievance procedures in, 606–607
  group norms and, 596
  lack of, 594
  leadership roles and management functions for, 595d,
    619
  marginal employees and, 594, 609–610
  reprimand form for, 599, 599d
  self-, 596
  with unionized employee, 607–609
Discipline, progressive, 598–601
  formal reprimand or written admonishment in, 599, 599d
  guide to, 601d
  informal reprimand or verbal admonishment in,
    598–599
  involuntary termination or dismissal in, 600
  suspension from work in, 599–600
Discrimination, 112
Disease management, 325–327, 326d
Disengagement, 242
Dismissal, 600, 605–606
Diversion programs, 616–618
Diversity, 61. *See also* Cultural diversity
  workforce, legal considerations in, 111–112
Doctrine of charitable immunity, 103
Documentation, of appraisal interview, 584–585, 585d
Downward communication, 449
Downward transfer, 250–251
Due process, 608
Dunham, J., 43
Duty-based reasoning, 73, 73t
Dynamic model of strategy, 145

E
Economic man, 19, 19t
Education, nursing, 244, 339–340
  requirements for, 354
  team building via, 390–391 (*See also* Team building)
  training *vs.*, 371–372
Educational needs, of culturally diverse staff,
    389–390
Education department responsibilities, 372
Education model, of differentiated nursing practice,
    327, 327d
Effectiveness
  leadership, Hollander on, 41
  organizational, 286–287
Effectiveness report, 571
Ego, politics and, 308

Elderly population, 148
Electronic health record (EHR), 448
e-mail (electronic mail), 447–448
Emotional intelligence, 55–57, 56d
Employee, problem. *See* Problem employees
Employee assessment, 244
Employee commitment, 595
Employee Free Choice Act, 523
Employee indoctrination, 359–362. *See also*
    Indoctrination, employee; Staffing
Employee motivation, performance appraisal for,
    570–572, 571d
Employee orientation, 360–362, 360d–362d
Employee placement, 357–359. *See also* Staffing
Employee recruitment, 251–252, 341–343. *See also*
    Staffing
Employee releases, 252
Employee selection, 354–357. *See also* Selection,
    employee; Staffing
Employee transfers, 249–251
Employment legislation, 525–532
  Age Discrimination and Employment Act (ADEA),
    530
  Americans with Disabilities Act, 532
  Civil Rights Act of 1964, 529
  equal employment opportunity laws, 528–529
  labor standards, 526–527
  leadership roles and management functions and, 514d,
    533
  minimum wages and maximum hours, 526–527
  Occupational Health and Safety Act, 532
  sexual harassment, 530–531
  state health facilities licensing boards, 533
  time clocks and, 527
  Veterans Readjustment Assistance Act,
    532
Empowerment
  definition and scope of, 299–300
  of others, 305
  of subordinates, 299–301
Energy
  maintaining personal, 303–306, 305d
  of managers, 433–434
Environment, in communication, 453
Environmental control, culture and, 479
Equal employment, 526
Equal Employment Opportunity Commission, U.S.
    (USEEOC), 530
Equal employment opportunity laws, 528–529
Equal Pay Act of 1963, 527
Errors, medical. *See* Medical errors
Essay appraisal method, 577
Essays, performance appraisal, 577
Ethical accountability, for staffing, 412–413
Ethical dilemma, 71

Ethical issues, 69–88
  ANA code of ethics and professional standards in, 77, 78d, 79d
  definitions in, 69
  ethical frameworks for decision making in, 72–73, 73t
  ethical problem solving and decision making in, 77–84
    MORAL decision-making model in, 82–84
    nursing process in, 80–82
    outcome in, 77–78
    structured problem solving in, 78
    traditional problem-solving process in, 79–80
    Wueste approach to, 84
  individual values, beliefs, and philosophy in, 72
  in leadership and management, 84–87
    collaborating for solutions in, 86–87
    creating ethical work environments in, 87
    ethical behavior as norm in, 86
    separating legal and ethical issues in, 86
    using institutional review boards appropriately in, 87
  leadership roles and management functions with, 71d, 88
  principles of ethical reasoning in, 73–76, 74d (See also Ethical principles)
  types of, 70–72
Ethical principles, 73–76, 74d
  autonomy (self-determination), 74, 74d
  beneficence (doing good), 74, 74d
  confidentiality (respecting privileged information), 74d, 76
  fidelity (keeping promises), 74d, 75–76
  justice (treating people fairly), 74d, 75
  paternalism, 74–75, 74d
  utility, 74d, 75
  veracity (truth telling), 74d, 75
Ethical relativism, 73
Ethical universalism, 73
Ethics
  ANA code of, 77, 78d
  applied, 69
  aspirational, 84
  consequential, 84
  definition of, 69
  deontological, 84
  teleological theory of, 72–73, 73t
Ethnic diversity, 62
Evidence-based medicine (EBM), 11–12
Evidence-based practice (EBP), 11–12, 12d
  clinical practice guidelines based on, 543
  vs. outcomes, 540
  shared responsibility for implementation of, 379
Exclusive provider organization (EPO), 225–226
Executive Order 10988, 516
Expectancy model, 426, 427f

Expectations for change, clarification of, 605
Expenses
  controllable vs. noncontrollable, 211, 213d
  fixed vs. variable, 211
  operating, 213d
  salary, 216
Experiential factors
  in decision making, 15–16, 17
  in learning, 374
Expert patient, 148
Expert power, 296
Experts, use of, 304
Express consent, 107
Expressed policies, 159
External climate, in communication, 444
Extrinsic motivation, 421
Eye contact, in communication, 453

F
Face-to-face communication, 450
Facial expression, in communication, 453–454
Fact finding, 504, 515
Fair Labor Standards Act (FLSA), 526–527
Fair rules, 597–598, 597d
False imprisonment, 105
Fayol, Henri, 35
Featherbedding, 528
Feedback, day-to-day, 586
Fee-for-service (FFS) system, 212d, 222
Felt conflict, 492
Feminist power, 297
Fidelity, 74d, 75–76
Fiedler, F., 40
Final offer approach, 504–505
First-level managers, 270, 271t
Fiscal accountability, for staffing, 412–413
Fiscal planning, 208–230
  balancing costs and quality in, 210
  budget types in, 214–218 (See also Budgets)
  budgetary process in, 211, 214
  budgeting methods in, 219–221 (See also Budgeting)
  critical pathways in, 221, 222
  forecasting in, 210
  health care milestones in, U.S., 229d–230d
  health care reimbursement in, 221–222
  leadership roles and management functions in, 209d, 230
  managed care in, 224–226
    future of, 228
    proponents and critics of, 226–227
  Medicare and Medicaid in, 223
  overview of, 208–209
  prospective payment system in, 223–224
  responsibility accounting in, 210
  terminology in, 212d–213d

5 Million Lives Campaign, 560
Fixed budget, 212*d*
Fixed costs, 212*d*
Fixed expenses, 211
Flat/flattened organizations, 270, 275, 275*f*
Flat-percentage increase method, 219
Flattery, 503
Flexibility, 305
Flexible budgeting, 220–221
Flextime, 403
Float pools, 403
Follett, Mary Parker, 36, 39–40
Followers, 53–54
Forced checklist, 577
Forecasting, 142–143, 210
Foreseeability of harm, 99
Forewarning, 597–598, 597*d*
Formal reprimand, 599, 599*d*
Formal structure, 265
Forming, 456, 457*t*
For-profit organization, 212*d*
Four-pronged approach
    to marginal employees, 610
    to medical errors, 559
Four-week cycle master time sheet, 402, 402*d*, 402*f*
Free-form review, 577
Free speech, 515
Full costs, 212*d*
Full-time equivalent (FTE), 212*d*
Functional foremen, 34
Functional nursing care, 317–319, 319*f*

G
Gardner, J.W., 44–45
Gatekeepers, 224
Gatekeeping positions, 277
Gellerman, Saul, 427–428
Gender
    in communication, 445–446
    conflict response and, 492
    on decision making, 14–15
    power and, 294–296
Generational diversity, 62
Generational work groups, 410–411, 410*d*
Generation X, 411*t*, 412
Generation Y, 411*t*, 412
Glass ceiling, 295
Goals, 156–157, 157*d*
Goal statements, 156–157, 157*d*
Good, doing, 74, 74*d*
Goodheim, L., 43
Good Samaritan laws, 109–110
Governance, shared, 280–283, 280*f*, 282*f*
Governmental immunity, 103
Grapevine communication, 277, 449

Great Man theory, 37, 38*d*
Grievance, 515
Grievance procedures, 606–607
Group building, 458
Group communication, 456, 457*t*
Group dynamics, 456–459, 458*d*
Group maintenance, 458
Group norms, 596
Group task roles, 457–458, 459*d*
Groupthink, 286
Guidance, in delegation, 472
Gulick, Luther, 35

H
Halo effect, 573
Hand-offs, 559
Happy people, 431
Harassment, sexual, 530–531
Hawthorne effect, 36
Hazard, moral, 227
HBR Breakthrough Ideas for 2007, 573
Health Care Financing Administration (HCFA), 553
"Healthcare in the Crossroads: Strategies for Improving
    the Medical Liability System and Preventing
    Injury," 101–102, 101*d*
Health care milestones, U.S., 229*d*–230*d*
Health care quality, 538–540
    vs. costs, 210
    definitions of, 538–540
    maintaining (*See* Quality control)
    nursing care hours and staffing mix in, 409–410
    quality assurance in, 548
Health care reimbursement, 221–222
Health Insurance Portability and Accountability Act of
    1996 (HIPAA), 110–111, 123
    confidentiality in, 459–460
Health maintenance organization (HMO), 213*d*, 225
Health Maintenance Organization Act of 1973, 225
Health Plan Employer Data and Information Set (HDIS),
    553–554
Hersey, P., 40
Herzberg, Frederick, 425–426, 426*t*
Heuristics, 5
Hidden agendas, 501
Hierarchy
    organizational (*See* Organizational structure)
    planning, 148, 149*f*, 151, 152*f*
High-performance teams, 41
HIPAA Privacy Rule, 111
HMO report cards, 556
Hollander, E. P., 40–41
Honeymoon phase, 384
Horizontal communication, 449
Horizontal violence, 490–491, 491*f*
Horns effect, 573

Hospital information system (HIS), 447–448
Hospital Quality Measures, 552–553
Hours, nursing care per patient-day (NCH/PPD),
    215–217, 216*f*
  calculating, 405, 405*f*
  on quality of care, 409–410
Hours per patient-day (HPPD), 213*d*
Human capital theory, 55
Human relations era, 36
Human relations management, 36–37, 36*t*
Humor, maintaining sense of, 305
100,000 Lives Campaign, 560
Hygiene factors, 425–426, 426*d*

I
IDEALS model, 8
Ignorance, as legal excuse, 99
Immediacy, 597, 597*d*
Immunity
  doctrine of charitable, 103
  governmental, 103
Impairment, 594
Impartiality, 597, 597*d*
Implied consent, 106–107
Implied policies, 159
Imprisonment, false, 105
Inactivism, 142
Inappropriate questioning, 503
Inappropriate transfers, employee, 250–251
Incentives, 429
Incident reports, 104
Incremental budgeting, 219
Independent practice association (IPA), 225
Indirect costs, 213*d*
Individual philosophies and values, 154–156
Indoctrination, employee, 359–362. *See also* Staffing
  content of, 359, 360*d*
  definition of, 359
  induction in, 359–360
  orientation in, 360–362, 360*d*–362*d*
Induction, 359–360
Industrial age leadership, transition to relationship age
    leadership from, 62–64, 63*f*, 63*t*
Informal reprimand, 598–599
Informal structure, 265
Information, expert handling of, 307
Informational power, 297
Informed consent, 106, 106*d*
Initial contact, in staffing, 343–344
Initiation, 381
Institute for Health Improvement (IHI), 560
Institutional licensure, 112–113
Institutional review boards (IRBs), appropriate
    use of, 87
Integrated leader–managers, 44–45

Integrity, transparent, 58
Intentional torts, 104–105
Interactional leadership theories, 40–42
Interactive planning, 142
Intergroup conflict, 490, 491*f*
Internal climate, in communication, 444
International Classification for Nursing Practice
    (ICNP), 546
International nurses, socialization of, 384
Internship, 384
Interpersonal conflict, 490–491, 491*f*
Interruptions, in time management, 194
Intervention programs, 616–618
Interview, appraisal. *See* Appraisal interview
Interviewing, 344–353
  acceptable and unacceptable inquiries in,
    351*t*–352*t*
  definition of, 344
  evaluation of, 350
  interviewee tips for, 352–353, 353*d*
  legal aspects of, 350–352
  limitations of, 344–345
  planning, conducting, and controlling, 348–350
  sample questions for, 348*d*
  structured, 344, 346*d*–347*d*
  unstructured, 344
Intrapersonal conflict, 490, 491*f*
Intrinsic motivation, 421
Intuitionist framework, 73, 73*t*
Intuitive decision-making model, 8–9
Intuitive thinking, 16
Involuntary termination, 600

J
Job dimension scales, 576, 576*d*
Job interview, conducting. *See* Interviewing
Job openings, posting, 243–244
Johns, C., 43
Joint Commission, 552–553
Joint liability, 102
Joint practice committees, 280
Joy, pathways to, 431–432, 432*d*
Just cause, 608
Justice, 74*d*, 75
Just-in-time ordering, 217

K
Kanter, R.M., 41, 42
Kasselbaum–Kennedy Act, 110–111
Kellerman, B., 44
Kennerly, S.M., 43
Klafehn, K.A., 43
Knowledge. *See also* Education, nursing; Training
  increasing professional, 304
  of results, 376

L

Labor intensive, 214
Labor–management relations, effective, 524–525
Labor relations, 526
Labor standards, 526
Laissez-faire leadership, 39
Language
  organizational, 304
  standardized nursing, 546
Latent conflict, 492
Lateral transfer, 249
Law
  Good Samaritan, 109–110
  sources of, 94–96, 95t
  types of, 96–97, 96t
Law of the situation, 39–40
Leaders, 32–33
  characteristics of, 32–33
  definition of, 32
  followers and, 53–54
Leadership
  authentic, 57–59, 58d
  authoritarian, 38
  behavioral theories of, 38–39
  characteristics associated with, 38d
  contingency theories of, 39–40
  definition of, 32
  democratic, 38–39
  integration with management of, 44–45
  interactional, 40–42
  laissez-faire, 39
  nondirected, 39
  quantum, 61
  relationship age, 62–64, 63f, 63t
  servant, 52–53, 53d
  situational theories of, 39–40
  thought, 59–60
  transactional, 42, 42t
  transformational, 42–44, 42t
Leadership and management, classical views, 31–45
  historical development of leadership theory in, 37–44
    (See also Leadership theory, historical
    development of)
  historical development of management theory in,
    33–37 (See also Management theory, historical
    development of)
  integrating leadership and management in, 44–45, 45t
  leaders in, 32–33, 32d
  managers in, 31–32
Leadership and management, 21st century, 52–66
  industrial age to relationship age transition in, 62–64,
    63f, 63t
  new thinking about, 52–62
    authentic leadership, 57–59, 58d
    cultural bridging, 61–62

  emotional intelligence, 55–57, 56d
  human and social capital theory, 55
  leaders and followers, 53–54
  principal agent theory, 54–55
  quantum leadership, 61
  servant leadership, 52–53, 53d
  thought leadership, 59–60
  for nursing's future, 64–65
  Stanley and Flumerfelt on, 52
Leadership roles, 32d
  ethics and, 71d, 88
  exercise on, 34
Leadership styles, 38–39
Leadership theory, historical development of, 37–44
  behavioral theories, 38–39
  Great Man theory and trait theories, 37, 38d
  interactional theories, 40–42
  situational and contingency theories, 39
  summary of, 45t
  theorists, 45t
  transactional and transformational leadership, 42–44,
    42t
Leapfrog Group and initiatives, 557–559, 558d
Learning, team building via, 390–391
Learning organizations (LOs), 370–371
Learning theories, 372–376
  adult, 373, 373d, 374t
  chunking, 376
  knowledge of results, 376
  motivation to learn, 375
  obstacles and assets, 373d
  overview, 372–373
  readiness to learn, 374
  reinforcement, 375
  social, 374, 375f
  span of memory, 376
  task learning, 375
  transfer of learning, 376
Left-brain thinkers, 16
Legal and legislative issues, 93–114
  avoiding malpractice claims in, 100–102, 101d
  chain of command in reporting inadequate care in, 105
  consent in, 106–107, 106d
  extending liability in, 102–104
  Good Samaritan laws in, 109–110
  Health Insurance Portability and Accountability Act of
    1996 in, 110–111
  incident reports in, 104
  intentional torts in, 104–105
  laws and courts in, 96–97, 96t
  leadership roles and, 94d
  leadership roles and management functions in,
    integrating, 113–114
  legal doctrines in, 97–98
  licensure in, 112–113, 113d

Legal and legislative issues (*continued*)
   management functions and, 94*d*
   in managing diverse workforce, 111–112
   medical records in, 108
   nursing's advocacy role in, 128–131, 130*d*
   Patient Self-Determination Act in, 109
   product liability in, 105–106
   professional negligence in, 98–100, 99*t*
   quality control in, 105
   reporting improper/substandard care in, 105
   sources of law in, 94–96, 95*t*
Legal doctrines, practice of nursing and, 97–98
Legal-rational authority, 265
Legislative law, 95, 95*d*
Legitimate power, 296
Lewin, Kurt, 38
Lewin's model of change, 167–169
   contemporary adaptation of, 169–170
   driving and restraining forces in, 170–171, 172*f*
Liability
   extending, 102–104
   joint, 102
   medical, reforms of, 101–102, 101*d*, 559
   product, 105–106
   vicarious, 102
Licensure and licensing boards
   professional *vs.* institutional, 112–113, 113*d*
   for state health facilities, 533
Life experience, on decision making, 15–16, 17
Line-and-staff structure, 268*f*, 273
Line positions, 268
Line structure/organization, 268*f*, 273
Lippitt, R., 38
Listening skills, 456
Lists, planning, 191–192
Lobbyists, nursing, 129
Lockout, 515
Logical thinking, 13–14
Logic models, 23
Longnecker, P.D., 42
Long-term career coaching, 245, 246*d*
Long-term planning, 146–148. *See also* Strategic
   planning
Love of work pathway, 431, 432*d*

M
Magnet status/magnetism, 283–284, 284*d*
Maintenance factors, 425–426, 426*d*
Malpractice, 98–100, 99*t*
Malpractice claims, avoiding, 100–102, 101*d*
Managed care, 213*d*, 224–226, 225*d*. *See also specific*
   types
   future of, 228
   proponents and critics of, 226–227
Managed care backlash, 228

Managed care organizations (MCOs), 225–226
Management
   classical views of (*See* Leadership and management,
      classical views)
   control in, 31
   definition of, 31–32
   effectiveness in, 31
   leadership integration with, 44–45
   participative, 36
   scientific, 33–35
   seven activities of, 35
   in 21st century (*See* Leadership and management,
      21st century)
Management by objectives (MBO), 573, 578–580
Management development, 253–254
Management functions, 31–32
   ethics in, 71*d*, 88–89
   exercise on, 34
Management process, 35, 35*f*
Management theory, historical development of,
   33–37
   human relations management, 36–37
   management functions identified, 35
   management process, 35, 35*f*
   scientific management, 33–35
   up to 1970, 36–37, 36*t*
Managerial decision-making models, 6
Managerial levels, 270–271
Manager power, 297
Managers, 31–32
Mandatory overtime, 411–412
Mandatory staffing requirements, 400–401, 401*d*
Manifest conflict, 492
Manojlovich, M., 42
Marginal employees, 594, 609–610
Marquis-Huston critical thinking teaching model,
   3–5, 4*f*
Maryland Hospital Association Quality Indicator
   Project, 554, 555*d*–556*d*
Maslow's hierarchy of needs, 424–425, 425*f*
Matrix structure, 274–275, 274*f*
Matthew effect, 573–574
Maturation, in learning, 374
Mayo, Elton, 36
McClelland, David, 427
McGregor, Douglas, 36, 38, 428–429
McGregor's hot stove, 597–598*d*
McGruie, E., 43
Media, nursing and, 131–132, 132*d*
Mediation–arbitration, 504, 515
Medicaid, 213*d*, 223
   Centers for Medicare and Medicaid Services and,
      553
   fiscal planning in, 223
   managed care in, 226

Medical errors, 557–560
  four-pronged approach to, 559
  future of, 559–560
  hand-offs in, 559
  hours worked and, 412
  Leapfrog Group on, 557–559, 558d
  overview of, 557
  reforming medical liability system and, 559
  reporting and analyzing, 557
  Six Sigma approach to, 559
Medical liability system reform, 559
Medical records, 108
Medicare, 213d, 223
  Centers for Medicare and Medicaid Services and, 553
  fiscal planning in, 223
  managed care in, 226
Medicare Quality Initiative (MQI), 553
Memos, 451
Memory span, 376
Mentors, 381–382, 382d, 386
Meperidine abuse, 611. See also Chemically impaired
    employee
Merit rating, 571
Middle-level managers, 270, 271t
Minimum Data Set, nursing, 546
Minimum wages, 526–527
Minorities. See also Cultural diversity
  in labor force, 111–112
Mission statements, 149–150, 150d, 156
Modular nursing, 321
MORAL decision-making model, 82–84
Moral dilemma, 71
Moral distress, 71
Moral hazard, 227
Moral outrage, 71
Moral uncertainty/conflict, 70–71
Morphine abuse, 611. See also Chemically impaired
    employee
Motivating climate, 421–434
  creating, 429–433, 432d
  individual vs. collective motivators in, 424
  joy at work in, 431–432, 432d
  leadership roles and management functions in, 423d,
    434
  positive reinforcement in, 430–431
  support systems for managers in, 433–434
Motivation, 421–424
  definition of, 422
  individual and collective motivators in, 424
  intrinsic vs. extrinsic, 421–424
  to learn, 375
  overcoming deficiencies in, 382
  performance appraisal for, 570–572, 571d
Motivational theory, 424–429
  Gellerman on, 427–428

Herzberg on, 425–426, 426t
  Maslow on, 424–425, 425f
  McClelland on, 427
  McGregor on, 428–429
  overview of, 424
  Skinner on, 425
  Vroom on, 426, 427f
Motivator factors, 425, 426t
Motivator–hygiene theory, 425–426, 426t
Motivators, individual vs. collective, 424
Mouton, J.S., 40
Multidisciplinary action plans (MAPs), 324
Multistate Nursing Home Case Mix and Quality
    Demonstration, 556

N
National Committee for Quality Assurance (NCQA),
    553–554
National drug code (NDC), 559
National Guideline Clearinghouse (NGC), 544, 545d
National Labor Relations Act (NLRA), 520
National Labor Relations Board (NLRB), 515, 523
Naturalistic decision making, 8
Needs, individual, motivation and, 429–430
Negative sanctions, 383
Negligence, professional, 98–100, 99t
Negotiation, 499–506, 500d. See also Conflict
    management
Nelson, L., 41
Network
  HMO, 225
  wireless, 448
Network groups, 131
Networking, 308
New performance budgeting, 220
Noncontrollable costs/expenses, 211, 213d
Nondirected leadership, 39
Nonmaleficence, 74, 74d
Nonproductive time, 216
Nonverbal communication, 450, 452–454
Normative–re-educative strategies, 175
Norming, 456, 457t
Norms, group, 596
Not-for-profit organization, 213d
Nurse–patient ratio, 400–401, 401d
Nurse Practice Act of 1903, 93
Nurse recruiter, 342
Nursing advocacy, 119–120
Nursing care hours (NCH), on quality of care,
    409–410
Nursing care hours per patient-day (NCH/PPD),
    215–217, 216f
  calculating, 405, 405f
  on quality of care, 409–410
Nursing care plan, 324

Nursing education enrollments, 339–340
Nursing Interventions Classification (NIC), 546
Nursing Minimum Data Set (NMDS), 546
Nursing process, 7–8, 7f, 7t. *See also specific topics*
    ethical issues and, 80–82
Nursing profession
    mobilizing power of, 301–303, 301d, 302d
    renewal of, 180
Nursing service philosophy, 150–151, 151d
Nursing shortage
    fundamentals of, 337–338 (*See also* Staffing)
    resolution of, 340–341, 341d
    on staffing, 411–412

O
Objectives, 10, 157–158. *See also* Mission statements
Occupational Safety and Health Act (OSHA), 532
Older workers, 338–339, 341, 341d
Ombudspersons, 505
Open shop, 515
Open systems thinking, 370
Operant conditioning, 426
Operating budget, 217–218
Operating expenses, 213d
Operational and strategic planning, 140–162
    forecasting in, 142–143
    goals in, 156–157, 157d
    individual philosophies and values in, 154–156
    leadership roles and management functions in,
        140–141, 141d, 161–162
    long-term planning in, 146–148
    mission statements in, 149–150, 150d, 156
    objectives in, 157–158
    overcoming barriers to, 161
    philosophy statement in, 150–153, 151d (*See also*
        Philosophy statement)
    planning hierarchy in, 148, 149f
    policies in, 158–160 (*See also* Policies)
    proactive planning in, 142
    procedures in, 160
    rules in, 160
    societal philosophies and values in, 153–154
    strategic planning in, 143–146 (*See also* Strategic
        planning)
    vision statements in, 148–149, 149d
Ordering, just-in-time, 217
Organizational accountability, 550–556. *See also* Quality
    control
Organizational aging, 179
Organizational change with nonlinear dynamics,
    171–174
    chaos theory in, 173–174
    complex adaptive systems theory in, 172–173, 173d
    complexity science in, 172
    overview of, 171–172

Organizational charts
    advantages of, 278d
    components of, 267, 268f
    limitations of, 277–278, 278d
Organizational climate, 279
Organizational communication. *See also*
        Communication
    integrating leadership and management in, 461
    overview of, 441–442
    strategies of, 446–447, 447d
    technology on, 447–448
    variables in, 445–446
Organizational culture, 278–280, 281d–282d
Organizational effectiveness, 286–287
Organizational philosophy, 150
    employee understanding of, 156
    manager changes in, 156
Organizational standards, 543
Organizational structure, 264–288
    committee responsibilities and opportunities in, 285–286
    committee structure in, 284–285, 285d
    components of
        centrality, 271–273
        managerial levels, 270–271, 271t
        organizational chart, 267, 268f
        relationships and chain of command, 268–269
        span of control, 269–270
    decision making within organizational hierarchy in,
        275–276
    definition and scope of, 265
    formal and informal structure in, 265
    leadership roles and management functions in, 266d,
        287–288
    magnet status and, 283–284, 284d
    organizational culture in, 278–280, 281d–282d
    organizational effectiveness in, 286–287
    organizational theory in, 265–267
    organization charts in, limitations of, 277–278
    shared governance in, 280–283, 280f, 282f
    stakeholders in, 276–277, 277d
    types of, 273–275
Organizational theory, 265–267
Organizing
    in management process, 35, 35f
    of patient care (*See* Patient care, organizing)
Orientation, employee, 360–362, 360d–362d, 384
ORYX, 552
ORYX Plus, 552
Ouchi, W.G., 41
Outcome audit, 545–546
Outcomes
    in ethical problem solving and decision making,
        77–78
    vs. evidence-based practice, 540
    in quality control, 539 (*See also* Quality control)

Outcomes accountability, 538. *See also* Quality control
Outlier, 223
Overdelegating, 470
Overgeneralizing, 13
Overload, role, 387
Overt conflict, 492
Overtime, mandatory, 411–412
Oxycodone abuse, 611. *See also* Chemically impaired employee

P
Participative decision making, 36
Participative management, 36, 282
Part learning, 375
Passive-aggressive people, 454
Passive communication, 454
Paternalism, 74–75, 74*d*
Patient
  expert, 148
  use of term for, 77
Patient acuity tools, 405
Patient advocacy, 121–123, 122*d*
Patient care, organizing, 315–331, 325
  differentiated nursing practice in, 327–328, 327*d*
  disease management in, 325–327, 326*d*
  future of patient delivery models and, 328–329
  leadership roles and management functions in, 316*d*, 331
  optimum mode for, selecting, 329–330
  terminology for, 315
  traditional modes of, 315–325
    case management, 323–325
    functional method, 317–319, 319*f*
    modular nursing, 321
    overview, 315–317, 316*d*
    primary nursing, 321–322, 322*f*, 329
    team nursing, 320–321, 320*f*
    total patient care nursing/case method nursing, 317
Patient care facilitator (PCF), 329
Patient classification system (PCS), 213*d*, 405–408, 406*t*–407*t*
Patient injury, in malpractice, 100
Patient rights. *See also* Advocacy
  bill of, 123, 124*d*
Patient Safety and Improvement Act, *557*
Patient safety officer, 550
Patient safety organizations, 557
Patient satisfaction, 550
Patient Self-Determination Act (PSDA), 109
Payoff tables, 21
Pedagogy, 373, 374t
Peer assistance programs, 616–618

Peer review, 580–582
Pentazocine abuse, 611. *See also* Chemically impaired employee
Perceived conflict, 492
Performance appraisal, 569–587
  accuracy and fairness in, 572–574, 575*d*
  coaching in, 586–587
  documentation of interview in, 584–585, 585*d*
  for employee motivation, 570–572, 571*d*
  interview in
    overcoming difficulties in, 583–585
    planning, 582–583
  leadership roles and management functions in, 570*d*, 587
  overview of, 569–570
  performance management *vs.*, 585–586
  tools in, 575–582 (*See also* Performance appraisal tools)
Performance appraisal tools, 575–582
  behaviorally anchored rating scales, 576–577
  checklists, 577
  essays, 577
  job dimension scales, 576, 576*d*
  management by objectives, 578–580
  peer review, 580–582
  self-appraisals, 578
  summary, 581*d*
  trait rating scales, 575, 576*d*
Performance deficiency coaching, 602, 603*d*–604*d*
Performance management, 585–586
Perpetual budget, 214
Personal digital assistants (PDAs), 448
Personal goals, organization and, 308
Personal philosophies and values, 154–156
Personal power base, building, 303–306, 305*d*
Personal resources, expanding, 307–308
Personal time inventory, 197, 198*d*
Personal time management, 196–197
Personal time wasters, 197
Personnel budgets, 214–217
  labor-intensive nature of, 214
  nursing care hours per patient-day in, 215–217, 216*f*
  staffing mix in, 214
  worked/productive time and nonproductive/benefit time in, 216
Personnel policies, 244
Peter Principle, 252
Philosophy, 150
  individual, 154–156
  nursing service, 150–151, 151*d*
  organizational, 150, 156
  societal, 153–154
  unit, 151–152

Philosophy statement, 150–153, 151*d*
  nursing service philosophy in, 150–151, 151*d*
  organizational philosophy in, 150, 156
  philosophical congruence in planning hierarchy in, 151, 152*f*
  sample, 151*d*
  unit philosophy in, 151–152
  working, 152–153
Physical examination, for hiring, 355
Placement, employee, 357–359. *See also* Staffing
Plaintiff, 98
Planned change, 166–181
  classic change strategies in, 174–175
  as collaborative process, 177–178
  definition of, 166–167
  leader-manager as role model in, 178–179
  leadership roles and management functions in, 168*d*, 180–181
  Lewin's driving and restraining forces in, 170–171, 172*f*
  Lewin's model (change theory) in, 167–169, 170*d*
  in nursing profession, 180
  organizational aging and, 179
  organizational change with nonlinear dynamics in, 171–174 (*See also* Organizational change with nonlinear dynamics)
  renewal from, 179
  resistance in, 176–177
Planning, 140. *See also* Operational and strategic planning
  daily actions in, 193
  effective, 140–141
  fiscal (*See* Fiscal planning)
  long-term, 146–148
  in management process, 35, 35*f*
  overcoming barriers to, 161
  proactive, 142
  reactive, 142
  short-term, 186 (*See also* Time management)
  succession, 253
  taking time for, 188–189
  in time management at work, 192–193
Planning hierarchy, 148, 149*f*
  philosophical congruence in, 151, 152*f*
Planning lists, 191–192
Point-of-service (POS), 225–226
Policies, 158–160
  expressed, 159
  implementation of, 159–160
  implied, 159
  value of, 160
Political action committees (PACs), 129
Political alliances, developing, 308
Political strategies, 305*d*

Politics
  definition of, 306
  effective strategies in, 307–308
  interdependence in, 307
  reading environment of, 306–307
Politics of power, 306–309
Population-based health care, 325–327, 326*d*
Portfolio, 256–257, 578
POSDCORB, 35
Position power, 296
Positive organizational scholarship, 57
Positive reinforcement, as motivator, 430–431
Positive sanctions, 383
Posture, in communication, 453
Power, 293–310
  authority–power gap in, 297–301 (*See also* Authority–power gap)
  building personal power base in, 303–306, 305*d*
  charismatic, 297
  coercive, 296
  definition of, 293
  expert, 296
  feminist, 297
  gender and, 294–296
  informational, 297
  leadership roles and management functions in, 294*d*, 309–310
  legitimate, 296
  manager, 297
  of nursing, mobilizing, 301–303, 301*d*, 302*d*
  politics of, 306–309
  referent, 296–297
  reward, 296
  types and sources of, 296–297, 297*t*
Power base, building personal, 303–306, 305*d*
Power–coercive strategies, 175
Power differentials, 584
Powerlessness, 296, 518
Power-oriented people, 427
Praise, as motivator, 430–431
Preceptors, 380–381
Preemployment testing, 355
Preferred provider organization (PPO), 213*d*, 226
Preponderance of evidence, 96
Primary nursing care model, 321–322, 322*f*, 329
Principal agent theory, 54–55
Principal syndrome, 271–272
Priority setting, 189, 189*d*
Privacy Rule, HIPAA, 111, 459–460
Privileged information, respecting, 74*d*, 76
Proactive decision making, 307
Proactive leader, 41
Proactive planning, 142
Problem-centered coaching, 602

Problem employees, 593–619. *See also* Discipline
  chemically impaired employee, 610–618, 612*d* (*See also* Chemically impaired employee)
  disciplinary strategies for, 602–606 (*See also* Disciplinary strategies)
  disciplining of, 594
    constructive *vs.* destructive, 594–596
    with unionized employee, 607–609
  fair and effective rules and, 597–598
  grievance procedures for, 606–607
  group norms and, 596
  leadership roles and management functions for, 595*d*, 619
  marginal employee, 594, 609–610
  progressive discipline in, 598–601, 601*d* (*See also* Progressive discipline)
  reprimand form, 599, 599*d*
  self-discipline of, 596
Problem solving, 487–488
  critical elements of, 9–14, 9*d*
  definition of, 2
  ethical, 77–84
  structured approach to, ethical issues and, 78
  theoretical approaches to, 5–9
    heuristics, 5
    IDEALS model, 8
    intuitive model, 8–9
    managerial models, 6
    nursing process, 7–8, 7*d*, 7*f*
    structured approach, 5–6
    traditional problem-solving process, 6
  traditional, ethical issues and, 79–80
  Wueste approach to, 84
Problem-solving process, traditional, 6
Process audit, 547
Procrastination, 190–191, 190*d*
Production hours, 213*d*
Productive time, 216
Product liability, 105–106
Professional advocacy, 127–128
Professional boundaries, 584
Professional code of ethics, ANA, 77, 78*d*
Professional licensure, 112–113, 113*d*
Professional negligence, 98–100, 99*t*
Professional Nurse Practice Model (PNPM), 283
Professional portfolio, 256–257
Professional specialty certification, 248–249, 248*d*
Professional standards, 77, 79*d*
Professional standards review organizations (PSROs), 551
Program evaluation and review technique (PERT), 23–24, 24*f*
Progressive discipline, 598–601
  formal reprimand or written admonishment in, 599, 599*d*
  guide to, 601*d*
  informal reprimand or verbal admonishment in, 598–599
  involuntary termination or dismissal in, 600
  suspension from work in, 599–600
Promises, keeping, 74*d*, 75–76
Promotions, 251–253
Prospective audits, 545
Prospective payment system (PPS), 213*d*, 223–224, 551
Public policy, nursing's advocacy role in, 128–131, 130*d*
Punctuality, 196–197
Punishment, 296, 594

Q
QI Project, 554, 555*d*–556*d*
Quality, *vs.* cost, 210
Quality assurance (QA), 548
Quality Compass, 554
Quality control, 537–561
  audits in, 545–547
  Centers for Medicare and Medicaid Services on, 553
  definition of, 538
  effective, 538, 538*d*
  external impacts on, 550–551
  Joint Commission on, 552–553
  leadership roles and management functions in, 539*d*, 560–561
  as legal responsibility, 105
  Maryland Hospital Association Quality Indicator Project for, 554, 555*d*–556*d*
  medical errors in, 557–560, 558*d* (*See also* Medical errors)
  Multistate Nursing Home Case Mix and Quality Demonstration on, 556
  National Committee for Quality Assurance on, 553–554
  nursing care hours and staffing mix in, 409–410
  as organizational mandate, 550–556
  outcomes in, 539
  participants in, 550
  as process, 540–542, 541*f*
  professional standards review organizations in, 551
  prospective payment system in, 551
  quality health care definition in, 538–540
  quality improvement models in, 548–549
  report cards in, 556
  standards development in, 543–545, 544*d*, 545*d*
Quality gap, 540
Quality health care, 538–540. *See also* Health care quality
  vs. costs, 210
  definitions of, 538–540
  maintaining (See Quality control)
  nursing care hours and staffing mix in, 409–410
  quality assurance in, 548
Quality improvement (QI), 548–549

Quality measurement, 538. *See also* Quality control
Quantum leadership, 61

R
Rational decision making, 19, 19*t*
Rational–empirical strategies, 174–175
Reactive leader, 41
Reactive planning, 142
Readiness to learn, 374
Reality shock, 384, 385
"Reasonable and prudent," 98
Recency effect, 573
Recognition pathway, 432, 432*d*
Recognition-Primed Decision (RPD) model, 8
Records, medical, 108
Recovery programs, State Board of Nursing,
        616–618
Recruitment, employee, 251–252, 341–343. *See also*
        Staffing
Redefinition, 381
Reference checks, 354–355
Referent power, 296–297
Reflective practice, 586
Reflective thinking. *See* Critical thinking
Refreezing, 169, 170
Rehabilitation Act of 1973, 532
Reimbursement, health care, 221–222
Reinforcement, 375, 430–431
Relationship age leadership, from industrial age
        leadership, 62–64, 63*f*, 63*t*
Relationship-based nursing, 321–322, 322*f*
Releases, employee, 252
Renewal, of nursing profession, 180
Report cards, 556
Reports
    effectiveness, 571
    on improper/substandard care, 105
    incident, 104
    of medical errors, 557
Reprimand
    formal, 599, 599*d*
    informal, 598–599
Reprioritizing, 190
Research, influencing health care policy with, 128
Resistance, to change, 176–177
Res judicata, 97
Resocialization, 380. *See also* Socialization
Respondeat superior, 102–103
Responsibility, 278
Responsibility accounting, 210
Responsibility charting, 498
Responsive leader, 41
Restraining forces, 170–171, 172*f*
Résumé, 254–256, 256*d*
    cover letter for, 255–256

    sample, 256*d*
    structure of, 255
Retention, 342–343
Retrospective audits, 545
Revenue, 213*d*
Revocation, of nursing license, 112–113, 113*d*
Reward power, 296
Rewards
    accomplishment, in delegation, 473
    as motivator, 430–431
Ridicule, 502
Right-brain thinkers, 16
Rights
    Civil Rights Act of 1964, 529
    patient (*See* Advocacy)
    patient bill of, 123, 124*d*
Rights-based reasoning, 73, 73*t*
Robotic technology, 148
Role ambiguity, 377
Role change, 380
Role demands, assistance in meeting of, 382
Role expectations, clarifying, 380–382, 382*d*
Role models
    in delegation, 472
    in planned change, 178–179
    in socialization, 380
Role overload, 387
Role status change, employee socialization with,
        385–387
Role stress, 387
Role theory, in socialization, 380
Role transition, assisting experienced nurse in, 387–388
Root cause analysis (RCA), 542
Rule breaking, 597–599
Rules
    fair and effective, 597–598, 597*d*
    in operational and strategic planning, 160

S
Salary expense, 216, 540
Sanctions, negative and positive, 383
Satisfaction, patient, 550
"Satisficing," 20, 470
SBAR, as communication tool, 446, 447*d*
Scalar chain, 275–276
Scales
    behavioral expectation, 576–577
    behaviorally anchored rating, 576–577
    job dimension, 576, 576*d*
    trait rating, 575, 576*d*
    weighted, 577
Scheduling, 402–405
    agency nurses and travel nurses in, 403
    developing policies on, 413–414, 414*d*
    flextime in, 403

float pools in, 403
  leadership roles and management functions in, 398*d*, 415
  overview of, 402–403
  self-scheduling in, 403–404
  shift bidding in, 404
Schein, E.H., 40
Schmidt, W., 40
Scientific management, 33–35
Scope and Standards for Nurse Administrators, 77, 79*d*
Scorecard, balanced, 144–145
Selection, employee, 354–357. *See also* Staffing
  educational and credential requirements in, 354
  finalizing selection in, 355–356
  internal applicants in, 355
  making the selection in, 355
  physical examination in, 355
  preemployment testing in, 355
  process overview in, 356*f*
  reference checks in, 354–355
Selective contracting, 224
Self-appraisal, 573, 578
Self-care, 434
Self-denial, 613
Self-determination, 74, 74*d*
Self-discipline, 596
Self-power, 297
Self-scheduling, 403–404
Sentinel events, 552
Separation, 381
Servant leadership, 52–53, 53*d*
Service Employees International Union (SEIU), 517
Service line organization, 275
Service rating, 571
Sexual harassment, 530–531
Shadow workforce, 242
Shared governance, 280–283, 280*f*, 282*f*
Shift bidding, 404
Shock, reality, 384, 385
Shortage, nursing. *See also* Staffing
  actions for resolution of, 340–341, 341*d*
  fundamentals of, 337–338
  on staffing, 411–412
Short-term wins, 176
Silent generation, 410, 411*t*
Situational leadership theory, 39–40
Situation-Background, Assessment-
    Recommendation/Request (SBAR), 446, 447*d*
Six Sigma approach, 559
Skills, increasing professional, 304
Skinner, B.F., 425
Smoothing, 495
Social capital theory, 55
Socialization, 379–383. *See also* Team building
  anticipatory, 384
  assistance in meeting role demands in, 382

clarifying role expectations in, 380–382, 382*d*
  definition and overview of, 380
  mentors in, 381–382, 382*d*
  negative sanctions in, 383
  overcoming motivational deficiencies in, 382
  positive sanctions in, 383
  preceptors in, 380–381
  role models in, 380
  team building via, 390–391
Socialization, employees with unique needs for,
    383–389
  coaching as teaching strategy in, 388–389
  experienced nurse in new position, 387
  experienced nurse in role transition, 387–388
  international nurses, 385
  new nurse, 383–384
  role status changes, 385–387
Social learning activities, 254
Social learning theory, 374, 375*f*
Societal philosophies and values, 153–154
Space, interpersonal, culture and, 479
Spaced practice, 375
Span of control, 269–270
Span of memory, 376
Staff development, 371–372
  assessing needs for, 376–377
  evaluation of activities for, 377–378
  socialization and, 390–391
Staffing, 335–363
  aging workforce and, 338–339
  centralized, 398–399
  closed-unit, 411
  decentralized, 398–399
  demand factors in, 340–341
  indoctrination in, 359–362, 360*d*–362*d* (*See also*
    Indoctrination, employee)
  initial contact in, 343–344
  interviewee tips in, 352–353, 353*d*
  interviewing as selection tool in, 344–353
    (*See also* Interviewing)
  leadership roles and management functions in, 337*d*,
    363
  in management process, 35, 35*f*
  mandatory requirements for, 400–401, 401*d*
  nursing education enrollments and, 339–340
  nursing shortage and, 337–338
  overview of, 335–336
  placement in, 357–359
  predicting needs for, 336–337
  recruitment for, 341–343
  selection in, 354–357 (*See also* Selection, employee)
  sequential steps in, 336*d*
  standards for, 215
  supply factors in, 338–340
  workforce budget in, 214–217

Staffing mix, 213*d*, 214, 410
Staffing needs, 397–401. *See also* Scheduling
  centralized *vs.* decentralized staffing in, 398–399
  complying with mandates on, 400–401, 401*d*
  developing policies for, 413–414, 414*d*
  diverse staff management in, 399–400
  fiscal and ethical accountability for, 412–413
  generations and, 410–411, 410*t*
  leadership roles and management functions in,
    398*d*, 415
  nursing care hours, staffing mix, and quality of care
    relationship in, 409–410
  nursing shortage on, 411–412
  scheduling options and, 402–405 (*See also*
    Scheduling)
  unit manager's responsibilities for, 397–398
  workload measurement systems in, 408
  workload measurement tools in, 405–408, 405*f*,
    406*t*–407*t* (*See also* Workload measurement
    tools)
Staff organization, 268*f*
Staff positions, 268
Stakeholder analysis, 276–277
Stakeholders, 276–277, 277*d*
Standardized clinical guidelines, 543
Standardized nursing language, 546
Standards
  development of, 543–545, 544*d*, 545*d*
  establishing, 540, 541*f*
  labor, 526
  organizational, 543
  professional, 77
Standards of care, 98, 543, 544*d*
Standards of practice
  for clinical nursing, 543, 544*d*
  for nurse administrators, 77, 79*d*, 543
Standards of Professional Performance, 543,
    544d
Stare decisis, 97
State Board of Nursing recovery programs, 616–618
State health facilities licensing boards, 533
Statutes, 95, 95*d*
Statutory law, 95, 95*d*
Storming, 456, 457*t*
Strategic planning, 143–146. *See also* Operational and
    strategic planning
  balanced scorecard in, 144–145
  as management process, 145
  participants in, 145–146
  SWOT analysis in, 143–144, 144*d*
Strategy, dynamic model of, 145
Stress, role, 387
Strike, 515
Structure audit, 547
Structure change, 498–499

Structured approach
  of decision making, 5–6
  ethical issues and, 78
Structured interview, 344, 346*d*–347*d*
Subordinate advocacy, 124–125
Subordinate empowerment, 299–301
Subordinate identification, promoting, 308
Substance misuse. *See* Chemically impaired employee
Succession planning, 253
Summative task patient classification system, 405
Supplies, 217–218
Support systems, for managers, 433–434
Supraordinate common goal, 495
Suspension
  of nursing license, 112–113, 113*d*
  from work, 599–600
SWOT analysis, 143–144, 144*d*
Symbols, organizational, 304
System, 40
Systematic soldiering, 33

T
Taft-Hartley Amendment, 528
Tannenbaum, R., 40
Tardiness, 196
Task learning, 375
Taylor, Frederick W., 33–34
Team building, 369–391
  culturally diverse staff educational needs in, 389–390
  evidence-based practice implementation in, shared
    responsibility for, 379
  leadership roles and management functions in, 370*d*,
    391
  learning organization in, 370–371
  learning theories in, 372–376 (*See also* Learning
    theories)
  socialization and resocialization in, 379–383 (*See also*
    Resocialization; Socialization)
  socialization in, employees with unique needs for,
    383–389
  staff development in, 371–372
    assessing needs for, 376–377
    evaluation of activities for, 377–378
    socialization and, 390–391
Team nursing, 320–321, 320*f*
Telecommunication, 447–448
Teleological theory of ethics, 72–73, 73*t*
Telephone communication, 450
Termination
  of group communication, 456
  involuntary, 600
Termination conference, 605–606
Theories of learning, 372–376. *See also* Learning theories
Theory X, 36, 428–429, 428*d*
Theory Y, 36, 428–429, 428*d*

Theory Z, 41
Thinking logically, 13–14
Thinking styles, on decision making, 16–18
Third-party consultation, 498
Third-party payment system, 213*d*
Thought leadership, 59–60
360-degree evaluation, 582
Time, culture and, 479
Time clocks, 527
Time inventory, 197, 198*d*
Time management, 186–199
  crisis in, 192
  definition of, 186
  leadership roles and management functions in, 187*d*,
    197–199
  three basic steps to, 187–192
    overview, 187, 188*f*
    planning lists, 191–192
    priority setting, 189, 189*d*, 191
    procrastination, 190–191, 190*d*
    reprioritizing, 190
    taking time to plan, 188–189
  at work, 192–197
    daily planning actions, 193
    interruptions, 194
    personal, 196–197
    planning, 192–193
    taking breaks, 194
    time inventory, 197, 198*d*
    time wasters, 195
Time wasters, 195, 197
Timing
  in communication, 454
  sensitivity to, 308
Title VII of Civil Rights Act, 111–112, 529
Top-level managers, 270, 271*t*
Tort law, 95*d*, 96
Torts, 104–105
Total patient care nursing, 317, 318*f*
Total quality management (TQM), 548
TOWS analysis, 143–144, 144*d*
Toyota Production System (TPS), 549
Trade-offs, 501
Tradition bearers, 176
Training, 37, 244. *See also* Team building
  vs. education, 371–372
  team building via, 390–391
Trait rating scales, 575, 576*d*
Trait theories, 37, 38*d*
Transactional leadership, 42, 42*t*
Transfer of learning, 376
Transfers, employee, 249–251
Transformational leadership, 42–44, 42*t*
Transparent integrity, 58
Travel nurses, 403

Truth telling, 74*d*, 75
Turnover ratio, 213*d*, 342–343
Two-factor theory, 425–426, 426*t*

U
Underdelegating, 469–470
Unfreezing, 167–168, 169
Union, 514–515
Union organizing/unionization, 514–525
  ANA and, 517–518
  disciplining with, 607–609
  effective labor–management relations and, 524–525
  employee motivation for joining, 518–519, 519*d*
  employee motivation for rejecting, 519–520, 519*d*
  historical perspective on, 515–517, 517*t*
  leadership roles and management functions in, 514*d*,
    533
  managers' role during, 521–523, 522*d*
  strategies in, 521, 521*d*
Union shop, 515
Unit goals
  organization and, 308
  quality control evaluation of, 542
Unit philosophy, 151–152
Unity of command, 269
Unlicensed assistive personnel (UAP), 319
  definition and scope of, 474
  delegation to, 474–476
  increased use of, 409
  on patient outcome, 476
Unstructured interview, 344
Upward communication, 448
U.S. Equal Employment Opportunity Commission
    (USEEOC), 530
Utilitarianism, 72–73, 73*t*, 75, 84
Utilization review, 224

V
Values
  on decision making, 15, 17
  definition of, 153
  in health care policy, 153
  individual, 154–156
  individual, motivation and, 429–430
  learning new roles and, 382
  societal, 153–154
Variable costs, 213*d*
Variable expenses, 211
Variance analysis, 221
Veracity, 74*d*, 75
Verbal admonishment, 598–599
Verbal communication. *See* Communication, verbal
Veteran generation, 410, 411*t*
Veterans Readjustment Assistance Act, 532
Vicarious learning, 3–5, 4*f*

Vicarious liability, 102
Violence, workplace, 491
Visibility, developing, 305
Vision statements, 148–149, 149*d*
Vocal expression, in communication, 454. *See also* Communication
Voice, developing, 305
Vroom, Victor, 426, 427*f*

W

Wages, minimum, 526–527
Wagner Act, 516, 528
Weber, Max, 34–35, 265–267
Weighted scale, 577
Whistle-blowing, 125–126
White, R.K., 38
Whole learning, 375
Win–win solution, 495, 499
Wireless, local area networking (WLAN), 448
Wolf, G.A., 42, 43

Workforce. *See also* Staffing
    aging, 148
    budget for, 214–217
Working philosophy, 152–153
Workload management, 405
Workload measurement systems, 408
Workload measurement tools, 405–408
    internal and external forces on, 407
    nursing care hours per patient-day in, 405, 405*f*
    patient classification systems in, 405–408, 406*t*–407*t*
    workload measurement systems and, 408
Workload units, 213*d*
Workplace aggression, 491
Workplace violence, 491
Written admonishment, 599, 599*d*
Written communication, 450–452
Wueste approach, 84

Z

Zero-based budgeting, 219–220, 219*d*